Molar Incisor Hypomineralisation: New Perceptions

Monographs in Oral Science

Vol. 32

Series Editors

M.A.R. Buzalaf Bauru

A. Lussi Bern and Innsbruck

Molar Incisor Hypomineralisation: New Perceptions

Daniela Rios Bauru
Lourdes Santos-Pinto Araraquara

134 figures, 124 in color, and 31 tables, 2024

Karger

Daniela Rios
Department of Paediatric Dentistry, Orthodontics and Public Health
Bauru School of Dentistry, University of São Paulo
Alameda Dr. Octávio Pinheiro Brisolla, 9-75, PO Box 73, Bauru, SP 17012-101 (Brazil)
danirios@usp.br

Lourdes Santos-Pinto
Department of Morphology and Pediatric Dentistry
Araraquara School of Dentistry, São Paulo State University (Unesp)
Rua Humaitá 1680, Araraquara, SP 14801-385 (Brazil)
lourdes.santos-pinto@unesp.br

Bibliographic Indices. This publication is listed in bibliographic services, including Current Contents® and Index Medicus.

www.karger.com
Printed in Germany on acid-free and non-aging paper (ISO 9706)
ISSN 0077–0892
e-ISSN 1662–3843
ISBN 978–3–318–07157–3
e-ISBN 978–3–318–07248–8

Contents

Published online: June 28, 2024
Rios D, Santos-Pinto L (eds): Molar Incisor Hypomineralisation: New Perceptions. Monogr Oral Sci. Basel, Karger, 2024, vol 32, pp IX–XI (DOI: 10.1159/000539493)

Preface

To introduce this book, it is essential to share two intertwined narratives that converged in addressing a common challenge: molar incisor hypomineralisation (MIH).

First Narrative: How and When Rios Discovered MIH

MIH is an enamel development defect that catches the attention of those who work with children, and my experience was no exception. While my research had always centered around erosive tooth wear, an invitation to join an international multicenter study on atraumatic restorative treatment led me down a different path. Treating over a thousand children as part of this study in 2012, I began systematically observing severely affected molars, despite most teeth exhibiting good oral health overall. Initially mistaking it for aggressive caries lesions, I soon realized these cases were distinct due to the unique presence of pain and challenges with anesthesia. Despite employing various treatment approaches and materials, none yielded satisfactory long-term outcomes. This prompted a deeper investigation, ultimately revealing that the underlying issue was MIH.

From that moment on, I embarked on a relentless quest to understand this alteration and find effective care alternatives, driven by the need to solve my patients' problems. I realized that, in addition to relying solely on the available scientific evidence, I needed more data, considering the relatively unexplored territory I was facing. Encouraged by this insight and with the assistance of a PhD student (Fernanda Lyrio Mendonça), I initiated a new research line on MIH – a significant challenge given my already established research background on erosion. However, I also saw an opportunity to contribute meaningfully. For instance, I questioned why the term "remineralisation" was applied to an enamel developmental defect, while a similar designation was not used for conditions like fluorosis, which also involve hypomineralisation. Additionally, I questioned the concept of dentin hypersensitivity, especially in cases where dentin may not be exposed in MIH scenarios. At the same time, I felt that my expertise in cariology could shed light on these nuances, while my clinical experience could offer new insights for advancing treatment-related research. The passion for the topic inspired several students to embark on their research projects in undergraduate, master, and PhD studies on MIH.

However, the narrative does not conclude here. In 2018, I found myself in the office of Professor Buzalaf, the general editor of *Monographs in Oral Science*, alongside Professor Lussi. Our focus was on planning a project concerning erosive tooth wear when Professor Buzalaf received an email from Professor Lussi. She mentioned her upcoming trip to Switzerland to strategize future editions of the book. In a moment of spontaneity, I proposed the idea of creating a book on MIH, recognizing its growing demand for evidence across various perspectives, crucial for both clinicians and further research. Her face lit up with enthusiasm as she replied, "Great idea! Submit a proposal for me to take to Switzerland; I'm leaving tomorrow." Leaving her office, I immediately compiled a comprehensive list of topics pertinent to MIH. Subsequently, I delved into PubMed, meticulously scrutinizing abstracts from papers published between 2001 and 2018, ensuring no vital aspect was overlooked. Despite a sleepless night, I successfully submitted the proposal. The news of its approval by Karger filled me with joy, albeit accompanied by the realization that I would be tasked with editing it. Despite my clinical experience, I still felt inadequately prepared, having only begun my studies on the subject. Consequently, I sought the guidance of one of the foremost authorities in MIH research, Professor Lourdes Santos-Pinto. Now we begin her part of the story.

Second Narrative: How and When Santos-Pinto Discovered MIH

In 2002, I signed up to present the results of research into new technologies at the 6th Congress of the European Academy of Pediatric Dentistry. With an intense commitment to the University where I work and two young children, the only opportunity I had to open the Congress program was when I sat on the plane on the way to Dublin, Ireland. I was feeling very uncomfortable as I had just seen a patient with an enamel defect that I had not been able to recognize. Not all the permanent molars were affected, and the clinical characteristics of the defect were very different in each tooth. As the patient had sensitivity in one of the upper molars, which had already fractured after eruption, I decided to place a glass ionomer cement as protection and investigate further when I returned from my trip. What struck me most was the asymmetry of the defect and the ineffectiveness of the anesthesia. When I read the congress program, I was surprised to see that there was a conference on Mineralization Defect of Permanent First Molars. Would this help me understand what I had just seen in my patient?

I attended Professor Karin Weerheijm's lecture and did not forget the three points she then made: achieving anesthesia, challenge to restore, and immediate and long-term restoration. I returned to my university determined to motivate my postgraduate students to start studying the subject.

In the search for more knowledge and already with some results from our preliminary studies, we attended the 6th EAPD Interim Seminar and Workshop on Developmental Defects of the Enamel – Comprehensive Clinical Approach, in Helsinki, Finland, in 2009, where we had the opportunity to take part in group discussions on the Prevalence and Diagnosis of Molar-Incisor Hypomineralization (MIH) with Dr. Birgitta Jälevik; Aetiology of Molar-Incisor Hypomineralization (MIH) with Professor Satu Alaluusua, and Treatment and Clinical Guidelines for Developmental Enamel Defects in Permanent Teeth with Dr. Nick Lygidakis.

Inspired by all the knowledge shared by this group of professors and researchers who, together with the EAPD, had taken this challenging subject to the world, we formed the long-dreamed-of group of professors and students interested in studying MIH, and within a few months, we already had some projects for master's theses. This was the origin of the MIH Research Group, registered with the National Council for Scientific and Technological Development, a body that belongs to the Brazilian Ministry of Science, Technology and Innovation, and which over time has added students and professors and become a multinational group with the participation of Universidade Estadual Paulista (Unesp) in Brazil and CES University in Colombia. The work of this group, which had its first article published in 2010, can be seen in more than 50 articles published in English, Spanish, and Portuguese, 1 book in Portuguese with a Spanish version and another 15 chapters on MIH in pediatric dentistry books. With the support of the Brazilian Association of Pediatric Dentistry and the Brazilian Group of Teachers of Orthodontics and Pediatric Dentistry, we were able to make pediatric dentists and orthodontists aware of MIH and the importance of early diagnosis. And so, during the pandemic, we started an interactive online course on differential diagnosis and treatment strategies for MIH. These courses were attended by professionals from all Latin American countries, Portugal, Spain, France, and Angola, and more than 700 professionals were trained. In face-to-face activities, one of the group's goals was to train professionals working in the public health network in various Brazilian cities to carry out early diagnosis. MIH has also been disseminated through more than 200 courses and conferences throughout Latin America.

In this journey of learning and teaching about MIH, the invitation to participate as coeditor of the Monographs in Oral Sciences volume was a gift and an unparalleled experience. This book brought us the opportunity to have gathered, in a single book, the researchers who are studying many interesting topics about MIH. All those nominated to be part of this group have demonstrated for years a long experience related to MIH. So, we thought that the title *Molar Incisor Hypomineralisation: New Perceptions* would be appropriate since new perception or acquisition are only possible to be highlighted by those who know the history and participated in the evolution of studies on the subject.

Last Narrative

Together, Rios and Santos-Pinto, we deeply appreciate everyone who has greatly contributed to this book and the editors for trusting our work. We hope to bring valuable knowledge to clinicians and innovative insights to researchers, enabling us to collaborate in the search for new solutions in the care of patients affected by MIH.

Daniela Rios
Lourdes Santos-Pinto

Published online: July 1, 2024
Rios D, Santos-Pinto L (eds): Molar Incisor Hypomineralisation: New Perceptions. Monogr Oral Sci. Basel, Karger, 2024, vol 32, pp XII
(DOI: 10.1159/000539494)

Editorial

Despite not being a recent condition, the terminology molar incisor hypomineralisation (MIH) was only coined in the early 2000s [1]. In recent years, researchers and clinicians worldwide have been devoting great attention to this developmental defect. The reason for such awareness is because MIH has a complex etiology, is difficult to diagnose, and increases the susceptibility of the affected teeth to fracture as well as their hypersensitivity, with a significant impact on the quality of life of the patients [2]. Additionally, given the complex and dynamic clinical presentation of MIH, managing these lesions continues to pose a challenge and might represent a significant burden on health care systems.

Due to this scenario, when I invited Professor Rios to write a volume for the *Monographs in Oral Science* series back in 2018, the topic "MIH" naturally arose. We then contacted Professor Santos-Pinto, one of the foremost experts on the topic, who promptly accepted our invitation to join the project. Six years later, looking at the finished volume, I acknowledge that we could not have chosen a better theme for this monograph.

Professors Rios and Santos-Pinto, the volume editors, were very fortunate to invite the most renowned researchers worldwide on each aspect related to MIH to contribute to this monograph. As a result, the volume includes a full range of state-of-the-art information necessary for those interested in the subject, covering aspects related to its etiology, prevalence, clinical features, differential diagnosis, histological and ultrastructural aspects of the lesions, scoring systems, patient assessment, management of the lesions and their consequences. The impact of the lesions on the quality of life of the affected patients and the cost-effectiveness of their treatment are presented as well. The quality of the available information on MIH is discussed. Some new concepts are also presented, with the appropriate background.

For readers interested in the subject, whether for educational purposes, research, or clinical practice, this volume will undoubtedly be considered essential.

Marília Afonso Rabelo Buzalaf
Bauru, Brazil

References

1 Weerheijm KL, Jälevik B, Alaluusua S. Molar-incisor hypomineralisation. Caries Res. 2001;35(5):390–1.
2 Jawdekar AM, Kamath S, Kale S, Mistry L. Assessment of oral health-related quality of life (OHRQoL) in children with molar incisor hypomineralization (MIH) – A systematic review and meta-analysis of observational studies. J Indian Soc Pedod Prev Dent. 2022;40(4):368–76.

Chapter 1

Published online: July 1, 2024
Rios D, Santos-Pinto L (eds): Molar Incisor Hypomineralisation: New Perceptions. Monogr Oral Sci. Basel, Karger, 2024, vol 32, pp 1–9
(DOI: 10.1159/000538843)

Molar Incisor Hypomineralisation: A Recent Condition or a New Perception?

Lourdes Santos-Pinto[a] Daniela Rios[b]

[a]Department of Morphology, Genetics, Orthodontics and Pediatric Dentistry, Araraquara School of Dentistry, São Paulo State University (Unesp), Araraquara, Brazil; [b]Department of Paediatric Dentistry, Orthodontics and Public Health, Bauru School of Dentistry, University of São Paulo, Bauru, Brazil

Abstract

The condition known as molar incisor hypomineralisation (MIH) has been featured in the dental literature for some time. However, the condition itself, characterized by demarcated opacities, had been observed and documented in various forms before the official terminology was coined. The awareness and understanding of MIH have increased over the years, and there has been ongoing research to explore its prevalence, etiology, clinical implications, care, and treatment. In summary, MIH is not a recent condition, but the terminology and recognition of this dental phenomenon have been refined and formalized in the relatively recent past. This chapter reflects on our clinical experience, juxtaposing it with information from scientific literature and personal insights, as well as identifying gaps in understanding this enamel defect. Furthermore, another aim was to foster contemplation for potential research advancements in the MIH field.

Introduction

Molar incisor hypomineralisation (MIH) was first described in the literature in the early 2000s [1]. At that time, scant attention was given to the subject due to a lack of comprehensive studies, and the developmental defect was not recognized as a significant clinical issue. Since then, there has been an increase in awareness and research, leading to a better understanding of its clinical characteristics and prevalence. Nowadays, MIH is acknowledged as a significant challenge to public health in many countries. The reason for this is that MIH affects a large number of children in various nations [2]. Affected teeth are more prone to enamel fractures and exhibit hypersensitivity, potentially resulting in discomfort and functional issues during chewing. This can have a significant impact on oral health and the quality of life for these children [3, 4]. MIH can be challenging to diagnose, and its complex and costly treatment poses a financial burden on health care systems.

This chapter aims to reflect on our clinical experience, juxtaposing it with information from scientific literature and personal insights. Drawing inspiration from a similar approach taken a decade ago concerning erosive tooth wear [5], we will identify crucial gaps in understanding, fostering contemplation for potential research advancements in the MIH field.

Change in Interest

Nearly 3 decades ago, MIH was either unknown or, at the very least, not recognized in the manner it is today. A search was conducted in PubMed literature using the terms "molar incisor hypomineralization" and "molar incisor hypomineralisation" (MeSH terms) for a number of publications from 1982 to 2023. There is a consistent rise evident in the quantity of published works over this time frame. Segmenting this period into three 10-year phases, we notice a 5- to 6-fold surge in the number of publications during the subsequent decade compared to the preceding one. Even though the term MIH was officially published in 2001 [1], PubMed identified research that had already utilized the term "hypomineralisation in molars" as early as 1982. From 1982 to 2003, 14 publications were found with the term "hypomineralisation" spelled with "z" and 20 with "s." Moving on to the period between 2004 and 2013, there were 79 publications with "z" and 132 with "s." Lastly, from 2014 to 2023, there were 443 publications with "z" and 584 with "s." This indicates that MIH is becoming increasingly significant, both in research and in clinical practice.

Despite the considerable advancements in understanding both the causes of and care/treatments to MIH, there remains much that requires clarification [6]. Recent studies involving students, general practitioners, and specialists have revealed significant heterogeneity in results [7–11]. While dental professionals seem more inclined to recognize and treat MIH, it is essential to emphasize that untrained dentists have a limited ability to perform differential diagnoses among enamel developmental defects [12]. In addition, there is unanimous agreement among the findings, highlighting the imperative for enhanced knowledge and training in clinical care/treatment procedures [7–11].

Change in Historical Interpretation

Since its first recognition, this enamel defect has been interpreted as a distinct phenomenon, different from other enamel defects. In 2004, it was asserted that MIH does not seem to be a recent phenomenon; rather, when caries prevalence was high, the developmental defect responsible for cavity initiation was likely not diagnosed [13]. The challenging identification of this enamel defect may be attributed to the fact that MIH can manifest differently in each patient. Some cases may be mild and not always easy to identify, while others are more severe and evident. Many professionals have not received specific training on MIH and may not be familiar with the signs and symptoms of the condition. Additionally, gaps in communication between parents, patients, and dental professionals may hinder the diagnoses.

Once trained for defect recognition, we reviewed orthodontic records of 2,000 Brazilian patients who underwent treatment from 1980 to 2020, separated into 3 blocks (1980–1989, 1990–1999, and 2000–2020). Based on the diagnostic criteria of the European Academy of Paediatric Dentistry (EAPD), we observed that patients treated in the 1980s presented multiple and extensive amalgam restorations, the most used material at the time to restore a population with a high prevalence of caries. However, it was not possible to identify opacities around the restorations or on other unrestored surfaces. There were no atypical restorations, and most restorations had been in place for several years with fully acceptable marginal adaptation (as shown in Fig. 1a).

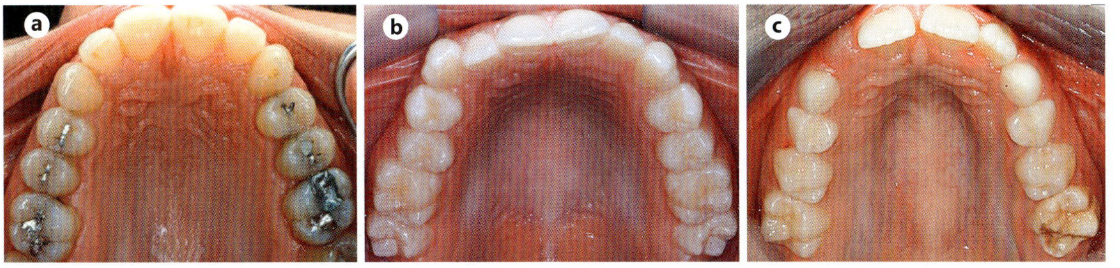

Fig. 1. **a** Oral condition that represents patients treated in the period 1980–1989: multiple and extensive amalgam restorations (no atypical restorations), without opacities around the restorations or on other unrestored surfaces. **b** 1990–1999: caries-free teeth, with sealants or small adhesive restorations and few enamel defects could be identified. **c** 2000–2010: little experience of caries, with the presence of opacities in molars and/or incisors or first permanent molars with posteruptive breakdown (MIH).

In the 1990s, most patients had caries-free teeth, with sealants or small adhesive restorations. One possible explanation for these changes in dental caries behavior was the introduction of preventive dentistry in Brazilian university curricula, as well as the strong influence of the Brazilian Association of Prevention, which not only introduced concepts of prevention and control of caries and periodontal diseases but also acted as a motivator, encourager, and paradigm shifter in the concept of dental caries. Additionally, the significant decline in decayed, missing, and filled teeth observed between 1980 and 2003 may be a result of increased access to fluoridated water and toothpaste, along with changes in the goals of public oral health programs. In that decade, dental caries was no longer a confounding factor for the early diagnosis of MIH. However, few defects could be identified [14] (as shown in Fig. 1b).

Patients who began treatment after the 2000s had little experience with caries; however, 1 in every 12 presented opacities in molars and/or incisors or first molars with atypical rapidly destructive caries (as shown in Fig. 1c). What changed? We still do not know how to explain it. However, the fact is that if the high prevalence of caries in the 1980s may have hindered the diagnosis of MIH in molar defects, it certainly would have not prevented us from diagnosing enamel defects in incisors (as shown in Fig. 2). On the other hand, it can be argued that teeth with characteristics akin to MIH have been identified in archaeological samples [15]. Nevertheless, the accuracy of these diagnoses has recently come under scrutiny due to the complexity of diagnosing MIH in archaeological collections. This complexity arises from confounding factors, such as taphonomic staining, dental wear, or other developmental enamel defects [15]. Therefore, several factors warrant clarification before establishing the historical context of MIH.

Change in Terminology

The process for selecting a name for a disease is a crucial undertaking that involves scientific, ethical, and practical considerations. The chosen nomenclature should be clear, precise, nonstigmatizing, and promote effective communication among health care professionals, researchers, and the public. In the context of enamel defects, there is no established criterion for naming. In the case of hypomineralisations, the predominant factors for nomenclature choice were the clinical characteristics of the defect and the teeth most frequently affected.

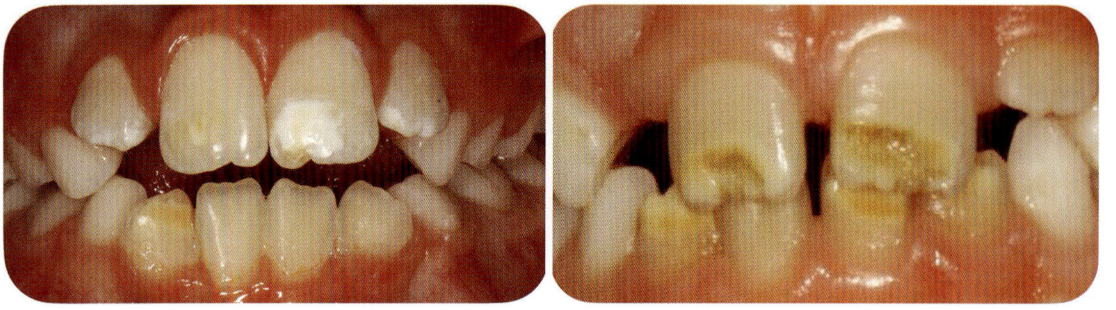

Fig. 2. Enamel defects in incisors (MIH) present in patients treated after the 2000s.

There is coexistence and similarity of clinical and structural characteristics among MIH, deciduous molar hypomineralisation (DMH), also referred to as hypomineralised second primary molars (HSPM), and hypomineralisation of other permanent teeth (HOPT) [16–19]. This observation leads us to hypothesize that these conditions may belong to the same spectrum of hypomineralisation. However, despite advancements in research on the subject, definitely establishing that these enamel defects are part of the same hypomineralisation spectrum remains intricate and requires a comprehensive analysis with an interdisciplinary approach involving dental professionals, medical geneticists, and other relevant specialists. Until we have a more thorough understanding of the MIH phenomenon, especially its etiology and risk factors, we continue to use different denominations that may refer to the same type of defect. Similarly, there is no uniformity among various classifications for the severity of MIH, a factor that likely contributed to the heterogeneity of research results.

In addition, prior to proposing a change in nomenclature, it is imperative to remember that the careful selection of a disease's name plays a crucial role in communication, research, and treatment. The chosen nomenclature can influence how patients perceive the disease, how health care professionals address it, and how society responds to it. Therefore, it is a process that should be undertaken with careful consideration of all relevant factors. Due to the lack of a consensus definition, before 2001, the literature on MIH was equally diffuse, making it challenging to ensure that different researchers were referring to the same defect. We agree with those who argue that the purpose of a scientific name, besides containing the maximum information about the disease, should also enable future investigators and physicians to find all available information gathered about it. Therefore, changing the designation of MIH more than 20 years after its identification should fulfill these objectives.

Achieving consensus on the nomenclature for hypomineralisation of multifactorial etiology, characterized by similar clinical features, continues to be challenging. However, there is a potential avenue for standardization in the English language, particularly in the spelling of hypomineralisation. In consideration of the initial publication of the term by European researchers [1], it is proposed that the term be spelled with an "s": molar-incisor hypomineralisation.

Change of Prevalence

Another gap identified in our clinical experience is related to the incidence of MIH. We cannot definitively state the extent to which there is a rising number of affected patients or if we have improved our ability to diagnose and recognize the defect in our patients. Understanding the prevalence (the frequency at which the defect is present) and the number of new cases occurring each year (incidence) allows dentists to tailor clinical decision-making, policymakers to define strategies and allocate resources appropriately, and dental schools to address the topic adequately in their curricula.

An estimate of the prevalence and incidence of MIH indicated a global increase of approximately 2% in cases between 2015 and 2016. Specifically for Brazil, the estimated increase was approximately 1.6% in new cases within a year [20]. These values are concerning, as the absolute number of new cases can be substantial in a large population. The disease has a significant impact on the quality of life of those affected [3], and an annual incidence rate of 2% can represent a significant burden on the health care system, requiring considerable personnel and financial resources for care/treatment, especially given that enamel defects necessitate long-term monitoring.

Drawing comparisons between prevalence studies is challenging due to differences in the studied population, encompassing factors, such as age, gender, socioeconomic status, ethnic origin, sample selection, and diagnostic criteria [21, 22]. However, studies conducted in the same population with absolute control of the variables responsible for variability in prevalence studies allowed for result comparison, revealing an evolution rate of MIH prevalence of 2% over a 6-year period [23]. These data suggest that, in addition to a lack of knowledge about the defect, utilizing the found incidence value to estimate the prevalence of the defect in the 1980s in the studied population was low. The prevalence was so low that it did not enable the identification of existing cases.

Change of Concepts

MIH Does Not Inherently Increase the Risk of Caries

In most articles outlining the characteristics and definition of MIH, a heightened risk of developing caries lesions is often reported. This is frequently attributed to existing data in the literature, suggesting a positive association between MIH and caries [24–27]. However, aligning with contemporary cariology concepts, the predominant factor influencing the development of caries lesions is dental plaque dysbiosis, specifically in the presence of sucrose [28, 29]. The mere presence of dental plaque is insufficient to cause lesion development unless it is unbalanced. How do we account for the observed positive association between caries and MIH in previous studies, considering that the etiological factor of caries is not directly linked to MIH?

Caries indexes frequently classify restorations as a treatment for caries lesions. However, when it comes to teeth affected by MIH, restorations may be linked to posteruptive breakdown, indicating rehabilitation from fractures rather than necessarily indicating prior caries lesions. According to the MIH classification, an atypical restoration is identified when (1) the shape and size do not align with a typical caries lesion, (2) it involves the buccal and palatal/lingual surfaces, (3) opacity is associated with the restoration margin, or (4) a patient lacks caries lesions in other teeth [30, 31]. Therefore, studies that categorize an atypical restoration as a prior caries lesion may lead to an overestimation of disease presence, potentially influencing the association between MIH and dental caries.

Therefore, we propose that MIH does not inherently elevate the risk of caries. This proposition is based on the premise that, in the absence of a cariogenic diet, caries development will not occur, even when faced with the presence of dental plaque resulting from MIH hypersensitivity or enamel breakdown. However, it is imperative to acknowledge the potential risks inherent in this statement, as individuals with MIH present enamel characteristics necessitating cations associated with dental caries. The compromised mineral content of the affected enamel (a host factor) and the potential for posteruptive breakdown (contributing to increased plaque accumulation, a biofilm factor) can exert influence on the manifestation of the caries lesions. Both these characteristics have the potential to expedite the speed and extent of caries lesion progression. Therefore, it is essential to focus on providing patients with information, education, and conditions conducive to preventing the development of caries.

Hypomineralised Enamel Opacities Cannot Be Remineralised

The concept of remineralisation comes from cariology. Initial noncavitated carious lesions, resulting from bacterial acid action over time, exhibit a demineralisation pattern attributed to distinct mineral phases in dental tissues. Acid production during sugar metabolism lowers saliva and biofilm fluid pH, causing subsurface carbonate hydroxyapatite dissolution and fluorhydroxyapatite formation in surface layers. Subsequent pH elevation leads to initial caries lesion remineralisation. Fluoride enhances remineralisation by increasing fluorhydroxyapatite supersaturation during carbonate hydroxyapatite dissolution. This process yields a less soluble and F-inclusive coating, more resistant to future acidic challenges. Demineralisation and remineralisation, governed by solubility constants, aim for a chemical balance in enamel [32].

MIH is a developmental defect in which during amelogenesis the enamel is formed with a reduced mineral content, less densely packed enamel crystals, thicker prism sheaths, and increased organic content, mainly protein [33]. Considering the information on the chemistry of de-remineralisation provided above and the inherent stability of hypomineralised enamel, where there is no existing loss that necessitates mineral gain, the feasibility of remineralising MIH opacities is questionable. Although the superficial enamel can undergo remineralisation following demineralisation episodes in the oral environment, contributing to posteruptive maturation [34], it is crucial to emphasize that defected hypomineralised enamel cannot transition to a normal state. However, its surface can undergo alterations through a more effective level of posteruptive mineralisation. It is important to clarify that this process does not necessarily restore the enamel's mechanical resistance, as remineralising agents do not affect the deeper layers of enamel.

Change the Rationale for Treatment

Since its inception, dentistry has evolved philosophies and techniques aimed at preserving or restoring oral health in the face of dental caries. Traditionally, rehabilitative materials and techniques have been designed to address decayed tooth structures. However, contemporary challenges, such as MIH, are introducing additional complexities to oral health. This enamel defect is acknowledged as a substantial public health challenge in numerous countries. The significance lies in the fact that MIH impacts a considerable number of children globally [2].

A prior investigation, which assessed the worldwide prevalence of MIH, indicated that a quarter of these affected teeth have experienced or will experience the necessity for care/treatment due to issues, such as pain, sensitivity, or post-eruptive breakdown [2]. Therefore, the need for care and restorative treatment is imperative. Currently, it is understood that adhesion to hypomineralised enamel is compromised, and posteruptive breakdown exhibits different patterns, which are entirely atypical compared to caries lesions [35, 36]. Furthermore, opacities in MIH cases cannot effectively seal and protect the dentin-pulp complex. Despite these distinctions, current treatment approaches for MIH largely mirror those employed for caries lesions. This conventional approach may be impeding progress in advancing MIH treatment over the past two decades. Perhaps, by adopting a more individualized perspective not only for different cases of MIH but also distinguishing MIH from caries, we could better grasp the unique requirements and explore new care and treatment alternatives.

Real-World Evidence for Establishing Scientific Validity

The choice of treatment for MIH depends on individual patient characteristics and needs, the dentist's expertise, and scientific evidence. While various treatments have been suggested for MIH treatment, there is currently insufficient high-quality scientific evidence to formulate a conclusive clinical treatment strategy for managing this condition [37]. Heterogeneities in treatment studies, including variations in design, defect severity, tooth preparation, and pretreatment procedures, pose methodological limitations that elevate the risk of bias and diminish the external validity of results. Consequently, treatment recommendations rely on best clinical practices [38], drawn from case reports with extended follow-up periods and real-world evidence (RWE). This RWE is derived from services provided in university dental clinics, where patients share similar characteristics with those in private clinical practice, enhancing the external validity of the results in real-world scenarios. Additionally, the RWE approach facilitates an understanding of the treatment's impact on patients and their families, generating research questions for further exploration in randomized controlled trials [39–41].

Conclusions

MIH has evolved into a significant global public health challenge, impacting numerous children, and affecting oral health. The increase in MIH-related publications reflects its growing importance in research and clinical practice. Challenges persist, however, requiring enhanced knowledge and training among dental professionals. It remains uncertain whether the rise in MIH cases is a result of improved diagnostic capabilities or an actual increase in the prevalence of the condition.

There are different terms used to refer to conditions with similar clinical characteristics, perpetuating terminology inconsistencies, which highlights the need for precise and standardized nomenclature. The conceptual association of MIH with caries risk requires reevaluation, emphasizing the role of a cariogenic diet in lesion development, even in the presence of MIH-related factors. In addition, the feasibility of remineralising MIH opacities is questioned, emphasizing surface alterations through effective posteruptive mineralisation rather than defect reversal to a normal state.

The rationale for MIH treatment challenges traditional paradigms, requiring individualized approaches distinct from caries treatment strategies to unveil new alternatives. In conclusion, the evolving landscape of MIH demands continuous scrutiny, collaborative interdisciplinary efforts, and targeted research to address persistent gaps and elevate clinical practices, ultimately improving oral health outcomes.

Acknowledgment

We express our gratitude to the Bauru School of Dentistry, University of São Paulo and Araraquara School of Dentistry, São Paulo State University (Unesp) for the invaluable support and resources, which played a crucial role in the development of this chapter.

Statement of Ethics

We state that the pictures of patients were obtained by patient's written informed consent for publication of the images.

Conflict of Interest Statement

The authors declare no conflicts of interest.

Funding Sources

D.R. is a researcher funded by CNPq (Productivity Program).

Author Contributions

L.S.-P. and D.R. conceived the chapter and were responsible for overall direction and planning. All authors actively participated in the writing process and reviewed the final version of the chapter.

References

1 Weerheijm KL, Jälevik B, Alaluusua S. Molar-incisor hypomineralisation. Caries Res. 2001;35(5):390–1.
2 Schwendicke F, Elhennawy K, Reda S, Bekes K, Manton DJ, Krois J. Global burden of molar incisor hypomineralization. J Dent. 2018;68:10–8.
3 Jawdekar AM, Kamath S, Kale S, Mistry L. Assessment of oral health-related quality of life (OHRQoL) in children with molar incisor hypomineralization (MIH) – a systematic review and meta-analysis of observational studies. J Indian Soc Pedod Prev Dent. 2022;40(4):368–76.
4 Villani F, Aiuto R, Re D, Paglia L, Garcovich D. Caries prevalence and molar and incisor hypomineralization (MIH) in children. Is there an association?: a systematic review. Int J Oral Health. 2023;3(1):1–6.
5 Lussi A, Carvalho TS. Erosive tooth wear: a multifactorial condition of growing concern and increasing knowledge. Monogr Oral Sci. 2014;25:1–15.
6 Lygidakis NA, Garot E, Somani C, Taylor GD, Rouas P, Wong FSL. Best clinical practice guidance for clinicians dealing with children presenting with Molar-Incisor-Hypomineralisation (MIH): an updated European Academy of Paediatric Dentistry policy document. Eur Arch Paediatr Dent. 2022;23(1):3–21.
7 Yehia AM, Abdelaziz AM, Badran A. Knowledge, clinical experience, and perceived need for training regarding molar-incisor hypomineralization among a group of Egyptian dental students: a cross-sectional study. BMC Oral Health. 2022;22(1):323.
8 Delgado RM, Botelho J, Machado V, Mendes JJ, Lopes LB. Knowledge, perception, and clinical experiences on molar incisor hypomineralization amongst Portuguese dentists. BMC Oral Health. 2022;22(1):250.
9 Serna-Muñoz C, Martínez-Beneyto Y, Pérez-Silva A, Poza-Pascual A, Ibáñez-López FJ, Ortiz-Ruiz AJ. Perception, knowledge, and attitudes towards molar incisor hypomineralization among Spanish dentists: a cross-sectional study. BMC Oral Health. 2020;20(1):260.
10 Hamza B, Karkoutly M, Papageorgiou SN, Bshara N. Molar-incisor hypomineralisation: knowledge and perception of Syrian undergraduate and postgraduate dental students. Eur J Dent Educ. 2023;27(2):343–52.
11 Gómez-Clavel JF, Sánchez-Cruz FY, Santillán-Carlos XP, Nieto-Sánchez MP, Vidal-Gutiérrez X, Pineda Á. Knowledge, experience, and perception of molar incisor hypomineralisation among dentists in the metropolitan area of Mexico City: a cross-sectional study. BMC Oral Health. 2023;23(1):1018.
12 Jälevik B, Szigyarto-Matei A, Robertson A. Difficulties in identifying developmental defects of the enamel: a BITA study. Eur Arch Paediatr Dent. 2019;20(5):481–8.
13 Weerheijm KL. Molar incisor hypomineralization (MIH): clinical presentation, aetiology and management. Dent Update. 2004;31(1):9–12.
14 Narvai P, Frazão P, Roncalli A, Antunes J. Cárie dentária no Brasil: declínio, iniqüidade e exclusão social. Rev Panam Salud Publica. 2006;19(6):385–93.
15 Garot E, Couture-Veschambre C, Manton D, Beauval C, Rouas P. Analytical evidence of enamel hypomineralisation on permanent and primary molars amongst past populations. Sci Rep. 2017;7(1):1712.
16 Elfrink MEC, Schuller AA, Weerheijm KL, Veerkamp JSJ. Hypomineralized second primary molars: prevalence data in Dutch 5-year-olds. Caries Res. 2008;42(4):282–5.
17 Vlachou C, Arhakis A, Kotsanos N. Distribution and morphology of enamel hypomineralisation defects in second primary molars. Eur Arch Paediatr Dent. 2021;22(2):241–6.
18 Alifakioti E, Arhakis A, Oikonomidis S, Kotsanos N. Structural and chemical enamel characteristics of hypomineralised second primary molars. Eur Arch Paediatr Dent. 2021;22(3):361–6.
19 Kevrekidou A, Kosma I, Kotsanos I, Arapostathis KN, Kotsanos N. Enamel opacities in all other than Molar Incisor Hypomineralisation index teeth of adolescents. Int J Paediatr Dent. 2021;31(2):270–7.
20 Schwendicke F, Elhennawy K, Krois J. Prevalence, incidence, and burden of molar incisor hypomineralization. In: Bekes K, editor. Molar incisor hypomineralization: a clinical guide to diagnosis and treatment. Cham: Springer International Publishing; 2020. p. 21–31.
21 Spronk I, Korevaar JC, Poos R, Davids R, Hilderink H, Schellevis FG, et al. Calculating incidence rates and prevalence proportions: not as simple as it seems. BMC Public Health. 2019;19(1):512.
22 Özükoç C, Balli Akgöl B, Patir Münevveroglu A. Prevalence of molar incisor hypomineralization: meta-analysis study. Med Sci Discov. 2020;7(10):652–8.

23 Damares Lago J, Restrepo M, Girotto Bussaneli D, Patrícia Cavalheiro J, Feltrin de Souza J, Santos-Pinto L, et al. Molar-incisor hypomineralization: prevalence comparative study in 6 years of interval. ScientificWorldJournal. 2022; 2022:4743252.
24 Kosma I, Kevrekidou A, Boka V, Arapostathis K, Kotsanos N. Molar incisor hypomineralisation (MIH): correlation with dental caries and dental fear. Eur Arch Paediatr Dent. 2016;17(2):123–9.
25 Americano GC, Jacobsen PE, Soviero VM, Haubek D. A systematic review on the association between molar incisor hypomineralization and dental caries. Int J Paediatr Dent. 2017;27(1):11–21.
26 Oreano MD, Santos PS, Borgatto AF, Bolan M, Cardoso M. Association between dental caries and molar-incisor hypomineralisation in first permanent molars: a hierarchical model. Community Dent Oral Epidemiol. 2023;51(3): 436–442.
27 Kühnisch J, Kabary L, Malyk Y, Rothmaier K, Metz I, Hickel R, et al. Relationship between caries experience and demarcated hypomineralised lesions (including MIH) in the permanent dentition of 15-year-olds. Clin Oral Investig. 2018;22(5):2013–9.
28 Ismail AI, Pitts NB, Tellez M, Banerjee A, Deery C, Douglas G, et al. The International Caries Classification and Management System (ICCMS™) an example of a caries management pathway. BMC Oral Health. 2015;15(suppl 1):S9.
29 Manzoor M, Lommi S, Furuholm J, Sarkkola C, Engberg E, Raju S, et al. High abundance of sugar metabolisers in saliva of children with caries. Sci Rep. 2021;11(1):4424.
30 Weerheijm KL, Duggal M, Mejàre I, Papagiannoulis L, Koch G, Martens LC, et al. Judgement criteria for molar incisor hypomineralisation (MIH) in epidemiologic studies: a summary of the European meeting on MIH held in Athens, 2003. Eur J Paediatr Dent. 2003;4(3): 110–3.
31 Ghanim A, Silva MJ, Elfrink MEC, Lygidakis NA, Mariño RJ, Weerheijm KL, et al. Molar incisor hypomineralisation (MIH) training manual for clinical field surveys and practice. Eur Arch Paediatr Dent. 2017;18(4):225–42.
32 Buzalaf MAR, Pessan JP, Honório HM, Ten Cate JM. Mechanisms of action of fluoride for caries control. Monogr Oral Sci. 2011;22:97–114.
33 Elhennawy K, Manton DJ, Crombie F, Zaslansky P, Radlanski RJ, Jost-Brinkmann PG, et al. Structural, mechanical and chemical evaluation of molar-incisor hypomineralization-affected enamel: a systematic review. Arch Oral Biol. 2017;83:272–81.
34 Cardoso CA, Magalhães AC, Rios D, Lima JE. Cross-sectional hardness of enamel from human teeth at different posteruptive ages. Caries Res. 2009; 43(6):491–4.
35 Krämer N, Bui Khac NN, Lücker S, Stachniss V, Frankenberger R. Bonding strategies for MIH-affected enamel and dentin. Dent Mater. 2018;34(2):331–40.
36 Lagarde M, Vennat E, Attal JP, Dursun E. Strategies to optimize bonding of adhesive materials to molar-incisor hypomineralization-affected enamel: a systematic review. Int J Paediatr Dent. 2020;30(4):405–20.
37 Weber KR, Wierichs RJ, Meyer-Lueckel H, Flury S. Restoration of teeth affected by molar-incisor hypomineralisation: a systematic review. Swiss Dent J. 2021; 131(12):988–97.
38 Antoine D, Hillson S. Enamel structure and properties. A companion to dental anthropology. Wiley Blackwell; 2015. p. 223–43.
39 Linner T, Khazaei Y, Bücher K, Pfisterer J, Hickel R, Kühnisch J. Comparison of four different treatment strategies in teeth with molar-incisor hypomineralization-related enamel breakdown – a retrospective cohort study. Int J Paediatr Dent. 2020;30(5):597–606.
40 Santos-Pinto L, Fragelli CMB, Girotto Bussaneli D, Restrepo M, Nogueira VKC, de Farias AL, et al. Real-world evidence in the context of molar incisor hypomineralization: a new perspective. Int J Paediatr Dent. 2021;31(4):483–5.
41 de Farias AL, Rojas-Gualdrón DF, Mejía JD, Bussaneli DG, Santos-Pinto L, Restrepo M. Survival of stainless-steel crowns and composite resin restorations in molars affected by molar-incisor hypomineralization (MIH). Int J Paediatr Dent. 2022;32(2):240–50.

Daniela Rios
Department of Paediatric Dentistry, Orthodontics and Public Health
Bauru School of Dentistry, University of São Paulo
Alameda Dr. Octávio Pinheiro Brisolla, 9-75, PO Box 73, Bauru, SP 17012-101 (Brazil)
danirios@usp.br

Published online: July 1, 2024

Rios D, Santos-Pinto L (eds): Molar Incisor Hypomineralisation: New Perceptions. Monogr Oral Sci. Basel, Karger, 2024, vol 32, pp 10–34 (DOI: 10.1159/000538850)

Developmental Defects of Enamel

Daiana da Silva Martins[a] Franciny Querobim Ionta[a, b]
Gustavo Pompermaier Garlet[c] Rafael Rodrigues Lima[d]
Aline de Almeida Neves[e] Daniela Rios[a] Adrian Lussi[f, g]

[a]Department of Pediatric Dentistry, Orthodontics and Public Health, Bauru School of Dentistry, University of São Paulo, Bauru, Brazil; [b]Department of Dentistry, University of Marília, Marília, Brazil; [c]Department of Biological Sciences, Bauru School of Dentistry, University of São Paulo, Bauru, Brazil; [d]Laboratory of Functional and Structural Biology, Institute of Biological Sciences, Federal University of Pará, Belém, Brazil; [e]Department of Paediatric Dentistry and Orthodontics, School of Dentistry, Federal University of Rio de Janeiro, Rio de Janeiro, Brazil; [f]University Hospital for Conservative Dentistry and Periodontology, Medical University of Innsbruck, Innsbruck, Austria; [g]School of Dental Medicine, University of Bern, Bern, Switzerland

Abstract

Amelogenesis, the intricate process governing enamel formation, is susceptible to a range of genetic, systemic, and environmental influences, resulting in distinct developmental defects of enamel (DDE), such as molar incisor hypomineralisation (MIH), enamel hypoplasia, dental fluorosis, and amelogenesis imperfecta (AI). This chapter aims to provide a comprehensive overview of amelogenesis and DDE, establishing correlations between histopathological findings and clinical manifestations. MIH, a qualitative enamel defect, occurs during the mineralisation and maturation phases, affecting first permanent molars and eventually incisors. Diagnostic challenges in MIH arise from the disorder's unique features, including variable tooth involvement and severity, influenced by a complex interplay of genetic, systemic, and environmental factors. Enamel hypoplasia, a quantitative defect, manifests in any tooth during enamel matrix secretion. Etiological factors include local, systemic, environmental, and genetic influences, with variable enamel matrix abnormalities depending on the stage of amelogenesis when aggression occurred. Dental fluorosis, a toxicological concern from chronic and excessive fluoride exposure, affects ameloblasts and compromises crystal growth of the homologous teeth during enamel development. Lastly, AI, an inherited condition, encompasses diverse phenotypes in enamel development. AI phenotypes, whether hypoplastic or hypomineralised, entail mutations in genes, such as AMELX, ENAM, MMP20, KLK4, WDR72, FAM83H, C4ORF26, amelotin, GPR68, and ACPT. Diagnosing AI involves considering family history and clinical observation. In conclusion, navigating the intricacies of amelogenesis, from MIH to AI, underscores the critical importance of accurate diagnosis for proper clinical management of DDE.

Introduction

Amelogenesis is a multifaceted and genetically controlled process responsible for enamel formation, characterized by distinct stages of a highly coordinated activity of ameloblasts, which are specialized epithelial cells at the core of enamel development. The ameloblasts are responsible for secretion of enamel matrix proteins, and later, for proteolytically degradation and removal, allowing the progressive mineral deposition. This tightly regulated process is susceptible to detrimental triggers from systemic or environmental factors, influenced by genetic variability. Hence, diverse pathological and medical conditions, such as fever, infection, trauma, fluctuations in oxygen levels, antibiotics, among others, have the potential to disrupt amelogenesis, leading to the developmental defects of enamel (DDE) with distinct clinical characteristics [1]. It is important to note that after enamel formation is complete, its biological remodeling is not possible. Consequently, these insults become permanently recorded as biomarkers within the mineral structure [2]. This chapter will address exclusive enamel defects, specifically those that involve only enamel and exclude other structures. For example, conditions like odontodysplasia, where both enamel and dentin are affected, will not be covered.

In fact, by combining histological and clinical analyses focusing on the location of the enamel defect, it is possible to establish the time at which the disturbance manifested in the teeth. This is facilitated by the discernible patterns of enamel deposition, progressing from the crown's top to its base. During the enamel formation process, microscopic formations known as the striae of Retzius gain prominence at birth, giving rise to neonatal lines. Identification of the neonatal lines and the location of the enamel defect allow determination of whether the injury occurred during the gestational period or after birth. It is noteworthy that each tooth follows a distinct developmental pattern; for instance, in deciduous incisors, the majority of enamel formation takes place before birth, whereas in deciduous canines, a significant portion of enamel development occurs in the postnatal period. The insights derived from this temporal diagnosis are very important to understand the etiological factors associated with DDE [3, 4].

Theoretically, any disruption of the physiological homeostasis along the various stages of amelogenesis can lead to hypoplasia, characterized by a reduction in enamel thickness/volume (quantitative defect) or in hypomineralisation or hypomaturation, characterized by deficiencies in mineral content (qualitative defect). If the insult occurs during the mineralisation and maturation phases, it can lead to hypomineralisation or hypomaturation. Noteworthy, it is not possible to clinically distinguish between these two. They are marked by enamel translucency, appearing as opacities that can be diffuse or demarcated, with varying severity. Therefore, throughout this chapter, they will be generically referred to as hypomineralisation. An example of hypomineralisation, with a known origin, is dental fluorosis (DF). The excessive ingestion of fluoride during amelogenesis may result in the formation of hypomineralised enamel, which exhibits a porous appearance and symmetrically affects the developing teeth. On the other hand, hypoplasia occurs when there is disturbance during the secretory phase, and therefore, on a clinical level, enamel will show a deficient amount.

Structural or functional disruption of ameloblasts may result from a diverse range of factors, despite the presence of similar clinical characteristics of impaired enamel. Causative factors can manifest locally, targeting an individual tooth, or systemically, affecting the group of teeth undergoing enamel formation in that period. When alterations in amelogenesis are of genetic origin, typically all teeth are affected; however, the compromised gene may be associated with the matrix deposition phase (hypoplasia) or enamel mineralisation (hypomineralisation), resulting in distinct clinical characteristics. The phase of ameloblast activity, the origin, duration, and severity of the disruption, might lead to temporary or permanent disturbance of the cells determining the appearance of DDE. Therefore, understanding the typical process of enamel formation is important in recognizing and comprehending these anomalies. Knowledge of the mechanisms and causes underlying these conditions is critical for early diagnosis and the effective management of these enamel disorders.

Amelogenesis

Understanding the process of enamel formation necessitates a comprehensive insight into the structural components pivotal to the development of this tissue. Therefore, this section delineates the initial phases of tooth formation, laying the foundational knowledge required [1, 5].

The genesis of a tooth is orchestrated by two primary embryonic layers: the ectoderm and the mesoderm. The ectoderm is instrumental in forming the enamel, while the mesoderm contributes to the development of the tooth's other structures. Initially, the ectoderm forms the oral epithelium. This epithelium engages in a critical interaction with mesenchyme, which is derived from the mesoderm, marking the commencement of the dental lamina phase [1, 5]. This phase is characterized by the oral epithelium folding and invading the underlying mesenchyme, resulting in the dental placode's formation. This event triggers the progression through the bud, cap, and bell stages. The bell stage is a critical juncture where histodifferentiation of the dental germ takes place, signifying the onset of enamel formation. It is during this stage that the crown's shape is established, and the enamel organ is first identifiable [1, 5].

The enamel organ is comprised of two distinct epithelial layers: the inner enamel epithelium and the outer enamel epithelium. The inner enamel epithelium consists of a single layer of cells that undergo differentiation to become ameloblasts, the cells responsible for enamel production. Similarly, the outer enamel epithelium is a single-layered structure. These layers converge at the cervical loop, a specialized region that maintains a reservoir of dental epithelium and undifferentiated cells. This reservoir is essential for the continuous enamel formation process, ensuring the dental crown's development to completion [1, 5].

Until the initial enamel formation, ameloblasts go through a series of transformations, establishing their phenotype, developing a prominent protein synthesis apparatus, and preparing to secrete the initial organic matrix of enamel [5]. The ameloblasts display distinct characteristics, including elongation and the polarized repositioning of their nuclei toward the stratum intermedium [5]. Furthermore, upon differentiation, these cells lose their ability to undergo further division [5].

Additionally, along its differentiation, ameloblasts develop an additional junctional complex with attachment forming at the distal and apical ends of the cell, creating a polarized cell structure with distinct regions, the body, and a distal process known as Tomes' process [5]. As a result, the ameloblast becomes a fully polarized cell, with most organelles positioned in the cell body, distal to the nucleus. Throughout this phase, ameloblasts align closely as a single epithelial layer, being connected by the junctional complexes, which are essential for keeping their structural integrity and to regulate movement of substances involved in the enamel formation process [5]. Indeed, the ameloblast layer features results in a region of relative impermeability since the substances in the underlying connective tissue only can reach the developing enamel through active control of the ameloblasts.

Noteworthy, the enamel organ presents a complex microvascular system, with fenestrated capillaries, probably involved in the control of lo-

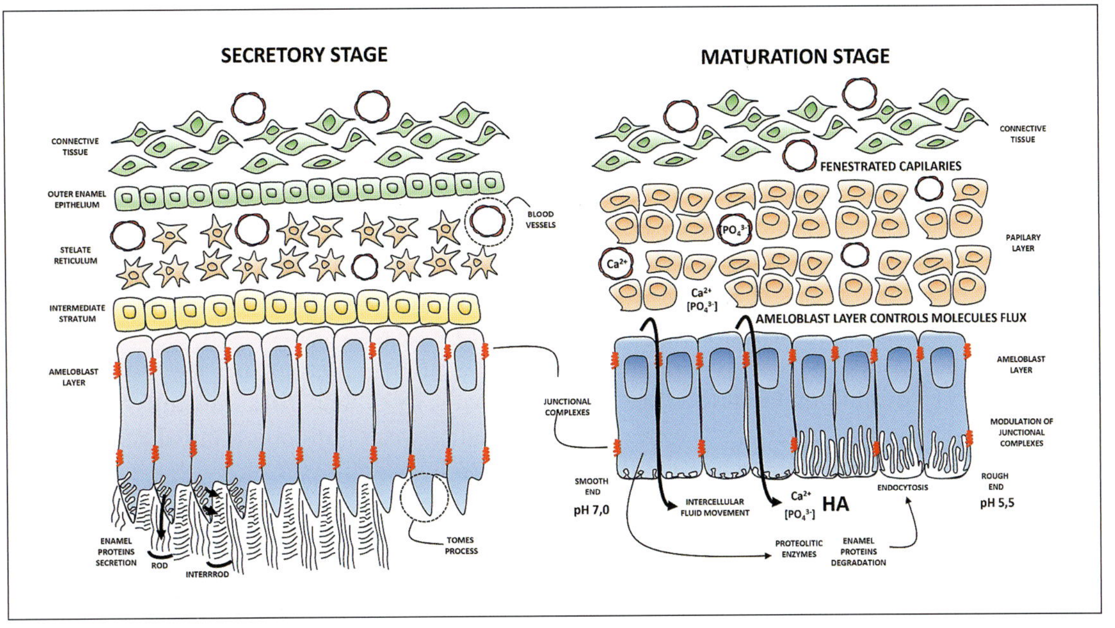

Fig. 1. Secretory stage (left) and maturation stage (right) of amelogenesis. Key structures and mechanisms within both phases are highlighted. During the secretory stage, ameloblasts are interconnected by junctional complexes and possess Tome's processes. Tome's processes are crucial for the directed exocytosis of secretory vesicles and the organization of enamel matrix protein deposition, shaping the rod and interrod enamel pattern. In the maturation stage, ameloblasts undergo shortening and lose Tome's processes. The intermediate stratum, stellate reticulum, and outer enamel epithelium reconfigure into papillary layer cells. In this phase, the membrane of the distal portion of ameloblasts undergoes cycling modulation between smooth-ended (SA) and ruffle-ended (RA) ameloblasts. SA ameloblasts feature incomplete junctional complexes that potentially enhance intercellular fluid movement, aiding in pH neutralization within the enamel matrix. RA cells exhibit proficiency in the endocytosis of remnants of enamel matrix proteins and demonstrate a robust capability for ion transport. Additionally, proteolytic enzymes are secreted by ameloblasts during this stage.

cal influx of molecules (proteins and ions) required for the distinct amelogenesis phases [6–8]. In this context, these localized vascular permeabilities associated with the selective permeability of the ameloblast layer are regarded as crucial factors in establishing a well-controlled microenvironment in the developing enamel region. This environment is believed to play a role in enamel formation by facilitating the regulation of local pH, which is essential for proper tissue development during various formative stages. From the differentiation of ameloblasts, the process of amelogenesis can be categorized into two main stages: the secretory stage, as ameloblasts secrete proteins into the enamel space, and the maturation stage, where ameloblasts facilitate the degradation and replacement of organic material with inorganic components [1].

During the secretory stage (shown in Fig. 1), also referred to as the formative stage, ameloblasts meticulously arrange and shape the enamel layer, leading to the formation of a well-structured tissue. At this stage, four distinct cell populations are typically observed within the enamel organ: secretory ameloblasts, organized in a single layer; the intermediate stratum, consisting of one or two layers of densely packed cells; the stellate reticulum, comprising a cluster of star-shaped cells; and the outer enamel epithelium, which is a single layer of cells [1].

Secretory ameloblasts are highly polarized cells with an intricate Golgi complex and rough endoplasmic reticulum occupying a significant portion of the cell's supranuclear compartment [5]. In this stage, ameloblasts synthesize and secrete a limited number of enamel matrix structural proteins, including amelogenin (AMELX), ameloblastin (AMBN), and enamelin (ENAM), all of which play a fundamental role in enamel development [1]. In addition to these well-recognized "enamel proteins," other key players, such as alkaline phosphatase, heat shock proteins, cofilin-1, calmodulin, and peptidyl-prolyl cis-trans isomerase, appear to participate in the amelogenesis process [9, 10].

In this stage, the ameloblasts' Tomes' processes are essential for the exocytosis of secretory vesicles. In addition, they help to define the orientation of enamel matrix deposition, which consequently will orientate mineral deposition and ultimately the prismatic structure [1]. Therefore, Tomes' processes play a significant role in the three-dimensional arrangement of enamel crystal deposition. As the distal portion of Tomes' process is formed, the secretion of enamel proteins becomes staggered and is confined to two sites. The proximal part of the process secretes proteins along the *c* axis, later forming a continuous layer known as interrod enamel. Secretion from the second site (distal portion of the Tomes' process) provides the matrix that participates in formation of the enamel rod, along the *z* axis, that later fills a pit. It is important to emphasize that the interrod enamel is typically formed first, and then the rod enamel is deposited in the spaces or gaps of interrods.

Secretory ameloblasts exhibit robust adhesion mediated by intercellular junctional complexes, with distinct arrangements. In the apical membrane region, these complexes tightly encircle the cell, creating a semipermeable barrier that regulates the diffusion of mineral ions into the enamel matrix. However, at the basal pole region, these complexes are incomplete or permeable, facilitating ion movement. As the enamel layer thickens, the distal Tomes' process stretches and gradually becomes thinner due to the pressure exerted by the growing enamel rods. Eventually, the Tomes' process disappears, leaving a space between the rod and interrod enamel filled with organic material, known as the rod sheath. Finally, as the ameloblast becomes shorter and loses the distal Tomes' process, the enamel layer comprises a prismatic layer with rods and interrods, sandwiched between thin rodless initial and final layers [5].

During the transition between the secretory and maturation phases, significant morphological alterations become evident. The secretory ameloblasts undergo a transformation, resulting in a reduction in their height, the loss of Tome's processes, while the other three populations of epithelial cells (intermediate stratum, stellate reticulum, and outer enamel epithelium) reconfigure themselves into papillary layer cells, characterized by a high degree of blood vascularization [1]. These transformations coincide with substantial changes in gene expression patterns. Genes responsible for encoding enamel matrix proteins (AMELX, AMBN, and ENAM) experience downregulation, whereas numerous other genes, particularly those involved in ion transport, proteolysis, and pH regulation, exhibit upregulation [5].

During the enamel maturation stage (shown in Fig. 1), ameloblasts play a crucial role in several key processes. These include ion transport [11], acid-base balance [12], the removal or endocytosis of enamel matrix protein remnants [13, 14], and apoptosis [1]. These activities collectively contribute to increasing the mineral content of the enamel to over 96% [5], enhancing its durability and hardness.

The primary function of ameloblasts during this stage involves the extensive removal of water and organic material from the enamel. This process allows for the incorporation of additional inorganic elements, thereby facilitating enamel's maturation. Ameloblasts exhibit two morphological forms: smooth-ended ameloblasts (SA) and ruffle-ended ameloblasts (RA), with their membrane adjacent to the enamel surface undergoing cyclic changes. An ameloblast spends approximately 20% of its lifetime in the SA form and 80% in the RA form [5]. RA cells are distinguished by their folded apical membrane, which enables a significant ion transport capacity. This capacity is crucial for the influx and efflux of ions across the enamel organ. Additionally, RA cells are adept at endocytosing remnants of enamel matrix proteins. In contrast, SA cells feature incomplete junctional complexes that facilitate the movement of intercellular fluid, aiding in pH neutralization within the enamel matrix. Thus, both RA and SA cells play vital roles in pH regulation and bicarbonate transport [5]. Hydroxyl ions within the enamel matrix can diffuse and be substituted by various ions, such as fluoride (F^-), carbonate ($CO32^-$), or chloride (Cl^-), from aqueous solutions. This adaptability in the apatite's composition reflects its ability to respond to environmental conditions.

The removal of the organic matrix during enamel maturation is predominantly achieved through the extracellular activity of enzymes secreted by ameloblasts, such as matrix metallopeptidases 20 (MMP20) during the secretory stage and kallikrein-related peptidase 4 (KLK4) during the maturation stage [1, 5]. These enzymes degrade matrix proteins into smaller fragments that can exit the enamel layer, highlighting a process distinct from the active resorption of intact proteins by ameloblasts [5]. These polypeptide fragments are believed to pass through the permeable distal junctions of SA cells, diffusing laterally among ameloblasts and being absorbed along their basolateral surfaces. As ameloblasts transition to the RA state, enhancing the permeability of the proximal junctional complex, some peptides may disperse into the papillary layer and potentially beyond [5]. Furthermore, the active incorporation of mineral ions into enamel crystals is primarily associated with RA cells. The current understanding is that calcium ions, essential for crystal growth, pass through the sealed distal junctions of RA cells, whereas they travel along the sides of the more permeable SA cells [5].

After elucidating the process of amelogenesis, the subsequent sections will delve into molecular processes and genetic mechanisms governing histopathological responses, thereby influencing the occurrence of different DDEs.

Molar Incisor Hypomineralisation

Recent studies have shown that hypomineralisation was present in the first permanent molars and permanent incisors among past populations, indicating that this condition is not exclusive to contemporary times [15, 16]. However, it was only in 2001 that the European Academy of Paediatric Dentistry officially coined the term molar incisor hypomineralisation (MIH) [17]. This term encompasses the qualitative DDE affecting at least one first permanent molar, potentially involving permanent incisors [17]. While other DDE, such as fluorosis, hypoplasia, and amelogenesis imperfecta (AI), have well-established etiological factors, the pathogenesis of MIH remains unclear, presenting a putative multifactorial etiological profile, which encompasses genetic, systemic, and environmental influences. Potential contributing factors for MIH are categorized into three distinct groups: (1) prenatal (pathologies and maternal diseases during pregnancy); (2) perinatal (time and type of delivering and complications during childbirth); and (3) postnatal factors (occurrence of infectious diseases or fever episodes in the first years of life).

An additional challenge, aside from elucidating the specific etiological determinants contributing to this condition, lies in comprehending the asymmetric distribution of MIH within the denti-

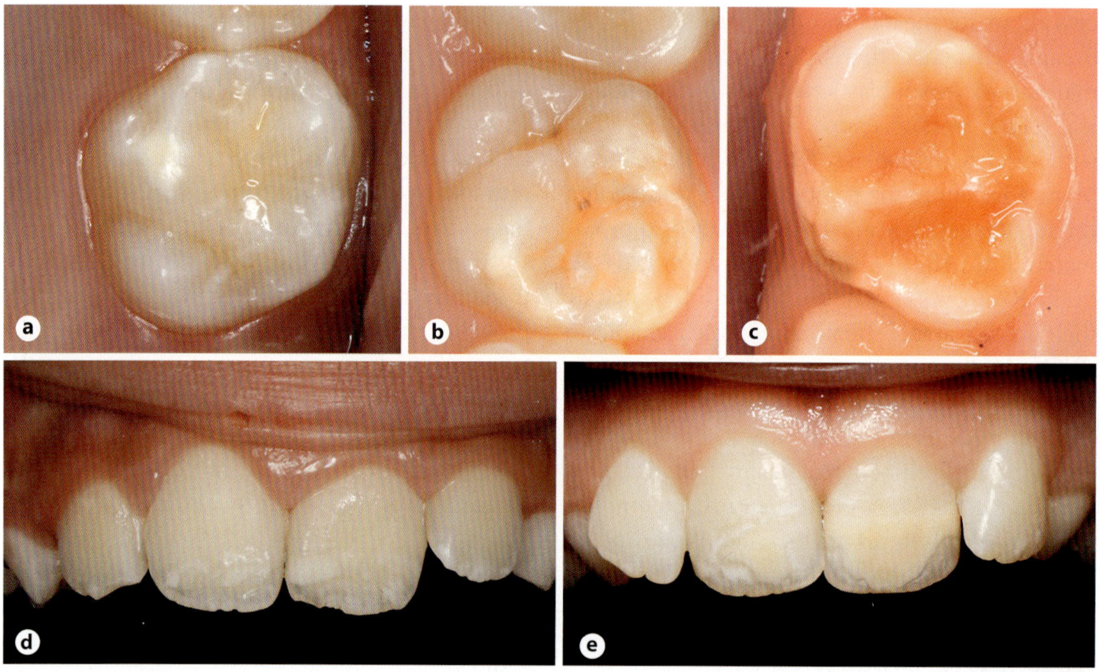

Fig. 2. Different clinical presentation of MIH on first permanent molars. **a** A localized white spot. **b** Localized white spot plus diffuse opacity alteration with a loss of structure. **c** Brown discoloration with a substantial loss of structure; and demarcated stains on central incisors in white spots (**d**) and yellow-brownish stain (**e**).

tion. These characteristics include (1) affected teeth: it may manifest in any number, ranging from one to four first permanent molars and could be concomitant with any permanent incisors; (2) severity: it can present significant variation within the same individual; and (3) nonuniform distribution of demarcated opacities, since they show variations in their location and severity among the affected teeth [18] (shown in Fig. 2, 3).

The variability of these defects among the same group of teeth in a single patient, and even the heterogeneity within individual teeth, can pose challenges not only in diagnosis but also in comprehending the etiology of the defect. The present challenge for researchers is to comprehend how MIH determinants influence the occurrence of clinically variable defects in specific regions of the dentition.

It has been proposed that differences in gene expression between the right and left sides, along with potential environmental/systemic disruptions, might disrupt the development of a specific permanent first molar, whereas the opposite permanent first molar may remain unaffected [18]. This hypothesis provides a potential explanation for the occurrence of a defect in only one permanent first molar. Furthermore, it has been also hypothesized that variations in the affected regions of the first permanent molars could stem from differences in genetic regulation and mechanical forces. They suggested that pressure within the connective tissues surrounding the enamel organ, particularly near the papillary layer, could induce disturbances during enamel development [18]. Considering this, we also propose that asymmetry in MIH may arise from asymmetric behavior in vascularization of a specific region. Vascular-

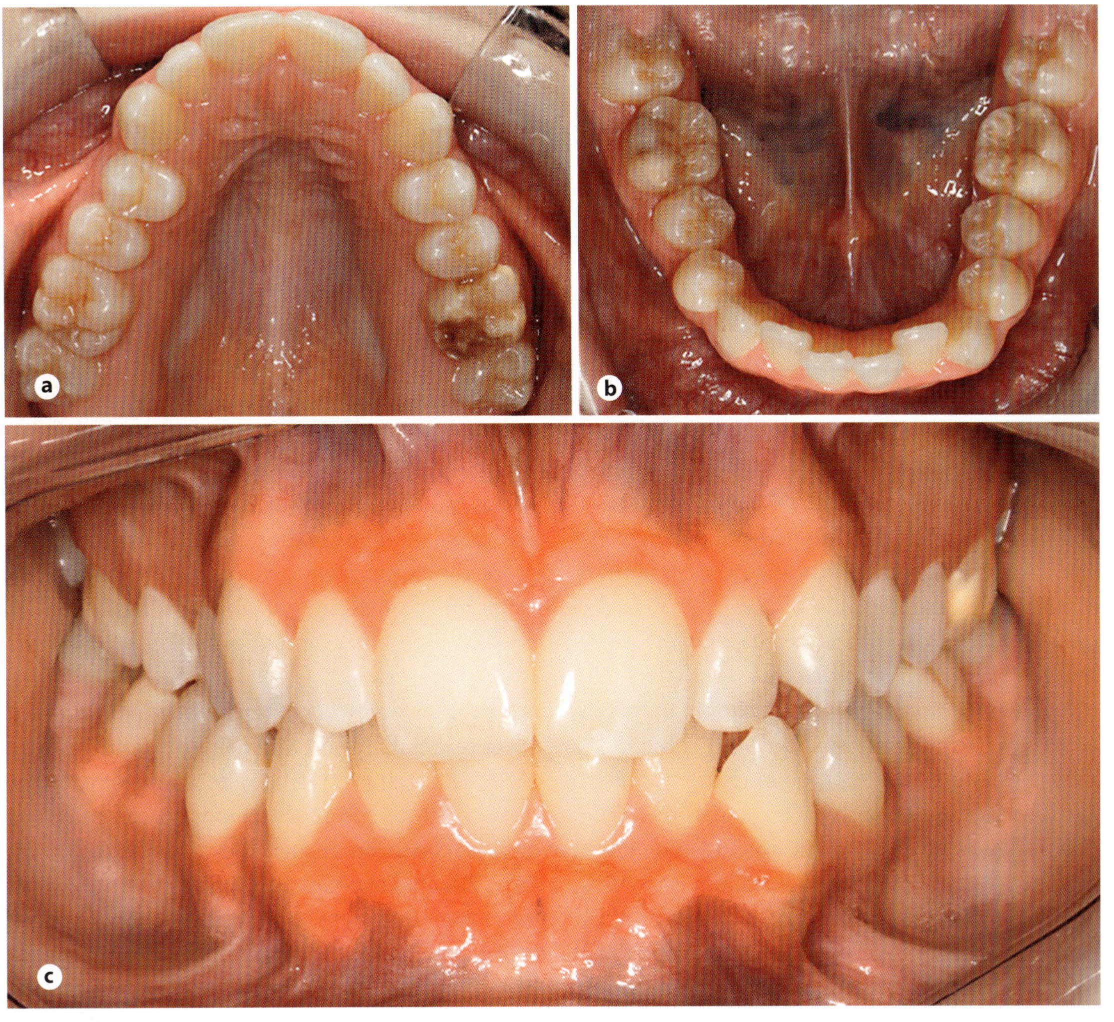

Fig. 3. The asymmetrical clinical presentation of a patient with MIH, showing structural loss only on tooth 26; yellow-brown stains on teeth 16, 36, and 46, and discrete white spots on teeth 11, 21, 22, and 12.

ization plays a pivotal role by supplying nutrients and mineral ions crucial for enamel development and may even transport aggressive factors near the enamel organ. In this context, it is essential to consider the presence of a complex microvascular system within the enamel organ. Theoretically, this system plays a role in regulating the local influx of molecules, including proteins and ions, necessary for various stages of amelogenesis. However, it can also serve as a local source of factors that may interfere with the normal progression of the amelogenesis process [6–8]. However, further studies are necessary to confirm whether this is an acceptable hypothesis.

Current research has primarily focused on etiological factors associated with compromised enamel mineralisation, but there is a significant gap in understanding the specific molecular events leading to this condition. While these aspects remain elusive, various research models are dedicated to unraveling the pathogenesis of hypomineralisation during the amelogenesis process [19–21]. Laboratory investigations involving rats and mice serve as primary sources for comprehending the mechanisms underlying enamel hypomineralisation, given the continued occurrence of amelogenesis in their continuously growing incisors throughout life [1]. Given that ameloblasts are only active during enamel formation phases, and human tooth eruption occurs years after amelogenesis is completed [1, 5], coupled with enamel's nonremodeling nature [1, 5], identifying and studying insults endured by the enamel organ during its development presents significant challenges. Additionally, establishing a causal link between insults related to amelogenesis and MIH through longitudinal studies in humans proves to be a complex task.

Indeed, the classical theory regarding the occurrence of MIH is primarily associated with the fragility of ameloblasts and how alterations in these cells are believed to be responsible for MIH [22]. During the maturation phase, morphological alterations in ameloblasts are primarily associated with oscillations of transporting mineral ions to the enamel matrix, particularly involving calcium and phosphate, as well as variations in pH within the cellular environment [1, 5, 23, 24]. It is widely accepted that crystal growth and proteinase activity in the extracellular space are pH-dependent phenomena, demanding a highly controlled coordination of cellular transport processes to regulate the pH of the extracellular fluid [11, 12]. During the process of amelogenesis, variations in pH are observed, typically being more acidic during the secretory stage and more alkaline during the maturation stage [12, 24]. While various factors contribute to the regulation of pH during enamel formation, recent findings suggest that gene regulation and protein expression are key players in this process [12]. Additionally, chloride channels, bicarbonate transporters, and carbonic anhydrases are recognized as crucial components in maintaining and regulating pH levels [12].

An acidified microenvironment presents challenges to the proteolytic activity of key enzymes, such as KLK4. The diminished ability of KLK4 to hydrolyze proteins, such as amelogenin, results in their persistence within the enamel matrix during mineralisation. This, in turn, exerts influence over the expansion of enamel prisms and the incorporation of minerals [25–27]. As infectious processes and the consequent inflammatory immune response often lead to acidification of the microenvironment, we hypothesize that acidifying the medium during an infection might impact pH regulation in amelogenesis. This could result in alterations in enamel crystal growth and proteinase activity. However, to validate this hypothesis, further investigations are necessary to explore the connection between infectious and/or inflammatory events during the amelogenesis process and how this might contribute to alter the enamel maturation.

Another way to explore the histopathology of MIH is the alteration of selective permeability of the ameloblast layer, since alterations of proteins in the tight junctions of ameloblasts can comprise a critical factor in the development of enamel [28, 29]. Claudins constitute the primary protein family comprising tight junctions, playing a crucial role in regulating their permeability [28]. Notably, recent findings have linked loss-of-function mutations in the encoding genes, specifically claudins 16 and 19, to cases of AI [28–30]. Additionally, a research study investigated the impact of administering amoxicillin to young mice on enamel mineralisation and the activity of specific proteins, such as KLK4 and tight junction proteins (claudin 1 – CLDN1, claudin 4 – CLDN4, and occludin – OCLN) in ameloblasts [31]. It was noted that administering amoxicillin resulted in increased gaps between mature ameloblasts, and "cyst-like" lesions were detected in the enamel matrix [31]. Noteworthy, the enamel chalky/white patches caused by amoxicillin experimental administration resembled the clinical appearance of hypomineralisation [31]. These findings revealed that rats treated with amoxicillin experienced a reduction in the expression of KLK4, CLDN1, CLDN4, and OCLN in mature ameloblasts. This suggests a noteworthy influence of amoxicillin on the mentioned proteins in the context of enamel development. Indeed, studies demonstrate that the exposure to 50 and 100 mg/kg per day of amoxicillin resulted in elevated instances of enamel chalky/white patches, reaching 58% and 100%, respectively. In contrast, the control group, which did not receive amoxicillin, exhibited such enamel changes in only 8.3% of mice [31]. While the use of amoxicillin affects the enamel formation process, other factors may also contribute to the occurrence of these enamel alterations.

Furthermore, the presence of unusual proteins in hypomineralised enamel, such as serum albumin, alpha-1-antitrypsin, antithrombin III, and type I collagen, beyond those typically found in amelogenesis, has been previously demonstrated [32–34]. These proteins appear to contribute to hypomineralisation through direct inhibition, either by albumin binding to minerals or by inhibition through KLK4, alpha-1-antitrypsin, and antithrombin [32–34]. The Mineralization-Poisoning Model proposed by Hubbard et al. [35] suggests that albumin, by binding to immature enamel crystals and resisting degradation during enamel maturation, disrupts the normal process of crystal growth. This interference could result in the development of porous and weakened enamel. This theory moves away from the conventional understanding of ameloblast injury to underscore the extracellular influence of albumin on the mineralisation process during enamel development.

Albumin is an abundant protein in blood plasma with multifunctional properties, characterized by its ligand-binding capacity, which is an important carrier/transporter in the human body for both endogenous and exogenous components. Consequently, albumin assumes a significant role in ion transport by binding to minerals like Ca^{2+}, Na^{+}, and K^{+}. Additionally, it acts as a potential drug carrier and can influence in vascular permeability [36]. Certain aspects pertaining to the mechanisms through which albumin permeates the enamel space remain incompletely understood [35]. Nevertheless, existing knowledge suggests that albumin accumulates in inflamed tissue, driven by extensive neovascularization in these areas. This accumulation is influenced by the combined effects of a permeable capillary network and impaired lymphatic drainage, known as the enhanced permeability and retention effect [36]. Additionally, a contributing factor facilitating the proximity of albumin to ameloblasts may be attributed to the presence of fenestrated capillaries, which is responsible for supplying blood to the papillary layer [6]. However, to elucidate this theory, further investigations are necessary.

We propose that disturbances in control of ameloblast layer permeability as well in the underlying enamel organ vascular system could be involved in MIH. Initially, the presence of fenestrated capillaries and the putative alterations in the local vascular flow by systemic and inflammatory factors can result in the presence of "unusual" proteins in the vicinity of the ameloblast layer. In parallel, alterations in ameloblast tight junction proteins, observed in response to amoxicillin, for example [31], may be a potential avenue through which albumin could be implicated. It could be hypothesized that changes in the permeability of tight junctions could affect movement of substances, including albumin, across the ameloblast layer, influencing enamel development. Moreover, the clinical manifestation of chalky or white patches in the enamel, reminiscent of hypomineralisation, aligns with the potential impact of albumin on mineralisation processes. The lesion-like cysts and intercellular spaces may be indicative of disturbances in the ameloblast capacity to control the flux of protein and mineral ions during enamel maturation, and consequently, result in local alterations due the presence of albumin in

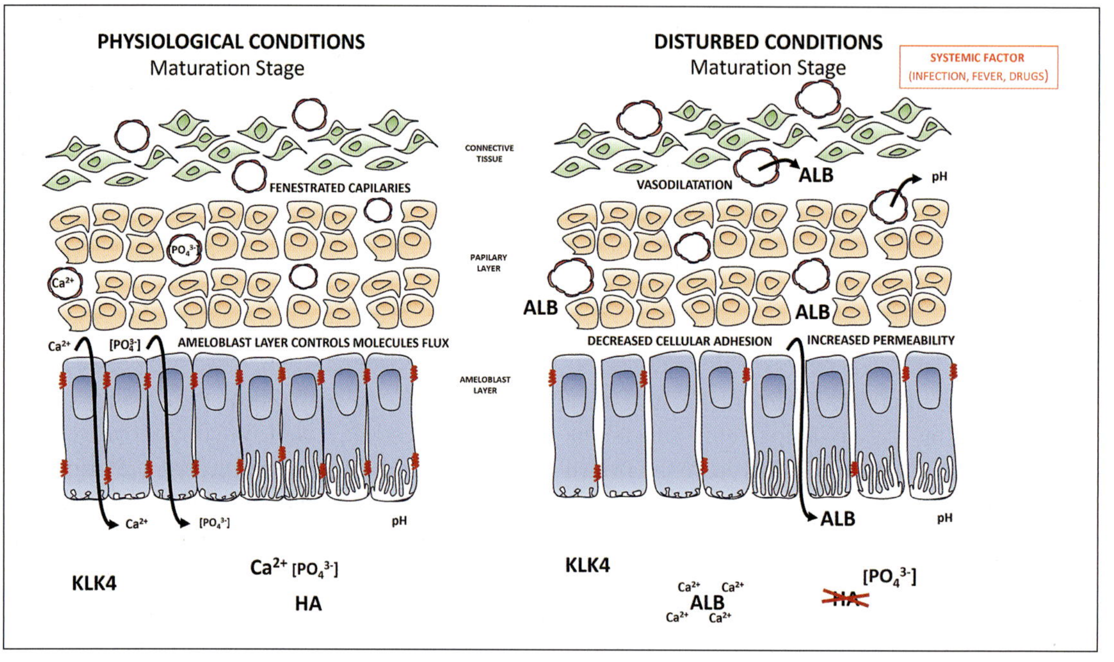

Fig. 4. Physiological conditions of maturation stage (left) and formulated hypotheses of disturbed conditions in the maturation stage that lead to MIH (right). Under physiological conditions, during the maturation stage, ameloblasts regulate the flow of ions and molecules. The binding of Ca^{2+} and [PO4] gives rise to the precursors of hydroxyapatite crystals, which, in turn, organize themselves within the amelogenin matrix. KLK4 is secreted by ameloblasts to enzymatically degrade amelogenin. Formulated hypotheses regarding disturbed conditions in the maturation stage that could lead to MIH: systemic and inflammatory factors may induce alterations in vascular flow, promoting vasodilatation, potentially allowing the presence of albumin in the ameloblast layer region. Furthermore, a decrease in the expression of tight junction proteins could lead to reduced cellular adhesion and increased permeability between ameloblasts, facilitating the entry of substances, such as albumin, into the enamel space. Albumin, due to its high affinity for calcium, binds to Ca^{2+}, inhibiting the formation of hydroxyapatite crystals. Additionally, a decrease in the expression of KLK4 may interfere with the proteolysis of enamel proteins, such as amelogenins. These hypotheses must be interpreted with caution, as further studies are necessary to confirm their validity.

the developing enamel, which in turn would affect the mineralisation process. Additional factors, such as the decreased KLK4 activity, must also be considered as putative elements underlying the enamel alteration. These formulated hypotheses of histopathology of MIH are shown in Figure 4. Thus, it seems interesting to investigate the interplay between factors that disturb host homeostasis (which can include infectious processes and its consequences, such as fever, and therapeutic elements such as some antibiotics), tight junctions, and albumin in the complex orchestration of enamel mineralisation. Lastly, we suggest that more research should be conducted studying the influence of gene expressions, especially those related to tight junctions, in shaping permeability and substance entry, with a keen focus on albumin.

The genetic and/or epigenetic influence is also an important factor to be considered in the causes of MIH. A recent systematic review delved into the identification of genetic variants and interactions among genes associated with critical processes like amelogenesis, immune response, aquaporins, vitamin D receptors, and other relevant factors [37]. The potential impact of single nucleotide polymorphisms in key amelogenesis-related genes, such as BMP2, BMP4, BMP7, AMTN, MMP20, AMBN, AMELX, ENAM, FAM83H, DLX3, and SCUBE1/TTLL1, could play a role in the development of MIH, impacting enamel mineralisation and crystal growth. Moreover, the study revealed genetic variations in ion transport-related genes (VDR, ORAI, STIM1, STIM2, SLC34A2, SLC34A3, PVALB, HSP90B1, SLC24A4, and TRPM7) associated with MIH, suggesting their involvement in enamel matrix mineralisation. The association of immune response genes (DEFB1, TGFBR1, TGFA, IL-4, IL-17A, IL-10, IL-1A, and STAT1) with MIH indicates a potential connection between inflammatory processes and DDE. This link may alter the expression profile, leading to increased vascularization and/or vasodilatation in dental germs upon inflammatory stimuli, and consequently to a higher risk of serum albumin leakage, ultimately affecting enamel formation. The study also explored the influence of aquaporin genes (AQP5) and the hypoxia-related HIF-1 gene on MIH, shedding light on their roles in enamel mineralisation and adaptation to hypoxic conditions [37]. Additionally, the review addressed single nucleotide polymorphisms not directly associated with amelogenesis or immune response (e.g., near PPARGC1A/MIR573, RMI1/SLC28A3, CDH5, and KCNG1/NFATC2), emphasizing the intricate nature of genetic factors contributing to MIH. However, the level of certainty in the evidence presented in this systematic review was very low due to methodological heterogeneity among the studies, underscoring the need for future research to elucidate the intricate genetic mechanisms underlying MIH [37].

In conclusion, while there have been advancements in understanding the causative mechanisms of MIH, there are still unresolved issues that require further clarification. For example, the asymmetric nature of MIH remains a mystery. The intricate interplay between genes and local disrupting factors, including environmental or systemic related, require exploring the pathogenesis of MIH via this multitude of factors and their interactions.

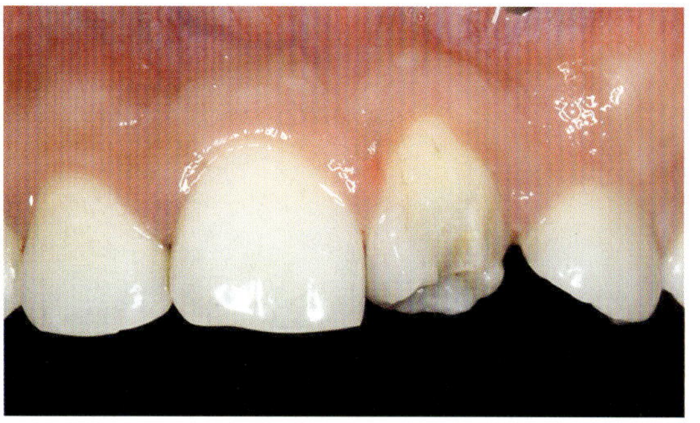

Fig. 5. Clinical aspect of enamel hypoplasia on upper left central incisor characterized by a reduced quantity of enamel.

Enamel Hypoplasia

Enamel hypoplasia (EH) has multiple causes and occurs at an earlier stage of enamel development compared to enamel hypomineralisation, specifically during the secretion of enamel matrix [38]. The disturbance in the secretory stage leads to hampered or inhibition of ameloblast function, resulting in a quantitative enamel defect [39–43]. Clinically, teeth affected by EH shows upon eruption lines, pits, grooves, or larger areas lacking enamel, which can be localized or generalized [38, 44–46] (shown in Fig. 5).

Local, systemic, environmental, or genetic disturbances are considered etiological factors associated to the occurrence of EH [38, 47–52]. This defect may affect deciduous or permanent teeth and occur due to pre-, peri-, and postnatal injuries [48–52]. As an example for local etiological factor, systematic reviews have highlighted that in cases of trauma in primary teeth, EH in the permanent successor tends to prevail, rather than other DDE [53, 54]. A common thread among

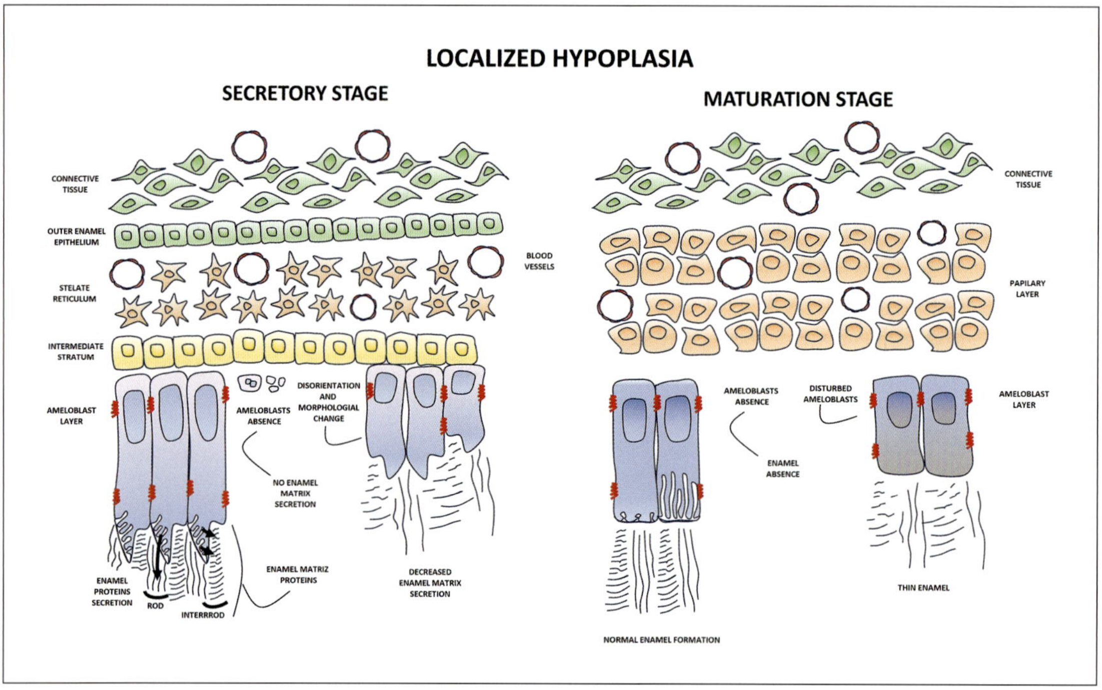

Fig. 6. Dysfunctions during the secretory (left) and maturation (right) stages of amelogenesis that lead to localized hypoplasia due to trauma. Disorientation and morphological changes in ameloblasts during the secretory stage interfere with the deposition of enamel matrix proteins, consequently promoting the formation of thin enamel during the maturation stage. Conversely, the degeneration/disappearance of ameloblasts during the secretory stage results in a lack of enamel in the subsequent stage.

various potential risk factors is their interference with the molecular regulation of amelogenesis [55]. In instances of enamel underdevelopment stemming from local and environmental factors, the formation of the defect is contingent upon the intensity, duration of the injury, and the number of ameloblasts affected by specific factors. These factors include the number and orientation of ameloblasts and their location in the crown [55]. Additionally, given that each tooth follows a distinct developmental pattern, the extent of involvement, location, and appearance of the defect can vary among different teeth. When clinical alteration impacts all teeth, the potential influence of genetic factors must be investigated [55].

The histopathological mechanism of EH may vary depending on the causal factor. Laboratory studies involving rats are essential for a comprehensive understanding of this process. Next, the histopathological mechanism of EH will be exemplified through four distinct causal factors: trauma, hypoxia, diabetes, and episodic stress. The findings of Taniguchi et al. [56] contribute to the understanding of how trauma in deciduous teeth can differentially affect the development of permanent successor teeth depending on the stage that the injury occurs. Trauma during the initiation stage (postnatal day 1) resulted in enamel matrix abnormalities, particularly in the traumatized area. This suggested direct injury to ameloblasts, leading to localized EH. Significant histological changes have occurred, including degenerative alterations in enamel matrix substances and immature dentin adjacent to ameloblasts and odontoblasts. Damage to the enamel organ and papillary layer has resulted in disfiguration of the cuspid shape. Subsequent days showed degeneration and disappearance of ameloblasts, the absence of enamel matrix formation, lack of ameloblast alignment after 10 days, and observation of EH and irregular dentin after 18 days [56]. Trauma at the thin layer of hard tissue stage (postnatal day 3) resulted in irregular arrangements of ameloblasts, distortion of the ameloblast layer, and failure of enamel matrix formation within a day of trauma. Subsequent days exhibited more significant failures, leading to a delayed and dilacerated crown eruption [56]. Trauma at the thick matrix formation stages (postnatal days 5 and 7) caused disturbances in enamel and matrix formation, affecting multiple cuspids. Although changes were less severe than those at postnatal day 3, a larger area of enamel was affected, likely due to increased resistance from hard tissues, suggesting a trauma in bloc [56]. Trauma during the mineralisation stage (postnatal day 10) resulted in minimal enamel defects, with observed EH at the cervical portion of the crown. This was attributed to the hardness of the enamel organ tissues at this stage [56]. A simplified illustration of the primary consequences of trauma to amelogenesis is presented in Figure 6. Another study observed that in rats whose mothers were subjected to 22 days of hypoxia during gestation, secretory ameloblasts exhibited disruptions [57]. The severity of these alterations varied, encompassing disorientation and morphological changes in ameloblasts to the formation of cyst-like lesions on enamel space and abnormal matrix formation [57].

It is important to highlight that clinically hypomineralisation can occur together with hypoplasia. Sidaly et al. [21] examined the impact of a short episode of induced hypoxia on enamel formation in adult mice. The study observed that the incisors of mice exposed to hypoxia exhibited hypoplastic and hypomineralised enamel. This research established that the induced injury significantly affected the secretory ameloblasts, resulting in EH and compromising ameloblast functions in the subsequent mineralisation/maturation stage of amelogenesis.

EH in primary teeth was observed in children born to diabetic mothers [49, 50, 58]. It is believed that the prolonged disturbance in ameloblast function or alterations in gene expression profiles are responsible for the alteration [58, 59]. A study conducted by Silva-Sousa et al. [60] examined structural alterations in the enamel organ of rats born to mothers with diabetes mellitus. In the group where diabetic mothers were untreated (without insulin), there was a thinning of the enamel matrix and ameloblasts. Additionally, the nuclear area of the ameloblasts was smaller. These characteristics may have led to a decrease in enamel matrix secretion [60]. In mothers who were treated (with insulin), the ameloblast nuclei had a more elliptical shape, and there was an increase in the interstitial area of the stellate reticulum [60]. Given the elevated permeability of the basement membrane in various tissues among diabetic patients, the expansion in the area corresponding to the stellate reticulum's interstitium may be attributed to an increase in fluid content facilitated by the heightened permeability of blood vessels in the region [60]. The expansion in this area may have prevented nutrients from reaching the secretory ameloblasts, resulting in alterations in enamel matrix secretion [60]. Finally, during stress episodes, the narrowing of blood vessels in the enamel organ hinders the differentiation of ameloblasts and odontoblasts, leading to the formation of shortened enamel prisms and decreased enamel matrix secretion [61–65].

It is important to disclose that the literature describes various possible causative factors for EH; however, the mechanisms involved in histopathogenesis require further clarification. Due to the reduced quantity of enamel in an irregular form, patients with EH may face difficulties in

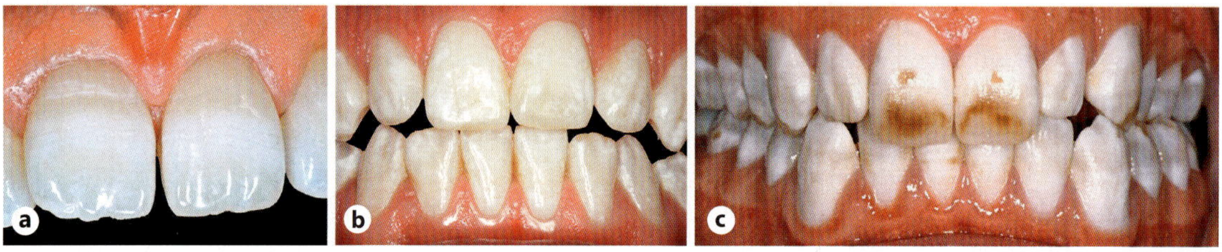

Fig. 7. Clinical aspects of dental fluorosis (DF). **a** DF with narrow white lines resembling the pericymatia. Confluent in a few places (grade 2). **b** DF with strongly merging lines with irregular cloudy-opaque areas. **c** DF with the whole area opaque white or brownish with single loss of enamel.

conducting efficient oral hygiene and may experience compromised aesthetics, which can impact their quality of life. Given these considerations, it is evident that the multifaceted nature of EH demands an adequate diagnostic and management.

Dental Fluorosis

DF is a toxicological issue that affects tooth enamel due to excessive exposure to fluoride during the development of enamel. Unlike changes caused by trauma, infections, or systemic health issues, DF occurs independently of such events. Researchers have comprehended this condition as a disorder arising from the developmental process of enamel, resulting from exposure to a xenobiotic. During amelogenesis, exposure to elevated levels of fluoride can affect the structure and crystallinity of enamel leading to alterations in the color, hardness, and mineral content. Clinically, the observed aspects may include a loss of enamel luster, chalk-colored patches, streak-like alterations, and areas displaying chalk-like discoloration with brown staining in more severe cases (shown in Fig. 7). Due to the soft nature of enamel, it is prone to chipping easily after eruption, which can result in pits and grooves [66, 67]. It is important to note that the severity of DF depends on the duration of exposure and the total amount of fluoride intake during enamel secretion. Moreover, there is no particular dose threshold that is responsible for causing tissue malformation [68].

Recognizing that amelogenesis has a finite duration within odontogenesis directs our attention to the chronological development of teeth, in which the fluoride exposure will only affect the dental elements that are still undergoing amelogenesis during exposure. Seeking greater precision and remembering that enamel formation occurs along the cusp/incisal edge and continues toward the cervical region, crown regions of the same dental element may have different magnitudes of this problem. Using the same logic as when considering enamel thickness, DF-related alterations can vary along this thickness, as enamel formation occurs in a direction from the dentin-enamel junction to the surface. In other words, in the same tooth, there are variations in the magnitude of these changes both along the surface and in its thickness. Another key consideration in understanding DF is that homologous teeth share a similar formation chronology. This explains why, for instance, the upper central incisors may display similar DF patterns, both in deep and superficial extension along the cervical-incisal edge direction.

However, how does this fluoride exposure interfere with amelogenesis? Reduced ameloblast proliferation, heightened ameloblast apoptosis, and increased Ca^{2+} intracellular in vitro have been associated with high fluoride exposure. Among the pathways that may play a role in the

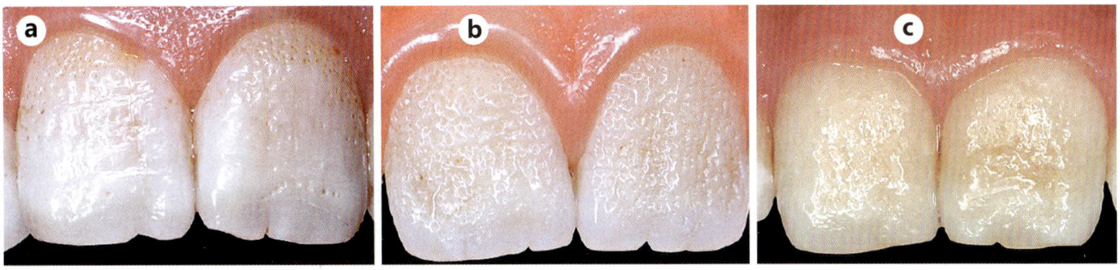

Fig. 8. Clinical aspect of hypoplastic AI. **a** Central anterior teeth in the mother (after bleaching). **b** Central anterior teeth in the first daughter (after bleaching). **c** Central anterior teeth in the second daughter (without bleaching). Note the indentations on the cutting edges of mother and daughters.

occurrence of apoptosis are endoplasmic reticulum stress (ERS), oxidative stress, and an increase in the phagocytic activity of mature ameloblasts [69, 70]. Zhang et al. [71] observed an increase in calcium concentration directly associated with the rise in fluoride concentration. The calcium overload can induce changes in ameloblasts, leading to ERS. In addition, ERS results in disruptions in ameloblast protein synthesis, affecting its functions, including the synthesis of proteins such as proteinases responsible for removing enamel matrix proteins (MMP20 and KLK4). In essence, the reduction in proteinase secretion results in a delayed hydrolysis of enamel matrix proteins. The failure to remove these proteins leads to hypomineralised enamel known as DF [70–72].

Amelogenesis Imperfecta

AI was first defined as a hereditary condition that significantly affects enamel development [73]. This genetic disorder may present either in isolation or as part of a syndrome [1, 74, 75] and is observable in both primary and permanent dentitions, even if not macroscopically evident [76]. Therefore, its definition was redefined to a group of conditions, with genomic origin, affecting the structure and clinical appearance of enamel of all (or nearly all) the teeth, and which may be associated with morphologic or biochemical changes elsewhere in the body [77].

The diagnosis of AI relies on factors such as family history, pedigree mapping, and meticulous clinical observation. However, the heterogeneity of phenotypes and the absence of a universally accepted nomenclature system can complicate the accurate diagnosis of AI. Initially, AI classification systems primarily involved assessing clinical appearance (phenotype) of the condition [78, 79]. However, Aldred et al. [77] proposed a refined system that classifies AI primarily based on inheritance, with the phenotype as a secondary consideration. This system categorizes AI according to the molecular basis (chromosomal localization/locus/mutation – when known), biochemical outcome (putative result of the mutation – when known), and phenotype (description of clinical and/or radiographic features and/or other relevant findings). Nonetheless, since this book is centered on the MIH topic, we will describe the condition based on phenotypic classification, aimed at facilitating the differentiation among enamel defects with different origins.

The phenotypes of DDE associated with AI are categorized as hypoplastic (shown in Fig. 8, 9), indicating a reduction or the absence of enamel formation (enamel agenesis), and hypomineralised (shown in Fig. 10), denoting an elevated protein content compared to normal enamel [1, 74, 80]. Mutations in various genes related to enamel ex-

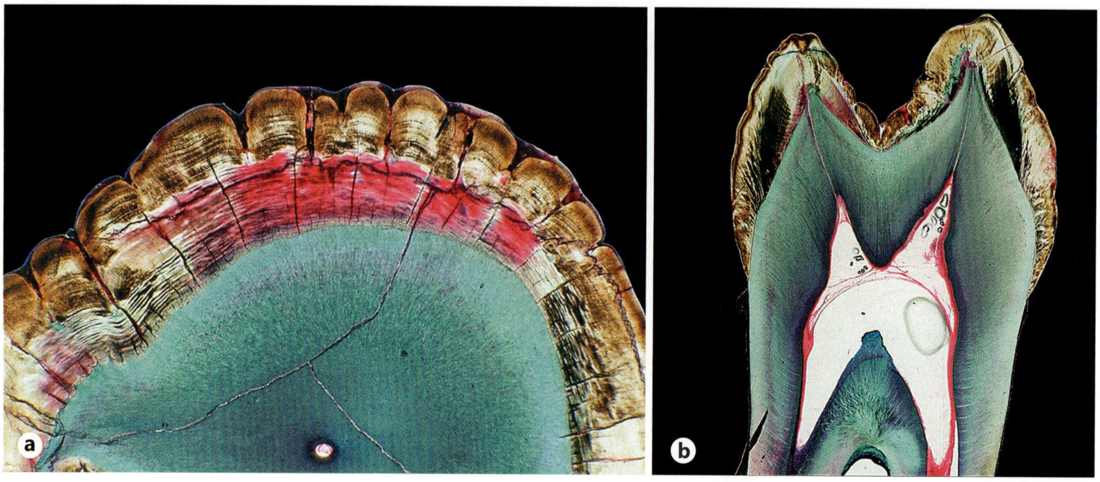

Fig. 9. Horizontal (**a**) and longitudinal (**b**) histological sections of human teeth with AI of the dimple-like type. The different characteristics and depth of the dimples are recognizable. The teeth were stained with fuchsin and acetic light green.

tracellular matrix proteins or proteinases, along with other gene types, have been linked to the occurrence of AI [1, 74, 75]. Following, we will explore key findings related to mutations that lead to the occurrence of isolated forms of AI.

Mutations linked to AI have been recognized in numerous enamel extracellular matrix proteins and proteinases as well as several other genes. The association between genetics (type of mutation) and phenotype (type of enamel problem) arises from the impact of mutations on protein function, which is essential in cellular processes such as self-aggregation of proteins, interactions between proteins and minerals, and alterations in the processing of the mutant protein [1, 81, 82].

AMELX, the gene that codes amelogenin, the most abundant enamel matrix protein, was associated with AI [1, 83–86]. Different alterations in the protein results in different phenotypes of AI caused by various allelic mutations in AMELX [1, 87]. If the mutation leads to the deletion of a specific segment (the carboxyl terminus) of the amelogenin protein, it is commonly associated with a hypoplastic enamel phenotype. The correlation between the type of mutation and enamel defects arises from the pivotal roles played by specific regions of the amelogenin protein in the formation and orientation of developing enamel crystals. For instance, the carboxyl terminus is crucial for the grouping and orientation of amelogenin during this process. When mutations occur in the amelogenin gene, leading to changes in a single amino acid, they are often associated with a hypomineralised enamel phenotype.

Certain phenotypes give rise to more localized enamel defects, while others are associated with generalized enamel defects affecting all teeth and enamel areas [88]. Different mutations can result in proteins having a dominant negative effect, while others cause haploinsufficiency. For example, the impact of mutations on the ENAM gene defines variations in the characteristics of AI. When a dominant negative effect occurs, it leads to generalized thin EH, whereas haploinsufficiency results in bands of pitted enamel [1, 89, 90]. The absence of organized and mineralised layers of enamel is observed in mice when the ENAM gene is knocked out, underscoring the

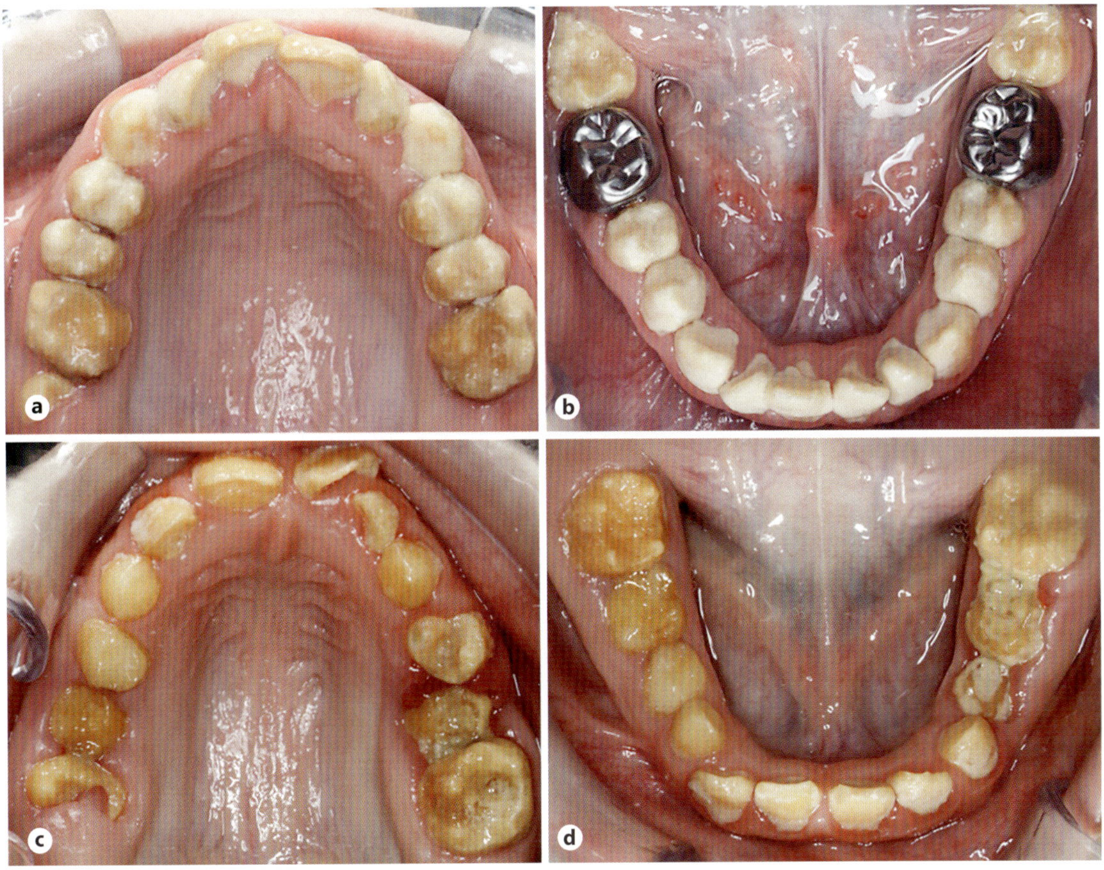

Fig. 10. Clinical aspect of hypomineralised AI affecting all teeth in two patients (brothers), highlighting the hereditary pattern. Occlusal views of upper and lower teeth for patient 1 (**a**, **b**) and patient 2 (**c**, **d**).

significance of ENAMELIN in crystal growth [1, 91].

It has been identified that mutations in genes encoding MMP20 and KLK4 lead to a decrease in the final mineral content in enamel, causing hypomineralisation. This occurs through a reduction in the processing and removal of enamel matrix proteins. Consequently, there is an increased retention of protein content in the affected enamel, leading to alterations in crystallite growth [1, 80, 92–94].

Although proteins, such as WDR72, FAM83H, and C4ORF26, have been linked as causative factor to develop AI [1, 95–100], their functions are not completely understood [1]. Mutations in the WDR72 gene lead to enamel hypomaturation defects. This arises from an irregular pathway involving endocytic vesicles transporting matrix proteins, impacting the subsequent mineralisation of the enamel [1, 95–97]. FAM83H interacts with casein kinase 1 and is believed to contribute to the organization of the keratin cytoskeleton and desmosomes in ameloblasts [1, 98]. Mutations in the FAM83H gene are associated with autosomal dominant inheritance of hypocalcified (hypomineralised) AI [99]. While the C4ORF26 gene is specific to teeth rather than enamel, its phosphorylated carboxy terminus suggests a potential contribution to enamel development dur-

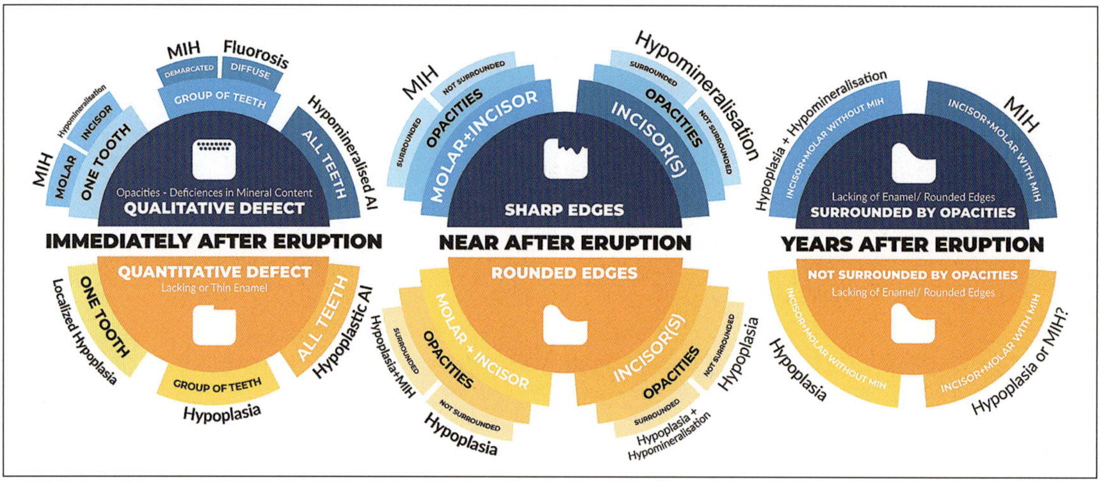

Fig. 11. Flowchart of the differential diagnosis of the developmental defects of enamel from a clinical perspective.

ing hydroxyapatite nucleation [100], mutations in proteins namely amelotin (Amtn) – expressed during the maturation stage of amelogenesis [101–103], GPR68 – a pH-sensing G protein-coupled receptor [104], and ACPT (testicular acid phosphatase) [105], have been associated with the occurrence of AI [1].

In summary, from a clinical perspective, AI phenotypes are classified as hypoplastic or hypomineralised, with different gene mutations linked to various DDE. Further research is needed to elucidate the functions of certain genes and their roles in enamel development, including the different pathways undertaken by genetic regulation in causing AI or MIH. Understanding the genetic basis of AI is crucial for accurate diagnosis and developing targeted interventions to manage the impact of this condition on dental health.

Differential Diagnosis from a Clinical Perspective

After discussing in this chapter several molecular and genetic mechanisms that regulate histopathological response of DDE that lead to different clinical characteristics, we present a flowchart outlining the differential diagnosis of DDE based on their most distinctive clinical aspects (shown in Fig. 11).

Immediately after eruption is the optimal time for performing differential diagnosis between quantitative defects, which occur during the organic matrix deposition phase (hypoplastic – lacking or thin enamel), and qualitative defects during the maturation and mineralisation phase (hypomineralised – deficiencies in mineral content). At this stage, these defects present in their original form, without transformation influenced by the oral environment. The number and types of teeth involved will determine the differentiation between locally caused defects affecting only one nonmolar tooth (hypomineralisation and hypoplasia), systemically environmentally caused defects, which may or may not be influenced by genetics, affecting a group of teeth (EH, DF, or MIH), or genetically caused defects affecting all teeth (AI). The opacity's characteristics can also aid in the differential diagnosis. Hypomineralisation impacting homologous groups of teeth, attributed to the toxic effects of fluoride (DF), exhibit a distinctive feature, characterized by the

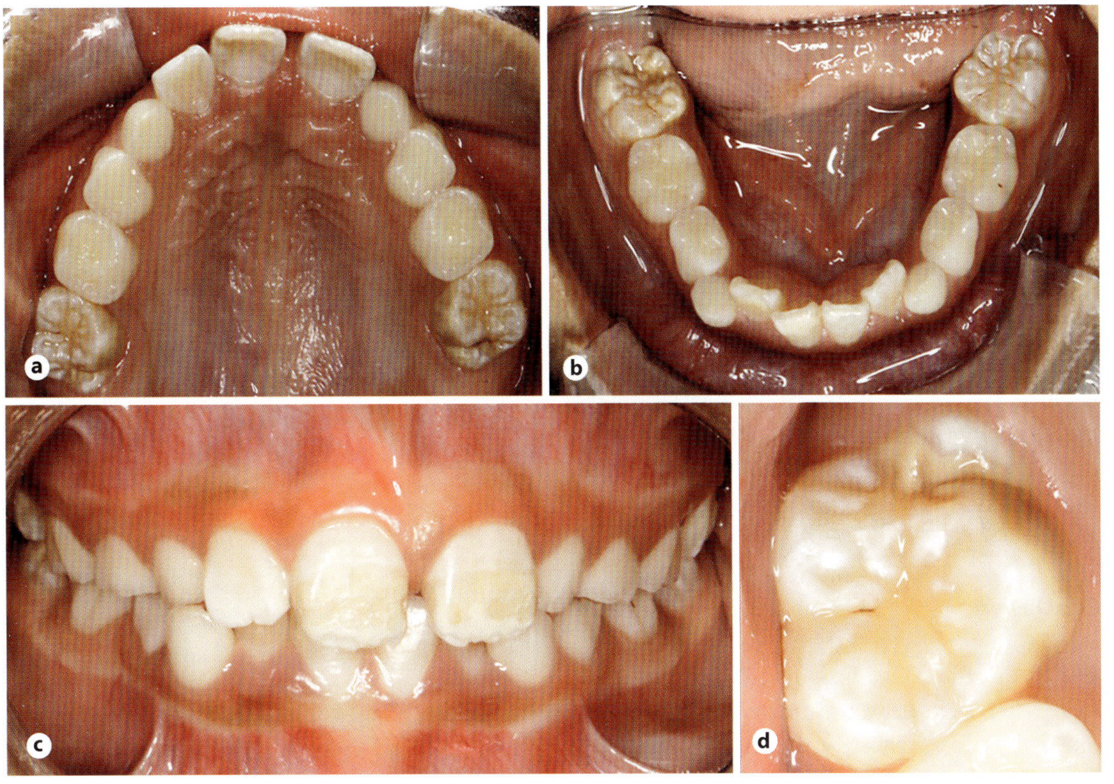

Fig. 12. Clinical representation of DF coupled with MIH. **a**, **b** Symmetrical manifestation of DF on homologous teeth and the asymmetrical presentation of MIH are evident in occlusal view. **c** Frontal view of central incisors with DF. **d** Occlusal view of MIH on palatal and distal cusps and DF on the occlusal edge.

presence of diffuse opacities instead of localized ones, as observed in MIH.

A second crucial period for differential diagnosis is the early years after eruption. During this time, enamel weakened by the presence of hypomineralisation may experience fractures and exhibit characteristics resembling EH, such as lacking enamel. In these conditions, clinical features determining the differential diagnosis include the edges and color of the remaining enamel. If the edges are irregular and sharp, it indicates hypomineralisation, which, if affecting molars, may be diagnosed as MIH. Conversely, if the edges are rounded, it suggests EH. However, the presence of opacity around the rounded absent enamel may suggest the coexistence of EH and hypomineralisation across the same tooth. This condition could manifest as EH combined with MIH in molars, or as EH plus hypomineralisation in incisors. It is important to recognize that both scenarios essentially reflect a combination of EH and hypomineralisation, whether classified as MIH or not.

Several years after eruption, in cases where hypomineralised enamel has undergone posteruptive fractures, over time, the remaining enamel undergoes natural wear, and its sharp edges become rounded. During this period, the differential diagnosis with respect to EH is determined by the presence of demarcated opacity and the characteristics of the molars. Thus, if there is rounded loss with opacity in the remaining enamel, when it occurs only in incisors, it is EH associated with hypomineralisation. However, when it occurs in both incisors and molars, it is then diagnosed as MIH. When there is no opacity, and the absence is only in incisors, it is EH, but in molars, it remains undefined, possibly being either EH or MIH.

Finally, despite the ongoing discussion regarding the nomenclature of MIH, the same defect can occur in deciduous molars (deciduous molar hypomineralisation – or hypomineralised second primary molars) or in other permanent teeth besides the first molars (hypomineralisation of other permanent teeth), and this flowchart (shown in Fig. 11) is applicable to all cases. It is important to highlight that different types of DDE may affect the same individual (shown in Fig. 12).

Conclusion

The histopathological insights into various DDE follow distinct trajectories and involve diverse etiological factors. Therefore, their knowledge is fundamental for accurate clinical diagnoses and adequate management. It is noteworthy that studies related to disturbances in amelogenesis are predominantly limited to animals, particularly rodents, and the extrapolation of these findings to human amelogenesis requires cautious consideration. Many hypotheses were formulated to explain certain aspects of the histopathology of MIH and other DDE; however, future investigations are warranted to scrutinize and validate them.

Acknowledgment

We express our gratitude to the Bauru School of Dentistry – University of São Paulo, Institute of Biological Sciences – Federal University of Pará and School of Dentistry – Federal University of Rio de Janeiro for their invaluable support and resources, which played a crucial role in the development of this chapter.

Statement of Ethics

We state that the pictures of patients were obtained with patients' written informed consent for publication of the images.

Conflict of Interest Statement

The authors declare no conflicts of interest.

Funding Sources

D.S.M. received a scholarship provided for CAPES. F.Q.I. received a scholarship provided for FAPESP. D.R., G.P.G., and R.R.L. are researchers funded by CNPq (Productivity Program). A.A.N. is a researcher funded by CNE and FAPERJ.

Author Contributions

A.L., D.R., D.S.M., and G.P.G. conceived the chapter and were responsible for overall direction and planning. D.R., D.S.M., and G.P.G. wrote the amelogenesis section. D.R., D.S.M., and F.Q.I. wrote the MIH and EH sections. R.R.L. wrote the DF section. D.R. wrote the differential diagnosis section. A.A.N. wrote the AI section. All authors actively participated in the writing process and reviewed the final version of the chapter.

References

1 Lacruz RS, Habelitz S, Wright JT, Paine ML. Dental enamel formation and implications for oral health and disease. Physiol Rev. 2017 Jul 1;97(3):939–93.
2 Collignon AM, Vergnes JN, Germa A, Azogui S, Breinig S, Hollande C, et al. Factors and mechanisms involved in acquired developmental defects of enamel: a scoping review. Front Pediatr. 2022;10:836708.
3 Purvis RJ, Barrie WJ, MacKay GS, Wilkinson EM, Cockburn F, Belton NR. Enamel hypoplasia of the teeth associated with neonatal tetany: a manifestation of maternal vitamin-D deficiency. Lancet. 1973 Oct;2(7833):811–4.
4 Skinner MF, Hung JT. Social and biological correlates of localized enamel hypoplasia of the human deciduous canine tooth. Am J Phys Anthropol. 1989 Jun;79(2):159–75.
5 Nanci A, TenCate AR. Ten Cate's oral histology: development, structure, and function. 9th ed. St. Louis, Missouri: Elsevier; 2018.
6 Garant PR, Gillespie R. The presence of fenestrated capillaries in the papillary layer of the enamel organ. Anat Rec. 1969 Jan;163(1):71–9.
7 El-Agroudi MA, Selliseth NJ, Selvig KA. Microvascular system of the rat incisor enamel organ. A scanning electron microscopic study of vascular corrosion casts. Eur J Oral Sci. 1998 Dec;106(6):1013–21. Erratum in: Eur J Oral Sci. 1999 Feb;107(1):73.
8 Prostak KS, Skobe Z. Ultrastructural study of tracer permeability through the cat and ferret enamel organ. Tissue Cell. 1990;22(5):681–96.
9 Pandya M, Liu H, Dangaria SJ, Zhu W, Li LL, Pan S, et al. Integrative temporo-spatial, mineralogic, spectroscopic, and proteomic analysis of postnatal enamel development in teeth with limited growth. Front Physiol. 2017 Oct 24;8:793.
10 Guo S, Yang H, Liu J, Meng Z, Sui L. Heat shock proteins in tooth development and injury repair. Int J Mol Sci. 2023 Apr 18;24(8):7455.
11 Smith CE. Cellular and chemical events during enamel maturation. Crit Rev Oral Biol Med. 1998;9(2):128–61.
12 Lacruz RS, Nanci A, Kurtz I, Wright JT, Paine ML. Regulation of pH during amelogenesis. Calcif Tissue Int. 2010 Feb;86(2):91–103.
13 Lacruz RS, Feske S. Diseases caused by mutations in ORAI1 and STIM1. Ann N Y Acad Sci. 2015 Nov;1356(1):45–79.
14 Simmer JP, Hu JC. Expression, structure, and function of enamel proteinases. Connect Tissue Res. 2002;43(2–3):441–9.
15 Garot E, Lopez Onaindia D, Couture C, Morales JI, Cebrià A, Oms X, et al. Insights into molar-incisor hypomineralisation in past populations: A call to anthropologists. Int J Paleopathol. 2023 Sep;42:18–26.
16 Garot E, Couture-Veschambre C, Manton D, Beauval C, Rouas P. Analytical evidence of enamel hypomineralisation on permanent and primary molars amongst past populations. Sci Rep. 2017 May 10;7(1):1712.
17 Weerheijm KL, Jälevik B, Alaluusua S. Molar-incisor hypomineralisation. Caries Res. 2001 Sep-Oct;35(5):390–1.
18 Vieira AR, Manton DJ. On the variable clinical presentation of molar incisor hypomineralization. Caries Res. 2019;53(4):482–8.
19 Tung K, Fujita H, Yamashita Y, Takagi Y. Effect of turpentine-induced fever during the enamel formation of rat incisor. Arch Oral Biol. 2006 Jun;51(6):464–70.
20 Yanagawa T, Itoh K, Uwayama J, Shibata Y, Yamaguchi A, Sano T, et al. Nrf2 deficiency causes tooth decolourization due to iron transport disorder in enamel organ. Genes Cells. 2004 Jul;9(7):641–51.
21 Sidaly R, Risnes S, Khan QE, Stiris T, Sehic A. The effect of hypoxia on the formation of mouse incisor enamel. Arch Oral Biol. 2015 Nov;60(11):1601–12.
22 Suga S. Enamel hypomineralization viewed from the pattern of progressive mineralization of human and monkey developing enamel. Adv Dent Res. 1989 Sep;3(2):188–98.
23 Pandya M, Diekwisch TGH. Amelogenesis: transformation of a protein-mineral matrix into tooth enamel. J Struct Biol. 2021 Dec;213(4):107809.
24 Kim HE, Hong JH. The overview of channels, transporters, and calcium signaling molecules during amelogenesis. Arch Oral Biol. 2018 Sep;93:47–55.
25 Martinović B, Ivanović M, Milojković Z, Mladenović R. Analysis of the mineral composition of hypomineralized first permanent molars. Vojnosanit Pregl. 2015 Oct;72(10):864–9.
26 Jeremias F, Koruyucu M, Küchler EC, Bayram M, Tuna EB, Deeley K, et al. Genes expressed in dental enamel development are associated with molar incisor hypomineralization. Arch Oral Biol. 2013 Oct;58(10):1434–42.
27 Nanci A, Zalzal S, Lavoie P, Kunikata M, Chen W, Krebsbach PH, et al. Comparative immunochemical analyses of the developmental expression and distribution of ameloblastin and amelogenin in rat incisors. J Histochem Cytochem. 1998 Aug;46(8):911–34.
28 Bardet C, Ribes S, Wu Y, Diallo MT, Salmon B, Breiderhoff T, et al. Claudin loss-of-function disrupts tight junctions and impairs amelogenesis. Front Physiol. 2017;24;8:326.
29 Bardet C, Courson F, Wu Y, Khaddam M, Salmon B, Ribes S, et al. Claudin-16 deficiency impairs tight junction function in ameloblasts, leading to abnormal enamel formation. J Bone Miner Res. 2016;31:498–513.
30 Yamaguti PM, Neves FA, Hotton D, Bardet C, de La Dure-Molla M, Castro LC, et al. Amelogenesis imperfecta in familial hypomagnesaemia and hypercalciuria with nephrocalcinosis caused by CLDN19 gene mutations. J Med Genet. 2017 Jan;54(1):26–37. Erratum in: J Med Genet. 2017 Nov;54(11):786.
31 Gao J, Li X, Gao L, Chen H, Baras BH, Liu X, et al. Effects of applying amoxicillin in juvenile mice on enamel mineralization and the expression of kallikrein-related peptidase 4 and tight junction proteins in ameloblasts. Int J Mol Med. 2020 Jul;46(1):179–190.
32 Farah RA, Monk BC, Swain MV, Drummond BK. Protein content of molar-incisor hypomineralisation enamel. J Dent. 2010 Jul;38(7):591–6.

33 Mangum JE, Crombie FA, Kilpatrick N, Manton DJ, Hubbard MJ. Surface integrity governs the proteome of hypomineralized enamel. J Dent Res. 2010 Oct; 89(10):1160–5.
34 Williams R, Perez VA, Mangum JE, Hubbard MJ. Pathogenesis of molar hypomineralisation: hypomineralised 6-year molars contain traces of fetal serum albumin. Front Physiol. 2020 Jun; 11:619.
35 Hubbard MJ, Mangum JE, Perez VA, Williams R. A breakthrough in understanding the pathogenesis of molar hypomineralisation: the mineralisation-poisoning model. Front Physiol. 2021 Dec 21;12:802833.
36 Sleep D. Albumin and its application in drug delivery. Expert Opin Drug Deliv. 2015 May;12(5):793–812.
37 da Silva Figueira R, Mustafa Gomes Muniz FW, Costa LC, Silva de Moura M, Moura LFAD, Mello de Oliveira B, et al. Association between genetic factors and molar-incisor hypomineralisation or hypomineralised second primary molar: a systematic review. Arch Oral Biol. 2023 Aug;152:105716.
38 Seow WK. Clinical diagnosis of enamel defects: pitfalls and practical guidelines. Int Dent J. 1997 Jun;47(3):173–82.
39 Clarkson J. Review of terminology, classifications, and indices of developmental defects of enamel. Adv Dent Res. 1989; 3(2):104–9.
40 Mahoney E, Ismail FS, Kilpatrick N, Swain M. Mechanical properties across hypomineralized/hypoplastic enamel of first permanent molar teeth. Eur J Oral Sci. 2004 Dec;112(6):497–502.
41 Suckling G, Thurley DC. Histological, macroscopic and microhardness observations of fluoride-induced changes in the enamel organ and enamel of sheep incisor teeth. Arch Oral Biol. 1984; 29(3):165–77.
42 Suckling GW. Developmental defects of enamel – historical and present-day perspectives of their pathogenesis. Adv Dent Res. 1989 Sep;3(2):87–94.
43 Suckling GW. History of the DDE indices. N Z Dent J. 1998 Mar;94(415):9–11.
44 Guatelli-Steinberg D. Dental stress indicators from micro- to macroscopic. In: A companion to dental anthropology. Wiley Blackwell; 2015. pp. 450–64.
45 Hillson S. Tooth development in human evolution and bioarchaeology. Cambridge, UK: Cambridge University Press; 2014.
46 Marchewka J, Skrzat J, Wróbel A. Analysis of the enamel hypoplasia using micro-CT scanner versus classical method. Anthropol Anz. 2014;71(4):391–402.
47 Seow WK. Developmental defects of enamel and dentine: challenges for basic science research and clinical management. Aust Dent J. 2014 Jun;59(suppl 1):143–54.
48 Xu S, Zhao C, Jia L, Ma Z, Zhang X, Shi H. Relationship between preterm, low birth weight, and development defects of enamel in the primary dentition: a meta-analysis. Front Pediatr. 2022 Nov; 10:975340.
49 Tolomeu JSO, Soares MEC, Mourão PS, Ramos-Jorge ML. Is gestational diabetes mellitus associated with developmental defects of enamel in children? A systematic review with meta-analysis. Arch Oral Biol. 2022 Sep;141:105488.
50 Pascon T, Barbosa AM, Cordeiro RC, Bussaneli DG, Prudencio CB, Nunes SK, et al. Prenatal exposure to gestational diabetes mellitus increases developmental defects in the enamel of offspring. PLoS One. 2019 Feb;14(2):e0211771.
51 Jacobsen PE, Haubek D, Henriksen TB, Østergaard JR, Poulsen S. Developmental enamel defects in children born preterm: a systematic review. Eur J Oral Sci. 2014 Feb;122(1):7–14.
52 Tapalaga G, Bumbu BA, Reddy SR, Vutukuru SD, Nalla A, Bratosin F, et al. The impact of prenatal vitamin D on enamel defects and tooth erosion: a systematic review. Nutrients. 2023 Sep; 15(18):3863.
53 Villasenín L, Serna-Muñoz C, Pérez-Silva A, Vicente-Hernández A, Poza-Pascual A, et al. Developmental dental defects in permanent teeth resulting from trauma in primary dentition: a systematic review. Int J Environ Res Public Health. 2022;19(2):754.
54 Gibbison R, Crozier R. Does primary trauma lead to developmental defects in permanent teeth? Evid Based Dent. 2022 Sep;23(3):112–3.
55 Lv P, Gao XJ. Phenotype analysis and the molecular mechanism of enamel hypoplasia. Beijing Da Xue Xue Bao Yi Xue Ban. 2009 Feb 18;41(1):121–3.
56 Taniguchi K, Okamura K, Hayashi M, Funakoshi T, Motokawa W. The effect of mechanical trauma on the tooth germ of rat molars at various developmental stages: a histopathological study. Endod Dent Traumatol. 1999 Feb;15(1):17–25.
57 Via WF Jr, Elwood WK, Bebin J. The effect of maternal hypoxia upon fetal dental enamel. Henry Ford Hosp Med Bull. 1959 Jun;7(2):94–101.
58 Silva-Sousa YT, Peres LC, Foss MC. Are there structural alterations in the enamel organ of offspring of rats with alloxan-induced diabetes mellitus? Braz Dent J. 2003A;14(3):162–7.
59 Chen G, Chen J, Yan Z, Li Z, Yu M, Guo W, et al. Maternal diabetes modulates dental epithelial stem cells proliferation and self-renewal in offspring through apurinic/apyrimidinicendonuclease 1-mediated DNA methylation. Sci Rep. 2017;7:40762.
60 Silva-Sousa YT, Peres LC, Foss MC. Are there structural alterations in the enamel organ of offspring of rats with alloxan-induced diabetes mellitus? Braz Dent J. 2003B;14(3):162–7.
61 Hillson SW. Dental enamel growth, perikymata and hypoplasia in ancient tooth crowns. J R Soc Med. 1992 Aug; 85(8):460–6.
62 Hillson S, Bond S. Relationship of enamel hypoplasia to the pattern of tooth crown growth: a discussion. Am J Phys Anthropol. 1997 Sep;104(1):89–103.
63 King T, Humphrey LT, Hillson S. Linear enamel hypoplasias as indicators of systemic physiological stress: evidence from two known age-at-death and sex populations from postmedieval London. Am J Phys Anthropol. 2005 Nov;128(3): 547–59.
64 Reid DJ, Dean MC. Variation in modern human enamel formation times. J Hum Evol. 2006 Mar;50(3):329–46.
65 Ritzman TB, Baker BJ, Schwartz GT. A fine line: a comparison of methods for estimating ages of linear enamel hypoplasia formation. Am J Phys Anthropol. 2008 Mar;135(3):348–61.
66 Newbrun E. Studies on the physical properties of fluorosed enamel – II: microhardness. Arch Oral Biol. 1960;2(1): 21–7.
67 Bronckers AL, Lyaruu DM, DenBesten PK. The impact of fluoride on ameloblasts and the mechanisms of enamel fluorosis. J Dent Res. 2009 Oct;88(10): 877–93.
68 Aoba T, Fejerskov O. Dental fluorosis: chemistry and biology. Crit Rev Oral Biol Med. 2002;13(2):155–70.

69 Yang T, Zhang Y, Zheng D, Hao Y, Snead ML, Duan X. High-fluoride promoted phagocytosis-induced apoptosis in a matured ameloblast-like cell line. Arch Oral Biol. 2015 Jan;60(1):84–90.
70 Wei W, Pang S, Sun D. The pathogenesis of endemic fluorosis: Research progress in the last 5 years. J Cell Mol Med. 2019 Apr;23(4):2333–42.
71 Zhang Y, Zhang K, Ma L, Gu H, Li J, Lei S. Fluoride induced endoplasmic reticulum stress and calcium overload in ameloblasts. Arch Oral Biol. 2016 Sep;69: 95–101.
72 Wei W, Gao Y, Wang C, Zhao L, Sun D. Excessive fluoride induces endoplasmic reticulum stress and interferes enamel proteinases secretion. Environ Toxicol. 2013 Jun;28(6):332–41.
73 Witkop CJ Jr. Heterogeneity in inherited dental traits, gingival fibromatosis and amelogenesis imperfecta. South Med J. 1971 Feb;64(suppl 1):16–25.
74 Dong J, Ruan W, Duan X. Molecular-based phenotype variations in amelogenesis imperfecta. Oral Dis. 2023 Sep; 29(6):2334–65.
75 Crawford PJ, Aldred M, Bloch-Zupan A. Amelogenesis imperfecta. Orphanet J Rare Dis. 2007 Apr 4;2:17.
76 Gadhia K, McDonald S, Arkutu N, Malik K. Amelogenesis imperfecta: an introduction. Br Dent J. 2012 Apr;212(8): 377–9.
77 Aldred MJ, Savarirayan R, Crawford PJ. Amelogenesis imperfecta: a classification and catalogue for the 21st century. Oral Dis. 2003;9(1):19–23.
78 Sundell S, Koch G. Hereditary amelogenesis imperfecta. I. Epidemiology and clinical classification in a Swedish child population. Swed Dent J. 1985;9(4):157–69.
79 Sundell S, Valentin J. Hereditary aspects and classification of hereditary amelogenesis imperfecta. Community Dent Oral Epidemiol. 1986 Aug;14(4):211–6.
80 Wright JT, Hall KI, Yamauche M. The enamel proteins in human amelogenesis imperfecta. Arch Oral Biol. 1997 Feb; 42(2):149–59.
81 Paine ML, Lei YP, Dickerson K, Snead ML. Altered amelogenin self-assembly based on mutations observed in human X-linked amelogenesis imperfecta (AIH1). J Biol Chem. 2002 May;10; 277(19):17112–6.
82 Shaw WJ, Campbell AA, Paine ML, Snead ML. The COOH terminus of the amelogenin, LRAP, is oriented next to the hydroxyapatite surface. J Biol Chem. 2004 Sep;279(39):40263–6.
83 Snead ML, Zeichner-David M, Chandra T, Robson KJ, Woo SL, Slavkin HC. Construction and identification of mouse amelogenin cDNA clones. Proc Natl Acad Sci U S A. 1983 Dec;80(23): 7254–8.
84 Snead ML, Lau EC, Zeichner-David M, Fincham AG, Woo SL, Slavkin HC. DNA sequence for cloned cDNA for murine amelogenin reveal the amino acid sequence for enamel-specific protein. Biochem Biophys Res Commun. 1985 Jun; 129(3):812–8.
85 Snead ML, Luo W, Lau EC, Slavkin HC. Spatial- and temporal-restricted pattern for amelogenin gene expression during mouse molar tooth organogenesis. Development. 1988 Sep;104(1):77–85.
86 Snead ML, Lau EC, Fincham AG, Zeichner-David M, Davis C, Slavkin HC. Of mice and men: anatomy of the amelogenin gene. Connect Tissue Res. 1989; 22(1–4):101–9.
87 Wright JT, Hart PS, Aldred MJ, Seow K, Crawford PJ, Hong SP, et al. Relationship of phenotype and genotype in X-linked amelogenesis imperfecta. Connect Tissue Res. 2003;44(suppl 1):72–8.
88 Wright JT. The molecular etiologies and associated phenotypes of amelogenesis imperfecta. Am J Med Genet A. 2006 Dec;140(23):2547–55.
89 Hart PS, Michalec MD, Seow WK, Hart TC, Wright JT. Identification of the enamelin (g.8344delG) mutation in a new kindred and presentation of a standardized ENAM nomenclature. Arch Oral Biol. 2003;48:589–96.
90 Kida M, Ariga T, Shirakawa T, Oguchi H, Sakiyama Y. Autosomal-dominant hypoplastic form of amelogenesis imperfecta caused by an enamelin gene mutation at the exon-intron boundary. J Dent Res. 2002;81:738–42.
91 Hu JC, Hu Y, Lu Y, Smith CE, Lertlam R, Wright JT, et al. Enamelin is critical for ameloblast integrity and enamel ultrastructure formation. PLoS One. 2014;9:e89303.
92 Hart PS, Hart TC, Michalec MD, Ryu OH, Simmons D, Hong S, et al. Mutation in kallikrein 4 causes autosomal recessive hypomaturation amelogenesis imperfecta. J Med Genet 2004;41:545–9.
93 Ozdemir D, Hart PS, Ryu OH, Choi SJ, Ozdemir-Karatas M, Firatli E, et al. MMP20 active-site mutation in hypomaturation amelogenesis imperfecta. J Dent Res. 2005 Nov;84(11):1031–5.
94 Wright JT, Hart TC, Hart PS, Simmons D, Suggs C, Daley B, et al. Human and mouse enamel phenotypes resulting from mutation or altered expression of AMEL, ENAM, MMP20 and KLK4. Cells Tissues Organs. 2009;189(1–4): 224–9.
95 Wang SK, Hu Y, Yang J, Smith CE, Nunez SM, Richardson AS, et al. Critical roles for WDR72 in calcium transport and matrix protein removal during enamel maturation. Mol Genet Genomic Med. 2015;3:302–19.
96 Katsura KA, Horst JA, Chandra D, Le TQ, Nakano Y, Zhang Y, et al. WDR72 models of structure and function: a stage-specific regulator of enamel mineralization. Matrix Biol. 2014;38:48–58.
97 El-Sayed W, Parry DA, Shore RC, Ahmed M, Jafri H, Rashid Y, et al. Mutations in the beta propeller WDR72 cause autosomal-recessive hypomaturation amelogenesis imperfecta. Am J Hum Genet. 2009 Nov;85(5):699–705.
98 Kuga T, Sasaki M, Mikami T, Miake Y, Adachi J, Shimizu M, et al. FAM83H and casein kinase I regulate the organization of the keratin cytoskeleton and formation of desmosomes. Sci Rep. 2016;6:26557.
99 Kim JW, Lee SK, Lee ZH, Park JC, Lee KE, Lee MH, et al. FAM83H mutations in families with autosomal-dominant hypocalcified amelogenesis imperfecta. Am J Hum Genet. 2008;82:489–94.
100 Parry DA, Brookes SJ, Logan CV, Poulter JA, El-Sayed W, Al-Bahlani S, et al. Mutations in C4orf26, encoding a peptide with in vitro hydroxyapatite crystal nucleation and growth activity, cause amelogenesis imperfecta. Am J Hum Genet. 2012 Sep;91(3):565–71.
101 Nakayama Y, Holcroft J, Ganss B. Enamel hypomineralization and structural defects in amelotin-deficient mice. J Dent Res. 2015 May;94(5):697–705.
102 Iwasaki K, Bajenova E, Somogyi-Ganss E, Miller M, Nguyen V, Nourkeyhani H, et al. Amelotin – a novel secreted, ameloblast-specific protein. J Dent Res. 2005;84:1127–32.

103 Smith CE, Murillo G, Brookes SJ, Poulter JA, Silva S, Kirkham J, et al. Deletion of amelotin exons 3–6 is associated with amelogenesis imperfecta. Hum Mol Genet. 2016 Aug;25(16):3578–87.

104 Parry DA, Smith CE, El-Sayed W, Poulter JA, Shore RC, Logan CV, et al. Mutations in the pH-sensing G-protein-coupled receptor GPR68 cause amelogenesis imperfecta. Am J Hum Genet. 2016 Oct;99(4):984–90.

105 Seymen F, Kim YJ, Lee YJ, Kang J, Kim TH, Choi H, et al. Recessive mutations in ACPT, encoding testicular acid phosphatase, cause hypoplastic amelogenesis imperfecta. Am J Hum Genet. 2016 Nov;99(5):1199–205.

Daniela Rios
Department of Pediatric Dentistry, Orthodontics and Public Health
Bauru School of Dentistry, University of São Paulo
Alameda Dr. Octávio Pinheiro Brisolla, 9–75, PO Box 73, Bauru, SP 17012-101 (Brazil)
danirios@usp.br

Published online: July 1, 2024
Rios D, Santos-Pinto L (eds): Molar Incisor Hypomineralisation: New Perceptions. Monogr Oral Sci. Basel, Karger, 2024, vol 32, pp 35–42 (DOI: 10.1159/000538853)

Clinical Characteristics and Differential Diagnosis of Hypomineralised Second Primary Molars and Molar Incisor Hypomineralisation

Marlies E.C. Elfrink[a, b, c] Karin Weerheijm[a]

[a]Paediatric REsearch Project (PREP), Barneveld, The Netherlands; [b]Mondzorgcentrum Nijverdal, Nijverdal, The Netherlands; [c]Mondzorgcentrum Wiranto&Go, Almelo, The Netherlands

Abstract

Molar incisor hypomineralisation (MIH) and hypomineralised second primary molars (HSPMs) are commonly seen dental developmental problems with a mean prevalence of around 14% and 9%, respectively, but with a large variability in the reported prevalences. From the dental development, we know that the enamel mineralisation of the second primary molar is taking place between the 19th week of pregnancy until 1 year of age. For the first permanent molars (FPMs) and incisors, the enamel mineralisation is taking place between birth until the age of 3–5. When there is a disturbance during this period, HSPM and/or MIH can occur. There is an overlap in the development of the second primary molars and the FPMs and incisors; the period between birth and the first birthday of the child. A disturbance in this period could cause both HSPM and MIH. There is a relation found in the occurrence of HSPM and MIH. Diagnosing HSPM and MIH can be challenging. All teeth present in the mouth need to be examined. The use of the European Association of Paediatric Dentistry scoring criteria is a good help. In these criteria also, the most common differential diagnoses are included.

Introduction

Molar incisor hypomineralisation (MIH) and hypomineralised second primary molars (HSPMs) are commonly seen dental developmental problems with a mean prevalence of around 14% and 9%, respectively, but with a high variability in the reported prevalences [1, 2].

The hypomineralisation we now know as MIH was initially described under many different names, such as cheese molars, hypomineralised permanent first molars, idiopathic enamel hypomineralisation in the permanent first molar and nonfluoride hypomineralisation of the permanent first molar [3]. After the congress of the European Association of Paediatric Dentistry (EAPD) in Bergen (2000), Weerheijm et al. [3] came up with the name MIH to describe the phenomenon. The definition of MIH published by Weerheijm et al. [3] in 2001 was a hypomineralisation of one to four permanent first molars frequently associated with affected incisors. In 2003, the EAPD published an article on the MIH scor-

Table 1. Dental development; changes in function of the ameloblasts [10]

Stage	Ameloblast function
Presecretory	The ameloblast cells get longer and develop processes in the direction of the developing dentin.
Secretory	The ameloblasts deposit the enamel. The process starts from the cusps to the more cervical region. Enamel matrix protein is formed, and the hydroxyapatite crystals grow in length.
Transition	The change of function from secretion to maturation
Maturation	The mineralisation takes place, and the enamel hardens.

ing criteria [4], and these criteria became the most used ones for MIH research [1, 5].

Later, the same clinical characteristics observed in teeth affected by MIH were seen in second primary molars, and this phenomenon was also described; at first as cheese-Es, MIH-deciduous teeth and deciduous molar hypomineralisation [6]. In 2008, Elfrink et al. [7] published the definition of HSPM, hypomineralised second primary molars. The term HSPM is used to describe the phenomenon in the primary dentition where 1 to 4 second primary molars show hypomineralisation [7].

Ghanim et al. [8] described in 2015 an index that provides scoring forms for both MIH and HSPM for research purposes. In this index, the differential diagnosis with other enamel defects can also be registered [8]. These other enamel defects are not included in the definition of neither HSPM nor MIH.

The variety of denominations often makes communication between professionals and the search for scientific evidence difficult. When looking for research on PubMed on hypomineralisation, we are still only having the MeSH (Medical Subject Headings) term dental enamel hypoplasia, which is nowadays not in line with the definitions we use. However, recent MeSH created a vocabulary thesaurus "Molar Hypomineralization" that can enhance the precision and relevance of your search in databases like PubMed [9].

Enamel Development

To get a better understanding of the clinical characteristics and differential diagnosis of HSPM and MIH, we need to take a look at the dental development. This development starts during pregnancy for the primary dentition. For the permanent dentition, it starts around birth [10].

The ameloblasts form the enamel during the tooth development in four different stages, as shown in Table 1. In the secretory phase, the enamel consists of 10–20% mineral, and the rest is protein and water. At the end of the development of the enamel in the mineralisation phase, the enamel contains up to 95% of mineral [11].

A hypomineralisation, like we see in HSPM and MIH, is a qualitative defect of the enamel. There has been an alteration in the transition or maturation phase of the enamel formation.

In case of an alteration in the (pre)secretion phase, a quantitative enamel defect will occur and this is known as a hypoplasia (shown in Fig. 1) [11, 12].

The enamel mineralisation of the second primary molar is taking place between the 19th week of pregnancy until 1 year of age, and for the first permanent molars (FPMs) and incisors, it is taking place between birth until the age of 3–5 at the latest. There is an overlap in the development of the second primary molars and the FPMs and incisors; the period between birth and the first birthday of the child [10]. Any risk factor present

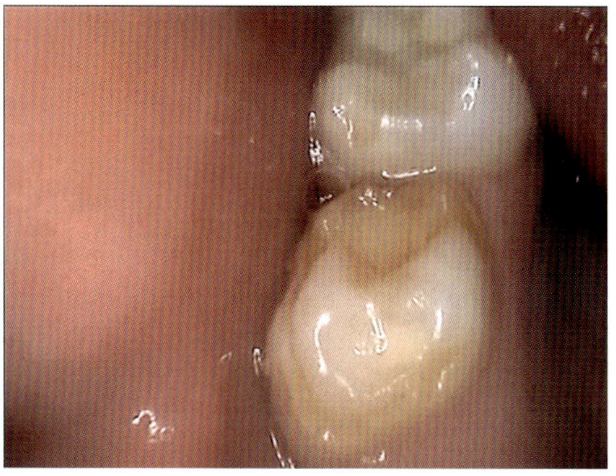

Fig. 1. Tooth 84 showing hypoplasia.

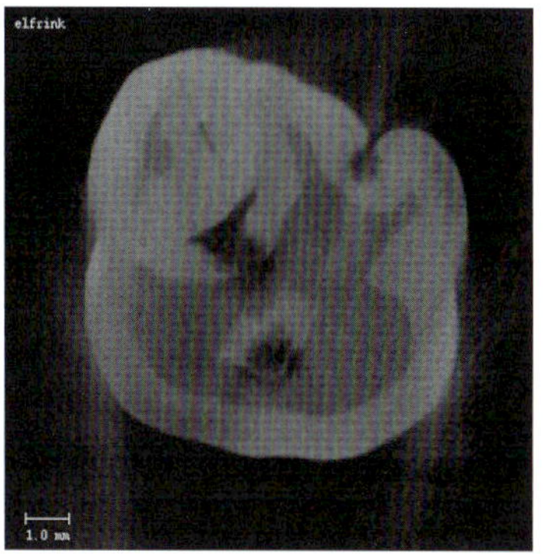

Fig. 2. MicroCT slide: the yellow opacities in the second primary molar can be seen as darker areas in the enamel.

during this period could cause both HSPM and MIH. This is also the period most research is focusing on.

Mineral Content of the Enamel

In both HSPM and MIH, hypomineralisation is identified as areas of demarcated opacities. The mineral content outcomes in HSPM and MIH molars are comparable [13–16]. The yellow and brown opacities show a statistically significant different mineral content compared to sound enamel. The white opacities contain around the same amount of mineral as sound enamel, but the darker opacities contain around 20% less mineral. The yellow opacities in the molar can be seen as darker areas in the enamel in a microCT slide (shown in Fig. 2).

The brown enamel showed a 15- to 21-fold higher protein content, and yellow and creamy-white enamel showed about 8-fold higher protein content in comparison to sound enamel [17]. In the enamel of MIH teeth, there are many different proteins found, but most frequently, albumin is found. In amelogenesis imperfecta enamel, most of the time, only one type of protein, amelogenin, is found [6, 17–19].

EAPD Scoring Criteria

The origin of HSPM and MIH is completely different from the origin of caries. The enamel defects in HSPM/MIH are already developing during the tooth development. In caries, the defects develop after eruption, caused by external influences.

The DDE (developmental defects of the enamel) and modified DDE index cannot be used for the good diagnosis of HSPM and MIH. The DDE index does not have a good opportunity to score posteruptive breakdown (PEB); it only has the option of hypoplasia. Also atypical caries, atypical restoration, and atypical extraction are not incorporated in DDE.

The first MIH scoring criteria were based on the modified developmental defects of the enamel index, but the adjustments made are essential to make a good differential diagnosis between HSPM/MIH and other DDE. Diagnosing HSPM and MIH can be challenging, especially when a child is seen for the first time, sometime after eruption, of the element without sufficient background. Early starting and frequent checkups can make it less difficult to diagnose. For a proper diagnosis, always examine all teeth. Diagnosing HSPM and or MIH can become a lot easier when

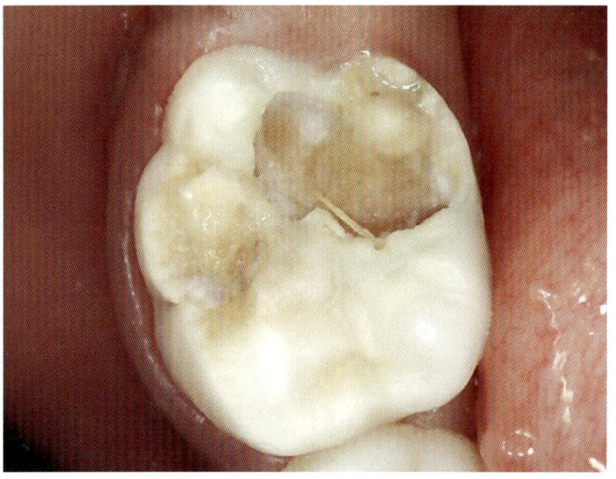

Fig. 3. HSPM in tooth 85, showing a combination of characteristics: opacities, PEB, and atypical caries (photo by J. Krikken).

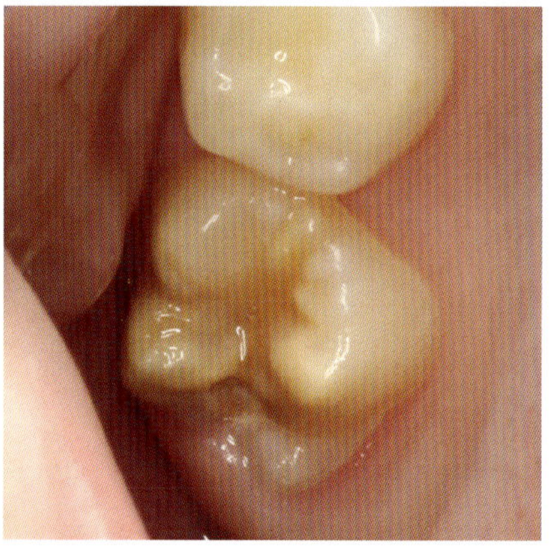

Fig. 4. MIH in tooth 16, showing a yellow demarcated opacity (photo by J. Heijdra).

a good overview over the caries activity and possible other enamel defects of the patient can be made.

Sometimes, one of the index teeth shows obvious characteristics of HSPM/MIH and another tooth gives doubt; in that case, a comparison should be made with the other characteristics in the teeth to be sure about the diagnosis on tooth level.

The EAPD scoring criteria not only give a good overview of the scoring criteria for HSPM and MIH but also include possible differential diagnosis. This makes it possible to properly compare research, also the ones that used the earlier scoring criteria of MIH. The EAPD clinical scoring criteria of MIH and HSPM as described by Ghanim et al. [8] help dentists and researchers for a comprehensive examination, diagnosis, and severity rating of MIH and HSPM.

It is important to highlight that a combination of the characteristics of HSPM/MIH can be seen in the same teeth as presented in tooth 85 (shown in Fig. 3). Demarcated opacities are seen as mild, the other criteria as severe [8]. The color and appearance of the opacity can be indicating of the risk of PEB. White shiny opacities are less at risk then dark-colored dull opacities. Petrou et al. [20] in Germany reported that the demarcated opacities (shown in Fig. 4) are the most common finding in both MIH and HSPM. In this study, HSPM had a lot of atypical restorations but that is also probably related to the age of the children in the study (mean age of 8.1 years). The number of hypomineralised molars per child is also associated with the severity of HSPM [21]. Table 2 shows some of the recent studies that are possible to compare results [20, 22–25].

White opacities due to hypomineralisation can sometimes look like caries white spots. The spot localization on the tooth where the opacity is located is the best indicator to make the difference between a hypomineralisation and caries. At the gingival border, it is more likely to have a white spot lesion. Diffuse opacities, for example, the opacities seen with fluorosis, can sometimes look like the white hypomineralisation opacities. The most important differences are the borders of the opacities: in diffuse opacities, the borders are not clear, and in hypomineralisation-related opacities, the borders are clear and demarcated.

The EAPD scoring criteria do not take into account the carious lesions, but sometimes it can be

Table 2. Scoring criteria seen in HSPM and MIH molars

	HSPM					MIH (FPMS)				
	opacity	posteruptive enamel breakdown	atypical caries	atypical restauration	atypical extraction	opacity	posteruptive enamel breakdown	atypical caries	atypical restauration	atypical extraction
Elfrink et al., 2012 [22]	64	24	9	13	9					
Petrou et al., 2014 [20]	62.1	5.5		33.4	0	77.5	12.7		9.6	0.2
Al-Nerabieah et al., 2023 [23]	51.4	9.5	31.6	4.7	2.5	54.9	13	20	9.9	2.1
Abdalla et al., 2021 [24]						56.3	40.5		1.2	2.0
Estivals et al., 2023 [25]						102.3		6.9	16.5	0.5

All numbers are percentages. One tooth can have more than one scoring criterion.

challenging to see the difference between, e.g., atypical caries and "normal" caries and posteruptive enamel loss (PEB) and "normal" caries because we do not always see the tooth just after eruption [19]. PEB can look like caries and/or hypoplasia. In case of PEB, it more likely to find signs of opacities at the edges of the breakdown, which indicates the relation to HSPM/MIH. Whereas in hypoplasia most often smoother edges in the areas next to the normal enamel can be noticed compared to irregular borders of the PEB. Posteruptive enamel breakdown most of the time involves a cusp; hypoplasia will show as a line of missing enamel.

Due to the rapid caries progression in severe HSPM/MIH cases in some lesions, the original opacity can be masked by caries, making the HSPM/MIH diagnosis more difficult. In most caries lesions, the affected dentine is softer compared to the dentine of HSPM/MIH-affected teeth. The atypical pattern of the caries can also be helpful in the diagnosis. In atypical caries also, most of the time opacities can be seen at the edges of the caries lesion.

Atypical caries is more often found at cusps or free surfaces, whereas "normal" caries is found at predilection sites. On the borders of the atypical caries lesion, sometimes opacities can be recognized.

Atypical restorations are recognized the same way as atypical caries lesions, but most of the time, the opacities are also covered by the restoration material. Atypical extractions are recognized based on the atypical caries pattern and atypical restorations.

Atypical extractions are difficult to diagnose because the teeth are not there anymore. If not all four index molars are taken out, you can probably have a hint that it is HSPM or MIH that caused the need of extraction. In case all four index molars are taken out, you have to base your diagnosis of atypical extraction more on the caries pattern of the child. The most favorable time to take out the FPMs is between the age of 8–10 years.

In this scoring criteria, the teeth that are, by definition, involved in HSPM/MIH are considered the index teeth. Therefore, for differential diagnosis of MIH and HSPM, it is important to look at not only the index teeth but also all teeth in the mouth. The other teeth that show hypomineralisation look like MIH and HSPM but are by definition excluded. In the index of Ghanim et al., they

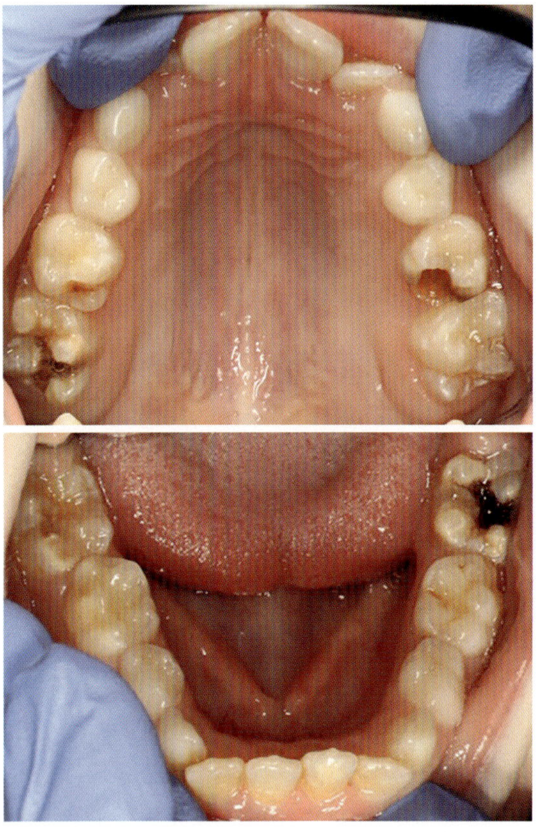

Fig. 5. Both the second primary molars as well as the first permanent molars are affected by HSPM and MIH, respectively. Many different scoring criteria can be seen in this patient. 16: white and yellow opacities and atypical caries, 55: brown opacity, 65: white opacity and atypical caries, 26: small white opacity, 36: white and yellow opacities and atypical caries, 75: creamy-white opacity, 31: creamy-white opacity, 85: creamy-white opacity, and 46: creamy-white opacity with PEB (photos by J. Heijdra).

are scored as hypomineralisation defects (not HSPM/MIH).

More difficult probably is to make the difference between amelogenesis imperfecta with hypomineralisation and HSPM/MIH. But amelogenesis imperfecta always is present on all teeth and not only on the index teeth. Amelogenesis imperfecta is a possible differential diagnosis of HSPM and MIH. The prevalence of amelogenesis imperfecta is between 1 in 700 till 1 in 1,500. It is a hereditary condition and can be autosomal dominant, recessive, or x-linked. This depends on the type of amelogenesis imperfecta.

Amelogenesis imperfecta is a specific group of enamel malformations and can include hypoplasia and/or hypomineralisation [26].

Especially the type that has hypomineralisation can be difficult to make the differential diagnosis with HSPM/MIH. In chapter 2, you can read more about amelogenesis imperfecta.

Relation of HSPM and MIH

Children with HSPM are more likely to have MIH. The meta-analysis from Garot et al. [27] shows that the possibility of having both HSPM and MIH is very common, more common than having only HSPM or MIH. Odds ratios vary a bit, but there is some evidence about the relation between HSPM and MIH [25, 28].

When a child is diagnosed with HSPM, be aware of MIH around the age of 6 (eruption moment of FPMs); as shown in Figure 5, a child with both HSPM and MIH.

Conclusion

Diagnosing HSPM and MIH can be challenging. All teeth present in the mouth need to be examined for a proper diagnosis. The use of the EAPD scoring criteria is a good help. In these criteria also, the most common differential diagnoses are included.

Acknowledgment

The authors like to thank their colleagues John Heijdra and Janneke Krikken for the clinical pictures.

Statement of Ethics

Informed consent was obtained from patients (or their parents/legal guardians/next-of-kin) for publication of the images.

Conflict of Interest Statement

The authors have no conflicts of interest to declare.

Funding Sources

There was no funding for the writing of this chapter.

Author Contributions

Both K.L. Weerheijm and M.E.C. Elfrink had a substantial contribution to the concept and writing/reviewing of this chapter. They both give approval for publication and agree to be accountable for all aspects of the work.

References

1 Elfrink ME, Ghanim A, Manton DJ, Weerheijm KL. Standardised studies on molar incisor hypomineralisation (MIH) and hypomineralised second primary molars (HSPM): a need. Eur Arch Paediatr Dent. 2015 Jun;16(3):247–55.
2 D3group. Available from: https://www.thed3group.org/prevalence.html.
3 Weerheijm KL, Jalevik B, Alaluusua S. Molar-incisor hypomineralisation. Caries Res. 2001 Sep-Oct;35(5):390–1.
4 Weerheijm K, Duggal M, Mejare I, Papagiannoulis L, Koch G, Martens LC, et al. Judgement criteria for molar incisor hypomineralisation (MIH) in epidemiologic studies: a summary of the European meeting on MIH held in Athens, 2003. Eur J Paediatr Dent. 2003;4:110–3.
5 Jälevik B. Prevalence and diagnosis of molar incisor hypomineralisation (MIH): a systematic review. Eur Arch Paediatr Dent. 2010;11(2):59–64.
6 Joshi M, Emmanuel BJ, Manzoor R, Manzoor M, Kumar M, Raja J. Hypomineralized second primary molar. Int J Dent Med Sci Res. 2021;3:895–7.
7 Elfrink ME, Schuller AA, Weerheijm KL, Veerkamp JS. Hypomineralized second primary molars: prevalence data in Dutch 5-year-olds. Caries Res. 2008;42(4):282–5.
8 Ghanim AM, Elfrink MEC, Weerheijm KL, Mariño R, Manton D. A practical method for use in epidemiologic studies of molar incisor hypomineralisation and hypomineralised second primary molars. Eur Arch Paediatr Dent. 2015 Jun;16(3):235–46.
9 What is new in MeSH? Available from: https://www.nlm.nih.gov/mesh/whatsnew.html.
10 ten Cate A. Oral histology, development, structure and function. 5th ed. St Louis: Mosby Inc.; 1998.
11 Alaluusua S. Aetiology of molar-incisor hypomineralisation: a systematic review. Eur Arch Paediatr Dent. 2010;11(2):53–8.
12 Suga S. Enamel hypomineralisation viewed from pattern of progressive mineralisation of human and monkey developing enamel. Adv Dent Res. 1989;3:188–98.
13 Elfrink MEC, ten Cate JM, van Ruijven LJ, Veerkamp JSJ. Mineral content in teeth with deciduous molar hypomineralisation (DMH). J Dent. 2013 Nov;41(11):974–8.
14 Farah RA, Swain MV, Drummond BK, Cook R, Atieh M. Mineral density of hypomineralised enamel. J Dent. 2010 Jan;38(1):50–8.
15 Fearne J, Anderson P, Davis GR. 3D X-ray microscopic study of the extent of variations in enamel density in first permanent molars with idiopathic enamel hypomineralisation. Br Dent J. 2004 May 22;196(10):634–8; discussion 625.
16 Farah R, Drummond B, Swain M, Williams S. Linking the clinical presentation of molar-incisor hypomineralisation to its mineral density. Int J Paediatr Dent. 2010;20:353–60.
17 Farah RA, Monk BC, Swain MV, Drummond BK. Protein content of molar-incisor hypomineralisation enamel. J Dent. 2010 Jul;38(7):591–6.
18 Gil-Bona A, Bidlack FB. Tooth enamel and its dynamic protein matrix. Int J Mol Sci. 2020 Jun 23;21(12):4458.
19 Bailleul-Forestier I, Molla M, Verloes A, Berdal A. The genetic basis of inherited anomalies of the teeth. Part 1:clinical and molecular aspects of non-syndromic dental disorders. Eur J Med Genet. 2008 Jul-Aug;51(4):273–91.
20 Petrou MA, Giraki M, Bissar AR, Basner R, Wempe C, Altarabulsi MB, et al. Prevalence of Molar-Incisor-Hypomineralisation among school children in four German cities. Int J Paediatr Dent. 2014 Nov;24(6):434–40.
21 Vlachou C, Arhakis A, Kotsanos N. Distribution and morphology of enamel hypomineralisation defects in second primary molars. Eur Arch Paediatr Dent. 2021 Apr;22(2):241–6.
22 Elfrink ME, ten Cate JM, Jaddoe VW, Hofman A, Moll HA, Veerkamp JS. Deciduous molar hypomineralization and molar incisor hypomineralization. J Dent Res. 2012 Jun;91(6):551–5.
23 Al-Nerabieah Z, AlKhouli M, Dashash M. Prevalence and clinical characteristics of molar-incisor hypomineralization in Syrian children: a cross-sectional study. Sci Rep. 2023 May 26;13(1):8582.
24 Abdalla HE, Abuaffan AH, Kemoli AM. Molar incisor hypomineralization, prevalence, pattern and distribution in Sudanese children. BMC Oral Health. 2021 Jan 6;21(1):9.

25 Estivals J, Fahd C, Baillet J, Rouas P, Manton DJ, Garot E. The prevalence and characteristics of and the association between MIH and HSPM in South-Western France. Int J Paediatr Dent. 2023 May;33(3):298–304.
26 Witkop CJ Jr. Amelogenesis imperfecta, dentinogenesis imperfecta and dentin dysplasia revisited: problems in classification. J Oral Pathol. 1988 Nov;17(9–10):547–53.
27 Garot E, Denis A, Delbos Y, Manton D, Silva M, Rouas P. Are hypomineralised lesions on second primary molars (HSPM) a predictive sign of molar incisor hypomineralisation (MIH)? A systematic review and a meta-analysis. J Dent. 2018 May;72:8–13.
28 da Silva Figueiredo Sé MJ, Ribeiro APD, Dos Santos-Pinto LAM, de Cassia Loiola Cordeiro R, Cabral RN, Leal SC. Are hypomineralized primary molars and canines associated with molar-incisor hypomineralization? Pediatr Dent. 2017 Nov 1;39(7):445–9.

Marlies E.C. Elfrink
Mondzorgcentrum Nijverdal
Stationsstraat 7
NL–7443 BX Nijverdal (The Netherlands)
marlieselfrink@gmail.com

Chapter 4

Published online: July 1, 2024
Rios D, Santos-Pinto L (eds): Molar Incisor Hypomineralisation: New Perceptions. Monogr Oral Sci. Basel, Karger, 2024, vol 32, pp 43–55 (DOI: 10.1159/000538865)

Implications of Histological and Ultrastructural Characteristics on the Chemical and Mechanical Properties of Hypomineralised Enamel and Clinical Consequences

Juliana de Lima Gonçalves Fabrício Kitazono de Carvalho
Alexandra Mussolino de Queiroz Francisco Wanderley Garcia de Paula-Silva
Department of Pediatric Clinics, School of Dentistry of Ribeirão Preto, University of São Paulo, Ribeirão Preto, Brazil

Abstract
Molar incisor hypomineralisation (MIH) is a qualitative type of enamel defect, which occurs due to a failure in the biomineralisation process of the enamel organic matrix during amelogenesis. The tooth enamel affected by MIH shows changes in its chemical, structural, and mechanical properties, leading to different clinical repercussions. The color of MIH opacities varies from opaque white to yellow/brown, and elemental analyses of these lesions show a lower calcium and phosphate content, minerals that are more abundant in sound enamel. Furthermore, the incorporation of other molecules occurs, such as carbonate, a component that provides a greater degree of solubility, thus making hypomineralised enamel more susceptible to posteruptive fractures. At a structural level, the layer of hydroxyapatite crystals appears to be disorganized, with morphological changes, implying a greater degree of porosity in the structure. The increase in porosity of the structure may be associated with dental hypersensitivity, a common clinical repercussion among patients with MIH. Among the mechanical properties, a decrease in hardness and modulus of elasticity occurs, and this also makes the enamel more fragile. Deficiency in biomineralisation can be caused by changes in the function of ameloblasts or by failures at the intercellular junction that result in lower activity of proteases such as MMP-20 and KLK4. The increase in proteins in the organic matrix of enamel impairs the growth and incorporation of minerals into the hydroxyapatite crystals, so that the enamel becomes hypomineralised and has larger organic content, thus having an impact on its properties. These changes present in the enamel with MIH help to explain the clinical repercussions caused by this condition.

Introduction

Enamel developmental defects are qualitative or quantitative changes in the enamel layer due to disorders that occur during amelogenesis, the process of tooth enamel formation. Amelogenesis, a complex process, depends on the presence of different molecules and signaling pathways that enable the enamel layer to form correctly [1–3]. To recognize changes in the chemical, mechanical, structural, and molecular properties of teeth with developmental defects, it is necessary to understand the process of formation and composition of healthy enamel, which will reflect on its final characteristics.

Tooth enamel is considered the hardest structure in the human body, due to the large quantity of minerals since it is composed of approximately 95% mineral content, and the remainder consists of organic content such as proteins and water [4–7]. Among the minerals present in enamel, calcium and phosphate are the most abundant elements, with the value of the Ca/P ratio indicating the degree of mineralisation of the enamel, and a high value would indicate a greater degree of mineralisation [8]. This unique composition of enamel will reflect on its mechanical properties, including high resistance to fractures and wear, and low porosity [7, 9]. In addition to the composition, another important factor in ensuring the high resistance of the enamel is its structural properties, such as the arrangement of enamel prisms. Enamel prisms have different shapes and can be rectangular or cuboidal, but the majority of them have a cylindrical shape [8]. They consist of hydroxyapatite crystals united by noncollagenous proteins and are positioned parallel to each other, extending from the dentin-enamel junction to the incisal/occlusal surface of the tooth [8, 10].

There are differences in the formation process and composition of enamel with developmental defects, and these imply different clinical repercussions [9, 11]. Molar incisor hypomineralisation (MIH) is a type of hypomineralisation in which the enamel of permanent molars and incisors has demarcated opacities, with a color that can vary from opaque white to yellow/brown. In enamel with MIH, there are differences in mineral density, structural, mechanical, and chemical properties, resulting from changes at the cellular and molecular levels during biomineralisation. These changes result in low resistance and a higher degree of porosity when compared with sound enamel, leading to clinical repercussions, such as esthetic damage, occurrence of posteruptive fractures, dental hypersensitivity, and failures in restorative processes, affecting the quality of the lives of children and their families [12–17].

Formation of Tooth Enamel – Molecular Mediators and Signaling Pathways

Mature tooth enamel is an acellular structure [18], nevertheless its formation is complex. Different molecules and signaling pathways are necessary for the apposition of organic content and biomineralisation [19–21]. Ameloblasts, cells responsible for deposition of the enamel organic matrix, are cells of ectodermal origin and undergo different morphological changes throughout amelogenesis [22]. Research to study the phases of amelogenesis in humans is extremely challenging since ameloblasts are cells that are only present during the phases of enamel formation that it occurs inside the jaw and maxilla bones and in most part of teeth occurs during intrauterine life and in the first years of life, except for permanent third molars. After the enamel is formed, they undergo apoptosis, thus limiting access to these cells in humans [1, 22]. The use of animal models, such as rodents and pigs, has become a feasible option for gaining better understanding of the mechanism of enamel formation, participation of molecules, and the signaling pathways activated during this process. Rodent incisors, specially, have a process of constant renewal and growth, which allow the evaluation of enamel formation throughout its life course. Interesting, in this model, incisor continuous eruption allows the observation of all phases of amelogenesis, thereby facilitating the study of this process [22, 23].

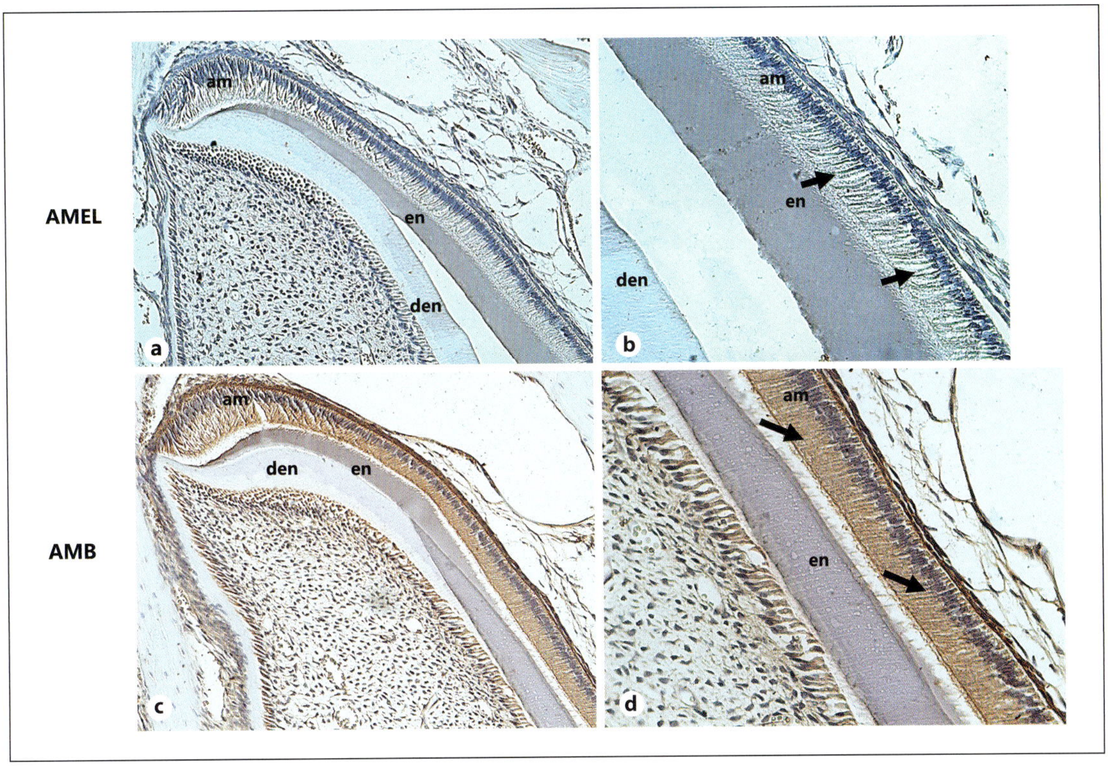

Fig. 1. The images show rodent incisors, in which the ameloblast layer and the newly secreted enamel layer are present. **a**, **b** Amelogenin is expressed throughout the ameloblast layer, one of the most abundant proteins in the organic enamel matrix (**a** ×20 magnification; **b** ×40 magnification). **c**, **d** The expression of ameloblastin, another protein also synthesized by ameloblasts. Like amelogenin, ameloblastin plays an important role during the secretion phase, as it is responsible for guiding the growth of hydroxyapatite crystals. This figure represents immunohistochemical staining, a technique used to detect different molecules in a given tissue using a chromogen such as 3,3′-diaminobenzidine tetrahydrochloride (DAB), which will result in a brown color in the regions where the molecule is present. Immunohistochemical staining occurs through the interaction of a specific antibody and the antigen, which may or may not be present in the tissue. When the antigen is present, the added antibody will bind to this antigen, and when the DAB is added, there will be a reaction that generates a brownish color. am, ameloblasts; den, dentine; en, enamel.

During the time of matrix secretion, ameloblasts appear as cells that have an elongated shape, with a nucleus positioned at the distal pole of the cell, and the presence of cytoplasmic processes at its other extremity. At the apical pole of the ameloblast, Tomes' process can be identified as a cellular projection that guides the formation of the prismatic enamel layer [24]. In the secretion stage, the ameloblasts secrete granules that contain proteins essential for amelogenesis. These proteins are responsible for forming a framework and thus guiding the growth of enamel prisms [5, 25]. In the matrix maturation phase, the morphology of ameloblasts changes, and the cells may show cytoplasmic extensions in the apical portion or even an apical base with the absence of these extensions. Oscillation in the morphology of these cells is related to the cellular microenvironment pH and to mineral ions being pumped into the enamel matrix [5, 22]. Occurrence of disturbances during the process of transporting ions such as Ca and P harms the biomineralisation of

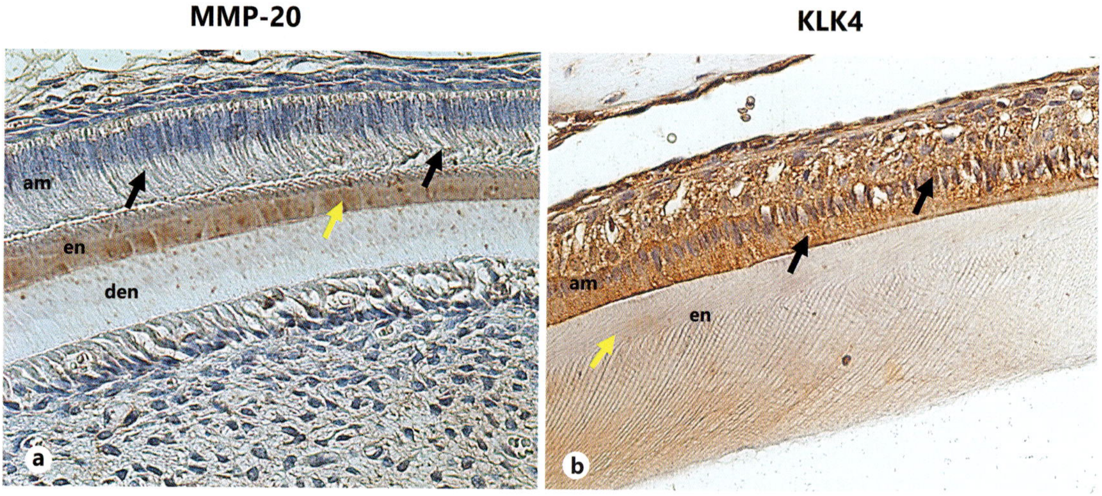

Fig. 2. Histological image of the ameloblast layer stained by immunohistochemistry for MMP-20 (**a**) and KLK4 (**b**), enzymes that are responsible for removing organic content during amelogenesis, which will allow minerals to be incorporated into hydroxyapatite crystals. The regions stained in brown represented by the black arrows indicate the presence of these enzymes in the ameloblasts. Yellow arrows show the expression of these enzymes in the presecreted layer of organic enamel. am, ameloblasts; den, dentine; en, enamel.

the tooth enamel matrix, resulting in hypomineralisation [5, 22, 26, 27].

Another factor to be taken into consideration relative to hypomineralised enamel is the increased protein content of this structure. During the secretory stage of enamel formation, a large quantity of proteins such as amelogenin and ameloblastin are released by the ameloblasts, and these serve as a guide for the formation and growth of hydroxyapatite crystals as shown in Figure 1. Subsequently, these proteins are removed by the action of proteases and thus allow the incorporation of minerals. Disturbances during the period of amelogenesis can impair mineralisation signaling, resulting in the formation of enamel with a higher protein content [7, 19–21]. Whereas developmental enamel defects such as amelogenesis imperfecta and dental fluorosis show changes in the quantity of amelogenin when compared with sound teeth, the tooth with MIH have a higher content of proteins, such as ameloblastin, albumin, hemoglobin, alpha-1-antitrypsin, anti-thrombin III, and serpin B3. Ameloblastin and enamelin represent around 10% of the enamel organic matrix, and the absence of these proteins is directly related to dental enamel malformation [22]. The presence of ameloblastin during the phase of organic matrix mineralisation can impact the expansion of enamel prisms and the incorporation of minerals [23, 28, 29]. Furthermore, MIH discoloration which is of a yellowish to brown color is characterized by the presence of ameloblastin in the lesion [22, 30]. Therefore, changes not only in gene expression and protein synthesis but also in matrix pH regulation are factors that impact molecular signaling during amelogenesis [27, 31].

Modulation of the expression and activity of proteases such as KLK4 and MMP-20 have been directly linked to the permanence of proteins in the enamel organic matrix as shown in Figures 2 and 3 [1, 7, 21]. MMP-20 is a matrix metalloproteinase expressed by odontoblasts and ameloblasts; in enamel formation, it cleaves amelo-

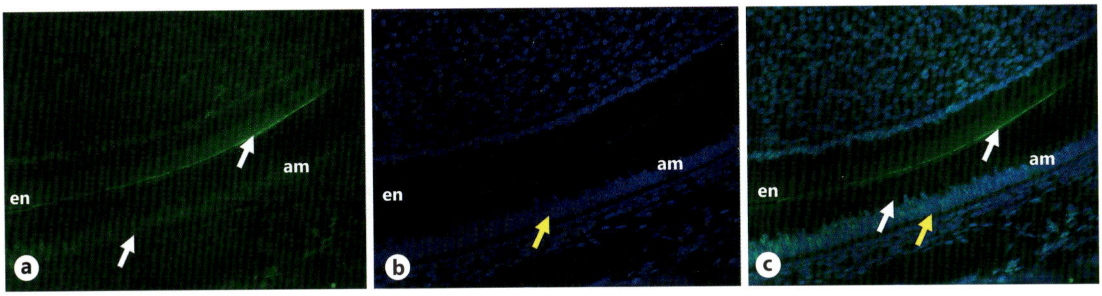

Fig. 3. a The activity of MMP in the ameloblast layer and in the organic enamel matrix using the FITC fluorophore (white arrows). This enzyme removes the protein content in the enamel layer. **b** DAPI is used to label the cell nucleus. It is possible to identify the nucleus of the ameloblasts, which are located at the distal pole, close to the stratum intermedium (yellow arrows). **c** shows a and b merged, where MMP activity can be seen in the cytoplasmic extensions of the ameloblasts and in the organic enamel matrix. In situ zymography is a technique that shows the proteolytic activity of metalloproteinases in cells using a fluorophore. am, ameloblasts; den, dentine; en, enamel.

genin. MMP-20 also plays a role in the cleavage of e-cadherin, a protein present in the cell membrane that promotes cell-cell adhesion [32–34]. E-cadherin cleavage results in the release of β-catenin into the cytoplasm and translocation to the nucleus of the ameloblast, acting as a transcription factor necessary for tooth enamel formation [34]. To investigate the direct effects of the absence of MMP-20 on enamel, one study used MMP-20 enzyme knockout rodents and performed qualitative and molecular analyses on the tissues [35]. Enamel of mice showed enamel rods with a lower level of minerals, in addition to a prismatic pattern that differed from that of wild-type animals. Furthermore, there was a greater content of organic molecules within the enamel prisms, showing that the lack of MMP-20 caused the entrapment of proteins within the hydroxyapatite crystals [35].

KLK4, another protease that also acts as an enamel protein removal, shows greater activity during the transition from the secretion to maturation stages of the organic matrix [20]. Studies have previously demonstrated that the lack of this enzyme impact enamel biomineralisation [24, 36, 37]. When visually analyzing the tooth enamel of KLK4-deficient mice ($KLK4^{-/-}$), incisor crowns showed demarcated white color opacities. For qualitative and quantitative analyses, microtomography of the mandibles, scanning electron microscopy, energy-dispersive X-ray spectroscopy for quantification of chemical elements, and microhardness were performed. No changes were found in the thickness and volume of the layer; however, a reduction in mineral density and hardness was reported. The outermost layer of the enamel had higher density and hardness values, and the innermost layers showed a reduction in these values [20].

The etiology of MIH is not yet fully known, despite the multifactorial nature of this condition [38]. The way in which genetic, systemic, and environmental factors affect amelogenesis has been the subject of studies in recent years [39–42]. As it is a process that requires the participation of different signaling pathways, changes in an individual's gene expression could directly impact amelogenesis, since mutations and single nucleotide genetic polymorphisms could impact the production of proteins and enzymes, and thus impair secretion and maturation of the enamel organic matrix [31]. Systemic factors, for example, childhood illnesses, such as fever, asthma, and hypoxia, are factors that may influence the activity of ameloblasts [39, 43]. Environmental factors have also been investigated, and they can be diverse, such as the mother's use of toxic substances during pregnancy, the use of certain medications, and toxic stress during early childhood [39, 41, 42].

Failures in tooth enamel formation that could lead to hypomineralisation might also occur due to an extracellular mechanism and not due to abnormal activity of ameloblasts [30, 44, 45]. This theory is supported by the presence of fetal albumin in teeth with MIH. Serum albumin, a protein present in the bloodstream, is found in two isoforms: fetal and adult albumin. The two isoforms were found in hypomineralised molars, showing that it was incorporated during the period of tooth enamel formation. The presence of albumin during enamel layer biomineralisation is harmful, as the presence of this protein inhibits biomineralisation. Furthermore, albumin is capable of resisting the activities of proteases such as MMP-20 and KLK4 and therefore remains incorporated into hydroxyapatite crystals, leading to the formation of a more porous enamel with a higher protein content. However, the mechanism of albumin entry during the formation of tooth enamel is not yet fully understood [44, 45].

Taking into consideration the theory that extracellular factors could be related to enamel defects, the study of claudins, present in tight junctions (TJs), has also been explored [1, 46, 47]. In ameloblasts, TJs are structures responsible for intercellular union, and that form a barrier separating the extracellular environment from the region in which the enamel matrix is being formed. TJs are responsible for promoting the epithelial permeability of cells by controlling the passage of molecules between cells. This type of cell junction is located in the basal region of the cell [46]. Claudins are proteins present in TJs, and according to their type, the epithelial permeability of the cells will be defined [46, 48]. Ameloblasts are cells of ectodermal origin, which form a continuous layer and are joined by TJs. During tooth enamel formation, claudins play an important role since it is their presence in the TJ that defines the permeability of the ameloblasts, and therefore, the transportation of mineral ions to the enamel organic matrix. The presence of at least 11 types of claudins in the tooth germ has previously been described in the literature, and changes in claudin-16 and -19 have been related to the occurrence of amelogenesis imperfecta [46]. An investigation was conducted on the impact that the absence of claudin-16 could have on tooth enamel formation in the incisors of rodents genetically deficient in this protein [46]. The authors reported that claudin-16 was a component in the TJ of secretory ameloblasts, and its expression was detected by immunohistochemical analysis of the protein. Those animals presented changes in the structure of the TJs, which appeared to be irregular. In situ zymography revealed a reduction in MMP-20 activity, with no impact in protein synthesis. These results demonstrated that the lack of claudin-16 would not impact the expression of MMP-20, but rather its activity, which might occur due to changes in the microenvironment, such as changes in pH, with values that were relatively lower in genetically deficient animals. Therefore, the absence of claudin-16, a component of the TJs of ameloblasts, impacted tooth enamel formation.

Chemical Properties and Mineral Density

The failure resulting in the formation of hypomineralised enamel occurs during the mineralisation stage of the enamel matrix [8]. In this stage, the ameloblasts are responsible for releasing proteases responsible for the removal of proteins present in the organic enamel matrix. At this moment, mineral ions such as Ca and P are released and incorporated into hydroxyapatite crystals $[Ca_{10}(PO_4)_6(OH)_2]$. Hypomineralised enamel has a mineral density around 20% lower than sound enamel [49, 50]. The difference in the mineral density of enamel with MIH is due to the change in chemical composition.

Teeth affected by MIH that have demarcated opacities not only have lower amounts of Ca and P, but also have a reduced Ca/P ratio, which indicates the degree of mineralisation [51]. Mineral ions will reach the enamel matrix via two pathways: the transcellular route, taken by ameloblasts, and paracellular route, which occurs in the extracellular environment through the passage between cells [52]. The lack of minerals in enamel may be related to different disturbances during the process of transporting mineral ions to the enamel matrix. The change in pH is a factor that has been considered to alter the activity of ameloblasts and inhibit the action of enzymes such as KLK4, which play an important role in removing proteins from the matrix during the maturation phase [26, 53, 54]. At the time of transition between the phases of secretion and maturation, the ameloblasts will show two distinct morphologies, one at the apical margin with cytoplasmic prolongations and the other with a flat margin as shown in Figure 4. Approximately 70% of the calcium in the enamel layer will be taken to the enamel matrix via transcellular ameloblasts with cytoplasmic prolongations, and the remainder will be taken via paracellular pathways of these cells [52, 54]. Calcium ions are transported to the enamel matrix by ameloblasts that have ion pathways in specific regions for performing this delivery. Among the ion pathways present in these cells, the PMCA-1 (plasma membrane Ca^{2+} ATPase-1) pathway is responsible for transporting intracellular Ca^{2+} to the extracellular environment, going from the least concentrated to the most concentrated environment by the expenditure of ATP molecules, and is present in the distal and lateral membranes of secretory ameloblasts. This pathway has a high affinity for the calcium molecule but a low transport speed. On the other hand, sodium/calcium exchanger pathways types 1 and 3 are present in secretory and maturing ameloblasts, but their exact location has not yet been described. The sodium/calcium exchanger pathway will exchange sodium ions for calcium across the plasma membrane, as there will be an electrochemical gradient in the extracellular fluid that attracts sodium. In spite of this channel having a low affinity for calcium, it has a rapid transport capacity [26].

pH regulation has a direct influence on the function of these ion pathways and thus affects the growth and incorporation of minerals into hydroxyapatite crystals [55]. In a recent study, the NCKX4 (sodium/potassium/calcium exchanger-4) ion pathway and its influence on the activity of the KLK4 enzyme was investigated. Incisors and molars from animals that were genetically deficient in NCKX4 ($NCKX4^{-/-}$) were used, and the activity of the KLK4 enzyme was analyzed. Moreover, elements of the enamel matrix and pH of this matrix were measured. Increased expression and lower activity of KLK4 in the enamel matrix were observed when the ion pathway did not perform its function adequately. Furthermore, the increase in pH was also related to the inhibition of enzyme activity. Acidification of the microenvironment was related to loss of KLK4 ability to hydrolyze proteins such as amelogenin, causing the accumulation of proteins in the enamel matrix [54]. The pH values alternate according to the degree of mineralisation of the matrix in the amelogenesis phases. In the secretory phase, in which there was a lower degree of mineralisation, lower pH values were found, indicating an acidic environment. Whereas, in more advanced stages of the maturation phase, in which there was a higher degree of mineralisation, pH values were higher, indicating an alkaline environment [56].

Another important point to emphasize is related to the incorporation of other chemical elements into the hypomineralised enamel, such as carbon and magnesium [5, 51]. Carbon is an element that is present in tooth enamel in a physiological form in the initial stages of amelogenesis. It is found in the form of carbonate, a compound with a high degree of solubility. As the enamel progressively advances through the mineralisa-

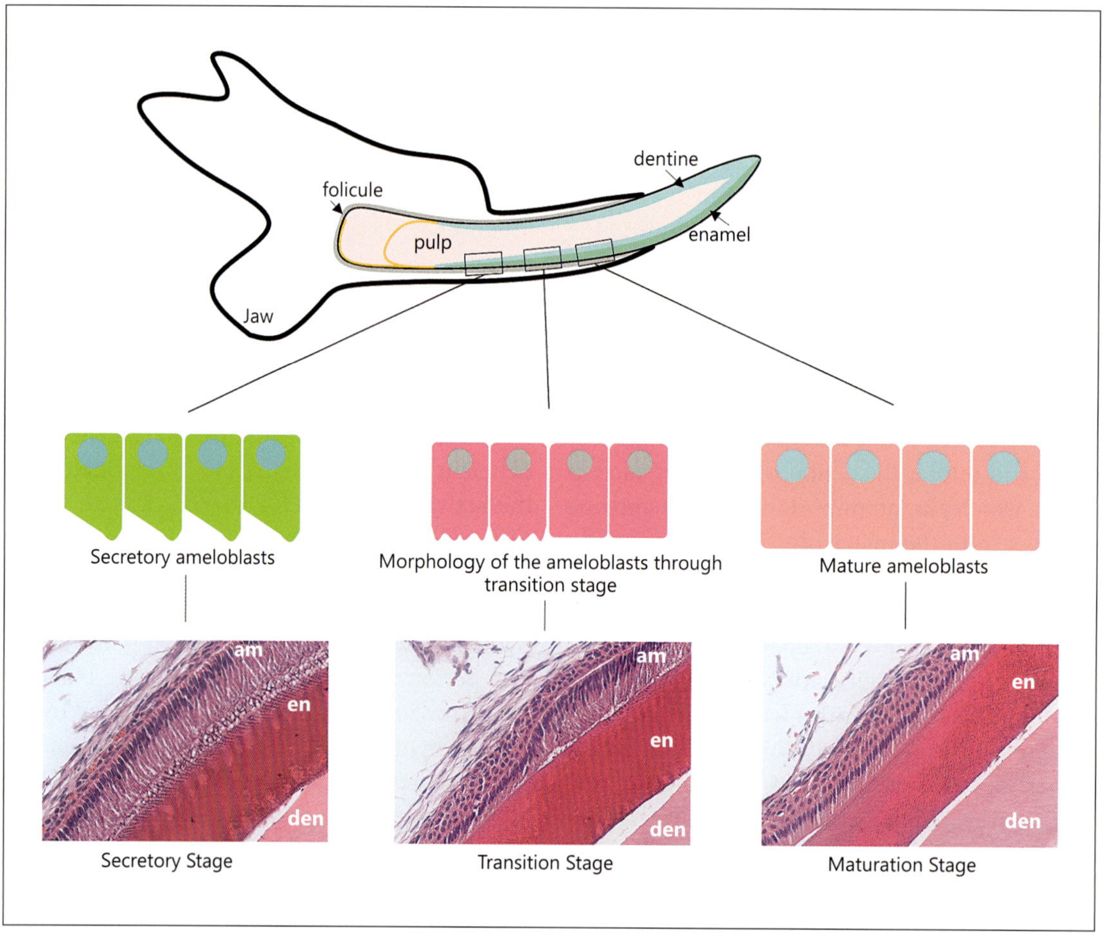

Fig. 4. The scheme shows the rat incisor, a tooth that has a continuous formation process, allowing all the phases of amelogenesis to be observed. During enamel formation, the ameloblast changes its shape according to the function to be performed at the time. In the secretory phase, the ameloblast has a cylindrical and elongated shape with a polarized nucleus, while at the other pole, there is a structure called the Tomes' process, which releases granules with proteins and mineral content. In the transition stage, between the secretory and maturation phase, it is possible to observe a change in the morphology of the ameloblasts, which no longer have the Tomes' process, and there is a loss of cytoplasmic extensions. During the maturation phase, the removal of proteins from the enamel matrix and the release of minerals such as Ca and P occurs, which will be incorporated into the hydroxyapatite crystals. am, ameloblasts; den, dentine; en, enamel.

tion process, the amount of carbonate is reduced. The larger quantity of carbon in hypomineralised enamel indicates higher amount of carbonate, resulting in an increase in organic components and thus a more fragile enamel [57]. With regard to the severity of MIH opacities, those that have an opaque white color show greater resistance than opacities that vary from yellow to brown, which would be associated with the quantity of minerals in the enamel (Table 1) [11].

The change in chemical composition of enamel with MIH results in loss of tissue strength, favoring the occurrence of posteruptive fractures. Furthermore, the adhesion of restorative materi-

Table 1. Mineral component analysis of an MIH tooth with brown spot

	Ca	P	O	C	Ca/P
Hypomineralised enamel	26.5	12.2	34.3	25.15	2.1
Transition area between hypomineralised and healthy enamel	29.4	14.8	41.4	13.3	1.9
Sound enamel	51.6	14.2	26.6	7.0	3.6

Energy-dispersive X-ray spectroscopy is an analysis that emits a beam of light under the tooth and analyzes the elements present in the sample and the relative quantity of these elements.

als is also affected [51]. There is a high failure rate of restorative treatment in teeth with MIH. This high value is related to the low quality of adhesion with the materials currently available, which were created to adhere to a structure with high mineral content [15].

Structural Properties

During tooth enamel formation, ameloblasts are arranged in a single layer, and each of them is responsible for the formation of one enamel prism. Throughout amelogenesis, these cells undergo different morphological changes and movements during the secretory stage, as they will connect with and disconnect from each other throughout this phase [1]. These movements cause the enamel prisms to expand, and form the enamel layer with the prismatic pattern, which guarantees the strength of the tissue. The enamel prisms are positioned parallel to each other, with a small space between each prism [58]. In studies that have evaluated the microstructure of the hypomineralised enamel layer, it was possible to observe differences, such as lower prism density, increase in the diameter of the prism sheath, larger interprismatic space, and loss of the prismatic pattern found in sound enamel as shown in Figure 5 [11, 14, 59–62]. Change in the prismatic pattern of hypomineralised enamel causes an increase in porosity since the structure has lower mineral and higher organic content [61].

Enamel affected by MIH has a higher degree of porosity (from 5 to 25%) when compared with sound enamel, and this change is directly related to mineral composition [14]. Studies have shown that higher degree of porosity of hypomineralised enamel is associated with the hypersensitivity of these teeth, a symptom commonly reported by people with MIH. Sound enamel is capable of preventing most external stimuli from arriving to dental pulp, and only more intense stimuli reach the connective tissue. This capacity is due to the high mineral content of enamel. When enamel is hypomineralised, the lower amount of mineral in its composition makes enamel more porous. Therefore, the enamel layer is not capable of preventing mild stimuli from reaching the dental pulp, which will overcome the enamel barrier, reach the dentinal tubules, and then the dental pulp. When stimuli constantly reach the pulp tissue, this might generate a state of chronic inflammation, exacerbating pain sensitivity in these patients [29, 63, 64].

Mechanical Properties

Teeth affected by MIH tend to have a lower degree of hardness when compared with sound teeth. Hardness of a tissue or a structure is mea-

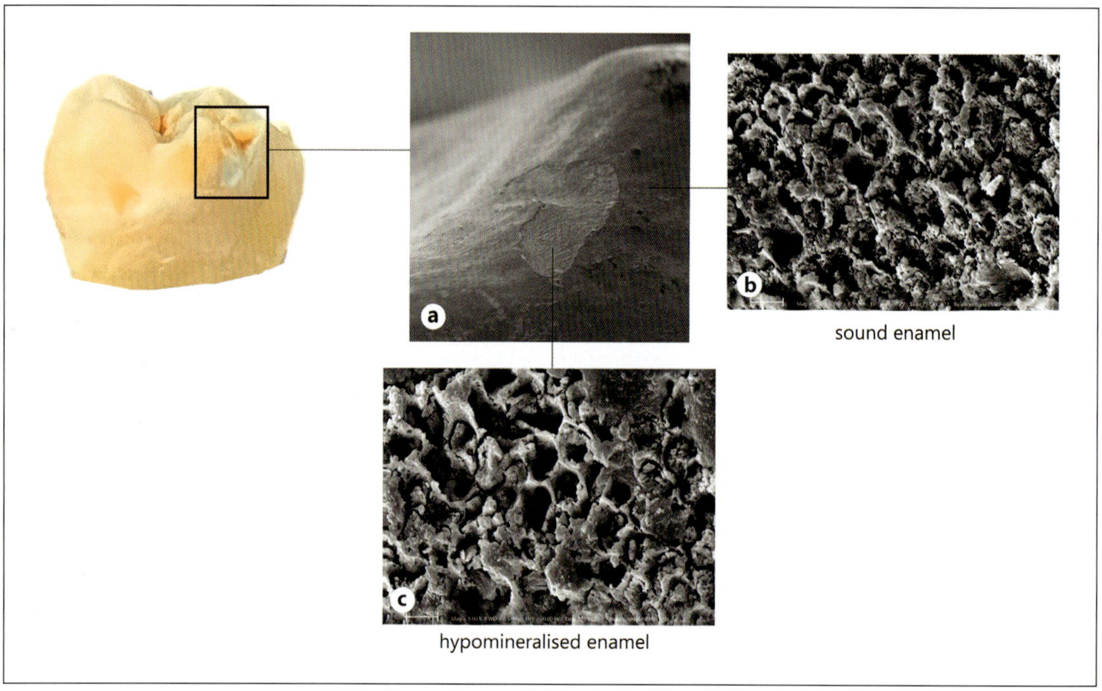

Fig. 5. Tooth with demarcated opacity of MIH with opaque white color seen in scanning electron microscopy. **a** The enamel surface at ×200 magnification and a loss of structure between the area of sound enamel and the hypomineralised area. At ×5,000 magnification, there is a change in the conformation of the enamel prisms between the two regions analyzed. In the sound enamel shown in **b**, it is possible to see a pattern of enamel prisms. **c** The enamel prisms in the hypomineralised enamel region show a disorganized structure with larger diameter enamel prisms, different from the region of sound enamel.

sured by the amount of force it is capable of resisting before fracturing. Tooth enamel is the most mineralised structure in the human body. It has the highest degree of hardness, and is, therefore, capable of resisting a high degree of force without rupture [58, 65]. When the degree of hardness of teeth from the cementoenamel junction to the cusp region was analyzed, a similar hardness with few variations in values was found, ranging between 2.71 and 4.13 kgf. When analyzing the hardness of teeth with MIH opacities of an opaque white color, studies have reported a greater degree of hardness found at the cementoenamel junction, while in the region of transition between sound and hypomineralised enamel, there is a gradual reduction in hardness. In the analysis performed directly in the area of the hypomineralised lesion, the hardness found was significantly lower, ranging from 0.27 to 1.74 kgf [65].

The modulus of elasticity of teeth affected by MIH was also found to be reduced [65, 66], similarly to hardness. Modulus of elasticity of mineralised tissue is related to the capacity of this tissue to flex under a given load and show deformation [63]. In sound teeth, dental enamel has an elastic modulus that varies from 40 to 100 GPa [60]. Teeth with MIH lesions show varying modulus of elasticity values, depending on the quantity of minerals present in the enamel layer. Studies have estimated that tooth enamel with 70% mineral content in its composition have an elastic modulus from 10 to 15 GPa [62, 65]. When tooth enamel has lower hardness and elastic modulus values, this means that this structure has a lower capacity to withstand chewing efforts and thus a greater tendency to fracture [67, 68]. In teeth with MIH, reduction of these properties is related to the lower mineral density, the reduction in the size of enamel prisms, the increase in the protein content in enamel matrix, and the incorporation of other chemical elements in the structure such as carbon. This results in an enamel with less resistance and, therefore, in the occurrence of posteruptive breakdowns, which is common in patients with MIH [13, 62]. Both the hardness and modulus of elasticity vary according to the severity of MIH. Opacities with an opaque white color have a higher mineral content, thus both hardness and modulus of elasticity show higher values than in opacities with a yellow or brownish color since teeth with these lesions have lower mineral content. A higher level of protein accumulation results in more significant tendency to posteruptive fracture occurrence [13]. The increase in proteins in the enamel ill affected their structural and mechanical properties, resulting in an enamel with a higher degree of porosity, a lower mineral content and degree of resistance and, therefore, with greater susceptibility to posteruptive breakdown [14].

Conclusion

Tooth enamel with MIH shows changes in chemical, mechanical, and structural properties resulting from molecular modulations that generate different clinical repercussions such as posteruptive fractures and tooth hypersensitivity. Recognizing the main changes in the structure of tooth enamel and the mechanisms related to the formation of these defects may help in the management of hypomineralised lesions. As these lesions occur in more fragile enamel, they require greater attention from the professional. Furthermore, studies related to the molecular etiology of MIH may have an impact on the discovery of future treatments for this clinical condition.

Acknowledgment

The authors are grateful to the faculty, staff, and graduate students of the Dental Enamel Clinic at the School of Dentistry of Ribeirão Preto at the University of São Paulo for providing the resources used in this manuscript.

Statement of Ethics

Images of subjects (or their parents or guardians) have not been used in this chapter. Therefore, written informed consent and study protocol approval was not obtained at the institute's committee on human research. Slides used were obtained from a databank from studies involving animals that were previously approved by the authors' Institutional Animal Care and Use Committee (IACUC) and followed internationally recognized ARRIVE guidelines.

Conflict of Interest Statement

The authors have no conflicts of interest to declare.

Funding Sources

This study was funded by FAPESP (2023/12014-8) and CAPES Foundation (Financial code 000).

Author Contributions

J.L.G. wrote the manuscript with support from F.K.C., A.M.Q., and F.W.G.P.-S. All authors revised the final version of the manuscript.

References

1 Bartlett JD. Dental enamel development: proteinases and their enamel matrix substrates. ISRN Dent. 2013;2013: 684607.

2 Salanitri S, Seow WK. Developmental enamel defects in the primary dentition: aetiology and clinical management. Aust Dent J. 2013;58(2):133–40.

3 Patel A, Aghababaie S, Parekh S. Hypomineralisation or hypoplasia? Br Dent J. 2019;227(8):683–6.

4 Pandya M, Diekwisch TGH. Enamel biomimetics-fiction or future of dentistry. Int J Oral Sci. 2019;11(1):8.

5 Pandya M, Diekwisch TGH. Amelogenesis: transformation of a protein-mineral matrix into tooth enamel. J Struct Biol. 2021;213(4):107809.

6 Gibson CW. The amelogenin proteins and enamel development in humans and mice. J Oral Biosci. 2011;53(3):248–56.

7 Chu Q, Gao Y, Gao X, Dong Z, Song W, Xu Z, et al. Ablation of Runx2 in ameloblasts suppresses enamel maturation in tooth development. Sci Rep. 2018;8(1): 9594.

8 Malmberg P, Norén JG, Bernin D. Molecular insights into hypomineralized enamel. Eur J Oral Sci. 2019;127(4):340–6.

9 Sarna-Boś K, Boguta P, Skic K, Wiącek D, Maksymiuk P, Sobieszczański J, et al. Physicochemical properties and surface characteristics of ground human teeth. Molecules. 2022;27(18):5852.

10 Sarna-Boś K, Skic K, Boguta P, Adamczuk A, Vodanovic M, Chałas R. Elemental mapping of human teeth enamel, dentine and cementum in view of their microstructure. Micron. 2023;172: 103485.

11 Fagrell TG, Dietz W, Jälevik B, Norén JG. Chemical, mechanical and morphological properties of hypomineralized enamel of permanent first molars. Acta Odontol Scand. 2010;68(4):215–22.

12 Arola DD, Gao S, Zhang H, Masri R. The tooth: its structure and properties. Dent Clin North Am. 2017;61(4):651–68.

13 Crombie FA, Manton DJ, Palamara JEA, Zalizniak I, Cochrane NJ, Reynolds EC. Characterisation of developmentally hypomineralised human enamel. J Dent. 2013;41(7):611–8.

14 Crombie FA, Cochrane NJ, Manton DJ, Palamara JEA, Reynolds EC. Mineralisation of developmentally hypomineralised human enamel in vitro. Caries Res. 2013;47(3):259–63.

15 Olmo-González B, Moreno-López R, Ribera-Uribe M. Dental management strategies for molar incisor hypomineralization. Pediatr Dent J. 2020;30(3): 139–54.

16 Vicioni-Marques F, Paula-Silva FWG, Carvalho MR, Queiroz AM, Freitas O, Duarte MPF, et al. Preemptive analgesia with ibuprofen increases anesthetic efficacy in children with severe molar: a triple-blind randomized clinical trial. J Appl Oral Sci. 2022;30:e20210538.

17 Houari S, DeRocher K, Thuy TT, Coradin T, Srot V, van Aken PA, et al. Multi-scale characterization of developmental defects of enamel and their clinical significance for diagnosis and treatment. Acta Biomater. 2023;169:155–67.

18 Histology, Tooth. StatPearls Publishing [Internet]; cited 2023 Sep 24. Available from: https://www.ncbi.nlm.nih.gov/books/NBK572055/.

19 Yamazaki H, Tran B, Beniash E, Kwak SY, Margolis HC. Proteolysis by MMP20 prevents aberrant mineralization in secretory enamel. J Dent Res. 2019;98(4): 468–75.

20 Núñez SM, Chun YHP, Ganss B, Hu Y, Richardson AS, Schmitz JE, et al. Maturation stage enamel malformations in Amtn and Klk4 null mice. Matrix Biol. 2016;52–54:219–33.

21 Hu Y, Smith, CE, Richardson AS, Bartlett JD, Hu JCC, Simmer JP. MMP20, KLK4, and MMP20/KLK4 double null mice define roles for matrix proteases during dental enamel formation. Mol Genet Genomic Med. 2015;4(2): 178–96.

22 Gil-Bona A, Bidlack FB. Tooth enamel and its dynamic protein matrix. Int J Mol Sci. 2020;21(12):4458.

23 Nanci A, Zalzal S, Lavoie P, Kunikata M, Chen W, Krebsbach PH, et al. Comparative immunochemical analyses of the developmental expression and distribution of ameloblastin and amelogenin in rat incisors. J Histochem Cytochem. 1998;46(8):911–34.

24 Smith CE, Richardson AS, Hu Y, Bartlett JD, Hu JCC, Simmer JP. Effect of kallikrein 4 loss on enamel mineralization. J Biol Chem. 2011;286(20):18149–60.

25 Guo J, Lyaruu DM, Takano Y, Gibson CW, DenBesten PK, Bronckers ALJJ. Amelogenins as potential buffers during secretory-stage amelogenesis. J Dent Res. 2015;94(3):412–20.

26 Bronckers ALJJ. Ion transport by ameloblasts during amelogenesis. J Dent Res. 2017;96(3):243–53.

27 Eckstein M, Aulestia FJ, Nurbaeva MK, Lacruz RS. Altered Ca^{2+} signaling in enamelopathies. Biochim Biophys Acta Mol Cell Res. 2018;1865(11 pt B):1778–85.

28 Ma P, Yan W, Tian Y, He J, Brookes SJ, Wang X. The importance of serine phosphorylation of ameloblastin on enamel formation. J Dent Res. 2016;95(12): 1408–14.

29 Jeremias F, Koruyucu M, Küchler EC, Bayram M, Tuna EB, Deeley K, et al. Genes expressed in dental enamel development are associated with molar-incisor hypomineralization. Arch Oral Biol. 2013;58(10):1434–42.

30 Farah RA, Monk BC, Swain MV, Drummond BK. Protein content of molar-incisor hypomineralisation enamel. J Dent. 2010;38(7):591–6.

31 Bussaneli DG, Restrepo M, Fragelli CMB, Santos-Pinto L, Jeremias F, Cordeiro RCL, et al. Genes regulating immune response and amelogenesis interact in increasing the susceptibility to molar-incisor hypomineralization. Caries Res. 2019;53(2):217–27.

32 Heymann R, About I, Lendahl U, Franquin JC, Obrink B, Mitsiadis TA. E- and N-cadherin distribution in developing and functional human teeth under normal and pathological conditions. Am J Pathol. 2002;160(6):2123–33.

33 Lynch CC, Vargo-Gogola T, Matrisian LM, Fingleton B. Cleavage of E-cadherin by matrix metalloproteinase-7 promotes cellular proliferation in nontransformed cell lines via activation of RhoA. J Oncol. 2010;2010:530745.

34 Bartlett JD, Yamakoshi Y, Simmer JP, Nanci A, Smith CE. MMP20 cleaves E-cadherin and influences ameloblast development. Cells Tissues Organs. 2011; 194(2–4):222–6.

35 Prajapati S, Tao J, Ruan Q, De Yoreo JJ, Moradian-Oldak J. Matrix metalloproteinase-20 mediates dental enamel biomineralization by preventing protein occlusion inside apatite crystals. Biomaterials. 2016;75:260–70.

36 Simmer JP, Hu Y, Lertlam R, Yamakoshi Y, Hu JCC. Hypomaturation enamel defects in Klk4 knockout/LacZ knockin mice. J Biol Chem. 2009;284(28):19110–21.
37 Perez VA, Mangum JE, Hubbard MJ. Direct evidence that KLK4 is a hydroxyapatite-binding protein. Biochem Biophys Res Commun. 2018;495(2):1896–900.
38 Juárez-López MLA, Salazar-Treto LV, Hernández-Monjaraz B, Molina-Frechero N. Etiological factors of molar incisor hypomineralization: a systematic review and meta-analysis. Dent J (Basel). 2023; 11(5):111.
39 Garot E, Rouas P, Somani C, Taylor GD, Wong F, Lygidakis NA. An update of the aetiological factors involved in molar incisor hypomineralisation (MIH): a systematic review and meta-analysis. Eur Arch Paediatr Dent. 2022;23(1):23–38.
40 Jedeon K, Dure-Molla M, Brookes SJ, Loiodice S, Marciano C, Kirkham J. Enamel defects reflect perinatal exposure to bisphenol A. Am J Pathol. 2013;183(1):108–18.
41 Shaffer IC, Nakano Y, Pham A, Short A, Nanci A, Zhang Y, et al. Effects of early life adversity on tooth enamel formation. Front Dent Med. 2022;3:894753.
42 Gonçalves JL, Duarte ACA, Almeida-Junior LA, Carvalho FK, Queiroz AM, Arnez MFM, et al. Enamel biomineralization under the effects of indomethacin and celecoxib non-steroidal anti-inflammatory drugs. Sci Rep. 2022; 12(1):15823.
43 Lee DW, Kim YJ, Kim SO, Choi SC, Kim J, Lee JH, et al. Factors associated with molar-incisor hypomineralization: a population-based case-control study. Pediatr Dent. 2020;42(2):134–40.
44 Perez VA, Mangum JE, Hubbard MJ. Pathogenesis of molar hypomineralisation: aged albumin demarcates chalky regions of hypomineralised enamel. Front Physiol. 2020;11:579015.
45 Williams R, Perez VA, Mangum JE, Hubbard MJ. Pathogenesis of molar hypomineralisation: hypomineralised 6-year molars contain traces of fetal serum albumin. Front Physiol. 2020;11: 619.
46 Bardet C, Ribes S, Wu Y, Diallo MT, Salmon B, Breiderhoff T, et al. Claudin loss-of-function disrupts tight junctions and impairs amelogenesis. Front Physiol. 2017;8:326.
47 Bardet C, Courson F, Wu Y, Khaddam M, Salmon B, Ribes S, et al. Claudin-16 deficiency impairs tight junction function in ameloblasts, leading to abnormal enamel formation. J Bone Miner Res. 2016;31(3):498–513.
48 Günzel D, Yu ASL. Claudins and the modulation of tight junction permeability. Physiol Rev. 2013;93(2):525–69.
49 Garot E, Rouas P, D'Incau E, Lenoir N, Manton D, Couture-Veschambre C. Mineral density of hypomineralised and sound enamel. Bull Group Int Rech Sci Stomatol Odontol. 2016;53(1):e33.
50 Elhennawy K, Manton DJ, Crombie F, Zaslansky P, Radlanski RJ, Brinkmann PGJ, et al. Structural, mechanical and chemical evaluation of molar-incisor hypomineralization-affected enamel: a systematic review. Arch Oral Biol. 2017; 83:272–81.
51 Martinović B, Ivanović M, Milojković Z, Mladenović R. Analysis of the mineral composition of hypomineralized first permanent molars. Vojnosanit Pregl. 2015;72(10):864–9.
52 Smith CE. Cellular and chemical events during enamel maturation. Crit Rev Oral Biol Med. 1998;9(2):128–61.
53 Nurbaeva MK, Eckstein M, Feske S, Lacruz RS. Ca^{2+} transport and signalling in enamel cells. J Physiol. 2017;595(10): 3015–39.
54 Chan B, Cheng CI, Rozita J, Gorshteyn I, Huang Y, Shaffer I, et al. Sodium/(calcium + potassium) exchanger NCKX4 optimizes KLK4 activity in the enamel matrix microenvironment to regulate ECM modeling. Front Physiol. 2023; 14:1116091.
55 Sui W, Boyd C, Wright JT. Altered pH regulation during enamel development in the cystic fibrosis mouse incisor. J Dent Res. 2003;82(5):388–92.
56 Lacruz RS, Nanci A, Kurtz I, Wright JS, Paine ML. Regulation of pH during amelogenesis. Calcif Tissue Int. 2010;86(2): 91–103.
57 Jälevik B. Enamel hypomineralization in permanent first molars. A clinical, histomorphological and biochemical study. Swed Dent J Suppl. 2001;149:1–86.
58 He LH, Swain MV. Understanding the mechanical behaviour of human enamel from its structural and compositional characteristics. J Mech Behav Biomed Mater. 2008;1(1):18–29.
59 Bozal CBB, Kaplan A, Ortolani A, Cortese SGG, Biondi AM. Ultrastructure of the surface of dental enamel with molar incisor hypomineralization (MIH) with and without acid etching. Acta Odontol Latinoam. 2015;28(2):192–8.
60 Chan YL, Ngan AHW, King NM. Degraded prism sheaths in the transition region of hypomineralized teeth. J Dent. 2010;38(3):237–44.
61 Jälevik B, Dietz W, Norén JG. Scanning electron micrograph analysis of hypomineralized enamel in permanent first molars. Int J Paediatr Dent. 2005;15(4): 233–40.
62 Xie ZH, Mahoney EK, Kilpatrick NM, Swain MV, Hoffman M. On the structure-property relationship of sound and hypomineralized enamel. Acta Biomater. 2007;3(6):865–72.
63 Raposo F, de Carvalho Rodrigues AC, Lia ÉN, Leal SC. Prevalence of hypersensitivity in teeth affected by molar-incisor hypomineralization (MIH). Caries Res. 2019;53(4):424–30.
64 Linner T, Khazaei Y, Bücher K, Pfisterer J, Hickel R, Kühnisch J. Hypersensitivity in teeth affected by molar-incisor hypomineralization (MIH). Sci Rep. 2021; 11(1):17922.
65 Mahoney E, Ismail FSM, Kilpatrick N, Swain M. Mechanical properties across hypomineralized/hypoplastic enamel of first permanent molar teeth. Eur J Oral Sci. 2004;112(6):497–502.
66 Farah RA, Drummond BK, Swain MV, Williams S. Relationship between laser fluorescence and enamel hypomineralisation. J Dent. 2008;36(11):915–21.
67 Chay PL, Manton DJ, Palamara JEA. The effect of resin infiltration and oxidative pre-treatment on microshear bond strength of resin composite to hypomineralised enamel. Int J Paediatr Dent. 2014;24(4):252–67.
68 William V, Burrow MF, Palamara JEA, Messer LB. Microshear bond strength of resin composite to teeth affected by molar hypomineralization using 2 adhesive systems. Pediatr Dent. 2006;28(3):233–41.

Francisco Wanderley Garcia de Paula-Silva
Department of Pediatric Clinics, School of Dentistry of Ribeirão Preto
University of São Paulo, Avenida do Café, s/n
Ribeirão Preto, SP 14040-904 (Brazil)
franciscogarcia@forp.usp.br

Published online: July 1, 2024
Rios D, Santos-Pinto L (eds): Molar Incisor Hypomineralisation: New Perceptions. Monogr Oral Sci. Basel, Karger, 2024, vol 32, pp 56–67 (DOI: 10.1159/000538867)

Challenges of Using Scoring Systems for the Assessment of Molar Incisor Hypomineralisation

Soraya Coelho Leal[a] Camila Fragelli[b] Fernanda Noal[c]
Eliana Mitsue Takeshita[a]

[a]Department of Dentistry, Faculty of Health Science, University of Brasília, Brasília, Brazil; [b]Online Training Program "Simplified Molar Incisor Hypomineralization", São Carlos, Brazil; [c]Division of Pediatric Dentistry, School of Dentistry, Scientific University of the South, Lima, Peru

Abstract

The dental professional is exposed to complex challenges daily, posed by molar incisor hypomineralisation (MIH). These range from understanding its etiology through to determining the most effective strategies for clinical management of the problem. Beyond any doubt, the choice of the diagnostic scoring system to be used for recording the condition is included among these challenges. To a certain degree, this is understandable since the development of specific diagnostic tools for recording the occurrence of MIH takes place parallel to the ongoing discoveries about the problem. Therefore, the aim of this chapter is to present different MIH scoring systems that have previously been proposed in the literature for detecting MIH and discuss their applications, advantages, and limitations.

Introduction

Since molar incisor hypomineralisation (MIH) was described as an entity for the first time in 2001 [1], this condition has drawn the attention of researchers, epidemiologists, and clinicians. At that time, it was, and up until now, it is still necessary to determine its prevalence, etiology, consequences, and the most cost-effective ways of clinically managing the problem. For this purpose, it is essential for the diagnosis of MIH to be performed in a reliable way, with the use of systematic and validated scoring systems that allow the comparison of data collected in different countries, populations, and clinical settings [2]. Moreover, understanding the dynamics of MIH in a specific population, which should be reflected in its evaluation criteria, is extremely relevant for the planning and formulation of public policies [3].

During a discussion meeting in Athens, a group of experts concluded that although there were some existent scoring systems for detecting development defects of the enamel (DDE), such as the FDI DDE index [4], they have shown some disadvantages relative to the diagnosis of MIH. This has made it necessary to develop a system that could specifically register the condition [5]. Therefore, a new system was proposed and has come to be known as "the EAPD (European Academy of Paediatric Dentistry) judgment criteria," which has proven to be easy to apply, mainly due to its simplicity. Whereas over the course of time, it has been observed that the criteria – precisely due to being simple – were incapable of portraying the entire spectrum of MIH. As a result, researchers have started to modify the criteria, in an attempt to record not only the different characteristics but also the severity of the condition. For example, the EAPD criteria [5] were used by da Costa-Silva et al. [6] and Leal et al. [7], but in both studies with modifications. In the first case, color was recorded separately (white, yellow, and brown), while in the second case, post-eruptive breakdown (PEB) was differentiated into two categories (restricted to enamel or already exposing dentin). This lack of consistency in data collection has hampered the comparison of results among reports.

The fact that MIH can evolve, and has a tendency worsen over time, is another aspect that should be taken into account at the time of its diagnosis, which justifies the selection of a standardized scoring system. From a clinical point of view, identifying the characteristics that make an affected tooth more prone to breakdown is extremely relevant since the literature has previously shown that the darker the opacity the greater the chances of breakdown in the long term [8, 9]. In other words, yellow/brown opacities are more likely to collapse than the white/creamy types over time. In possession of this information, the clinician can establish a more individualized follow-up visit plan for each patient and instruct parents about the need for careful and continuous monitoring of the tooth in question.

Since the limitations of using the EAPD criteria [5] were observed, different MIH scoring systems have been proposed, as shown in Table 1. It is interesting to observe that the way in which they are structured varies greatly, as some include sensitivity as part of the evaluation [10–13], while others include assessment of the extension of the defect [3, 11, 12]; other different types of DDEs [3] or severity of the MIH [9, 10]. With so many options, a question arises: *which is the most appropriate system to use?* Relative to this question, there are many factors that influence the response such as the aim of the investigation (epidemiological survey; clinical follow-up); the possibility of accurately measuring hypersensitivity; and the need for determining other DDEs.

Other aspects, which are not the aim of this chapter, also play a major role in the diagnosis of MIH and are, therefore, worth mentioning. These are the age of the child under investigation, minimum size of the opacity (>1 mm or >2 mm), calibration of the examiner(s), and the condition in which the tooth is assessed (wet or dry) [14]. All these aspects may interfere in the results and may, at least partly, explain divergences in the prevalence reported by different studies even when they have used the same assessment scoring system (Table 1).

MIH Assessment Scoring Systems

As mentioned above, as soon as MIH was reported in the literature [1], comparable and representative prevalence studies were urgently needed. Thus, surveys began to be conducted, mainly using the EAPD criteria [5]. According to the criteria, the four first permanent molars (FPMs) and eight permanent incisors (PIs) should be examined. Moreover, cleaned and wet teeth should be individually assessed, and five different conditions can be recorded as shown in Table 1. Un-

Table 1. MIH assessment scoring systems and their description by year of publication

Scoring system	Description	Severity
EAPD [5, 13]	• Demarcated opacity • Posteruptive enamel breakdown • Atypical restoration • Tooth sensitivity[a] (report) • Extracted molar due to MIH • Unerupted	• Mild[a] (demarcated opacities without PEB; occasional sensitivity and only mild aesthetic concern) • Moderate[a] (PEB, caries, persistent sensitivity, and strong aesthetic concern)
HSI [10]	• Presence FPM unerupted FPM erupted • Extent of hypomineralization 0: None 1: Mild (white cream opacity) 2: Moderate/severe • Sensitivity (parents are questioned) 0: None 1: Sensitive • Number of restorative procedures 0: None 1: One 2: Two 3: Three or more	• Mild (white cream opacity) • Moderate/severe (yellow/brown discoloration and/or PEB)
MHSI[b] [11]	• Eruptive status Unerupted Erupted • Color of most severe defect None White/cream Yellow Brown • Location of the most severe defect None Smooth surface Occlusal surface (1st permanent molars) Incisor edge (PIs) Cuspal involvement (1st permanent molars) • Restorations placed/replaced (prior to the exam) None One Two or more • Atypical restorations (prior to exam) None Present • Sensitive to temperature (child report) None Sensitive • Sensitive to toothbrushing (child report) None Sensitive	Severity is calculated according to the weights given to each of the MIH characteristics, in tooth and dentition levels. **Severity in tooth level** Mild: Intact colored defects, usually on smooth or occlusal surfaces Moderate: Yellow or brown defects on occlusal or cuspal surfaces, which may have atypical or previous restorations, PEB, or sensitivity Severe: Brown or yellow defects with a combination of PEB, sensitivity, and atypical restorations or previous restorations **Severity in dentition level** Mild: Dentitions ranging from one to four mildly affected FPMs, or one severely affected FPM. Moderate: Dentitions with two to four mild/moderately affected FPMs, or up to two severely affected FPMs. Severe: Dentitions with four severely affected FPMs.
Mittal [16]	a. MH: hypomineralization affecting only 1st permanent molars without affecting any other tooth in the dentition b. IH: hypomineralization affecting only PIs without affecting any other tooth in the arch; excluding those with a history of trauma/infection of primary incisors c. MH + IH: hypomineralization affecting only 1st permanent molars and PIs simultaneously but not any other tooth in the dentition d. MHO: hypomineralization affecting 1st permanent molars and at least one of the canines, premolars, or 2nd molars. PIs may be affected simultaneously. Those with a history of trauma/infection to primary teeth are excluded e. No FPM: hypomineralization affecting at least one of the canines, premolars, or 2nd molars. PIs may be affected simultaneously. Those with a history of trauma/infection to primary teeth are excluded	Measured by the number of surfaces affected and surfaces with PEB

Table 1 (continued)

Scoring system	Description	Severity
Ghanim et al.[c] [3]	• Eruption status criteria A = not visible or less than one-third of the occlusal surface or of the crown length of incisor is visible • Clinical status criteria 0. No visible enamel defect 1. Enamel defect, non-MIH/HSPM 11. Diffuse opacities 12. Hypoplasia[d] 13. Amelogenesis imperfecta[d] 14. Hypomineralization defect (not MIH/HSPM)[d] 2. Demarcated opacities 21. White or creamy[d] 22. Yellow or brown[d] 3. Posteruptive enamel breakdown 4. Atypical restoration 5. Atypical caries 6. Missing due to MIH/HSPM 7. Cannot be scored • Lesion extension criteria (scores 2–6) I = less than one-third of the tooth affected II = at least one-third but less than two-thirds of the tooth affected III = at least two-thirds of the tooth affected	Represented by both the stage of visible enamel destruction and the amount of tooth surface area affected
MIH-TNI[e] [12]	1. MIH without hypersensitivity, without defect 2. MIH without hypersensitivity, with defect 2a. <1/3 defect extension 2b. >1/3 <2/3 defect extension 2c. >2/3 defect extension or/and defect close to the pulp or extraction or atypical restoration 3. MIH with hypersensitivity, without defect 4. MIH with hypersensitivity, with defect 4a. <1/3 defect extension 4b. >1/3 <2/3 defect extension 4c. >2/3 defect extension or/and defect close to the pulp or extraction or atypical restoration	MIH diagnosis is performed according to the EAPD criteria
MIH-SSS [9]	0. Normal enamel translucency 1. White/creamy opacity 2. Yellow/brown opacity 3. Breakdown restricted to the enamel related to white opacity 4. Breakdown restricted to the enamel related to yellow opacity 5. Dentin breakdown (hard dentine) 6. Dentin breakdown (soft dentine) 7. Satisfactory atypical restoration 8. Unsatisfactory atypical restoration 9. Extraction due to MIH	• Mild (demarcated opacities) • Moderate (PEB restricted to enamel) • Severe (PEB exposing dentin; atypical (un) satisfactory restorations; lost due to MIH

[a]Included in the updated version of the EAPD criteria 2010 [13]. [b]Weights are assigned to each characteristic. [c]Lesion extension is recorded for scores 2–6 in three categories. [d]Only accounted for in the long form sheet. [e]In epidemiological studies, examinations by sextant and for individual assessment, by tooth (all primary and permanent teeth should be assessed).

doubtedly, the EAPD criteria [5], due to being the first MIH scoring system used in epidemiological research, has shed some light on the different aspects of this challenging condition. However, with the knowledge acquired over time, it has been observed that the criteria, although simple and replicable, were incapable of providing a detailed description of some important characteristics of MIH, such as the location and color of the opacity, and could not assess the severity of the condition. This became obvious in 2010 [13], when an updated version of the criteria was published including "tooth sensitivity" and recognizing that the defects could also be observed in other teeth such as second primary molars (Fig. 1).

In an attempt to develop an MIH severity index, Chawla et al. [10] analyzed the records of 182 children affected by MIH, which contained information about their treatment, medical histories, and dental condition. Based on this analysis, the "hypomineralization severity index (HSI)" was proposed with the aim of assisting professionals with the decision-making process for managing hypomineralised FPMs. To calculate the HSI, four aspects should be taken into account: the presence of the FPM; extent of the hypomineralisation area; presence of tooth sensitivity (air syringe and child's report); and the number of restorations placed and replaced in each FPM (Table 1). The final score is obtained for each FPM, by adding up the points from all categories and dividing the result by the number of erupted FPMs. Results can range from 1.25 to 10.00. However, this index has some drawbacks worth mentioning. First, up to date, there are no studies that have used the index, and therefore, its prognostic value in treatment planning could not be confirmed. Furthermore, it does not encompass important characteristics that are already known to be related to MIH severity, such as the presence or absence of PEB, atypical restorations, and the color of the opacity.

Another index, not only with the aim of assessing MIH severity, but also of guiding clinicians with developing a treatment plan, is the molar hypomineralisation severity index (MHSI) [11]. According to the MHSI, treatment needs of a child should be based on the clinical appearance of the most severe defects. The total score is calculated taking into account hypersensitivity, color, and location of the most severe defect, presence of atypical restoration, and PEB. MIH severity is then categorized as mild (scores 3–6), moderate (scores 7–9), and severe (scores 10–13). As expected, the authors have shown that low scores were associated with preventive care and few invasive treatments, while high scores were related to less preventive care and more invasive treatments. A limitation of MHSI is that the extension of the defect was not measured and included. The authors suggested that the location of the most severe MIH defects combined with other clinical characteristics could be the basis for a new MIH severity index. Up to the end of this publication, only one clinical trial [15] has used the MHSI to classify the severity of MIH but used the EAPD criteria [5] for MIH diagnosis.

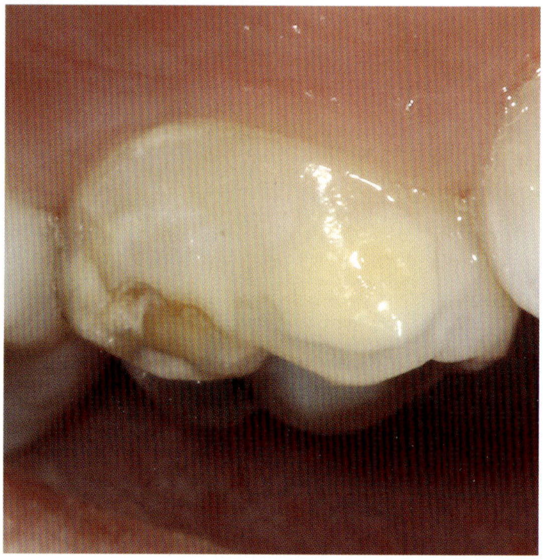

Fig. 1. Presence of demarcated opacity and PEB on the secondary primary molar, known as hypomineralisation of secondary primary molar (HPSM).

Over the years, researchers have observed that the main feature of MIH, which is the demarcated opacity, can manifest in other teeth, such as permanent canines, premolars and second molars, as well as primary teeth. As a result, the recommendation of Lygidakis et al. [13] was that to enable the full pattern of manifestation of enamel hypomineralisation to be portrayed, all primary and permanent teeth should be assessed. This represented one step ahead in the diagnosis of MIH considering the proposals made by the EAPD criteria in 2003 [5] that only describes two possible phenotypes: cases affecting only FPMs without affecting any other tooth in the dentition and cases affecting FPMs and PIs simultaneously but not any other tooth in the dentition.

In order to report different manifestations of hypomineralisation characterized by demarcated opacities, Mittal [16], in a cross-sectional observational study that included 1,726 adolescents, analyzed the extent and severity of enamel hypomineralisation in occlusal, buccal, lingual/palatal surfaces of all erupted permanent teeth using the EAPD criteria [5]. Five different phenotypes were identified and are presented in Table 1. By comparing the extent and severity of enamel hypomineralisation amongst all phenotypes, the author observed that the most significant severity occurred in patients presenting MIH and the least severity was reported for those with incisor hypomineralisation. To date, to the best of our knowledge, this classification scheme has not been used in any clinical study.

Although the EAPD criteria [5, 13] have been widely used, MIH prevalence rates still vary considerably when studies that have used the system are compared [3]. This was one of the reasons that Ghanim et al., after the workshop at the 12th EAPD Congress in 2014, proposed a grading method that allows demarcated hypomineralisation lesions to be classified according to their color and extension, and as categories, also includes "atypical caries" and "defects other than MIH" [3]. The criteria offer two ways of assessment: a short form for simple screening and a long form for community or clinical studies, or when more detailed information is required, as shown in Table 1. In the short form, FPMs, PIs, and primary second molars are evaluated, while in the long form, all erupted teeth and surfaces are assessed, both in the permanent and primary dentition. Another difference between the two forms refers to the fact that in the long form, items such as recording enamel defects other than MIH/hypomineralised second primary molar and dichotomization of cream/white and brownish/yellow opacities were added. Moreover, according to the system, the extent of MIH as well as the tooth eruption status should be assessed. Although this scoring system has been developed for epidemiological, clinical, and hospital-based studies, in practice, it becomes a differential in comparison with other scoring methods, only when the long form is applied.

It is important, however, to mention some difficulties that the examiner might face when using the system long form. When registering the condition, either by surface or tooth, 2 codes are used: a number and a Roman numeral – indicating the MIH clinical feature and the extent of the defect, respectively. To illustrate the use of these codes, the vestibular surface of the secondary primary molar shown in Figure 1 is analyzed. The condition, according to the system, is recorded as 3-II (PEB extending to more than one one-third of the surface and less than two thirds). However, if it had been used as a reference, the manual developed to assist researchers in epidemiological studies, published by the same authors in 2017 [17], the use of a letter would have been mandatory. That is, in addition to the letter A, the letter B would have been added (A – fully erupted or B – at least one third but less than the total crown length of the incisor is visible) in the charting criteria published in 2017. In this case, the tooth shown in Figure 1 would have been recorded as B-3-II. If the first version of the criteria was being used, the inclusion of the letter A would not be needed as it is used only for those situations in which the tooth/surface is not visible or less than one-third of the occlusal surface or of the crown length of the incisor is visible. As clearly shown in this example, the way of registering the criteria is quite complex, which may lead to errors in annotation, tabulation, and analysis.

Differently from the scoring systems described so far, Steffen et al. [12] developed a system, of which the main aim was to provide an easy and standardized MIH assessment focused on treatment needs. Therefore, according to the authors, MIH diagnosis (yes or no) should previously be performed using the EAPD criteria [5] and can be applied to both primary and permanent dentitions. The index, known as MIH-TNI (MIH treatment need index), that has previously been used in some studies [18–20], primarily takes two aspects into account: defect (posteruptive structural loss) and hypersensitivity (Table 1). During the examination, the mouth is divided in sextants (maxilla right, front and left and mandible right, front and left), and the highest value per sextant is recorded. However, although the index is also focused on treatment, it does not provide essential information to enable preventive measures to be established, such as the localization and the color of opacity. In this regard, the MIH-TNI dissociate prevention from treatment, which, according to the Minimum Intervention Dentistry philosophy, is not recommended. On the other hand, it is worth mentioning that the MIH-TNI index was the first classification system to take into account hypersensitivity as a key factor in the MIH diagnosis.

Furthermore, researchers concerned about MIH severity followed up children who, at the baseline, presented at least one FPM affected by MIH with demarcated opacity, with the aim of observing the pattern of transition of a mild condition into a severe type [9]. After 36 months of observation, the findings formed the basis of the MIH-SSS, which is presented in Table 1. It is interesting to note that the system is the only one that differentiates soft and hard dentine in relation to a PEB. This is relevant information, not only to identify the severity of the defect but also for the development of the treatment plan. Moreover, when the system is applied, it is possible to determine the status of the atypical restoration (satisfactory or not), which, once again, is crucial for the clinical management of the affected tooth. This scoring system showed high reliability and has previously been used in field [21, 22]. It has been proved, in a hierarchical way, to be capable of capturing the different levels of severity associated with MIH. However, the scope of the system covers neither the extent of the enamel alteration nor the presence of hypersensitivity.

MIH Assessment Scoring Systems and Severity

Once MIH has been detected, the next step is to determine the severity of the condition. Some of the systems presented in Table 1 encompass this aspect. Chawla et al. [10], for example, make a distinction between mild and moderate/severe conditions, whereas the codes of the MIH-SSS [9] are listed in a hierarchical way, indicating that as code values go up, from 1 to 9, so does the severity of MIH. Although other scoring systems are organized in such a manner, moving from the mildest condition (demarcated opacity) to the worst type (loss due to MIH), they do not cover all the transition patterns into which an opacity can evolve in the long term. In other words, depending on the scoring system selected for use, some of the stages of MIH progression cannot be registered. This may be visualized in Figure 2d, e. These teeth are obviously not comparable in terms of severity, but depending on the scoring system used, this difference is not noticeable. If the Ghanim et al. [3] system or the EAPD criteria [5, 13] are used, the tooth shown in Figure 2d would be classified as presenting PEB; however, just by reading this information, it is not possible to identify whether the PEB is restricted to enamel or whether it has already exposed the dentin; as it is in the case of the tooth shown in Figure 2e. With respect to the Ghanim et al. [3] criteria, the extent of the lesion would also been recorded, but even so, it would not provide any information relative to whether the breakage is in enamel or in dentin. In clinical practice, it is important to differentiate the PEB status, not only to guide the professional in the decision-making process

	Clinical condition			
	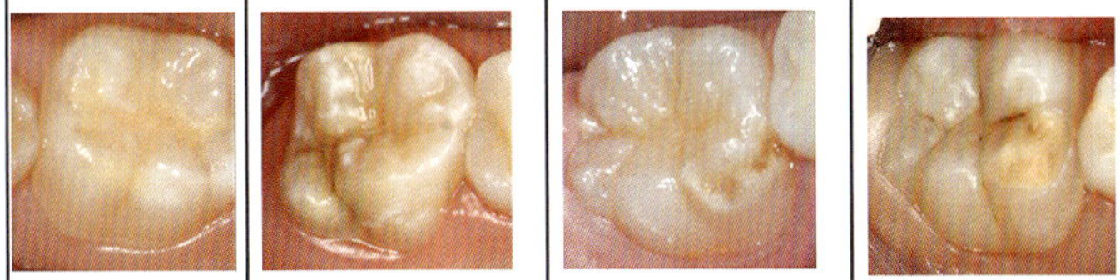			
	a	b	c	d
MIH scoring system	**Classification**			
EAPD criteria [5, 13]	Demarcated opacity	Demarcated opacity	PEB	PEB
Ghanim et al. [3] – short form	Demarcated opacity	Demarcated opacity	PEB	PEB
Ghanim et al. [3] – long form	White/creamy demarcated opacity	Yellow/brown demarcated opacity	PEB	PEB
MIH-SSS [9]	White/creamy opacity	Yellow/brown opacity	PEB restricted to the enamel related to a white opacity	PEB restricted to enamel related to a yellow opacity
	Clinical condition			
	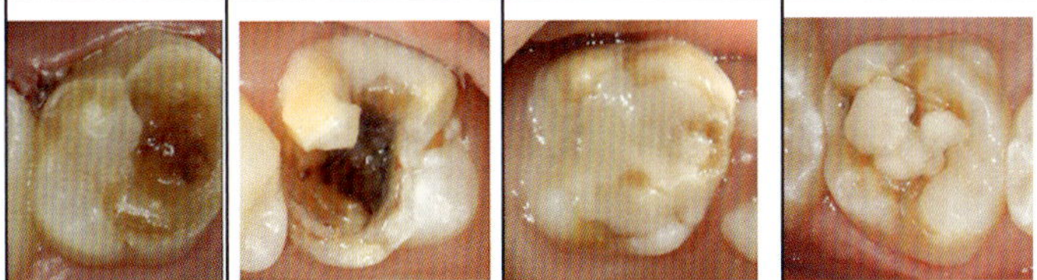			
	e	f	g	h
MIH scoring system	**Classification**			
EAPD criteria [5, 13]	PEB	PEB	Atypical restoration	PEB/atypical restoration (?)
Ghanim et al. [3] – short form	PEB	Atypical caries	Atypical restoration	PEB/atypical restoration (?)
Ghanim et al. [3] – long form	PEB	Atypical caries	Atypical restoration	PEB/atypical restoration (?)
MIH-SSS [9]	PEB exposing hard dentin	PEB exposingsoft dentin	Satisfactory atypical restoration	Unsatisfactory atypical restoration

Fig. 2. Classification of teeth affected by MIH according to different MIH assessment scoring systems.

about treatment (a fracture restricted to enamel requires clinical management that differs from the type that involves dentin) but also to enable policymakers to understand the seriousness of the problem in a specific population.

Apart from the scoring system used, the most common ways to clinically categorize MIH severity are to describe it either as mild and severe or mild, moderate, and severe. This variation is primarily related to the definition of what the moderate and severe forms are since it seems to be a consensus among researchers that demarcated opacities without PEB characterize a mild condition [9, 13, 14]. Relative to the "moderate/severe" categories, the divergence is mostly related to how to classify a PEB restricted to enamel. For some, it is already a severe characteristic of MIH [11, 23], while for others, it is a moderate condition [24, 25]. Moreover, Lygidakis et al. [13] suggested that strong aesthetic concerns (although no indication whether the aesthetic perception taken into account in this analysis is from the professional, parents, or children is provided by the authors), and the report of persistent/spontaneous hypersensitivity should also be considered signs of severe MIH.

Since hypersensitivity is associated with an MIH tooth, one of the greatest challenges is to establish the pain threshold, which refers to the lowest intensity at which a given stimulus (thermal, chemical, or pressure) is perceived as painful. In fact, some children with MIH report pain during their meals and even when smiling.

Considering the scoring systems listed in Table 1, four of them register hypersensitivity [10–13]. In all cases, the assessment is based on the child's or parents' reports and/or clinical examination but without measuring its intensity. In this regard, two questions arise: *is it important to record the intensity of hypersensitivity?* and, *will this information bring any benefit in terms of clinically managing the problem?* As the literature has shown, children with MIH show a higher frequency of hypersensitivity when compared with nonaffected children, but only a few report/show high levels of intensity [20, 25]. Therefore, it is believed that knowing the intensity of hypersensitivity could assist the professional in establishing strategies to manage pain during treatment. However, another question arises: *which is the best way to measure hypersensitivity in children?* Other than self-reporting, which is considerably subjective, studies that have assessed hypersensitivity associated with MIH used specific tools to measure it, such as the Schiff Cold Air Sensitivity Scale and the Visual Analog Scale [21, 26, 27]. However, to incorporate this into epidemiological studies, in the field, may be unrealistic, as it increases the examination time and requires extra equipment/material. As an alternative to overcome this issue, Steffen et al. [12] suggested analyzing hypersensitivity by sextants in epidemiological surveys. However, since the system does not record caries lesions (only extension of the defect), it is difficult to establish the cause of pain in cases in which MIH is associated with carious lesions and/or exposed dentin since both conditions are considered confounding factors for the diagnosis of hypersensitivity.

Furthermore, it is interesting to note that the majority of the scoring systems that cover hypersensitivity associate it with the size of the MIH defect, irrespective of its intensity, which might be a problem, since a less severe condition (i.e., opacity) does not necessarily mean lower intensity of sensitivity.

Applying Different MIH Assessment Scoring Systems

In view of the many different options of scoring systems, may be useful to identify the objective of registering MIH in order to assist professionals with deciding on one system or another. If the sole purpose is to run a screening session to identify the prevalence of MIH in a certain population, the use of a simplified assessment tool might be advantageous over a more detailed type. However, if the objective is to follow up the transition pattern of an opacity over time, detailed information about its condition at baseline is essential. In Figure 2, different clinical conditions of MIH are shown with their respective evaluation according to different assessment scoring systems. The same MIH feature has been observed to be recorded differently, depending on the scoring system used. An aspect that causes even more concern is that some clinical conditions, even when using the same scoring system, may be classified differently, depending on the examiners' interpretation. For example, the occlusal surface of the FPM in Figure 2h was judged as being an unsatisfactory restoration by the MIH-SSS [9]. However, when using both the EAPD [5, 13] and Ghanim et al. [3] criteria, it is possible to score it as an atypical restoration or as a PEB. This is because both criteria do not provide clear instructions on how to classify an atypical restoration, which presents partial loss of the restorative material exposing enamel/dentin but without association with a caries lesion. Translating this information into clinical practice, it means that, without the clinical image, one cannot really visualize the real condition of the tooth according to the EAPD criteria [5, 13] and Ghanim et al. [3]. This is a problem not only from a management point of view but also in terms of epidemiology. In the first case, recording the surface as PEB or atypical restoration does not give a correct indication on how to clinically manage the condition, which in this situation would be only a restoration repair. In the second case, the possibility of judging it in two different ways will impact the overall results, over or underestimating either the frequency of PEB or atypical restorations in the population studied. In addition, it is interesting to note that both the EAPD criteria [5, 13] and the Ghanim et al. [3] short form do not distinguish white/creamy to yellow/brown opacity (Fig. 2a, b, respectively), since both are classified as demarcated opacity. Using the Ghanim et al. [3] long form and the MIH-SSS [9], a more accurate prognosis can be achieved, as the literature has previously shown that yellow/brown opacities present a higher risk of breakdown compared with white/creamy opacities [8, 9].

As observed above, all the MIH assessment scoring systems presented have their strengths and limitations. Nonetheless, the use of a specific diagnostic tool, chosen according to the professionals' needs and/preference, undoubtedly assists them in recording MIH in a systematic way, which in turn allows for a better understanding of progression (or not) of the problem over time. According to a publication that compared the performance of the Ghanim et al. [3] and the MIH-SSS [9] systems for MIH detection in epidemiology surveys, the choice of the scoring system should take into account the characteristics of each of system and their alignment with the research objectives [28]. The authors reported that the MIH-SSS [9] had a shorter application time and provided more detailed information about MIH spectrum, while using the Ghanim et al. [3] long form, the recording of other DDE was possible [28]. On the basis of these findings, and primarily focusing on MIH diagnosis, the use of the MIH-SSS not only gathers essential information for the development of a care plan but also tailored follow-ups.

Final Remarks

The relevance of using validated scoring systems for an accurate diagnosis of MIH and, consequently, the adoption of the most effective treatment strategies is unquestionable. Considering that all assessment scoring systems for MIH diagnosis that have previously been proposed in the literature present advantages and limitations, the choice of the type to use should be made within the context of the examiners' objectives, whether they involve screening, longitudinal tracking, or a more comprehensive assessment of MIH. However, irrespective of this, it is important for system chosen to be capable of portraying the main clinical characteristics of the condition and its severity.

Since hypersensitivity is a factor that cannot be measured by visual inspection, but is an important item of information to determine MIH severity, it is believed that its evaluation can be incorporated into any of the MIH diagnostic tools available. The main question in this respect, therefore, refers to how hypersensitivity should be evaluated.

Although the majority of the MIH assessment scoring systems do not recommend the examination of all primary and/or permanent teeth, the knowledge accumulated over time indicates that this should be done.

The lack of consensus among researchers about which MIH assessment scoring system is the ideal type is an indication that more prognostic studies are still needed to determine which relevant MIH features should be maintained or added to the existent assessment scoring systems.

Statement of Ethics

Children's parents gave their consent for the publication of their children's teeth photographs for educational purposes.

Conflict of Interest Statement

Soraya C. Leal is one of the authors of the MIH-SSS assessment scoring system that have been discussed in the paper. The remaining authors have no conflict of interest to declare.

Author Contributions

All authors confirm contribution to the paper as follows: study design, conception, and manuscript preparation.

References

1 Weerheijm K, Jälevik B, Alaluusua S. Molar-incisor hypo-mineralisation (MIH). Caries Res. 2001;35(5):390–1.
2 Elfrink MEC, Ghanim A, Manton DJ, Weerheijm KL. Standardised studies on molar incisor hypomineralisation (MIH) and hypomineralised second primary molars (HSPM): a need. Eur Arch Paediatr Dent. 2015;16(3):247–55.
3 Ghanim A, Elfrink M, Weerheijm K, Mariño R, Manton D. A practical method for use in epidemiological studies on enamel hypomineralization. Eur Arch Paediatr Dent. 2015;16(3):235–46.
4 Commission on Oral Health, Research & Epidemiology. A review of the developmental defects of enamel index (DDE Index). Commission on Oral Health, Research & Epidemiology. Report of an FDI Working Group. Int Dent J. 1992;42(6):411–26.
5 Weerheijm KL, Duggal M, Mejare I, Papagiannoulis L, Koch G, Martens LC, et al. Judgment criteria for molar incisor hypomineralisation (MIH) in epidemiologic studies: a summary of the European meeting on MIH held in Athens. Eur J Paediatr Dent. 2003;4(3):110–3.
6 da Costa-Silva CM, Jeremias F, de Souza JF, Cordeiro RCL, Santos-Pinto L, Zuanon ACC. Molar incisor hypomineralization: prevalence, severity and clinical consequences in Brazilian children. Int J Paediatr Dent. 2010;20(6):426–34.
7 Leal SC, Oliveira TRM, Ribeiro APD. Do parents and children perceive mola-incisor hypomineralization as an oral health problem? Int J Paediatr Dent. 2017;27(5):372–9.
8 Neves AB, Americano GCA, Soares DV, Soviero VM. Breakdown of demarcated opacities related to molar-incisor hypomineralization: a longitudinal study. Clin Oral Investig. 2019;23(2):611–5.
9 Cabral RN, Nyvad B, Soviero VLVM, Freitas E, Leal SC. Reliability and validity of a new classification of MIH based on severity. Clin Oral Investig. 2020; 24(2):727–34.
10 Chawla N, Messer LB, Silva M. Clinical studies on molar-incisor-hypomineralization part 2:development of a severity index. Eur Arch Paediatr Dent. 2008; 9(4):191–9.
11 Oliver K, Messer LB, Manton DJ, Kan K, Ng F, Olsen C, et al. Distribution and severity of molar hypomineralisation: trial of a new severity index. Int J Paediatr Dent. 2014;24(2):131–51.
12 Steffen R, Krämer N, Bekes K. The Würzburg MIH concept: the MIH treatment need index (MIH TNI). Eur Arch Paediatr Dent. 2017;18(5):355–61.

13 Lygidakis NA, Wong F, Jälevik B, Vierrou AM, Alaluusua S, Espelid I. Best clinical practice guidance for clinicians dealing with children presenting with molar-incisor-hypomineralisation (MIH): an EAPD policy document. Eur Arch Paediatr Dent. 2010;11(2):75–81.
14 Jälevik B. Prevalence and diagnosis of molar incisor hypomineralisation (MIH): a systematic review. Eur Arch Paediatr Dent. 2010;11(2):59–64.
15 Dhareula A, Goyal A, Gauba K, Bhatia SK, Kapur A, Bhandari S. A clinical and radiographic investigation comparing the efficacy of cast metal and indirect resin onlays in rehabilitation of permanent first molars affected with severe molar incisor hypomineralisation (MIH): a 36-month randomised controlled clinical trial. Eur Arch Paediatr Dent. 2019;20(5):489–500.
16 Mittal N. Phenotypes of enamel hypomineralization and molar incisor hypomineralization in permanent dentition: identification, quantification and proposal for classification. J Clin Pediatr Dent. 2016;40(5):367–74.
17 Ghanim A, Silva MJ, Elfrink MEC, Lygidakis NA, Mariño RJ, Weerheijm KL, et al. Molar incisor hypomineralization (MIH) training manual for clinical field surveys and practice. Eur Arch Paediatr Dent. 2017;18(4):225–42.
18 Joshi T, Rahman A, Rienhoff S, Rienhoff J, Stamm T, Bekes K. Impact of molar incisor hypomineralization on oral health-related quality of life in 8–10-year-old children. Clin Oral Investig. 2022;26(2):1753–9.
19 Butera A, Pascadopoli M, Pellegrini M, Trapani B, Gallo S, Radu M, et al. Biomimetic hydroxyapatite paste for molar-incisor hypomineralization: a randomized clinical trial. Oral Dis. 2023;29(7): 2789–98.
20 Olczak-Kowalczyk D, Krämer N, Gozdowski D, Turska-Szybka A. Developmental enamel defects and their relationship with caries in adolescents aged 18 years. Sci Rep. 2023;13(1):4932.
21 Raposo F, Lia E, de Carvalho RAC, Lia EN, Leal SC. Prevalence of hypersensitivity in teeth affected by molar-incisor hypomineralization. Caries Res. 2019; 53(4):424–30.
22 Duarte MBS, Carvalho VR, Hilgert LA, Ribeiro AD, Leal SC, Takeshita EM. Is there an association between dental caries, fluorosis, and molar-incisor hypomineralization? J Appl Oral Sci. 2021; 29:e20200890.
23 Lygidakis NA, Garot E, Somani C, Taylor GD, Rouas P, Wong FSL. Best clinical practice guidance for clinicians dealing with children presenting with molar-incisor-hypomineralization (MIH): an update European Academy of Paediatric Dentistry policy document. Eur Arch Paediatr Dent. 2022;23(1):3–21.
24 Leppäniemi A, Lukinmaa PL, Alaluusua S. Nonfluoride hypomineralizations in the permanent first molars and their impact on the treatment need. Caries Res. 2001;35(1):36–40.
25 Mathu-Muju K, Wright T. Diagnosis and treatment of molar incisor hypomineralization. Compend Contin Edu Dent. 2006;27(11):604–10.
26 de Castro CRN, Lima CCB, Costa LC, Silva RNC, Pascotto RC, de Moura MS, et al. Hypomineralized teeth have a higher frequency of dental hypersensitivity. Pediatr Dent. 2021;43(3):218–22.
27 Linner T, Khazaei Y, Bücher K, Pfisterer J, Hickel R, Kühnisch J. Hypersensitivity in teeth affected by molar-incisor hypomineralization (MIH). Sci Rep. 2021; 11(1):17922.
28 Mendonça FL, Regnault FGC, Grizzo IC, Martins DS, Fragelli C, Leal SC, et al. Comparison of two molar incisor hypomineralization detection criteria in epidemiological surveys. Int J Paed Dent. 2023. doi: 10.1111/ipd.13127.

Soraya Coelho Leal
Department of Dentistry, Faculty of Health Science, University of Brasília
Campus Darcy Ribeiro, Asa Norte
Brasília, DF 70710.900 (Brazil)
sorayaodt@yahoo.com

Published online: July 1, 2024

Rios D, Santos-Pinto L (eds): Molar Incisor Hypomineralisation: New Perceptions. Monogr Oral Sci. Basel, Karger, 2024, vol 32, pp 68–78 (DOI: 10.1159/000538872)

Molar Incisor Hypomineralisation Patient Assessment: Comprehensive Oral, Clinical Records and Behavior Evaluation

Manuel Restrepo[a] Aline Leite de Farias[a] Juan Manuel Cárdenas[a] Diego G. Bussaneli[b] Kasandra Verónica Yupanqui[b] Lourdes Santos-Pinto[b]

[a]Department of Pediatric Dentistry, CES University, Medellin, Colombia; [b]Department of Morphology and Pediatric Dentistry, São Paulo State University (Unesp), Araraquara, Brazil

Abstract

Comprehensively evaluating molar incisor hypomineralisation (MIH) involves the integration of anamnesis and clinical data to diagnose, create a care plan, and predict prognoses. Anamnesis reveals relationships between defects and time, patient expectations, and impacts on the quality of life. Clinical studies emphasize posteruptive breakdown in yellow-brown opacities, highlighting the importance of identifying risk factors. The classification and recording of the clinical features associated with MIH are essential and allow for the longitudinal follow-up of the patient. Assessment of dental caries lesions, oral hygiene, and pain guides the care plan. Depending on the severity of MIH and associated symptoms, intraoral radiographs and cone beam computed tomography may be necessary. In cases of scheduled extractions, extraoral radiographs, photographs, and study models are indicated. Evaluations of the quality of life, aesthetic perception, and dental fear and anxiety provide valuable insights into the patient's emotional status and guide empathetic practice. A positive dental experience is based on communication with the patient, trust, and the proper use of behavior guidance techniques.

Introduction

Following the recommendations of Minimum Intervention Dentistry [1], the comprehensive evaluation of patients involves amalgamating data garnered from both anamnesis and clinical examinations alongside diagnostic aids. This chapter discusses the tools that clinicians may use to establish diagnoses, determine objectives, propose care plans, and predict the prognosis for patients with molar incisor hypomineralisation (MIH). The choice of tools will depend on the clinical setting (public, private, or mixed) as well as the individual characteristics and needs of the patient. Collecting information in a standardized manner can be beneficial for research, education, and evaluating service quality.

Anamnesis

There is currently no consensus in the scientific literature on the causes of MIH. However, data obtained from the anamnesis can indicate the relationship between the defect, time, and possible associated medical events (see Chapter 10). Additionally, it can unveil patient expectations, details regarding prior treatments, behavioral tendencies, impacts on quality of life, emotional well-being, and communication proficiency.

Clinical Examination

The clinical characteristics of a demarcated opacity may change over time and evolving to posteruptive breakdowns, worsening the severity of the defect. Clinical studies have shown that yellow-brown opacities tend to fracture more frequently than white opacities [2–5], and that these posteruptive breakdowns are more likely to occur shortly after tooth eruption, especially in molars [5].

Posteruptive fractures may contribute to the development of dental caries lesions; however, it is unknown whether, in cases of MIH, the presence of carious lesions could increase the likelihood of the tooth experiencing posteruptive breakdown. The risk of a patient with MIH presenting caries in the permanent dentition can be almost 5 times higher than a child without the defect [6] and, when classifying the caries lesion present in affected teeth, the scores increase in proportion to the severity of MIH [7–10].

For the diagnosis, treatment decision, and longitudinal monitoring of defects, it is necessary to classify the different forms of MIH according to their clinical characteristics, extent, the presence of hypersensitivity, and aesthetic alterations.

Despite the heterogeneity and methodological limitations of longitudinal studies in classifying defects or defining analysis units and evaluation periods, some risk factors related to the worsening severity of defects have been identified. However, no treatment strategy (i.e., fluorides, sealants, or resin infiltration) has proven truly effective in maintaining the structural integrity of the affected teeth (Table 1).

Clinically, it is a challenge to predict the risk of enamel opacity posteruptive breakdown in patients with MIH. Identifying risk factors helps the dentist to define early treatment and the interval for return visits, and it is of the utmost importance to detect any break in the surface of the affected tooth as early as possible to intervene and prevent the potential development and progression of caries lesions. Thus, monitoring of permanent first molars should be carried out during their eruption, at 5–6 years of age, since posteruptive breakdown can occur in the early periods of eruption [5]. The color of the opacity plays an important role in the occurrence of fracture and should be considered as a potential predictor, since there is a positive correlation between worsening MIH and the dark color of the defects [2–5, 11–13].

The intraoral clinical examination, the recording, and classification of MIH (see Chapter 5), is just one of several pieces of information needed to fully assess the patient. This examination can be complemented with an assessment of the depth of opacity (transillumination), caries risk assessment (CRA), classification of dental caries lesions, and pain assessment.

Transillumination

The detection of demarcated opacities associated with MIH is generally carried out by visual clinical examination under reflected light conditions [14]. However, this is a subjective method limited to assessing the color and extent of the defect and susceptible to variations due to lighting conditions, experience, age, and visual fatigue on the part of the examiner [14]. For this reason, very slight or mild defects in enamel translucency can go unnoticed by the naked eye. To overcome this limitation, visual clinical examination can be sup-

Table 1. Risk factors related to worsening defect severity and treatment strategies to maintain the structural integrity of the affected enamel

Author (year)	Follow-up, months	Patient characteristics					Defect						Treatment[a]
		age (years)	sex	oral hygiene	dental caries	housing, urban vs. rural	tooth				color, light vs. dark	extension	
							number of teeth affected	molar vs. incisor	molars (upper vs. lower)	surface exposed to masticatory forces			
Da Costa-Silva et al. (2011) [2]	18	(6–12) <10 ✕ >10 ✓	✕		✓	✕		Molars		✓	Dark		
Bullio Fragelli et al. (2015) [3]	6–12	(6–9)	✕		✓			Molars			Dark		Fluoride
Cabral et al. (2019) [5]	12, 18, 24–36	(7–12)						Molars			Dark		
Neves et al. (2019) [4]	12	(6–12) ✕	✕							✕	Dark		
Arslanagić et al. (2021) [11]	12	(6–9)					✕	Molars		✓	Dark	✕	
Schraverus et al. (2021) [12]	6–12	(5–9)		✕	✓				✕		Dark	✕	Glass ionomer sealant
Nogueira et al. (2021) [13]	18	(6–12) 6–8 ✓ 9–12 ✕	✕	✕	✓		✕	Molars		✓	Dark		Infiltrant (79.8% PEB) Fluoride (90.3% PEB)

PEB, posteruptive breakdown. ✓: Factor associated with the exacerbation of severity. ✕: Factor not related to the worsening of severity. [a]None of the treatments were effective in preventing PEB.

plemented with more sensitive methods for detecting small changes in enamel, such as transillumination. Transillumination is based on the principle of light scattering to increase the contrast between healthy and hypomineralised teeth. In anterior teeth, the light source is applied to the palatal/lingual surface and, as a result, the hypomineralisation appears dark due to light scattering, which is a product of increased demineralisation and porosity [14]. Although the scientific evidence for transillumination is limited, and its use is restricted to anterior teeth, it is a method with the potential to longitudinally monitor lesions associated with MIH, improve the detection of enamel development defects, provide quantitative information on lesions (extent and depth), and objectively assess the effectiveness of preventive and restorative treatments [14–16]. Until now, transillumination has been used in anterior teeth with MIH, and its application in affected molars could be limited due to the structural configuration of the enamel and the presence of demarcated opacities on various surfaces, which could affect the incidence and dispersion of the light source.

Caries Risk Assessment

Due to the association between dental caries and MIH [6], the CRA is recommended within a personalized and precision clinical practice. The aim of this step is to assess the likelihood that a patient will develop new dental caries lesions in the near future and the likelihood that these existing lesions will evolve. CRA also makes it possible to understand why the patient has disease activity and provides guidance on the strategies that should be taken to improve the risk state. From a behavioral point of view, understanding the level of risk of dental caries allows the patient to motivate, adhere to, and modify their behavior to improve their oral health. The patient's risk level is derived from social, medical, and behavioral history related to oral hygiene, diet (with emphasis on fermentable and cariogenic carbohydrates such as sucrose), and dental factors, together with a clinical oral examination. Currently, there are different tools and strategies for CRA with limited validation, but they can be used in clinical practice. These range from an informal subjective assessment to structured protocols/formats in paper or digital format. The most common tools are NUS-CRA, Cariogram, ADA, CAMBRA, and ICCMS™ [17]. Even though they use three or more risk categories to be more accurate (i.e., low, moderate, and high), this can generate variability and, eventually, lower accuracy. In clinical practice, it is quicker, easier, and more sufficient to focus on the extremes of the risk spectrum, i.e., those at "low risk" of dental caries and "high risk" of dental caries, once the treatment needs are clear [18]. From the point of view of prediction (future caries risk), scientific evidence suggests that the best individual indicators are dental caries experience and carious lesion activity [19].

Dental Caries Lesions and Oral Hygiene

Clinical diagnostic methods categorize dental caries lesions according to their stage of development and/or lesion activity. These include the Nyvad criteria, which assess the severity and activity of the lesion [20]; and the International Caries Detection and Assessment System (I–II) [21], which can be used in clinical practice, research, or public health services. The use of standardized criteria enables clinical monitoring and facilitates the determination of whether the caries lesion has progressed or not. Considering the changes in the structure and composition of teeth affected by MIH, the association with dental caries and biofilm accumulation, assessing oral hygiene is also important during the clinical examination. The Visible Occlusal Plaque Index is a validated method for predicting the activity of dental caries lesions at the level of molar pit and fissure systems using a scale: (0) no visible plaque identified when carefully running a dental probe on the groove-fossa system; (1) thin plaque: hardly detectable plaque, which is restricted to the groove-fossa

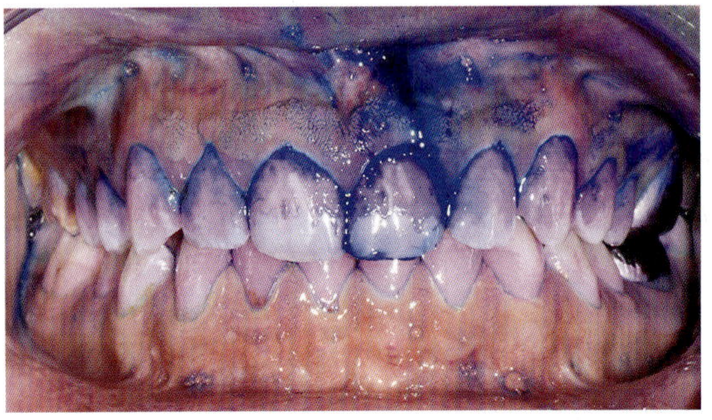

Fig. 1. Clinical evidence of significant accumulation of dental plaque in a patient affected by MIH, especially on the upper anterior teeth. Note the demarcated yellow opacity on the vestibular surface of the permanent upper right first molar. The pink color indicates young dental plaque; the purple/blue color indicates mature dental plaque (at least 48 h old); and light blue color indicates mature and acid-producing dental plaque. Courtesy of Dr. Restrepo M., CES University.

system and identified by carefully running a dental probe on the groove-fossa system; (2) thick plaque: easily detectable plaque on the groove-fossa system identifiable with the naked eye; and (3) heavy plaque: occlusal surfaces partially or totally covered with thick and heavy plaque accumulation identifiable with the naked eye [22, 23]. In addition, it is recommended to use a plaque revealer so that the patient and family can recognize the sites with poor oral hygiene (shown in Fig. 1).

Pain Assessment

Pain is a condition frequently associated with MIH [24]. However, it is important for the clinician to make the differential diagnosis of dental hypersensitivity with reversible or irreversible pulpitis, particularly in cases of demarcated opacities associated with atypical dental caries lesions and/or atypical restorations. Pain induced by thermal, physical, and mechanical stimuli can be assessed using the face scale, the Visual Analog Scale using numerical reference, and the Schiff Cold Air Sensitivity Scale (see Chapter 13).

Radiographic Examination and 3D Volumetric Tomography

Radiographic examination is important for diagnosis, treatment planning, reassessment, and patient follow-up [25]. Although the diagnosis and detection of MIH are not carried out radiographically, they do allow for the assessment and diagnosis of other associated conditions. Among intraoral radiographic techniques, periapical radiography is indicated when examining a tooth with necrosis or irreversible pulpitis associated with posteruptive breakdown, dental caries lesions, and/or restorations (shown in Fig. 2). Another intraoral technique is bitewing radiography, which is indicated to determine the presence and extent of dental caries lesions on the proximal and occlusal surfaces. It also provides information on the condition of restorations (overcontouring and distance from the dentin-pulp complex). In teeth with posteruptive breakdown, it also serves to determine the distance to the dental pulp, as well as the level of the alveolar bone.

In severe cases of MIH, as well as in cases in which scheduled tooth extraction is part of the treatment plan, panoramic and lateral cephalometric radiographs are essential. Panoramic radiography allows for the assessment of all bone and tooth structures in the maxilla and mandible. This image facilitates the determination of the developmental stages of all teeth (shown in Fig. 3) and the angulation of the second permanent molar. Lateral cephalometric radiography is primarily employed to evaluate the position, size, and rotation of the maxilla and mandible, intermaxillary relationships, as well as the sagittal and vertical inclination and position of the teeth (shown in Fig. 4) [26].

High-quality 3D images to assess structures in the axial, sagittal, and coronal planes are possible thanks to cone beam computed tomography (CBCT). The ability to examine different sections of the image from various angles is another positive feature of this type of diagnostic aid [27]. Ac-

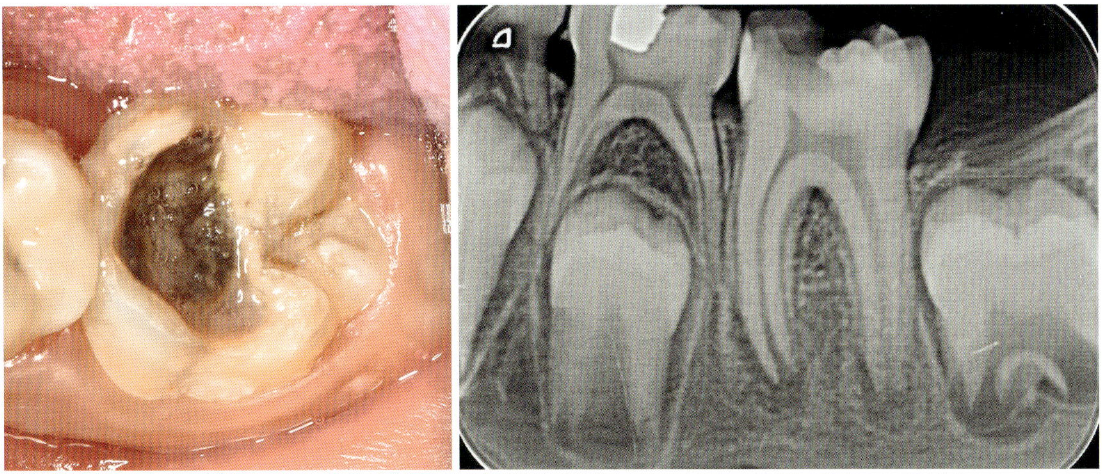

Fig. 2. Clinically, a posteruptive breakdown associated with active and cavitated caries lesion is observed. Based on the patient's pain characteristics, further examination was necessary to check for the presence of a periapical lesion (note the periapical region of the mesial and distal roots of the permanent first molar). Courtesy of Dr. Restrepo, CES University.

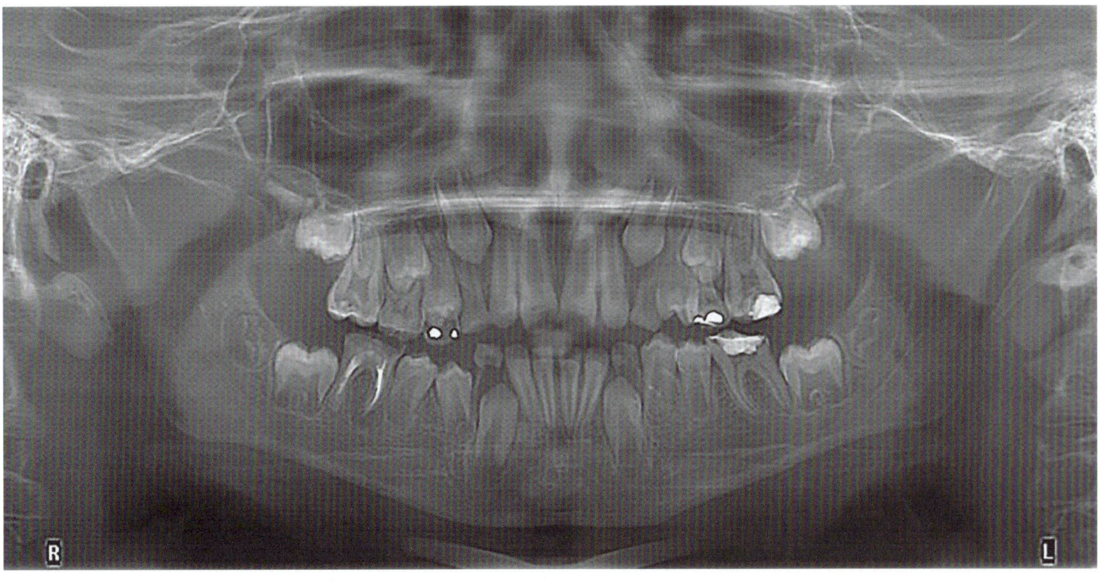

Fig. 3. Panoramic radiograph of a 9-year-old patient with severe MIH used for scheduled tooth extraction and orthodontic treatment planning. Note the stage of development and angulation of the permanent second molars and the presence of third molars. Courtesy of Dr. de Farias A. and Parajón K., CES University.

cording to Walshaw et al. [28], MIH can be associated with hypodontia, ectopic eruption of the first permanent molar, and morphological anomalies. Neboda et al. [29] reported that, in patients with MIH, maxillary molars can present anatomical variations in the mesiobuccal canal. Depending on the diagnostic conditions and care plane, the use of CBCT may be indicated in some patients with MIH. For example, when the patient presents contradictory or nonspecific clinical signs and symptoms, there is suspicion of unusual anatomy, or intraoral pain persists after endodontic treatment [30]. It is important for the clinician to consider the benefits and risks of CBCT especially regarding the cumulative effect of ionizing radiation and that children are more susceptible to radiation-induced carcinogenesis compared to adults. Therefore, the use of CBCT must be justified on the basis of the individual needs of the patient [25] affected by MIH.

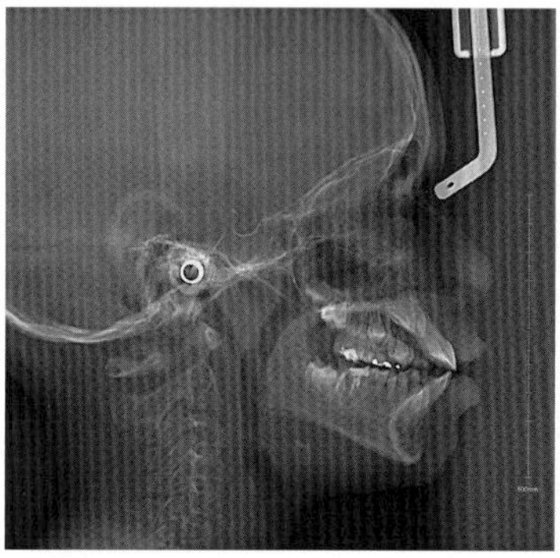

Fig. 4. Lateral cephalic radiograph of a 9-year-old patient with severe MIH used for scheduled tooth extraction and orthodontic treatment planning. Note that the patient presents skeletal class III relationship and buccally displaced and protruded incisors. Courtesy of Dr. de Farias A. and Parajón K., CES University.

Photographs and Study Models

Extraoral and intraoral photographs are useful tools in dentistry and are an essential part of contemporary clinical practice, helping with diagnosis, treatment planning, and patient communication. In addition, they can be used in training and calibration for MIH classification, serving as a source of secondary data for research [31, 32]. Similar to extraoral radiographs, photographs (shown in Fig. 5) and study models are necessary for orthodontic planning when scheduled extractions are considered within the care plan [26]. Intraoral photographs can be used to classify the shape of the arch, identify anomalies in the size, position, and number of teeth, the magnitude of crowding and record the clinical characteristics and extent of MIH [33, 34]. These photographs can be taken with professional photographic equipment, intraoral cameras, or smartphones. Study models are also an important diagnostic aid, especially those in digital format. 3D images obtained with an intraoral scanner are used for clinical monitoring of defects and digital planning of restorative and orthodontic treatments (shown in Fig. 6). In order to establish an appropriate diagnosis and treatment, it is essential to correlate the findings of the diagnostic aids with the clinical and radiographic examination.

Assessment of Quality of Life and Emotional State

Assessing quality of life, aesthetic perception, and emotional state in patients affected by MIH is important for structuring and reassessing the care plan, understanding the needs of the patient and family, prioritizing certain treatments, and making dental appointments effective and efficient. As described in Chapter 7, MIH has a negative impact on patients' quality of life because the associated pain can compromise oral hygiene, chewing, speech, and school performance [35]. Scientific evidence shows that both children and their parents perceive MIH as an oral health problem [35–37]; however, there is a difference in this

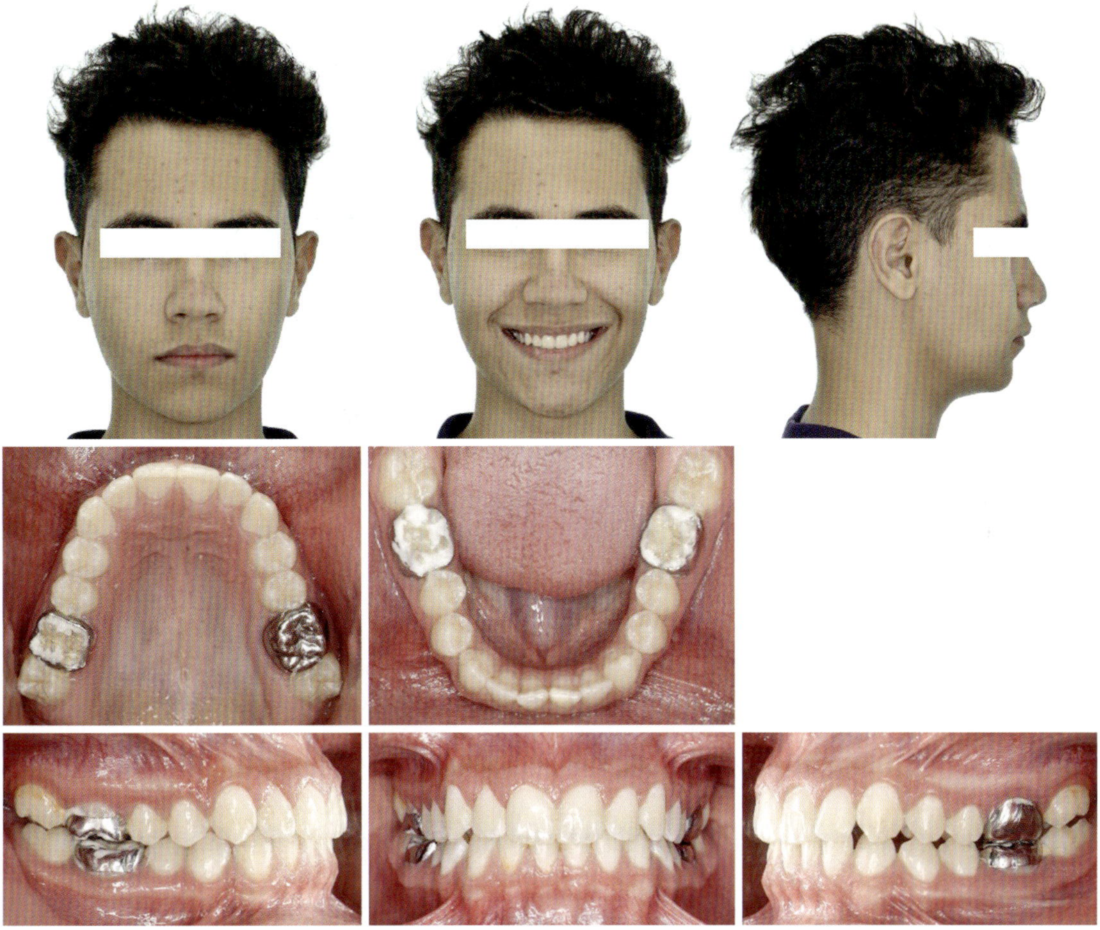

Fig. 5. Extraoral and intraoral photographs of a patient affected by MIH used for orthodontic planning. Extraoral photographs allow determining the profile, analyzing the smile, and evaluating the vertical and transversal proportions that establish the bilateral symmetry of the patient. Intraoral photographs serve to evaluate soft tissues, periodontal tissues, and dental structures (dental formula, type of dentition, shape and symmetry of the arches, and alterations in size, shape, and position). They are also useful for evaluating occlusion in the transversal plane (dental midline and transversal arch relationships), sagittal plane (molar and canine relationships), and vertical plane (overbite). Courtesy of Dr. Restrepo, CES University.

perception. While children report greater concern about the social domain, parents are more concerned about the physical domain [36]. Using questionnaires for children (CPQ 8–10 and CPQ 11–14) and for parents (P-CPQ), it is possible to measure and learn about the impact of MIH on the manifestation of oral symptoms, functional limitations, and emotional and social well-being [38]. The aesthetic impairment associated with MIH can interfere with socialization with other children, generate low self-esteem, and be a cause for bullying at school. Using the Child Perceptions Questionnaire About Tooth Appearance, it is possible to understand how patients perceive dental aesthetics (the appearance of the position, shape and color of their teeth) and how this can

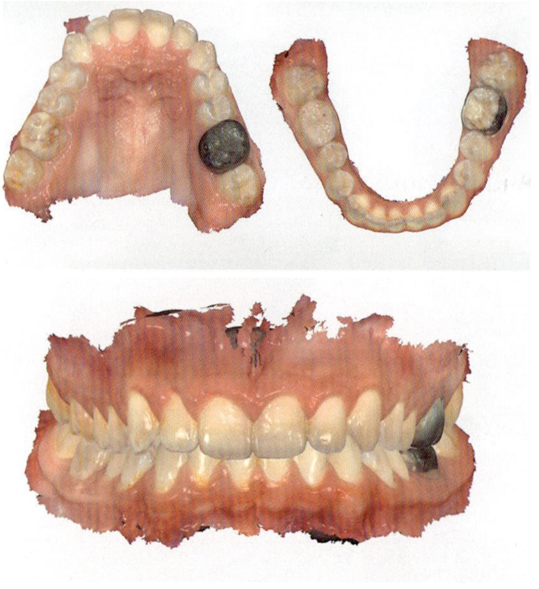

Fig. 6. Digital models of a patient affected by MIH. Note in the permanent upper right first molar the demarcated yellow opacity, loss of structure (posteruptive breakdown), and restoration on the occlusal surface. The permanent upper left first molar has a stainless-steel crown, and the permanent lower left first molar has an orthodontic band. Courtesy of Dr. Parra-Villegas M.A. and Restrepo M., CES University.

influence their psychosocial quality of life [39, 40]. Emotional assessment, specifically dental fear and anxiety, can be carried out using the Children's Fear Survey Schedule-Dental Subscale [41] or the modified Corah Dental Anxiety Scale [42]. Understanding and addressing dental fear and anxiety in patients with MIH is fundamental to offering a dental experience within an empathetic and patient-centered clinical practice.

Considering the biopsychosocial approach of MIH, the dental experience is a common factor between patient, parents, and clinician, and includes all moments of interaction between the patient and their family and the professional team [43]. Thus, during the dental experience offered, the clinician must have the sensitivity to identify the expectations of the patient and their family and be aware of the fact that these expectations are not always convergent. A new layer of complexity is added when we consider that the perception of aesthetic impairment is greater for the professional than for the patient themselves [44], which can result in more invasive procedures to solve problems not reported by the patient. The challenge for the clinician is to address the individual's needs, both functional and social, making sure that the treatment needs are not overestimated, considering both the child and their family [45].

Defining strategies to guide the behavior of patients with MIH is part of comprehensive management and is just as important as rehabilitative treatment, since there is often anxiety associated with pain, difficulty eating or drinking cold or hot food, and high expectations of dental treatment. Parents can also be anxious, especially when there is aesthetic impairment, which can be associated with self-esteem problems and feelings of guilt. In this context, it is essential for the clinician to communicate adequately with the family and the patient in order to jointly determine treatment strategies, as well as appropriate behavior guidance techniques.

Conclusion

A comprehensive approach to MIH patients involves a thorough clinical examination, integration of diagnostic aids, and consideration of emotional and psychosocial factors. The recording of clinical characteristics, affected surfaces, and associated pain related to MIH is crucial for documenting, making treatment decisions, and following up with patients over time. It is ideal for the care plan to be personalized based on the risk of dental caries. In managing severe cases, additional diagnostic aids such as X-rays, photographs, and study models may be necessary. Understanding the aesthetic perception and impact of MIH on the patient can be helpful when prioritizing aesthetic and restorative treatments.

Statement of Ethics

Written informed consent was obtained from patients/caregivers for publication of the details of their medical case and accompanying images. The patients and their caregivers signed the informed consent from the School of Dentistry/CES University for the acquisition of diagnostic aids.

Conflict of Interest Statement

The authors have no conflicts of interest to declare.

Author Contributions

All authors contributed equally to the conceptualization and writing of the review article.

References

1 Frencken JE, Peters MC, Manton DJ, Leal SC, Gordan VV, Eden E. Minimal intervention dentistry for managing dental caries – a review: report of a FDI task group. Int Dent J. 2012;62(5):223–43.

2 Da Costa-Silva CM, Ambrosano GM, Jeremias F, De Souza JF, Mialhe FL. Increase in severity of molar-incisor hypomineralization and its relationship with the colour of enamel opacity: a prospective cohort study. Int J Paediatr Dent. 2011;21(5):333–41.

3 Bullio Fragelli CM, Jeremias F, Feltrin de Souza J, Paschoal MA, de Cássia Loiola Cordeiro R, Santos-Pinto L. Longitudinal evaluation of the structural integrity of teeth affected by molar incisor hypomineralisation. Caries Res. 2015;49(4):378–83.

4 Neves AB, Americano GCA, Soares DV, Soviero VM. Breakdown of demarcated opacities related to molar-incisor hypomineralization: a longitudinal study. Clin Oral Investig. 2019;23(2):611–5.

5 Cabral RN, Nyvad B, Soviero VLVM, Freitas E, Leal SC. Reliability and validity of a new classification of MIH based on severity. Clin Oral Investig. 2020;24(2):727–34.

6 Americano GC, Jacobsen PE, Soviero VM, Haubek D. A systematic review on the association between molar incisor hypomineralization and dental caries. Int J Paediatr Dent. 2017;27(1):11–21.

7 Villani FA, Aiuto R, Dioguardi M, Paglia L, Caruso S, Gatto R, et al. Caries prevalence and molar incisor hypomineralisation (MIH) in children. Is there an association? A systematic review. Eur J Paediatr Dent. 2023;24(4):312–20.

8 Mazur M, Corridore D, Ndokaj A, Ardan R, Vozza I, Babajko S, et al. MIH and dental caries in children: a systematic review and meta-analysis. Healthcare (Basel). 2023;11(12):1795.

9 Ben Salem M, Chouchene F, Masmoudi F, Baaziz A, Maatouk F, Ghedira H. Are molar-incisor hypomineralization and hypomineralized second primary molars predictive of dental caries?: a systematic review. Eur J Dent. 2023;17(1):7–15.

10 Quintero Y, Restrepo M, Rojas-Gualdrón DF, Farias AL, Santos-Pinto L. Association between hypomineralization of deciduous and molar incisor hypomineralization and dental caries. Braz Dent J. 2022;33(4):113–9.

11 Arslanagić A, Marković N, Bajrić E, Burnazović Ristić L. Demarcated opacities as predictors of progression of the molar incisor hypomineralisation: a pilot study. Acta Stomatol Croat. 2020;54(4):420–30.

12 Schraverus MS, Olegário IC, Bonifácio CC, González APR, Pedroza M, Hesse D. Glass ionomer sealants can prevent dental caries but cannot prevent posteruptive breakdown on molars affected by molar incisor hypomineralization: one-year results of a randomized clinical trial. Caries Res. 2021;55(4):301–9.

13 Nogueira VKC, Mendes Soares IP, Fragelli CMB, Boldieri T, Manton DJ, Bussaneli DG, et al. Structural integrity of MIH-affected teeth after treatment with fluoride varnish or resin infiltration: an 18-month randomized clinical trial. J Dent. 2021;105:103570.

14 Marouane O, Douki N. The use of transillumination in detecting subclinical extensions of enamel opacities. J Esthet Restor Dent. 2019;31(6):595–600.

15 Marouane O, Manton DJ. The use of transillumination in mapping demarcated enamel opacities in anterior teeth: a cross-sectional study. Int J Paediatr Dent. 2022;32(1):49–55.

16 Marouane O, Manton DJ. The influence of lesion characteristics on application time of an infiltrate applied to MIH lesions on anterior teeth: an exploratory in vivo pilot study. J Dent. 2021;115:103814.

17 Cagetti MG, Bontà G, Cocco F, Lingstrom P, Strohmenger L, Campus G. Are standardized caries risk assessment models effective in assessing actual caries status and future caries increment? A systematic review. BMC Oral Health. 2018;18(1):123.

18 Martignon S, Pitts NB, Goffin G, Mazevet M, Douglas GVA, Newton JT, et al. CariesCare practice guide: consensus on evidence into practice. Br Dent J. 2019;227(5):353–62.

19 Campos MS, Fontana M. Risk assessment: considerations for coronal caries. Monogr Oral Sci. 2023;31:115–28.

20 Nyvad B, Machiulskiene V, Baelum V. Reliability of a new caries diagnostic system differentiating between active and inactive caries lesions. Caries Res. 1999;33(4):252–60.

21 Ismail AI, Sohn W, Tellez M, Amaya A, Sen A, Hasson H, et al. The International Caries Detection and Assessment System (ICDAS): an integrated system for measuring dental caries. Community Dent Oral Epidemiol. 2007;35(3):170–8.

22 Carvalho JC, Mestrinho HD, Oliveira LS, Varjão MM, Aimée N, Qvist V. Validation of the Visible Occlusal Plaque Index (VOPI) in estimating caries lesion activity. J Dent. 2017;64:37–44.

23 Carvalho JC, Mestrinho HD, Aimée NR, Bakhshandeh A, Qvist V. Visible occlusal plaque index predicting caries lesion activity. J Dent Res. 2022;101(8):905–11.
24 Raposo F, de Carvalho Rodrigues AC, Lia ÉN, Leal SC. Prevalence of hypersensitivity in teeth affected by molar-incisor hypomineralization (MIH). Caries Res. 2019;53(4):424–30.
25 American Academy of Pediatric Dentistry. Prescribing dental radiographs for infants, children, adolescents, and individuals with special health care needs. In: The Reference Manual of Pediatric Dentistry. Chicago, Ill: American Academy of Pediatric Dentistry; 2023. p. 308–11.
26 Laverde-Giraldo M, Mejía-Roldán J, Johnson-Giraldo N, Santos-Pinto L, Restrepo M. Diagnostic considerations for extraction of first permanent molars severely affected by molar-incisor hypomineralization. Rev CES Odont. 2021; 34(2):22.
27 Yiğit T, Yüksel HT, Evirgen Ş, Kaçmaz I, Türkmenoğlu A. Evaluation of use of cone beam computed tomography in paediatric patients: a cross-sectional study. Int J Paediatr Dent. 2023;33(5): 468–76.
28 Walshaw EG, Noble F, Conville R, Anne Lawson J, Hasmun N, Rodd H. Molar incisor hypomineralisation and dental anomalies: a random or real association? Int J Paediatr Dent. 2020;30(3): 342–8.
29 Neboda C, Anthonappa RP, Engineer D, King NM, Abbott PV. Root canal morphology of hypomineralised first permanent molars using micro-CT. Eur Arch Paediatr Dent. 2020;21(2):229–40.
30 Ríos-Osorio N, Quijano-Guauque S, Briñez-Rodríguez S, Velasco-Flechas G, Muñoz-Solís A, Chávez C, et al. Cone-beam computed tomography in endodontics: from the specific technical considerations of acquisition parameters and interpretation to advanced clinical applications. Restor Dent Endod. 2023;49:e1.
31 Restrepo M, Rojas-Gualdrón DF, de Farias AL, Escobar A, Vélez LF, Bussaneli DG, Santos-Pinto L. Development of undergraduate students' diagnostic accuracy for the classification of molar incisor hypomineralization. Eur J Dent Educ. 2024;28(1):154–160.
32 Hanan SA, de Farias AL, Santos-Pinto L. Molar incisor hypomineralization in adolescents and adults and its association with facial profile and occlusion. Clin Oral Investig. 2023;27(3):1243–53.
33 de Farias AL, Rojas-Gualdrón DF, Girotto Bussaneli D, Santos-Pinto L, Mejía JD, Restrepo M. Does molar-incisor hypomineralization (MIH) affect only permanent first molars and incisors? New observations on permanent second molars. Int J Paediatr Dent. 2022;32(1):1–10.
34 Restrepo M, Rojas-Gualdrón DF, de Farias AL, Girotto-Bussaneli D, Santos-Pinto L. Association between frequency and severity of dental fluorosis and molar incisor hypomineralization. J Clin Pediatr Dent. 2022;46(1):30–4.
35 Dantas-Neta NB, Moura LF, Cruz PF, Moura MS, Paiva SM, Martins CC, et al. Impact of molar-incisor hypomineralization on oral health-related quality of life in schoolchildren. Braz Oral Res. 2016;30(1):e117.
36 Leal SC, Oliveira TRM, Ribeiro APD. Do parents and children perceive molar-incisor hypomineralization as an oral health problem? Int J Paediatr Dent. 2017;27(5):372–9.
37 Portella PD, Menoncin BLV, de Souza JF, de Menezes J, Fraiz FC, Assuncao L. Impact of molar incisor hypomineralization on quality of life in children with early mixed dentition: a hierarchical approach. Int J Paediatr Dent. 2019; 29(4):496–506.
38 Jokovic A, Locker D, Tompson B, Guyatt G. Questionnaire for measuring oral health-related quality of life in eight- to ten-year-old children. Pediatr Dent. 2004;26(6):512–8.
39 Martínez-Mier EA, Maupomé G, Soto-Rojas AE, Ureña-Cirett JL, Katz BP, Stookey GK. Development of a questionnaire to measure perceptions of, and concerns derived from, dental fluorosis. Community Dent Health. 2004;21(4): 299–305.
40 Fragelli C, Barbosa TS, Bussaneli DG, Restrepo M, Cordeiro RCL, Santos-Pinto L. Aesthetic perception in children with molar incisor hypomineralization. Eur Arch Paediatr Dent. 2021;22(2):227–34.
41 Cuthbert MI, Melamed BG. A screening device: children at risk for dental fears and management problems. ASDC J Dent Child. 1982;49(6):432–6.
42 Humphris GM, Morrison T, Lindsay SJ. The Modified Dental Anxiety Scale: validation and United Kingdom norms. Community Dent Health. 1995;12(3):143–50.
43 Bussaneli DG, Vieira AR, Santos-Pinto L, Restrepo M. Molar-incisor hypomineralisation: an updated view for aetiology 20 years later. Eur Arch Paediatr Dent. 2022;23(1):193–8.
44 Mehl CJ, Harder S, Kern M, Wolfart S. Patients' and dentists' perception of dental appearance. Clin Oral Investig. 2011;15(2):193–9.
45 Large JF, Hasmun N, Lawson JA, Elcock C, Vettore MV, Rodd HD. What children say and clinicians hear: accounts relating to incisor hypomineralisation of cosmetic concern. Eur Arch Paediatr Dent. 2020;21(2):185–91.

Manuel Restrepo
Department of Pediatric Dentistry, CES University
Calle 10A # 22-04
Medellin, Antioquia 050021 (Colombia)
mrrestrepo@ces.edu.co

Published online: July 1, 2024
Rios D, Santos-Pinto L (eds): Molar Incisor Hypomineralisation: New Perceptions. Monogr Oral Sci. Basel, Karger, 2024, vol 32, pp 79–87 (DOI: 10.1159/000538873)

Impact of Molar Incisor Hypomineralisation on Quality of Life

Marina Deus Moura Lima[a] Lúcia Fátima Almeida Deus Moura[a]
Saul Martins Paiva[b] Cacilda Castelo Branco Lima[a] Marcoeli Silva Moura[a]
Marco Aurélio Benini Paschoal[b]

[a]Department of Pathology and Dentistry Clinic, Federal University of Piauí, Teresina, Brazil; [b]Department of Pediatric Dentistry, Federal University of Minas Gerais, Belo Horizonte, Brazil

Abstract

Oral health-related quality of life (OHRQoL) is a multifaceted concept that surpasses an exclusively clinical perception and includes functional, social, emotional, and environmental issues. The measure of OHRQoL represents a holistic approach for research and clinical practice. Negative impacts of oral conditions on OHRQoL in childhood can reflect on health development, especially in a life stage marked by social and cognitive maturation. Therefore, such problems can impact negatively on the daily lives of the individuals and their families. Individuals with molar incisor hypomineralisation (MIH) experience more frequent posteruptive breakdown, an elevated risk of tooth decay, filling failures, the need for recurrent dental treatment, and a higher prevalence of dental hypersensitivity. Children with severe MIH may struggle with everyday activities, such as brushing their teeth, speaking, smiling, chewing, and consuming hot or cold foods. MIH-affected incisors may exhibit opacities that can impact the aesthetics of their smiles. This condition may discourage children from smiling and can indirectly affect their parents as well. The management modalities are focused on solving functional, aesthetic, and hypersensitivity problems and to evaluate OHRQoL values before and after therapies. Therefore, this chapter aims to discuss how MIH affects the OHRQoL of children and the questionnaires that can be used to evaluate that impact.

Introduction

Oral health-related quality of life (OHRQoL) is a multifaceted and intricate concept that encompasses an individual's assessment of their oral health, functional, emotional, and social well-being [1]. In recent times, the significance of evaluating OHRQoL has grown, becoming essential for assessing oral health status in children, adolescents, and adults. The definition of quality of life was initially based on traditional definitions of health based on the physical state of health, restricted only to a biological model. However, just as there was an update in the definition of health, the definition of quality of life also expanded and began to include functional, social, and psychological aspects, as well as emotional domains of people's lives [1–3]. It is important to note that clinical indicators alone do not provide a complete picture of the psychosocial impact of oral conditions on a patient's well-being. The subjective assessment of OHRQoL encompasses factors such as "people's comfort while eating, sleeping, and participating in social interactions; their self-esteem; and their contentment regarding their oral health" [2, 3].

Patient-centered outcomes related to OHRQoL are important in decision-making processes, resource allocation, and the development/evaluation of public health policies. They can be used as a significant measure of patient-centered outcomes in clinical trials, cost-effectiveness analysis of treatments, monitoring treatment protocols, and facilitating decision-making in the face of different treatment options [4].

Instruments for Evaluating Oral Health-Related Quality of Life in Children and Adolescents

Instruments have been developed and cross-culturally adapted to evaluate the impact of oral conditions on the OHRQoL of children, adolescents, and their families. Some features distinguish these instruments and influence their selection, such as self or proxy-report, generic or specific condition, long or short-form, and less or more established used in the literature.

The diversity of measures indicates the evolution of OHRQoL studies, but there are methodological issues still in need to be improved in future developments or cross-cultural adaptations, according to current psychometric evidence. Especially when applied in children, some challenges may be faced such as age (especially in very young children) that tend to be unreliable informants, while their ongoing social and cognitive development meant that it was likely that different measures would be needed for different ages. Moreover, consideration also had to be given to the readability and formatting of the child questionnaires to ensure that the language was age-appropriate and they were designed and constructed to be easily and reliably completed (such as through using appropriate font sizes and alternate line colors) [5].

To date, there is no valid instrument specifically aimed at measuring the impact of molar incisor hypomineralisation (MIH) on OHRQoL. Previous studies using validated instruments to measure the impact of MIH on OHRQoL in different populations found no impact [6, 7], whereas other studies found a negative impact mainly related to oral symptoms, dental appearance, and functional limitations [8, 9]. The instrument most used in these studies was the Child Perceptions Questionnaire (CPQ).

Table 1 summarizes some of the most usual instruments to measure the OHRQoL of child, adolescent, and families supported by its different approaches, theoretical frameworks, and applications as follows.

Early Childhood Oral Health Impact Scale

The Early Childhood Oral Health Impact Scale (ECOHIS) was the first questionnaire developed to assess the negative impact of oral conditions on the OHRQoL of young children and their families [10]. Although it had been originally validated for 3- to 5-year-old children, some cross-cultural adaptations have extended this age range, and versions for children between 0 and 6 years of age have been developed. Both sections are answered by parents/caregivers (proxy-report). The ECOHIS contains 13 items corresponding to four domains for items included in the child impact section: symptoms – 01 item; function – 04 items; psychological – 02 items; self-image/social interaction – 02 items; and

Table 1. OHRQoL instruments for use with children, adolescents, and families

Instrument	Reference	Age group, years	Respondent	Number of items	Dimensions
Early Childhood Oral Health Impact Scale (ECOHIS)	Pahel et al., 2006 [10]	2–5	Parent/caregiver	13	Child impact section: -Symptoms -Functional -Psychological -Self-image/social interaction Family impact section: -Parental distress -Family functioning
Family Impact Scale (FIS)	Jokovic et al., 2003 [11]	2–14	Parent/caregiver	14	-Family functioning -Emotion of the parents -Family conflict
Parental-Caregiver Perceptions Questionnaire (P-CPQ)	Jokovic et al., 2003 [11]	2–14	Parent/caregiver	31	-Oral symptoms -Functional limitation -Emotional well-being -Social well-being
Parental-Caregiver Perceptions Questionnaire – Short version (SF:13 – B-P-CPQ)	Goursand et al., 2013 [12]	2–14	Parent/caregiver	13	-Oral symptoms -Functional limitation -Social well-being
Pediatric Quality of Life Inventory™ Oral Health Scale™ (PedsQL™ Oral Health Scale™)	Steele et al., 2009 [13]	2–18	Parent/caregiver, child or adolescent	5	Unidimensional: -Child/adolescent versions -Parent/caregiver version
Scale of Oral Health Outcomes for 5-year-old Children (SOHO-5)	Tsakos et al., 2012 [14]	5	Parent/caregiver and/or child	7	Unidimensional: -Child version -Parent/caregiver version
Child Perceptions Questionnaire 11–14 – Short version (CPQ_{11-14} SF:16–SF:8)	Jokovic et al., 2006 [15]	11–14	Adolescent	16	-Oral symptoms -Functional limitation -Emotional well-being -Social well-being
Child Perceptions Questionnaire 8–10 (CPQ_{8-10})	Jokovic et al., 2003 [11]	8–10	Child	29	-Oral symptoms -Functional limitation -Emotional well-being -Social well-being

two domains for the family impact section: parent distress – 02 items and family function – 02 items. The responses of each item of the S-ECOHIS are coded as follows: 0 = never; 1 = almost never; 2 = sometimes; 3 = often; 4 = very often; 5 = don't know. The total S-ECOHIS scores are calculated as the sum of the response's codes. The answers "do not know" were counted but excluded from the total ECOHIS score for each patient. Both sections are answered by parents/caregivers (proxy-report).

The ECOHIS can be self-administered or administered as face-to-face interviews or telephone interviews. For purposes of reliability, the same method should be used from the beginning to the end of the study.

A self-report questionnaire is the primary method for assessing health-related quality of life [16]. However, self-report instruments can be limited when investigating OHRQoL of preschoolers. There is reasoning for the adoption of the proxy-report approach in ECOHIS: individual's abstract thinking ability is developed at about 6 years of age; preschool children would be unable to understand the items; children younger than 6 years of age would be unable to accurately recall both every day and unique events beyond 24 h.

Family Impact Scale

The questionnaires that make up the Child Oral Health Quality of Life (COHQoL) Questionnaire are the CPQ, Parental-Caregivers Perceptions Questionnaire (P-CPQ), and the Family Impact Scale. The Family Impact Scale was developed as one component of the COHQoL instrument. This instrument was designed to assess the OHRQoL of children aged 6–14 years with oral and orofacial conditions and their families [17]. It consists of 14 items divided into four subscales: parental/family activity, parental emotions, family conflict, and financial burden. The global rating has a five-point response format ranging from "never = 0" to "every day or almost every day = 4." Higher scores indicate worse OHRQoL.

Parental-Caregiver Perceptions Questionnaire

P-CPQ is one of the instruments included in the COHQoL Questionnaire, developed to measure parents'/caregivers' perceptions of the impact of children's oral conditions on their OHRQoL in the previous three months. The questionnaire contains 31 items distributed across four domains: oral symptoms, functional limitations, emotional well-being, and social well-being. The P-CPQ also has two global questions; one rating children's oral health (How would you rate the health of your child's teeth, lips, jaws, and mouth?) and the other assesses the relationship between children's oral health and their overall well-being (How much is your child's overall well-being affected by the condition of his/her teeth, lips, jaws, or mouth?) [11]. The P-CPQ was designed to be analogous to the CPQ, enabling the practitioner or the researcher to obtain supplemental information about children's OHRQoL. Alongside CPQ, it allows to investigate agreement between child and parent/caregiver.

Short forms of the P-CPQ, such as the 8-, 13-, and 16-item scales have been developed [18]. They simplify the evaluation of the condition/problem due to the reduced number of items or domains, minimize the burden on the respondent, and mitigate the chance of missing data. Versions with 16- and 8-item scales have been the most used tools among all the P-CPQ short-form versions. The 13-item scale developed in Brazil has three domains (oral symptoms, functional limitations, and well-being) [12].

Pediatric Quality of Life Inventory™ Oral Health Scale

The Pediatric Quality of Life Inventory™ Oral Health Scale (PedsQL-OH) was developed in view of the criticisms of scholars for whom the assessment of oral health should be included in pediatric generic health-related quality of life (HRQoL) measurements [13]. Therefore, the PedsQL-OH is used along with a generic HRQoL instrument (PedsQL™ 4.0 Generic Core Scales – 23 items; PedsQL™ 4.0 Generic Core Scales Short Form – 15 items). The PedsQL-OH contains five items in two parallel forms for child self-report and parent proxy-report. Child and adolescent self-reports include ages 5–7, 8–12, and 13–18 years. Parent proxy-report includes ages 2–4 (toddler), 5–7 (young child), 8–12 (older child), and 13–18 (adolescent), assessing parental perceptions of their children's oral health. The forms are quite similar, differing in the use of age-specific language and the use of first or third person. A 5-point response scale is used in the child-, adolescent-, and parent proxy-reports. For the young child self-report (ages 5–7), response scale is simplified to a 3-point scale, using three pictures (ranging from a happy face to a sad face) portraying response to the impacts.

Scale of Oral Health Outcomes for 5-Year-Old Children

The Scale of Oral Health Outcomes for 5-year-old children (SOHO-5) was developed to assess the OHRQoL of young children through both self- and parental/caregiver reports [14]. SOHO-5 comprises two versions (child version and parental/caregiver version). Each version has seven items. The meaning of most items is similar in both versions, but there are differences in language and response scale: a 5-point Likert response scale was used in the parental/caregiver version and a 3-point Likert response scale was used in the child version.

Although there are limitations for preschool children to self-report issues related to abstract domains, evidence shows that 4- to 6-year-old children can reliably report on more concrete domains of their general health and quality of life, such as pain and dysfunction. Moreover, parents/caregivers may have an incomplete knowledge about their children's health due to their work routine, social life, or the amount of time children stay at day care facilities. However, the proxy measure by parents/guardians must be considered together with the self-report of children, since children may not be aware of issues concerning some psychosocial domains or may have difficulty in understanding emotions that require greater cognitive development. Given that parental and child reports measure different realities, SOHO-5 can evaluate both perspectives of the OHRQoL of preschool children [14].

Child Perceptions Questionnaire

The CPQ is one of the instruments included in the COHQoL, developed to measure child' perceptions of the impact of their oral conditions on their OHRQoL in the previous three months. The CPQ_{11-14} is a COHQoL questionnaire and is composed of 37 items that assess the repercussions of oral health problems on the quality of life of children between 11 and 14 years of age. The questionnaire contains four domains: oral symptoms, functional limitations, emotional well-being, and social well-being.

Short-form versions of the CPQ_{11-14}, such as the 8- and 16-item scales, have been developed [18]. They simplify the evaluation of the condition/problem due to the reduced number of items or domains, minimize the burden on the respondent, and mitigate the chance of missing data. However, the questionnaire may have lower internal consistency when compared to the full version. The scale version with 16 items has been the most used tool among the two CPQ short-form versions. The 16-item scale developed in Brazil has four domains (oral symptoms, functional limitations, emotional well-being, and social well-being).

How Can MIH Affect the Child/Adolescent and Their Family?

One of the big challenges in Pediatric Dentistry is treating children with MIH because the affected patients present frequently clinical problems such as posteruptive breakdown, increased susceptibility to caries, failure of fillings, recurrent dental treatment, and higher prevalence of hypersensitivity (e.g., severe MIH) [19, 20]. So, frequently children with severe MIH find it challenging to perform everyday tasks like brushing their teeth, speaking, smiling, and consuming hot or cold foods [21]. According to a systematic review with meta-analysis, children with MIH are about 17–25 times more likely to have negative impacts on the OHRQoL [22]. Furthermore, hypomineralised teeth are recognized for their tendency to pose challenges in responding effectively to local anesthesia, with a gradual need of approaches in both behavioral and technical aspects of their management [23].

In this context, MIH presents a significant negative impact on children's OHRQoL [24–26]. The results including physical/emotional function and the overall scale score were the most affected. Children with MIH and hypersensitivity who exhibited responsiveness to stimuli demonstrated poor OHRQoL, both from their own perspective and as reported by their parents. In addition, less mature teeth and younger children were more prone to have hypersensitivity [26].

Severe MIH is frequently associated with a greater negative impact on OHRQoL than mild phenotype (e.g., only opacities) [27]. The position of an MIH-affected tooth has a strong impact on perceived OHRQoL. Hypomineralised molars caused the most severe oral symptoms and functional limitations. These teeth are used during mastication, therefore leading to hypersensitivity and limitations in function as well. Hypomineralised incisors had the prominent negative effect on OHRQoL in the emotional well-being and social well-being subscales. As anterior MIH teeth are visible during human interaction, children tend to experience more socioemotional problems [24].

Considering "functional limitations" (difficulties in chewing, eating, speech, sleep, oral hygiene activities, pain, discomfort, and functional limitations in daily life), children with severely affected MIH teeth tend to exhibit a lower OHRQoL compared to children with carious lesions, which is attributed to the process of chronicity. In cases of dental caries, tertiary dentin formation acts as a protective barrier, delaying pulp irritation and potentially allowing for asymptomatic periods, even in teeth with advanced carious lesions and large cavities. Consequently, untreated MIH teeth result in significant impairments in the masticatory process, and treatment tends to alleviate these issues to a greater extent than in cases of severe caries [21]. In addition, MIH with its severe phenotype frequently presents hypersensitivity contributing to decrease the scores of OHRQoL.

Patients with MIH also exhibit a poorer OHRQoL in the "emotional well-being" domain (psychological and emotional impact of oral health conditions on an individual's mental state), indicating that they experience higher levels of emotional distress. MIH teeth present asymmetrical demarcated opacity with clear and defined limits, which affects the aesthetics. This can discourage children from smiling and impact their parents/family as well. In addition to resulting in have a ripple effect on the child's well-being, which can be improved through the restoration of satisfactory aesthetics [21] (shown in Fig. 1).

How to Improve the OHRQoL in Children and Adolescents with MIH?

Since the main issues with MIH teeth are functional, aesthetics, and hypersensitivity, the management modalities are focused on solving these problems and comparing the OHRQoL values before and after the employed therapies. Indirectly, the treatments improve oral hygiene (i.e., the ability to keep teeth clean) and minimize problems with food intake (e.g., hot, cold drinks, and solid food) [28].

In mild cases of MIH teeth generating improvement of OHRQoL, the treatments vary in fluoride varnish application and resin-based fluoride releasing [28, 29]. Related to severe MIH-affected molars, the use of direct filling (e.g., glass

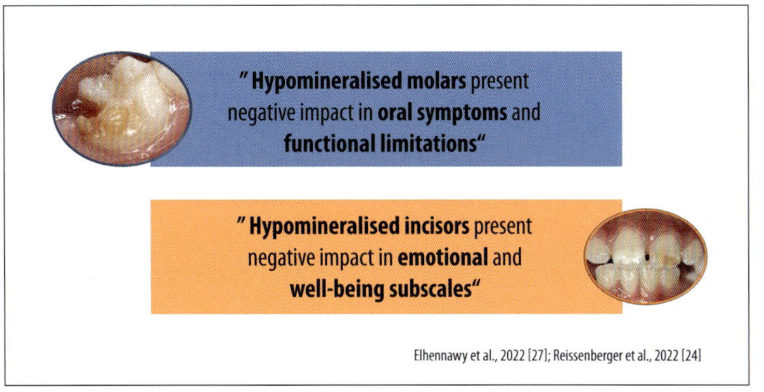

Fig. 1. Impacts of MIH on OHRQoL.

hybrid restorations, composite restorations) and metal crowns are the most investigated [7, 28, 30], whereas in MIH-affected incisors, the use of microabrasion, teeth whitening, resin infiltration, and direct restorations known as "camouflage technique" [31]. For the treatment of hypersensitivity, promising tools such as specific toothpaste, fluoride varnishes, and lasers can be used [32, 33].

MIH-affected molars restored with glass hybrid materials after selective caries removal improved these children's OHRQoL [30]. Sealing of hypersensitive MIH-affected molars with either a composite resin or a glass ionomer cement has shown a significant improvement in OHRQoL [29]. Some children present negative psychosocial impacts because of their visible enamel opacities that may have lifetime consequences. Children who express concern should be treated with minimally invasive and timely interventions (please see Chapters 18 and 19), with the expectation that these may measurably improve their well-being. Psychosocial factors and dental clinical characteristics were associated with changes in children's OHRQoL following minimal interventions for incisor opacities [31].

Therapy for MIH-damaged teeth can reduce hypersensitivity and improve the ability to ensure oral hygiene. Additionally, the number of dietary restrictions decreased after therapy. More severely damaged teeth are in greater need of invasive therapy than mildly damaged ones [28].

Conclusion

MIH can have a significant impact on various aspects of an individual's life, both functionally and aesthetically. Therefore, it is essential for dentists to undergo training in the early diagnosis and management of MIH, because detecting this enamel defect at an early stage can help mitigate the severity of the condition and reduce its impact on an individual's OHRQoL.

Statement of Ethics

Children's parents gave their consent for the publication of their children's teeth photographs for educational purposes.

Conflict of Interest Statement

The authors have no conflicts of interest to declare.

Author Contributions

All authors contributed to the conception and writing of this chapter.

References

1 Perazzo MF, Martins-Júnior PA, Abreu LG, Mattos FF, Pordeus IA, Paiva SM. Oral health-related quality of life of preschool children: review and perspectives for new instruments. Braz Dent J. 2020; 31(6):568–81.

2 McGrath C, Broder H, Wilson-Genderson M. Assessing the impact of oral health on the life quality of children: implications for research and practice. Community Dent Oral Epidemiol. 2004; 32:81–5.

3 Omara M, Stamm T, Bekes K. Four-dimensional oral health related quality of life impact in children: a systematic review. J Oral Rehabil. 2020;48:293–304.

4 Clementino LC, de Souza KSC, Castelo-Branco M, Perazzo MF, Ramos-Jorge ML, Mattos FF, et al. Top 100 most-cited oral health-related quality of life papers: bibliometric analysis. Community Dent Oral Epidemiol. 2022;50(3):199–205.

5 Thomson WM, Broder HL. Oral-health-related quality of life in children and adolescents. Pediatr Clin North Am. 2018;65(5):1073–84.

6 Arrow P. Dental enamel defects, caries experience and oral health-related quality of life: a cohort study. Aust Dent J. 2017;62(2):165–72.

7 Portella PD, Fraiz FC, Soares RC, Nagata AG, Tomaz COT, Assunção LRS. Molar-incisor hypomineralization and associated factors: a case-control study. Pesq Bras Odontoped Clin Integr. 2018; 18(1):e4320.

8 Dantas-Neta NB, Moura LF, Cruz PF, Moura MS, Paiva SM, Martins CC, et al. Impact of molar-incisor hypomineralization on oral health-related quality of life in schoolchildren. Braz Oral Res. 2016;30(1):e117.

9 Velandia LM, Álvarez LV, Mejía LP, Rodríguez MJ. Oral health-related quality of life in Colombian children with molar–incisor hypomineralization. Acta Odontol Latinoam. 2018;31(1):38–44.

10 Pahel B, Rozier RG, Slade G. Parental perceptions of children's oral health: The Early Childhood Oral Health Impact Scale (ECOHIS). Health Qual Life Outcomes. 2007;5(1):6.

11 Jokovic A, Locker D, Stephens M, Kenny D, Tompson B, Guyatt G. Measuring parental perceptions of child oral health-related quality of life. J Public Health Dent. 2003;63:67–72.

12 Goursand D, Ferreira MC, Pordeus IA, Mingoti SA, Veiga RT, Paiva SM. Development of a short form of the Brazilian Parental-Caregiver Perceptions Questionnaire using exploratory and confirmatory factor analysis. Qual Life Res. 2013;22(2):393–402.

13 Steele MM, Steele RG, Varni JW. Reliability and validity of the PedsQLTM Oral Health Scale: measuring the relationship between child oral health and health-related quality of life. Child Health Care. 2009;38:228–44.

14 Tsakos G, Blair YI, Yusuf H, Wright W, Watt RG, Macpherson LMD. Developing a new self-reported scale of oral health outcomes for 5-year-old children (SOHO-5). Health Qual Life Outcomes. 2012;10(1):62.

15 Jokovic A, Locker D, Guyatt G. Short forms of the Child Perceptions Questionnaire for 11–14-year-old children (CPQ11–14): development and initial evaluation. Health Qual Life Outcomes. 2006;4:4.

16 Ellert U, Ravens-Sieberer U, Erhart M, Kurth B-M. Determinants of agreement between self-reported and parent-assessed quality of life for children in Germany-results of the German Health Interview and Examination Survey for Children and Adolescents (KiGGS). Health Qual Life Outcomes. 2011;9:102.

17 Locker D, Jokovic A, Stephens M, Kenny D, Tompson B, Guyatt G. Family impact of child oral and oro-facial conditions. Community Dent Oral Epidemiol 2002; 30:438–48.

18 Thomson WM, Foster Page LA, Gaynor WN, Malden PE. Short-form versions of the parental-caregivers perceptions questionnaire and the family impact scale. Community Dent Oral Epidemiol. 2013;41(5):441–50.

19 Raposo F, de Carvalho Rodrigues AC, Lia ÉN, Leal SC. Prevalence of hypersensitivity in teeth affected by molar-incisor hypomineralization (MIH). Caries Res. 2019;53(4):424–30.

20 Castro CRN, Lima CCB, Costa LC, Silva RNC, Pascotto RC, Moura MS, et al. Hypomineralized teeth have a higher frequency of dental hypersensitivity. Pediatr Dent. 2021;43(3):218–22.

21 Altner S, Ebel M, Ritschl V, Stamm T, Hirsch C, Bekes K. Treatment of severe caries and molar incisor hypomineralization and its influence on oral health-related quality of life in children: a comparative study. Int J Environ Res Public Health. 2022;19(5):2983.

22 Jawdekar AM, Kamath S, Kale S, Mistry L. Assessment of oral health-related quality of life (OHRQoL) in children with molar incisor hypomineralization (MIH): a systematic review and meta-analysis of observational studies. J Indian Soc Pedod Prev Dent. 2022;40(4): 368–76.

23 Lygidakis NA, Garot E, Somani C, Taylor GD, Rouas P, Wong FSL. Best clinical practice guidance for clinicians dealing with children presenting with molar-incisor-hypomineralisation (MIH): an updated European Academy of Paediatric Dentistry policy document. Eur Arch Paediatr Dent. 2022;23(1):3–21.

24 Reissenberger T, Ebel M, Klode C, Hirsch C, Bekes K. Hypomineralized teeth and their impact on oral-health-related quality of life in primary school children. Int J Environ Res Public Health. 2022;19(16):10409.

25 Amrollahi N, Hashemi S, Heidari Z. Impact of molar incisor hypomineralization on oral health-related quality of life in 8–10 years old children: a systematic review and meta-analysis. J Evid Based Dent Pract. 2023;23(3):101889.

26 Kisacik S, Ozler CO, Olmez S. Molar incisor hypomineralization and oral health-related quality of life: a sample of 8–12-years-old children. Clin Oral Investig. 2024;28(1):105.

27 Elhennawy K, Rajjoub O, Reissmann DR, Doueiri MS, Hamad R, Sierwald I, et al. The association between molar incisor hypomineralization and oral health-related quality of life: a cross-sectional study. Clin Oral Investig. 2022;26(5): 4071–7.

28 Fütterer J, Ebel M, Bekes K, Klode C, Hirsch C. Influence of customized therapy for molar incisor hypomineralization on children's oral hygiene and quality of life. Clin Exp Dent Res. 2020;6(1):33–43.

29 Bekes K, Amend S, Priller J, Zamek C, Stamm T, Krämer N. Changes in oral health-related quality of life after treatment of hypersensitive molar incisor hypomineralization-affected molars with a sealing. Clin Oral Investig. 2021;25(11):6449–54.
30 Tugcu N, Sezer B, Caliskan C, Durmus B, Kargul B. Changes in oral health-related quality of life after treatment of molar incisor hypomineralisation using Glass Hybrid Restorations. J Pak Med Assoc. 2022;72(10):1977–82.
31 Hasmun N, Vettore MV, Lawson JA, Elcock C, Zaitoun H, Rodd HD. Determinants of children's oral health-related quality of life following aesthetic treatment of enamel opacities. J Dent. 2020; 98:103372.
32 da Silva FG, de Almeida SB, de Campos PH, Abrantes RM, de Oliveira AVA, Guaré RO, et al. Low-level laser therapy for management of hypersensitivity in molar-incisor hypomineralization and oral health-related quality of life: case report. J Clin Pediatr Dent. 2022;46(2): 107–11.
33 Paschoal MAB, Costa HE, Santos-Pinto L, Ferreira MC. Photobiomodulation therapy for hypersensitivity associated with molar-incisor hypomineralization: a case report. Gen Dent. 2021;69(6):50–3.

Marina Deus Moura Lima
Department of Pathology and Dentistry Clinic, Federal University of Piauí (UFPI)
Campus Universitário Ministro Petrônio Portella, Bloco 5, Ininga
Teresina, PI 64049-550 (Brazil)
mdmlima@gmail.com

Published online: July 1, 2024
Rios D, Santos-Pinto L (eds): Molar Incisor Hypomineralisation: New Perceptions. Monogr Oral Sci. Basel, Karger, 2024, vol 32, pp 88–99 (DOI: 10.1159/000538871)

Understanding the Enamel Disintegration and Posteruptive Breakdown of Demarcated Opacities on Molar Incisor Hypomineralisation

Roberta Costa Jorge[a, b] Patrícia Papoula Gorni dos Reis[a, b]
Vera Mendes Soviero[a, b]

[a]Department of Preventive and Community Dentistry, Faculty of Dentistry, Rio de Janeiro State University, Rio de Janeiro, Brazil; [b]Dental School, Arthur Sá Earp Neto University, Petrópolis, Brazil

Abstract

This review aims to present scientific knowledge regarding the demarcated opacities of molar incisor hypomineralisation (MIH) and factors that clarify the occurrence of posteruptive enamel breakdown. The demarcated opacities have distinct boundaries with the adjacent nonaffected enamel and may vary in color among white, creamy, yellow, and brownish. The hypomineralised enamel is more porous and less organized than the nonaffected enamel. As a result of the reduced mineral content and higher protein content, the hypomineralised enamel shows a progressive reduction in its mechanical properties according to the opacity feature. Chemically, the protein content of MIH opacities is abnormally high, mainly composed by albumin, which is a serum protein usually not found in mature enamel. The highest protein content is seen in brown opacities, followed by yellow and white opacities, both with higher protein content than nonaffected enamel. The fact that the hypomineralised enamel is more fragile than the nonaffected enamel is supported not only by laboratorial findings but also by clinical prospective studies that observed an aggravation of MIH over time, as well as the correlation between the color of the demarcated opacities and the risk of posteruptive enamel breakdown. A better understanding about the microstructure of the hypomineralised enamel has relevant implications for the clinical approach of the condition. In the clinic, besides a comprehensive assessment of anamnesis and clinical data, it is advisable to record the color and the location of the opacities by tooth surface in order to support the treatment decisions and estimate a prognosis for MIH patients.

Introduction

Enamel hypomineralisation is recognized as a qualitative developmental defect of dental enamel characterized by a lower mineral content compared to nonaffected enamel [1, 2]. Clinically, hypomineralised enamel exhibits abnormal translucency, which can be diffuse or demarcated [3]. Diffuse and demarcated opacities differ in clinical features, morphological features, and etiology [4].

The diffuse opacities, such as fluorosis, are linked with fluoride intake and similarly affect homologous teeth [3, 4]. The demarcated opacities result from a disturbance in mineralisation caused by local factors such as trauma or periapical infection in the predecessor tooth, usually affecting a single tooth, or they have a multifactorial/systemic origin, affecting one or a group of teeth symmetrically [4].

The clinical condition characterized by demarcated opacities affecting first permanent molars, often combined with affected permanent incisors, was first named molar incisor hypomineralisation (MIH) in 2001 [5]. However, it has been observed that other permanent teeth besides the first permanent molars and permanent incisors might also be affected by the same type of enamel hypomineralisation [6–9]. When the same pattern of enamel defect is present in primary teeth, it usually affects mainly the second primary molars and is called hypomineralised second primary molars [10].

MIH has been extensively studied in the last two decades. Regarding etiology, many studies have focused on environmental factors, such as perinatal complications, diseases, and medicines intake during the first years of life. This focus is because the enamel of the most affected teeth (first permanent molars and permanent incisors) is maturated during this period [11]. However, considering that the same type of enamel hypomineralisation has been observed both in primary and permanent teeth, affecting from the first permanent molars and incisors to the third permanent molars in the latter, the etiological factors may be present longer in life [8–10]. More recently, it has been suggested that the etiology of MIH is multifactorial, combining genetic predisposition with environmental factors [12, 13].

Regardless of the type of affected teeth, the demarcated opacity is the clinical manifestation of a defective mineralisation of the enamel [14]. The poorly mineralised enamel is a consequence of disturbances in the maturation/mineralisation phase of amelogenesis [15]. Depending on the severity of the hypomineralisation, the enamel can be highly porous, fragile, and prone to breakdown under physiological forces [16]. The clinical implications resulting from the abnormal enamel may include hypersensitivity, higher caries risk, and increased need for restorative treatment [17–19]. With an estimated worldwide prevalence of 14.2%, MIH and its clinical consequences became a relevant issue when dealing with pediatric dental patients [20]. A better understanding of the prognosis for demarcated opacities affecting both primary and permanent teeth is of major importance for a proper treatment plan and monitoring of patients with MIH.

What Do the Demarcated Opacities Tell Us about the Chemical and Mechanical Properties of the Enamel in MIH?

The demarcated opacities have distinct boundaries with the adjacent nonaffected enamel and may vary in color among white, creamy, yellow, and brownish [21]. Several in vitro studies have analyzed the chemical and mechanical properties of hypomineralised enamel in extracted human teeth using various methods of analysis. Despite limitations regarding the variability of the clinical characteristics, severity of the condition, and the limited number of available teeth for analysis, these studies greatly contribute to understanding the correlation between the clinical and ultrastructure aspects of hypomineralised enamel.

Highly porous subsurface zones, which can be seen in the hypomineralised enamel in the polarized light microscope, in the scanning electron microscopy, and in the micro-tomography (micro-CT) are not present in nonaffected enamel [1, 22–24]. The more affected areas can reach higher than 20% increased porosity [22, 23]. Moreover, an increased pore volume is seen in the darker opacities (yellow-brownish) in comparison with the light ones (white-creamy) [1, 22, 25].

In scanning electron microscopy and transmission electron microscopy, hypomineralised enamel shows indistinct and less organized enamel prisms [25–30]. The crystals appear less dense, loosely packed, and with wide interrod zones [24, 31, 32]. A significantly lower mineral content, below 60 vol% on average, was observed using transverse microradiograph [23]. This lower mineral content was also evidenced by decreased values of mineral density in the micro-CT in hypomineralised enamel in comparison with control nonaffected enamel. The difference in relation to nonaffected enamel may range from 5 to 25% in the white-creamy opacities to almost 40% in the yellow-brownish opacities [22, 33, 34]. A correlation between the mineral density and the color of the opacity was clearly observed. The darker the opacity, the lower is the mineral density, characterizing the darker opacities as the most severe ones in terms of hypomineralisation. This correlation was seen using micro-CT and laser fluorescence [35].

A tendency for lower levels of Ca and P in hypomineralised enamel in comparison with nonaffected enamel is reported by some studies, particularly in the yellow-brownish opacities, although not always statistically significant [25, 30, 31]. Higher protein content and reduced phosphate levels were observed in hypomineralised enamel through the Raman spectroscopy, represented by the ratio between amide I and phosphate. Comparisons among white, yellow, and brown lesions showed that the brown opacities had slightly higher amide I/phosphate ratios [36]. Due to the combination of lower mineral content, higher protein content, and increased porosity, the mechanical properties of hypomineralised enamel are drastically reduced. Values of microhardness, flexural strength, and modulus of elasticity are significantly lower in hypomineralised enamel in comparison with nonaffected enamel [23, 28, 29, 37].

The chemical characterization of hypomineralised enamel using energy-dispersive spectroscopy and Fourier-transform infrared spectroscopy shows an increased organic content, represented by a higher concentration of carbons and carbonates, and a decrease in apatite [23, 25, 26]. The protein content of MIH opacities is abnormally high [36, 38–40], mainly composed by albumin, a serum protein usually not found in mature enamel [38]. The highest protein content is seen in brown opacities, followed by yellow and white opacities, all with higher protein content than nonaffected enamel [36, 38, 39]. Besides the color of the opacities, the protein profile is influenced by surface integrity [40]. Hemoglobin was one of the major components in broken lesions, while serum albumin predominated in intact ones [40]. Certain chemical components, such as Mg, Fe, Zn, and/or Rb, which were scarce or absent in healthy enamel, were detected in hypomineralised enamel, specifically in brown opacities [25, 29, 30, 32].

Several laboratorial studies confirm that the hypomineralised enamel has markedly inferior mechanical properties in comparison with unaffected enamel. These studies are important for understanding the nature of demarcated opacities, thereby supporting proper management of the condition in clinical practice [41]. Table 1 summarizes the ultrastructure of hypomineralised enamel explored by several studies, using different methods of analysis. The lower mineral content and higher protein content explain the reduced hardness of the enamel. Consequently, the hypomineralised enamel may be fragile and prone to breakdown. The correlation between the color of the opacities and their chemical and mechanical properties supports the understanding that yellow-brownish opacities are at higher risk of developing posteruptive breakdown (PEB) in comparison with white-creamy opacities [22, 41].

A better understanding of the microstructure of hypomineralised enamel has relevant implications for the clinical approach to the condition. The fact that the hypomineralised enamel is more fragile than nonaffected enamel is supported by

Table 1. Chemical and mechanical properties of hypomineralised enamel and methods of analysis and studies

Chemical or mechanical property	Method of analysis	Author/year
Increased porosity	PLM	Jälevik and Norén, 2000 [1] Crombie et al., 2013 [23]
	Micro-CT	Gambetta-Tessini et al., 2017 [22]
	SEM	Jälevik et al., 2005 [24]
Less organized prismatic structure	SEM	Mahoney et al., 2004 [28] Jälevik et al., 2005 [24] Bozal et al., 2015 [25] Taube et al., 2015 [26] Melin et al., 2015 [30] Houari et al., 2023 [32]
	TEM	Xie et al., 2008 [27]
Lower mineral content	TMR	Crombie et al., 2013 [23]
	Micro-CT	Fearne et al., 2004 [33] Farah et al., 2010 [34] Farah et al., 2010 [35] Gambetta-Tessini et al., 2017 [22]
	LF	Farah et al., 2010 [35]
	EDS	Bozal et al., 2015 [25]
	Raman spectroscopy	Fraser et al., 2015 [36]
Lower level of Ca	EDS	Bozal et al., 2015 [25] Alifakioti et al., 2021 [31]
Lower level of P	EDS	Bozal et al., 2015 [25] Alifakioti et al., 2021 [31]
	Raman spectroscopy	Fraser et al., 2015 [36]
Lower microhardness	Microindentation	Mahoney et al., 2004 [28] Mahoney et al., 2004 [29] Chan et al., 2010 [37] Crombie et al., 2013 [23] Houari et al., 2023 [32]
Lower flexural strength	FIB	Chan et al., 2010 [37]
Lower modulus of elasticity	Microindentation	Mahoney et al., 2004 [28] Mahoney et al., 2004 [29] Chan et al., 2010 [37]
Increased carbon and carbonate	Weight percentage	Crombie et al., 2013 [23]
	EDS	Bozal et al., 2015 [25]
	FTIR	Taube et al., 2015 [26] Alifakioti et al., 2021 [31]
Decreased apatite content	FTIR	Taube et al., 2015 [26]
Higher level of Mg	EDS	Mahoney et al., 2004 [29] Bozal et al., 2015 [25]
	XRMA	Melin et al., 2015 [30]
Higher protein content in general	Electrophoresis	Farah et al., 2010 [38] Mangum et al., 2010 [40]
	Raman spectroscopy	Fraser et al., 2015 [36]
	Mass spectrometry	Mukhtar et al., 2022 [39]
High level of albumin specifically	Proteomic analysis	Mangum et al., 2010 [40]
	Mass spectrometry	Farah et al., 2010 [38] Mukhtar et al., 2022 [39]

EDS, energy-dispersive spectroscopy; FIB, focused ion beam; FTIR, Fourier-transform infrared spectroscopy; LF, laser fluorescence; micro-CT, microtomography; PLM, polarized light microscopy; SEM, scanning electron microscopy; TEM, transmission electron microscopy; TMR, transverse microradiograph; XRMA, X-ray microanalysis.

the literature and is explained by the differences observed in its chemical composition and topography. It is reasonable to state that the risk of enamel disintegration is higher as more severe is the hypomineralisation. Hence, it would be very useful to have a clinical indicator of its severity. When in vitro studies correlate the clinical appearance of opacities with their severity, showing that darker opacities have lower mineral content, they provide valuable information for clinical practice. Therefore, the color of the opacity may serve as a useful clinical characteristic to estimate the risk of breakdown and to suggest a prognosis.

Is the Color of MIH Demarcated Opacities a Predictor of Their Clinical Behavior over Time?

The typical MIH demarcated opacities are clearly distinguished from the surrounding nonaffected enamel by their well-defined borders. The abnormal enamel translucency is seen as an opacity that may vary in color among white, creamy, yellow, or brown [5]. The guideline proposed by the European Academy of Paediatric Dentistry in 2010 [42], updated in 2021 [21], recommends recording the severity of MIH at the patient level based on the clinical features of the opacities combined with symptoms and aesthetic concerns reported by the patient. Hence, MIH is classified into one of the two categories of severity: mild (demarcated opacity without PEB, induced sensitivity to cold air or water, and mild aesthetic concerns) or severe (demarcated opacity associated with PEB, spontaneous hypersensitivity affecting function, and strong aesthetic concerns) [21]. The classification of severity proposed by the European Academy of Paediatric Dentistry is a valuable guide for proposing a treatment plan. A major advantage is that it considers the patient as whole and pays special attention to symptoms and concerns reported by the patient. However, as it focuses on current signs and symptoms of the condition, it does not give indications for estimating prognosis. Is there any chance that a mild case becomes a severe one? Is this chance the same for all patients? Do different opacities in a same patient have the same chance to progress to PEB? Answers to these questions would be helpful in estimating prognosis and doing a monitoring plan.

If the analysis of the microstructure has shown that the hypomineralisation is more severe in the yellow-brownish opacities in comparison with the white-creamy ones [1, 22, 25, 33, 35, 36, 38, 39, 41], it is reasonable to consider including the color of the opacity among the criteria for classifying the severity of MIH. Therefore, in addition to classifying the patient, it may be valuable to classify each tooth or tooth surface according to the severity of the enamel defect. The developmental defects of enamel index modified in 1989 [3] and updated in 1992 [2], although not specifically developed for MIH, already suggests differentiation between white-creamy and yellow-brownish demarcated opacities. After the consensus on the MIH definition, other indices were proposed to assess the presence and severity of MIH, trying to overcome certain limitations of developmental defects of enamel index, such as the lack of scores to record PEB and atypical caries/restorations/extractions [43]. In general, these indices focused more on the integrity of the tooth surface (absence or presence of PEB) and extent of the enamel defect [44, 45] or in the type of affected teeth [6]. However, Ghanim et al. [46] proposed a more detailed criteria, where two different scores were suggested to differentiate the white-creamy opacities from the yellow-brownish ones. Later, Cabral et al. [47] validated an MIH severity scoring system, demonstrating reliability and validity of differentiating between yellow-brownish and white-creamy opacities. According to the study, classification by color successfully discriminated opacities at higher risk of PEB over time.

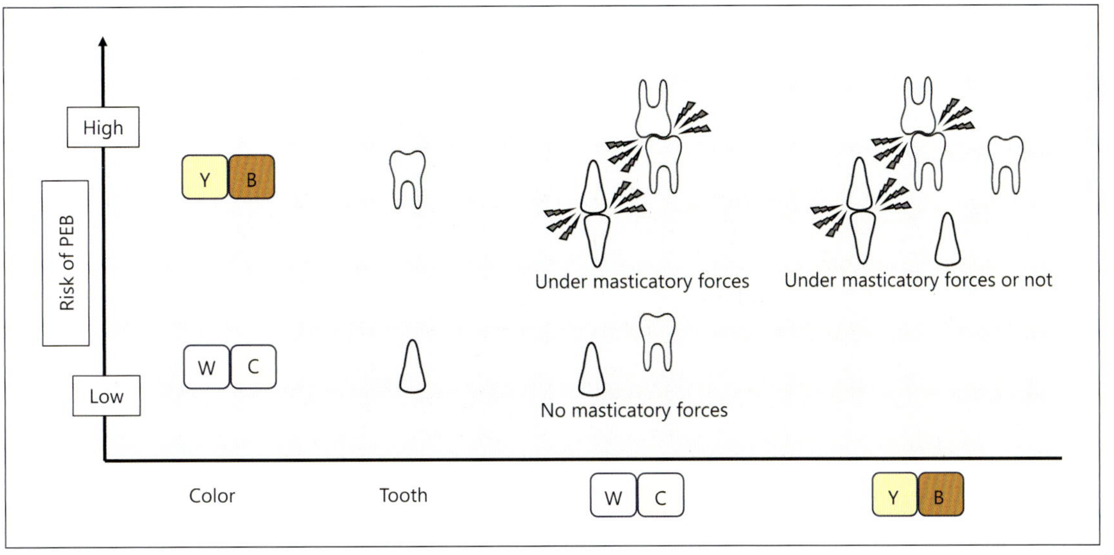

Fig. 1. Schematic representation of the risk of PEB according to the clinical characteristics of the demarcated opacity. Based on the available clinical data, in general, yellow-brownish (YB) opacities and first permanent molars are at higher risk of PEB in comparison with white-creamy (WC) opacities and permanent incisors, respectively. Among the WC opacities, the risk of PEB seems to be higher when located in areas exposed to masticatory forces. Among the YB opacities, the risk of PEB seems to be high independently of the presence of masticatory forces.

The higher risk of PEB in yellow-brownish opacities finds support not only on the results of several studies that evaluated the ultrastructure of the hypomineralised enamel but also on longitudinal prospective clinical studies that followed patients with MIH [16]. An increase in the severity of MIH was evaluated in 147 children who were examined twice over an 18-month interval by Costa-Silva et al. [48]. From 398 teeth, including 262 first permanent molars and 136 permanent incisors with demarcated opacities at baseline, 48 presented PEB at follow up. Six (9.2%) of 65 incisors with yellow or brown opacities presented PEB, while none of the 71 incisors with white opacity progressed to PEB. Among the molars, PEB was significantly more frequent in yellow or brown opacities (38/179–21.2%) than in white ones (4/83–4.8%) [48]. In another clinical study, Fragelli et al. [49] followed 45 children with MIH for 12 months and observed 6 (8.7%) PEB in 69 yellow or brown opacities, compared to only 1 (0.86%) case of PEB in 116 white opacities after 12 months. The correlation between the color of the opacity and tooth surface disintegration was also confirmed by Neves et al. [50]. The evaluation of demarcated opacities affecting first permanent molars in 58 children showed that 16.3% (14/72) of white opacities and 41.8% (38/91) of yellow or brown opacities aggravated to PEB after 15 months. In accordance with previous studies, Arslanagić et al. [51] observed that the proportion of PEB after 12 months was higher in dark opacities (5/8–62.5%) as compared to light ones (2/35–5.7%). From 29 permanent incisors and 14 first permanent molars in 25 children, PEB was also more frequent in the molars.

These clinical findings were supported by Cabral et al. [47] in a longer follow-up study. In the validation of the severity scoring system, 181 children with MIH were included, and 150 completed the 36-month follow-up period. Among the first permanent molars, 226 white-creamy and

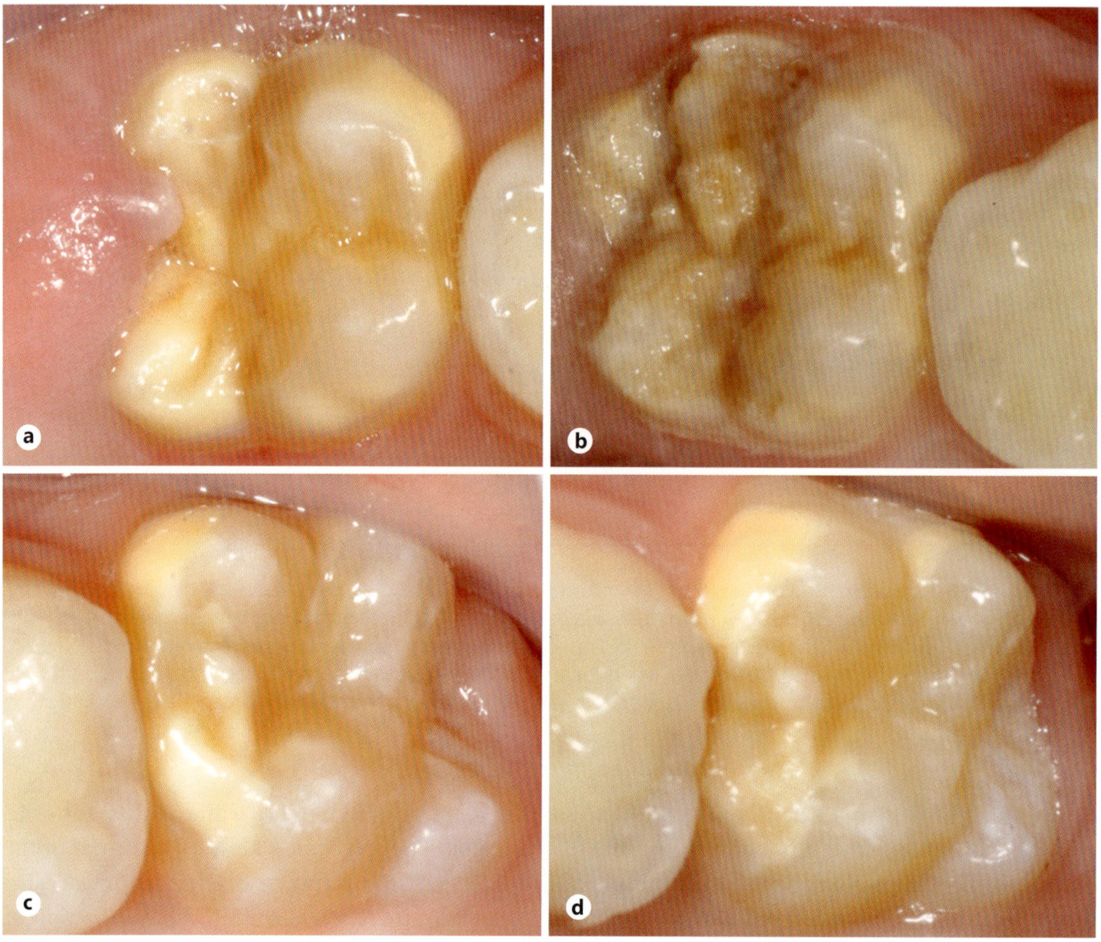

Fig. 2. A lower first permanent molar (**a** and **b**) and an upper first permanent molar (**c** and **d**) are shown with an interval of 12 months. In the lower first permanent molar, yellow-brownish opacity and an initial enamel disintegration (**a**) aggravated to a severe PEB affecting the occlusal, buccal, and lingual surfaces (**b**). In the upper first permanent molar, a creamy opacity in the mesial-lingual cusp (**c**) progressed to PEB (**d**).

130 yellow-brown opacities were included. After 36 months, the rate of PEB was 28.1% (54/192) and 52.7% (59/112) for white-creamy and yellow-brownish, respectively. Similar to previous clinical prospective studies [48, 49], the lower rate of PEB in incisors was confirmed. At the end of 36 months, the rate of PEB in the incisors was 3.2% (3/93) and 24.1% (7/29) for white-creamy and yellow-brownish opacities, respectively.

The association between the color of the opacity and the risk of PEB appears unequivocal. Darker opacities are at a higher risk of PEB [47–51]. A greater presence of PEB in yellow-brownish opacities was also observed in cross-sectional studies [52–54]. The higher frequency of PEB in molars [47–49, 51], particularly in the occlusal surface [48], suggests that masticatory forces play a relevant role in the aggravation to fracture, although this is not a consensus [50, 51]. In the study by Arslanagić et al. [51], 43 demarcated opacities were followed for 12 months, primarily white (35/43–81.4%) and located in incisors (29/43–

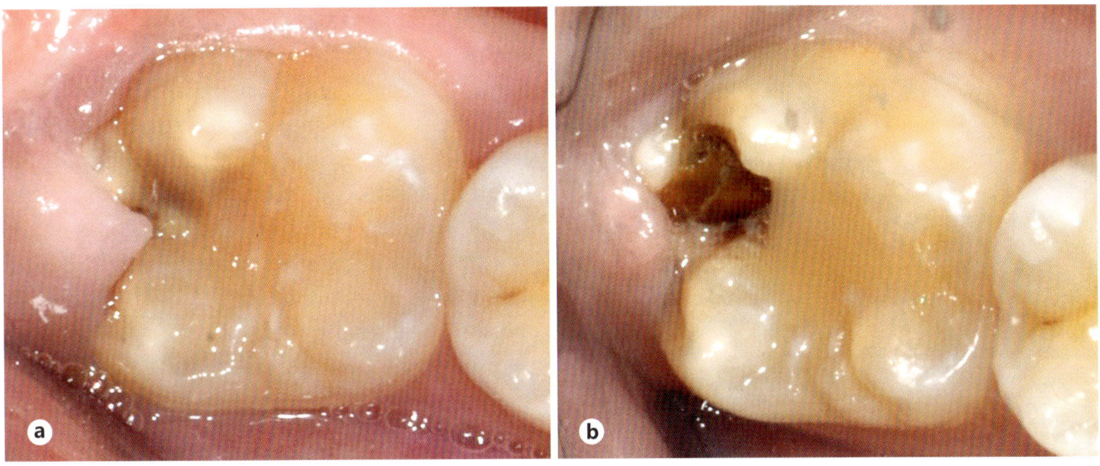

Fig. 3. A yellow-brownish opacity in a lower first permanent molar (**a**) aggravated to PEB and atypical caries (**b**) in 13 months.

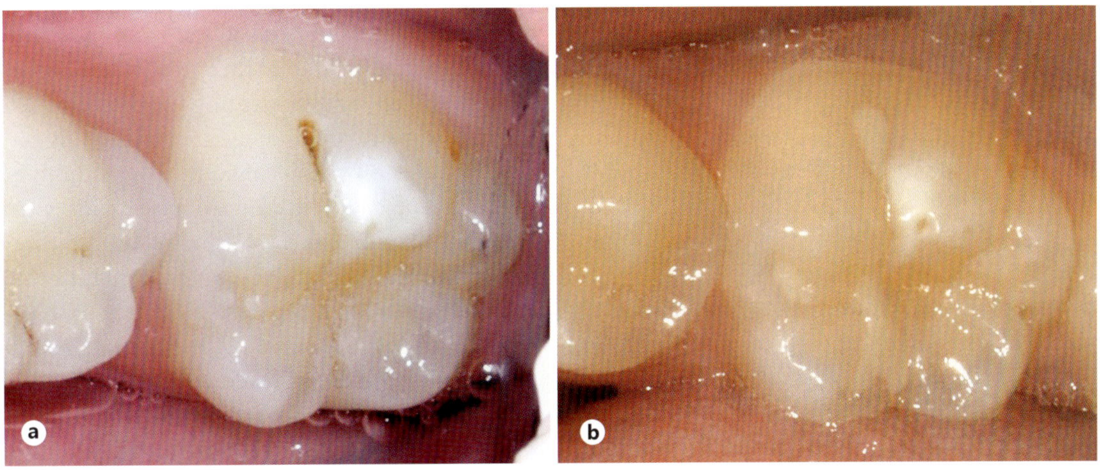

Fig. 4. A white opacity in a lower first permanent molar (**a**) remained practically unchanged over 3 years (**b**). An initial disintegration on the tip of cusp became slightly more visible.

67.4%). PEB occurred only on the occlusal/incisal surfaces, classified by the authors as areas exposed to masticatory forces. Neves et al. [50] observed an increase from 9.1% (3/33) to 20.8% (11/53) among white opacities not exposed and exposed to masticatory forces, respectively. However, a tendency of a higher rate of fracture in areas of masticatory stress was not seen among yellow-brownish opacities. The percentage of PEB in yellow-brownish opacities was 44.0% (22/50) and 36.8% (16/41) when not exposed or exposed to masticatory forces, respectively [50]. However, an important aspect that is not clearly addressed in studies investigating PEB is the conceptualization or understanding of the term "masticatory forces." It is crucial to distinguish between a tooth not being in

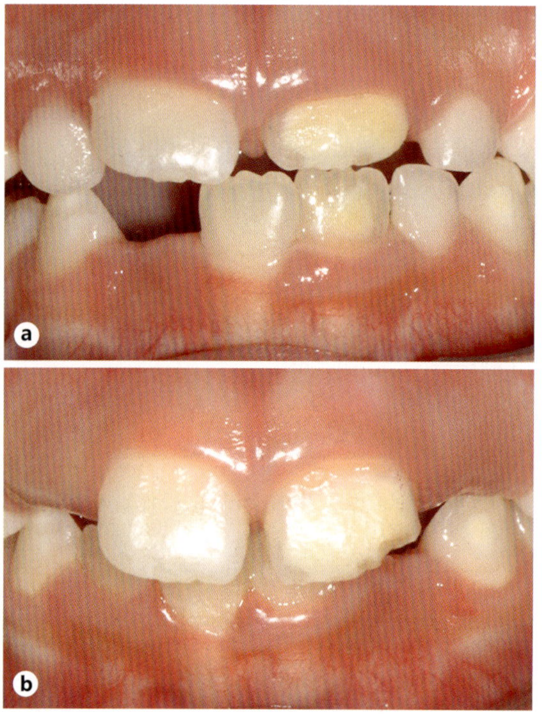

Fig. 5. The upper central permanent incisors are shown with an interval of 7 months. The yellowish opacity in the left incisor (**a**) aggravated to PEB (**b**).

occlusion and one not receiving any masticatory force. In our understanding, even an erupting tooth, which is not in occlusion, can experience mechanical force, such as from a popcorn kernel, whether it comes between the tooth with MIH (enamel hypomineralisation) and the opposing tooth. Figure 1 shows a schematic representation of the risk of PEB according to the clinical characteristics of the demarcated opacities. Figures 2 and 3 display clinical pictures of first permanent molars with yellow-brownish opacities that broke during a 12- and 13-month follow-up, respectively. Figure 4 shows a clinical case where a white opacity in a first permanent molar remained unchanged over a period of almost 3 years. Figure 5 shows a PEB in permanent incisor.

The relatively high frequency of PEB among the yellow-brownish opacities in incisors [47] and the similar rate of fracture in molars regardless of the presence of chewing forces [50] are suggestive that the darker opacities may be so fragile that they may be prone to break independently of direct exposure to masticatory stress. Dentists should be aware that MIH opacities tend to worsen over time, that the color of the opacity plays a key role in predicting PEB, and that molars are more often affected by PEB than incisors. Currently, there are no available data regarding the occurrence of PEB in other permanent teeth affected by enamel hypomineralisation besides first permanent molars and permanent incisors.

Conclusion

Although it is not possible to state that the specimens analyzed in the in vitro studies are representative of all teeth presenting hypomineralised enamel, some of the findings are consistently observed and confirmed using different methods of analysis. The data obtained from several in vitro studies are sufficient to conclude that the lower mineral content and higher protein content in the hypomineralised enamel result in a fragile structure. Moreover, the chemical profile and the mechanical properties correlate with the color. The darker the demarcated opacity, the lower its mechanical properties.

The susceptibility of hypomineralised enamel to fracture has been confirmed in prospective clinical studies, as has the correlation between the color of demarcated opacities and the risk of PEB. Therefore, the clinical findings available to this point corroborate with the laboratorial analyses reporting the mechanical properties of the hypomineralised enamel. Additionally, the increased fragility observed in yellow-brownish opacities as compared to white-creamy ones is substantiated by clinical findings suggesting a higher susceptibility to PEB.

In a clinical setting, identifying potential risk factors for PEB associated with demarcated opacities related to MIH is crucial to support treatment decisions and estimate the prognosis. Therefore, besides a comprehensive assessment of anamnesis and clinical data, it is valuable to record the color and the location of the opacities on each tooth surface.

Acknowledgment

The authors acknowledge the Rio de Janeiro State University (UERJ), the Centro Universitário Arthur Sá Earp Neto (UNIFASE), the Coordenação de Aperfeiçoamento de Pessoal de Nível Superior (CAPES), and the Rio de Janeiro Research Foundation (FAPERJ) for the support to our research group.

Statement of Ethics

Informed consent for publication of images was obtained from the patients' parents or guardians.

Conflict of Interest Statement

The authors have no conflicts of interest to declare.

Funding Sources

No specific funding was provided for this manuscript.

Author Contributions

All authors, R.C.J., P.P.G.R., and V.M.S., contributed to the conception and writing of the manuscript. V.M.S. drafted a first version that was substantially improved by inputs from R.C.J. and P.P.G.R. All authors reviewed and approved the final version of the manuscript.

References

1 Jälevik B, Norén JG. Enamel hypomineralization of permanent first molars: a morphological study and survey of possible aetiological factors. Int J Paediatr Dent. 2000;10(4):278–89.
2 FDI. A review of the developmental defects of enamel index (DDE Index). Commission on Oral Health, Research & Epidemiology. Report of an FDI Working Group. Int Dent J. 1992;42(6):411–26.
3 Clarkson J, O'Mullane D. A modified DDE index for use in epidemiological studies of enamel defects. J Dent Res. 1989;68(3):445–50.
4 Denis M, Atlan A, Vennat E, Tirlet G, Attal JP. White defects on enamel: diagnosis and anatomopathology: two essential factors for proper treatment (part 1). Int Orthod. 2013;11(2):139–65.
5 Weerheijm KL, Jälevik B, Alaluusua S. Molar–incisor hypomineralisation. Caries Res. 2001;35(5):390–1.
6 Mittal N. Phenotypes of enamel hypomineralization and molar incisor hypomineralization in permanent dentition: identification, quantification and proposal for classification. J Clin Pediatr Dent. 2016;40(5):367–74.
7 Farias AL de, Rojas-Gualdrón DF, Bussaneli DG, Santos-Pinto L, Mejía JD, Restrepo M. Does molar-incisor hypomineralization (MIH) affect only permanent first molars and incisors? New observations on permanent second molars. Int J Paediatr Dent. 2022;32(1):1–10.
8 Hanan SA, Farias AL de, Santos-Pinto L. Molar incisor hypomineralization in adolescents and adults and its association with facial profile and occlusion. Clin Oral Investig. 2023;27(3):1243–53.
9 Kevrekidou A, Kosma I, Kotsanos I, Arapostathis KN, Kotsanos N. Enamel opacities in all other than molar incisor hypomineralisation index teeth of adolescents. Int J Paediatr Dent. 2021;31(2):270–7.
10 Elfrink MEC, Cate JM ten, Jaddoe VWV, Hofman A, Moll HA, Veerkamp JSJ. Deciduous molar hypomineralization and molar incisor hypomineralization. J Dent Res. 2012;91(6):551–5.
11 Lopes LB, Machado V, Botelho J, Haubek D. Molar-incisor hypomineralization: an umbrella review. Acta Odontol Scand. 2021;79(5):1–11.
12 Vieira AR, Kup E. On the etiology of molar-incisor hypomineralization. Caries Res. 2016;50(2):166–9.

13 Teixeira RJPB, Andrade NS, Queiroz LCC, Mendes FM, Moura MS, Moura LFAD, et al. Exploring the association between genetic and environmental factors and molar incisor hypomineralization: evidence from a twin study. Int J Paediatr Dent. 2017 Aug 22;28(2):198–206.
14 Fagrell TG, Dietz W, Jälevik B, Norén JG. Chemical, mechanical and morphological properties of hypomineralized enamel of permanent first molars. Acta Odontol Scand. 2010;68(4):215–22.
15 Fagrell TG, Salmon P, Melin L, Norén JG. Onset of molar incisor hypomineralization (MIH). Swed Dent J. 2013;37(2):61–70.
16 Jorge RC, GorniReis P dos P, Marañón-Vásquez GA, Masterson D, Maia LC, Soviero VM. Are yellow-brownish opacities in hypomineralized teeth more prone to breakage than white-creamy ones? A systematic review. Clin Oral Investig. 2022;26(9):5795–808.
17 Americano GCA, Jacobsen PE, Soviero VM, Haubek D. A systematic review on the association between molar incisor hypomineralization and dental caries. Int J Paediatr Dent. 2017;27(1):11–21.
18 Linner T, Khazaei Y, Bücher K, Pfisterer J, Hickel R, Kühnisch J. Hypersensitivity in teeth affected by molar-incisor hypomineralization (MIH). Sci Rep. 2021;11(1):17922.
19 Biondi AM, Cortese SG, Babino L, Ortolani AM. Follow-up of first permanent molar restorative treatment with and without molar hypomineralization. Acta Odontol Latinoam. 2022;35(2):75–9.
20 Zhao D, Dong B, Yu D, Ren Q, Sun Y. The prevalence of molar incisor hypomineralization: evidence from 70 studies. Int J Paediatr Dent. 2017 Jul 21;28(2):170–9.
21 Lygidakis NA, Garot E, Somani C, Taylor GD, Rouas P, Wong FSL. Best clinical practice guidance for clinicians dealing with children presenting with molar-incisor-hypomineralisation (MIH): an updated European Academy of Paediatric Dentistry policy document. Eur Arch Paediatr Dent. 2022;23(1):3–21.
22 Gambetta-Tessini K, Mariño R, Ghanim A, Adams GG, Manton DJ. Validation of quantitative light-induced fluorescence-digital in the quantification of demarcated hypomineralized lesions of enamel. J Investig Clin Dent. 2017;8(4):e12259.
23 Crombie FA, Manton DJ, Palamara JEA, Zalizniak I, Cochrane NJ, Reynolds EC. Characterisation of developmentally hypomineralised human enamel. J Dent. 2013;41(7):611–8.
24 Jälevik B, Dietz W, Norén JG. Scanning electron micrograph analysis of hypomineralized enamel in permanent first molars. Int J Paediatr Dent. 2005;15(4):233–40.
25 Bozal CB, Kaplan A, Ortolani A, Cortese SG, Biondi AM. Ultrastructure of the surface of dental enamel with molar incisor hypomineralization (MIH) with and without acid etching. Acta Odontol Latinoam. 2015;28(2):192–8.
26 Taube F, Marczewski M, Norén JG. Deviations of inorganic and organic carbon content in hypomineralised enamel. J Dent. 2015;43(2):269–78.
27 Xie Z, Kilpatrick NM, Swain MV, Munroe PR, Hoffman M. Transmission electron microscope characterisation of molar-incisor-hypomineralisation. J Mater Sci Mater Med. 2008;19(10):3187.
28 Mahoney E, Ismail FSM, Kilpatrick N, Swain M. Mechanical properties across hypomineralized/hypoplastic enamel of first permanent molar teeth. Eur J Oral Sci. 2004;112(6):497–502.
29 Mahoney EK, Rohanizadeh R, Ismail FSM, Kilpatrick NM, Swain MV. Mechanical properties and microstructure of hypomineralised enamel of permanent teeth. Biomaterials. 2004;25(20):5091–100.
30 Melin L, Lundgren J, Malmberg P, Norén JG, Taube F, Cornell DH. XRMA and ToF-SIMS analysis of normal and hypomineralized enamel. Microsc Microanal. 2015;21(2):407–21.
31 Alifakioti E, Arhakis A, Oikonomidis S, Kotsanos N. Structural and chemical enamel characteristics of hypomineralised second primary molars. Eur Arch Paediatr Dent. 2021;22(3):361–6.
32 Houari S, DeRocher K, Thuy TT, Coradin T, Srot V, Aken PA van, et al. Multi-scale characterization of Developmental Defects of Enamel and their clinical significance for diagnosis and treatment. Acta Biomater. 2023;169:155–67.
33 Fearne J, Anderson P, Davis GR. 3D X-ray microscopic study of the extent of variations in enamel density in first permanent molars with idiopathic enamel hypomineralisation. Br Dent J. 2004;196(10):634–8.
34 Farah RA, Swain MV, Drummond BK, Cook R, Atieh M. Mineral density of hypomineralised enamel. J Dent. 2010;38(1):50–8.
35 Farah R, Drummond B, Swain M, Williams S. Linking the clinical presentation of molar-incisor hypomineralisation to its mineral density. Int J Paediatr Dent. 2010;20(5):353–60.
36 Fraser SJ, Natarajan AK, Clark ASS, Drummond BK, Gordon KC. A Raman spectroscopic study of teeth affected with molar–incisor hypomineralisation. J Raman Spectrosc. 2015;46(2):202–10.
37 Chan YL, Ngan AHW, King NM. Degraded prism sheaths in the transition region of hypomineralized teeth. J Dent. 2010;38(3):237–44.
38 Farah RA, Monk BC, Swain MV, Drummond BK. Protein content of molar-incisor hypomineralisation enamel. J Dent. 2010;38(7):591–6.
39 Mukhtar U, Goyal A, Luthra-Guptasarma M, Gauba K, Kapur A, Thakur AK. Label-free quantitative proteomics reveals molecular correlates of altered biomechanical properties in molar incisor hypomineralization (MIH): an in vitro study. Eur Arch Paediatr Dent. 2022;23(1):179–91.
40 Mangum JE, Crombie FA, Kilpatrick N, Manton DJ, Hubbard MJ. Surface integrity governs the proteome of hypomineralized enamel. J Dent Res. 2010;89(10):1160–5.
41 Elhennawy K, Manton DJ, Crombie F, Zaslansky P, Radlanski RJ, Jost-Brinkmann PG, et al. Structural, mechanical and chemical evaluation of molar-incisor hypomineralization-affected enamel: A systematic review. Arch Oral Biol. 2017;83:272–81.
42 Lygidakis NA, Wong F, Jälevik B, Vierrou AM, Alaluusua S, Espelid I. Best Clinical Practice Guidance for clinicians dealing with children presenting with Molar-Incisor-Hypomineralisation (MIH). Eur Arch Paediatr Dent. 2010;11(2):75–81.
43 Elfrink MEC, Ghanim A, Manton DJ, Weerheijm KL. Standardised studies on molar incisor hypomineralisation (MIH) and hypomineralised second primary molars (HSPM): a need. Eur Arch Paediatr Dent. 2015;16(3):247–55.
44 Ghanim A, Mariño R, Manton DJ. Validity and reproducibility testing of the Molar Incisor Hypomineralisation (MIH) Index. Int J Paediatr Dent. 2019;29(1):6–13.

45 Bekes K, Steffen R, Krämer N. Update of the molar incisor hypomineralization: Würzburg concept. Eur Arch Paediatr Dent. 2023;24(6):807–13.
46 Ghanim A, Silva MJ, Elfrink MEC, Lygidakis NA, Mariño RJ, Weerheijm KL, et al. Molar incisor hypomineralisation (MIH) training manual for clinical field surveys and practice. Eur Arch Paediatr Dent. 2017;18(4):225–42.
47 Cabral RN, Nyvad B, Soviero VLVM, Freitas E, Leal SC. Reliability and validity of a new classification of MIH based on severity. Clin Oral Investig. 2020; 24(2):727–34.
48 Costa-Silva CMD, Ambrosano GMB, Jeremias F, Souza JFD, Mialhe FL. Increase in severity of molar-incisor hypomineralization and its relationship with the colour of enamel opacity: a prospective cohort study. Int J Paediatr Dent. 2011;21(5):333–41.
49 Fragelli CMB, Jeremias F, Souza JF de, Paschoal MA, Cordeiro R de CL, Santos-Pinto L. Longitudinal evaluation of the structural integrity of teeth affected by molar incisor hypomineralisation. Caries Res. 2015;49(4):378–83.
50 Neves AB, Americano GCA, Soares DV, Soviero VM. Breakdown of demarcated opacities related to molar-incisor hypomineralization: a longitudinal study. Clin Oral Investig. 2019;23(2):611–5.
51 Arslanagić A, Marković N, Bajrić E, Ristić LB. Demarcated opacities as predictors of progression of the molar incisor hypomineralisation: a pilot study. Acta Stomatol Croat. 2020;54(4):420–30.
52 Abdalla HE, Abuaffan AH, Kemoli AM. Molar incisor hypomineralization, prevalence, pattern and distribution in Sudanese children. BMC Oral Heal. 2021; 21(1):9.
53 Mittal NP, Goyal A, Gauba K, Kapur A. Molar incisor hypomineralisation: prevalence and clinical presentation in school children of the northern region of India. Eur Arch Paediatr Dent. 2014; 15(1):11–8.
54 Rai PM, Jain J, Raju AS, Nair RA, Shashidhar K, Dsouza S. Prevalence of molar incisor hypomineralization among school children aged 9 to 12 years in Virajpet, Karnataka, India. Open Access Maced J Med Sci. 2019; 7(6):1042–6.

Vera Mendes Soviero
Department of Preventive and Community Dentistry
Faculty of Dentistry, Rio de Janeiro State University
Boulevard Vinte e Oito de Setembro, 157, Rio de Janeiro 20551-030 (Brazil)
verasoviero@gmail.com

Published online: July 1, 2024
Rios D, Santos-Pinto L (eds): Molar Incisor Hypomineralisation: New Perceptions. Monogr Oral Sci. Basel, Karger, 2024, vol 32, pp 100–116 (DOI: 10.1159/000538876)

Prevalence of Enamel Hypomineralisation/Molar Incisor Hypomineralisation: A Scoping Review

Jan Kühnisch Karl-Ferdinand Fresen

Department of Conservative Dentistry and Periodontology, University Hospital, Ludwig-Maximilians Universität München, Munich, Germany

Abstract

The aim of this scoping review was to provide an up-to-date assessment of the prevalence of enamel hypomineralisation (EH) and, in particular, molar incisor hypomineralisation (MIH). Epidemiological studies published from 2010 to 2023 were analyzed. After screening the primary literature, a total of 139 studies were included. According to the available epidemiological trials of children and adolescents from Europe (*n* = 39), the average prevalence of EH/MIH was 16.74%. The data from Asian studies (*n* = 50) showed an average prevalence of 15.6%. For South America (*n* = 33 studies), the mean prevalence of EH/MIH was 16.7%. The mean prevalence rates for North America (*N* = 9 studies), Africa (*N* = 6), and Australia (*N* = 2) were 25.9%, 11.4%, and 16.8%, respectively. Taken together, these data indicate that EH/MIH is a prevalent condition worldwide. With the aim of standardizing and generating comparable prevalence data, the use of the currently established criteria by the European Academy of Paediatric Dentistry (EAPD) for the detection of EH/MIH may support consistent reporting in epidemiological trials. However, other EH/MIH indices and phenotypes do exist. As the determination of EH/MIH prevalence depends on the correct use of index teeth, meticulous attention must be given to their correct application.

Introduction

While the prevalence of caries among children and adolescents has decreased, the prevalence of enamel hypomineralisation (EH) – in particular, molar incisor hypomineralisation (MIH) – has increased in recent decades. EH is a developmental disorder of enamel formation that is likely caused by multiple, still unknown systemic noxious agents [1–7]. The causative factor(s) or substance(s) lead to a disruption of regular enamel formation by the ameloblasts, and as a result, both hypomineralisation (qualitative deviations from the norm) and hypoplasia (quantitative enamel defects) can be observed. While the per-

1

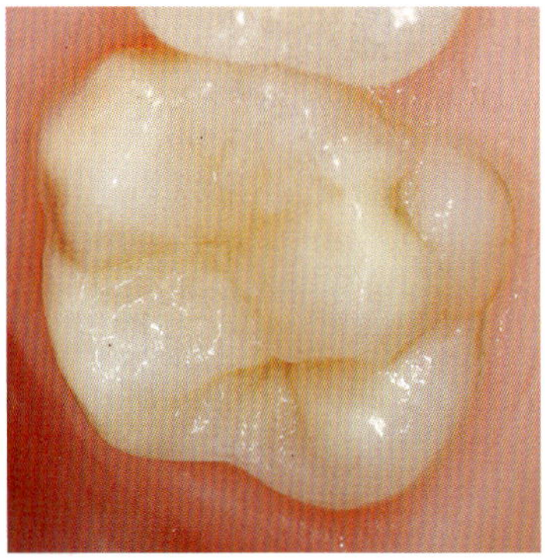

2

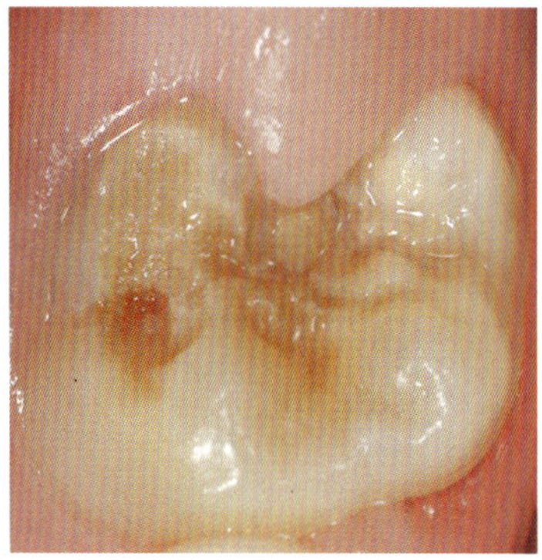

Fig. 1. Clinical appearance of a demarcated opacity.
Fig. 2. Enamel breakdown in a molar tooth with extensive enamel hypomineralisation.

manent incisors and first permanent molars are most frequently affected by EH/MIH, the disorder can occur in any deciduous and permanent teeth [8, 9].

Clinical Appearance

The main clinical symptoms of EH/MIH are demarcated opacities of white, yellowish, or brown color in the enamel (demarcated opacities), as shown in Figure 1. These enamel disturbances can potentially be associated with pre-eruptive defects and/or post-eruptive enamel breakdowns or enamel disintegrations, as shown in Figure 2. Teeth with pre-eruptive defects already break through into the oral cavity with partially missing enamel and/or dentin. However, this requires early dental assessment from the initial tooth eruption onward. Conversely, post-eruptive enamel breakdowns most often occur during occlusion after full eruption. The occlusal surfaces of the first permanent molars are predisposed to localize here; they often require restorative treatment and are located outside the typical caries locations in fissures, pits, or proximal spaces. Therefore, the term "atypical restorations," as shown in Figure 3, has been established for MIH-related restorations [3, 7]. In addition to these clinical signs, which are easy to assess visually, hypersensitivities of varying degrees of severity to thermal, chemical, or mechanical stimuli are recurring concomitant symptoms. In particular, the symptom complex of enamel breakdown and hypersensitivity can lead to limited functionality, restrictions in oral hygiene, and the need to treat the affected teeth.

Indices for EH Detection and Diagnosis

The identification of developmental defects in teeth has undergone methodological changes in recent decades. With the aim of developing a standardized terminology and a simple classification and documentation system, the Developmental Dental Defects of Enamel (DDE) index was established in 1982 [10]. Clarkson and O'Mullane [11] created a simplified version of the index due to the time required for documentation and the difficulty of interpretation. In March 1988, the DDE index was revised for FDI. The defect types were grouped into categories, and possible combinations were recoded. The work group replaced defect localization with defect extent. Other categories, such as need for treatment, etiology, and anamnestic data, were considered to be negligible and were removed. The group published the modified DDE (mDDE) index in 1992 [12]. In 2003, the DDE index was judged to be inadequate by the European Academy of Paediatric Dentistry (EAPD) and too time consuming for

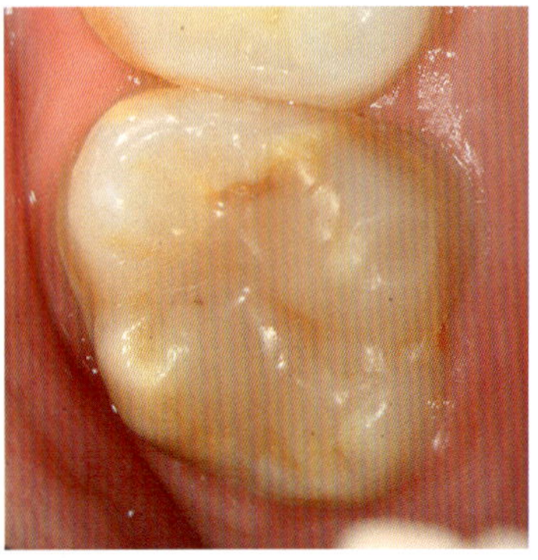

Fig. 3. Atypical restoration due to an enamel breakdown in a permanent molar.

the diagnosis of EH/MIH. In the course of the discussion, the diagnostic criteria for EH/MIH, which consisted of demarcated opacities, enamel breakdowns, atypical restorations, and extraction due to MIH, were formulated and published by Weerheijm et al. [13–15]. These criteria enabled an exact description of EH/MIH and were confirmed to be largely unchanged by the EAPD as diagnostic criteria in 2010 and 2022 [3, 7]. A further index was presented by Ghanim et al. [16], which combined elements of the EAPD criteria and the mDDE index. Steffen et al. [17] introduced the MIH treatment need index (MIH-TNI), which was updated in 2023, to capture hypersensitivities in particular [18]. It should also be noted that other developmental disorders of the teeth, such as fluorosis, Turner teeth, amelogenesis, or dentinogenesis imperfecta, represent independent diseases and must always be differentiated from EH/MIH.

Spectrum of EH/MIH Phenotypes

In principle, clinicians can diagnose typical EH/MIH symptoms in all teeth of primary or permanent dentition. Its clinical appearance suggests that it is the same clinical entity. However, this assumption is to some extent contradicted by the different names given to the primary and permanent dentition. For the primary dentition, the diagnostic terms "deciduous molar hypomineralisation" (DMH) [19, 20] and "hypomineralisation on second primary molars" (HSPMs) [21, 22] were proposed; these terms use the index teeth mentioned for diagnosis. The term "MIH" has been used exclusively for permanent dentition; based on the empirical definition of the EAPD, the term "MIH" is only applicable if a demarcated opacity, enamel breakdown, or atypical breakdown can be found on at least one first permanent molar [3, 7]. In addition, the MIH frequency is occasionally determined according to the naming convention [8, 9] in that EH must be diagnosable on the first permanent molars and permanent incisors (M + IH). The term "severe MIH" is mostly used to describe cases in which at least one enamel breakdown is present [3, 7]. In addition, Cabral et al. [23] proposed the MIH scoring severity system (MIH-SSS), which aims to predict the prognosis of MIH teeth more reliably. Here, yellow/brown opacities had a greater risk of disintegration than white/creamy opacities. The authors concluded that the MIH-SSS might be a valid instrument with high reliability. Furthermore, the clinical importance of enamel breakdowns is underlined.

Another plausible epidemiological determinant would be the number of individuals who are affected by at least one EH, regardless of the specific distribution pattern in the permanent (EH ≥1) or primary dentition [8, 9]. This phenotype includes both MIH children and those with a nonspecific distribution of EH. The prevalence of EH is typically higher than the MIH prevalence. This phenotype differs slightly from that of children with hypomineralisation on other permanent teeth, which was solely described by Kevrekidou et al. [24]. This index considers EH in nonindex teeth and broadens the perspective on EH/MIH prevalence. However, multiple phenotypes are linked to diverging prevalence rates and, therefore, need to be applied correctly by dental epidemiologists and researchers.

Aim of the Scoping Review

The aim of this report was to systematically search the available literature for cross-sectional epidemiological studies that reported EH/MIH prevalence data in relation to frequently reported phenotypes and to summarize the findings.

Materials and Methods

The reporting of this scoping review followed the corresponding PRISMA statement [25]. For this type of study, no statement of ethics was necessary.

Search of the Literature

PubMed was searched for articles published from January 1, 2010, to October 31, 2023; epidemiological studies that were published before 2010 were summarized by Jälevik [26]. Before conducting the systematic search of the literature, a PICO question ("What is the global prevalence of EH/MIH?") was formulated, and the search strategy was developed ("Molar Incisor hypomineral*" OR "Molar-Incisor-hypomineral*" OR "Demarcated opacity" OR "MIH") AND (Prevalence OR "Epidemiological study" OR "Cross-sectional study" OR "Systematic review" OR "Meta-analysis")). The identified papers were screened systematically for relevance by a work group (K.-F.F. and J.K.). The studies eligible for inclusion were epidemiological studies that reported the prevalence of EH/MIH. Studies containing information on MIH, M + IH teeth, and EH ≥1 prevalence were considered relevant. Trials in which epidemiological information about other EH/MIH phenotypes, including DMH, HSPM, or rare dental diseases, was published were not considered and excluded.

Study Selection

The electronic search yielded 550 abstracts from PubMed. All records were exported to the Rayyan platform (https://www.rayyan.ai/). Then, the titles and abstracts of all identified studies were systematically examined according to predefined inclusion and exclusion criteria. The review authors (K.-F.F. and J.K.) were not blinded to the names of the authors or institutions, to the journal of publication, or to the results of the studies. Records that were not relevant were excluded, and the full texts of all the remaining records were obtained. If relevant information for meeting the inclusion criteria was not available from the abstract and/or title, we obtained the full text. In this way, 165 studies were selected for full-text reading and were assessed independently by the same two reviewers (K.-F.F. and J.K.). Any doubts or disagreements were resolved by discussion with an experienced researcher (J.K.). Articles that did not meet all inclusion criteria after the full-text assessment (n = 26) were excluded from further reading, and the reasons for their exclusion were documented. The study selection process is illustrated in Figure 4.

Data Extraction and Statistics

The data from the included studies were extracted using a structured examination form. Any disagreements were resolved through discussion with an expert (J.K.) until a consensus was reached. If necessary, the trial authors were contacted for clarification or missing information. In brief, the following data were extracted from the included studies: (1) the region and country of the study, (2) population details, including the number of subjects, age of the population, and index used for EH/MIH recording, and (3) prevalence data for EH ≥1, MIH, and M + IH. In addition to the data extracted from the included reports, the mean MIH prevalence rates were calculated using an Excel spreadsheet (Excel 2019; Microsoft, Redmond, WA, USA).

Prevalence of EH/MIH

After reviewing the primary literature, a total of 139 epidemiological studies were included, as shown in Figure 4. All the extracted data are summarized in Tables 1–6 in relation to continents. The majority of all the surveys were conducted in children and adolescents in Europe (Table 1), Asia (Table 2), and South America (Table 3). From 2010 onward, the Weerheijm/EAPD diagnostic criteria were used in the majority of the studies. Only a few work groups have used other indices. An overview of the prevalence of EH/MIH in European children and adolescents (Table 1; 39 studies) revealed a heterogeneous appearance of affected individuals, with frequencies between 6.2% and 37.3%, provided that the

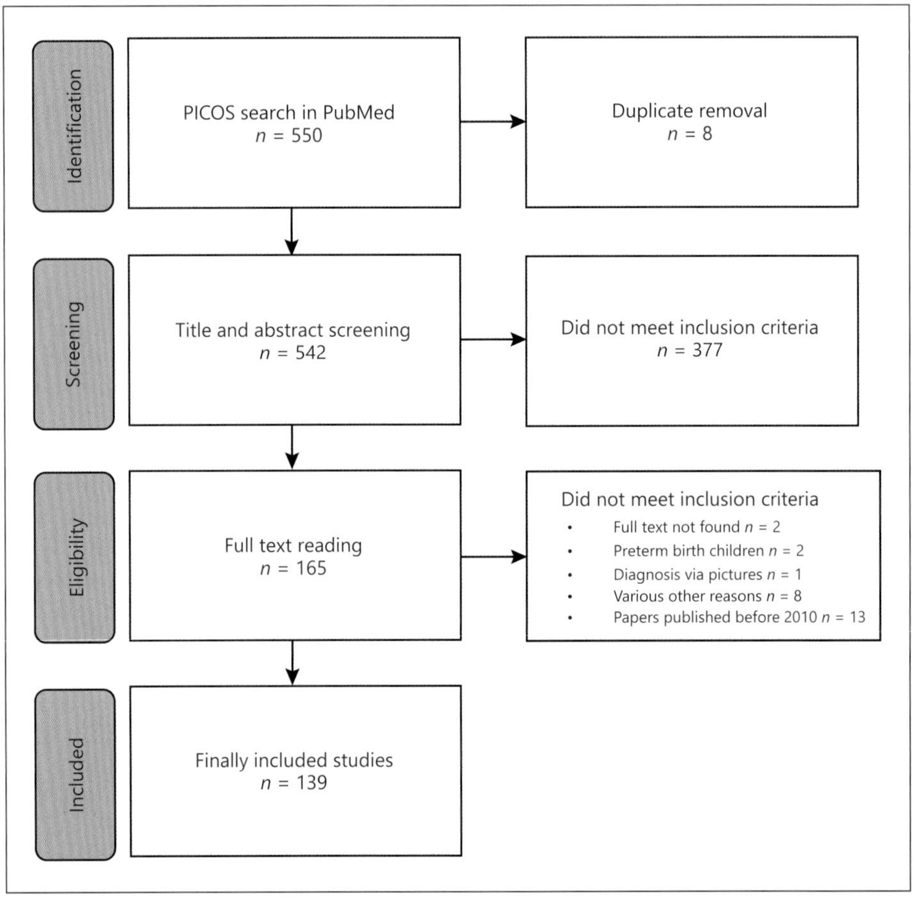

Fig. 4. Flowchart of the systematic search of the literature.

Weerheijm [13–15] and EAPD [3, 7] criteria were mostly applied (Table 1). When considering only those 29 studies that used the Weerheijm/EAPD criteria, the average MIH prevalence was 16.5%, and the mean MIH prevalence – irrespective of the methodology used – was 16.4% (Table 1). The data from Asian studies can be found in Table 2. Here, 50 scientific reports were identified, which also revealed a heterogeneous prevalence between 0.5% and 52.9% when the Weerheijm/EAPD criteria were applied (Table 2); according to these 44 references, the mean MIH prevalence was 15.2%. In general, the overall MIH prevalence was 15.6% (Table 2). The studies from South America are listed in Table 3, and a total of 33 reports were identified. According to the Weerheijm/EAPD criteria, between 6.5% and 45.6% of the included children and adolescents were affected by MIH (Table 3); the average MIH prevalence was 16.6%. When considering all identified studies, the MIH prevalence was 16.7%. The data for North America (Table 4; 9 studies), Africa (Table 5; 6 studies), and Australia (Table 6; 2 studies) can be taken from the mentioned tables, and the mean prevalence rates of MIH were 27.5%, 11.4%, and 16.8%, respectively. It is striking that the mean frequency for North America was approximately 10% greater than the mean values for the other continents.

Table 1. Published MIH prevalence data from epidemiological studies in Europe between 2010 and 2023

Reference	Country	Age, years	Scoring index	Children, *N*	EH ≥1, %	MIH, %	M + IH, %
Wogelius et al. (2010) [27]	DNK	6–8	Weerheijm	647	-	37.3	-
Gomez et al. (2012) [28]	ESP	6–14	Weerheijm	505	-	17.9	-
Condo et al. (2012) [29]	ITA	0–14	n.r.	1,500	-	7.3	-
Balmer et al. (2012) [30]	GBR	12	mDDE	3,233	-	15.9	-
Heitmüller et al. (2013) [31]	DEU	10	EAPD	693	36.5	14.7	9.4
Robles et al. (2013) [32]	ESP	3–12	mDDE	1,414	-	45.9	-
Groselj and Jan (2013) [33]	SVN	6–11.5	EAPD	308	-	21.4	-
Jankovic et al. (2014) [34]	BIH	8	Weerheijm	141	18.4	12.8	-
Garcia-Margarit et al. (2014) [35]	ESP	8–9	EAPD	840	-	21.8	-
Petrou et al. (2014) [36]	DEU	7–10	EAPD	2,395	-	10.1	-
Kühnisch et al. (2014) [8]	DEU	10.2	EAPD	693	36.5	14.7	9.4
Wuollet et al. (2014) [37]	FIN	7–13	EAPD	818	-	17.1	-
Kevrekidou et al. (2015) [38]	GRC	8–9/13–14	EAPD	2,335	-	21.0	-
Opydo-Szymaczek and Gerreth (2015) [39]	POL	6–8/12–14	mDDE	225/245	-	25.7	12.6
Schmalfuss et al. (2016) [40]	NOR	16	EAPD	794	-	13.9	-
Wuollet et al. (2016) [41]	FIN	7–12	EAPD	287	-	11.5	6.3
Hysi et al. (2016) [42]	ALB	8–10	Weerheijm	1,575	-	14.0	-
Kühnisch et al. (2018) [9]	DEU	15	EAPD	1,302	40.2	17.2	9.8
Mulic et al. (2017) [43]	BIH	8–9	Weerheijm	103	-	11.7	-
Buchgraber et al. (2017) [44]	AUT	6–12	EAPD	1,111	-	7.0	5.8
Hernandez et al. (2018) [45]	ESP	6–14	EAPD	705	-	7.9	-
Negre-Barber et al. (2018) [46]	ESP	8–9	EAPD	414	-	24.2	-
Wuollet et al. (2018) [47]	FIN	8–13	EAPD	636	-	18.1	-
Glodkowska and Emerich (2019) [48]	POL	6–12	Weerheijm	1,437	-	6.4	-
Muratbegovic et al. (2020) [49]	BIH	6–9	Weerheijm	444	-	11.5	-
Amend et al. (2021) [50]	DEU	6–12	Wetzel&Reckel	2,103	-	?	-
Glodkowska and Emerich (2020) [51]	POL	6–12	EAPD	2,354	-	9.3	-
Abdelaziz et al. (2022) [52]	CHE	4–12	New system	32,142	7.5	6.6	-
Wogelius et al. (2020) [53]	DNK	9	Weerheijm	1,837	-	29.5	-
Jurlina et al. (2020) [54]	HRV	8	EAPD	729	-	13.0	-
Nisii et al. (2022) [55]	ITA	7–8	MIH-SSS	346	-	18.2	-
Grieshaber et al. (2023) [56]	CHE	7/13/16	EAPD	1,252	-	14.8	-
Vanhee et al. (2022) [57]	BEL	8–9.5	Ghanim et al.	290	-	18.6	-
Ilczuk-Rypula et al. (2022) [58]	POL	8–12	EAPD	613	-	6.2	-
Afzal et al. (2023) [59]	NOR	7–9	EAPD	3,013	-	28.2	-
Stoica et al. (2023) [60]	ROU	5–12	n.r.	87	-	40.2	-
Estivals et al. (2023) [61]	FRA	7–9	EAPD	856	-	18.7	-
Olczak-Kowalczyk et al. (2023) [62]	POL	18	MIH-TNI	1,611	-	0.6	-
Ciocan et al. (2023) [63]	ROU	8–11	EAPD	266	-	14.3	-
Mean					27.8	16.4	8.9

Table 2. Published MIH prevalence data from epidemiological studies in Asia between 2010 and 2023

Reference	Country	Age, years	Scoring index	Children, *N*	EH ≥1, %	MIH, %	M + IH, %
Ghanim et al. (2011) [64]	IRQ	7–9	EAPD	823	21.5	18.6	-
Zawaideh et al. (2011) [65]	JOR	7–9	EAPD	3,241	-	17.6	-
Ghanim et al. (2012) [66]	IRQ	7–9	EAPD	823	-	18.6	-
Parikh et al. (2012) [67]	IND	8–12	EAPD	1,366	-	9.2	-
Ahmadi et al. (2012) [68]	IRN	7–9	DDE	433	-	12.7	-
Ghanim et al. (2014) [69]	IRN	9–11	EAPD	810	-	20.2	-
Mittal et al. (2014) [70]	IND	6–9	EAPD	1,792	-	6.3	-
Sönmez et al. (2013) [71]	TUR	7–12	Weerheijm	4,018	-	7.7	-
Pitiphat et al. (2014) [72]	THA	6–7	EAPD	484	-	20.0	-
Shrestha et al. (2014) [73]	NPL	7–12	EAPD	749	-	13.7	-
Pitiphat et al. (2014) [74]	THA	7–8	EAPD	282	-	27.7	-
Allazzam et al. (2014) [75]	SAU	8–12	EAPD	267	-	8.6	-
Ng et al. (2015) [76]	SGP	7.7	EAPD	1,083	-	12.5	-
Mittal and Sharma (2015) [77]	IND	6–8	EAPD	978	-	7.4	-
Krishnan et al. (2015) [78]	IND	9–14	EAPD	4,989	-	7.7	-
Hussein et al. (2015) [79]	MYS	7–12	EAPD	154	-	16.9	-
Kirthiga et al. (2015) [80]	IND	11–16	Cho et al.	2,000	-	8.9	-
Mittal et al. (2016) [81]	IND	6–12	EAPD	886	-	7.1	-
Yannam et al. (2016) [82]	IND	8–12	EAPD	2,864	-	9.7	-
Ravindran and Saji (2016) [83]	IND	12–15	mDDE	2,500	-	32	-
Mishra and Pandey (2016) [84]	IND	8–12	Weerheijm	1,369	-	13.9	-
Subramaniam et al. (2016) [85]	IND	7–9	Weerheijm	2,500	-	0.5	-
Mittal (2016) [86]	IND	12–16	EAPD	1,726	13.2	9.8	-
Salem et al. (2016) [87]	IRN	6–13	EAPD	553	-	18.4	-
Hussain et al. (2018) [88]	ARE	8–12	EAPD	342	-	27.2	-
Rai et al. (2018) [89]	IND	7–9	mDDE	992	-	21.4	-
Saitoh et al. (2018) [90]	JPN	7–9	EAPD	4,496	-	19.8	-
Koruyucu et al. (2018) [91]	TUR	8–11	EAPD	1,511	-	14.2	-
Padavala and Sukumaran (2018) [92]	IND	7–12	EAPD	170	-	12.9	-
Ahmad et al. (2019) [93]	ARE	7–9	EAPD	779	-	7.6	-
Goswami et al. (2019) [94]	IND	6–12	EAPD	1,026	-	1.2	-
Rai et al. (2019) [95]	IND	9–12	EAPD	1,600	-	13.1	-
Kilinc et al. (2019) [96]	TUR	9–10	EAPD	1,237	-	11.5	-
Owlia et al. (2020) [97]	IRN	8–9	Weerheijm	606	-	52.9	-
Yi et al. (2021) [98]	CHN	12–15	EAPD	6,523	-	10.0	-
Elzein et al. (2020) [99]	LBN	7–9	Ghanim et al.	659	-	26.7	-
Emmatty et al. (2020) [100]	IND	8–15	EAPD	5,318	-	4.1	-
Thakur et al. (2020) [101]	IND	8–16	EAPD	2,000	-	2.9	-
Almuallem et al. (2022) [102]	SAU	8–12	EAPD	1,562	-	15.2	-
Mariam et al. (2022) [103]	IND	8–12	EAPD	3,176	-	11.7	-
Tarannum et al. (2021) [104]	IND	8–14	EAPD	2,250	-	2.1	-
Alhowaish et al. (2021) [105]	SAU	8–10	EAPD	893	-	40.5	-
Elzein et al. (2021) [106]	LBN	10–13	Ghanim et al.	682	-	22.9	-
Khanmohammadi et al. (2022) [107]	IRN	7–12	n.r.	1,028	-	25.6	-
Khan et al. (2022) [108]	IND	8–12	EAPD	2,300	-	4.0	-
Verma et al. (2022) [109]	IND	8–16	DDE	5,585	-	7.6	-
Berenstein Ajzman et al. (2023) [110]	ISR	3–13	EAPD	1,209	-	10.3	-
Al-Nerabieah et al. (2023) [111]	SYR	8–11	EAPD	1,138	-	39.9	-
Shah et al. (2023) [112]	IND	8–13	EAPD	3,000	-	9.5	-
Brejawi et al. (2023) [113]	ARE	7–9	Ghanim et al.	162	-	38.9	-
Mean					17.4	15.6	-

Table 3. Published MIH prevalence data of MIH from epidemiological studies in South America between 2010 and 2023

Reference	Country	Age, years	Scoring index	Children, *N*	EH ≥1, %	MIH, %	M + IH, %
Da Costa-Silva et al. (2010) [114]	BRA	6–12	EAPD	918	-	19.8	-
Biondi et al. (2011) [115]	ARG	11.3	DDE	1,098	-	15.9	-
Biondi et al. (2012) [116]	ARG	11.6	Weerheijm	975	-	6.5	-
Souza et al. (2012) [117]	BRA	6–12	EAPD	903	-	19.8	-
Souza et al. (2013) [118]	BRA	7–12	EAPD	1,151	-	12.3	-
Jeremias et al. (2013) [119]	BRA	6–12	EAPD	1,157	-	12.3	-
De Lima et al. (2015) [120]	BRA	11–14	EAPD	594	-	18.4	-
Dantas-Neta et al. (2016) [121]	BRA	11–14	EAPD	594	-	18.4	-
Tourino et al. (2016) [122]	BRA	8–9	EAPD	1,181	-	20.4	-
Figueiredo et al. (2017) [123]	BRA	9.6	EAPD	858	-	14.7	-
Reyes et al. (2019) [124]	BRA	8	EAPD	731	-	12.1	-
Raposo et al. (2019) [125]	BRA	8	MIH-SSS	631	-	16.1	-
Portella et al. (2019) [126]	BRA	8	EAPD	728	-	12.1	-
Mejia et al. (2019) [127]	COL	6–15	EAPD	1,075	-	11.2	-
Gambetta-Tessini et al. (2019) [128]	CHL	6–12	EAPD	577	-	15.8	-
Fatturi et al. (2020) [129]	BRA	8	Weerheijm	731	-	12.0	-
Laureano et al. (2020) [130]	BRA	8–10	Ghanim et al.	466	-	12.0	-
Argote Quispe et al. (2021) [131]	PER	7–10	mDDE	404	-	19.8	-
Bonzanini et al. (2021) [132]	BRA	11.6	EAPD	513	-	19.7	-
Rodriguez-Rodriguez et al. (2021) [133]	VEN	6–12	EAPD	142/121	-	25.4/25.6	-
Dourado et al. (2021) [134]	BRA	8–14	EAPD	246	-	46.6	-
Saldarriaga et al. (2021) [135]	COL	8–12	EAPD	77	-	14.4	-
Farias et al. (2021) [136]	BRA	8–10	Ghanim et al.	471	-	9.8	-
Freitas Fernandes et al. (2021) [137]	BRA	11–14	Ghanim et al.	463	-	10.8	-
Reis et al. (2021) [138]	BRA	8	EAPD	450	-	28.7	12.7
Fernandes et al. (2021) [139]	BRA	6–12	EAPD	610	-	9.8	-
Duarte et al. (2021) [140]	BRA	11–14	MIH-SSS	400	-	18	-
Damares Lago et al. (2022) [141]	BRA	6–12	Weerheijm	545	-	14.3	-
Quintero et al. (2022) [142]	COL	6–7	Ghanim et al.	450	-	25.1	-
Oreano et al. (2023) [143]	BRA	8–10	EAPD	1,342	-	7.7	-
Barros et al. (2023) [144]	BRA	8–9	EAPD	1,181	-	20.2	-
Vicioni-Marques et al. (2023) [145]	BRA	6–12	Ghanim et al.	1,830	-	16.9	-
Harz et al. (2023) [146]	CHL	6–12	EAPD	1,270	-	12.8	-
Mean						16.7	12.7

Discussion

According to the results of this scoping review, the average MIH prevalence was between 11.4% (Africa) and 27.5% (North America). The prevalence of MIH in Europe was 16.5%. The majority of epidemiological surveys reported prevalence rates between ~10 and ~20%. In principle, the reported EH/MIH prevalence rates are similar to the ~14% rate reported by Schwendicke et al. [164] in a comparable systematic review.

When interpreting the epidemiological data, it must be highlighted that the documented EH/MIH prevalence rates from the various studies must be assessed as heterogeneous. Prevalence rates of approximately 30–50% are not uncommon; therefore, further discussion is required. Differences between epidemiological study re-

Table 4. Published MIH prevalence data from epidemiological studies in North America between 2010 and 2023

Reference	Country	Age, years	Scoring index	Children, *N*	EH ≥1, %	MIH, %	M + IH, %
Gurrusquieta et al. (2017) [147]	MEX	6–12	EAPD	1,156	-	15.8	-
Villanueva-Gutierrez et al. (2019) [148]	MEX	8–12	EAPD	506	-	42.4	-
Gutierrez et al. (2019) [149]	MEX	8–10	EAPD	411	-	40.4	-
Davenport et al. (2019) [150]	USA	7–12	EAPD	375	-	9.6	-
Villanueva-Gutierrez et al. (2019) [151]	MEX	9.0	EAPD	686	-	35.4	-
Irigoyen-Camacho et al. (2020) [152]	MEX	6–8	EAPD	232	-	20.3	-
Irigoyen-Camacho et al. (2020) [152]	MEX	6–8	EAPD	317	-	31.9	-
Sidhu et al. (2020) [153]	CAN	n.r.	Ghanim et al.	233/429	-	12.4	5.6
Sosa-Soto et al. (2022) [154]	MEX	8	Ghanim et al.	613	-	12.4	-
Garcia-Perez et al. (2022) [155]	MEX	8–10	EAPD	663	-	38.6	-
Mean					-	25.9	5.6

Table 5. Published MIH prevalence data from epidemiological studies in Africa between 2010 and 2023

Reference	Country	Age, years	Scoring index	Children, *N*	EH ≥1, %	MIH, %	M + IH, %
Temilola et al. (2015) [156]	NGA	8–10	Kemoli et al.	236	-	9.7	-
Oyedele et al. (2015) [157]	NGA	8–10	EAPD	469	-	17.7	-
Saber et al. (2018) [158]	EGY	8–12	Ghanim et al.	1,001	-	2.3	-
Folayan et al. (2018) [159]	NGA	6–16	EAPD	853	7.6	2.9	-
Abdalla et al. (2021) [160]	SDN	8–11	EAPD	568	-	20.1	12.5
Arheiam et al. (2021) [161]	LBY	8–10	Ghanim et al.	1,047	-	15.5	-
Mean					7.6	11.4	12.5

Table 6. Published MIH prevalence data from epidemiological studies in Australia/Oceania between 2010 and 2023

Reference	Country	Age, years	Scoring index	Children, *N*	EH ≥1, %	MIH, %	M + IH, %
Mahoney and Morrison (2011) [162]	NZL	7–10	Weerheijm	234	-	18.8	-
Gambetta-Tessini et al. (2018) [163]	AUS	6–12	EAPD	327	26.9	14.7	-
Mean					26.9	16.8	-

sults can, in principle, be due to the selected study sample. Regional deviations or urban-rural differences are possible here. The sampling method – representative or convenient – is also likely to have a potential influence on the results obtained. Another aspect to be discussed is age. The EAPD consented during a workshop in Helsinki, Finland, a minimum age of 8 years for recording EH/

MIH to ensure complete eruption and thus the assessment of the first permanent molars and permanent incisors [26]. However, a fully correct diagnosis of EH/MIH in the permanent dentition can be made only after the age of 12 with regard to dental eruption status, as all permanent teeth except the third molars are typically present. The inclusion of 6- to 8-year olds is likely to lead to an underestimation of EH/MIH prevalence, as not all permanent index teeth have erupted and can, therefore, not be assessed at this age. With regard to the lack of new EH/MIH formations after tooth eruption, it should also be noted that there can no longer be an increase in prevalence after the age of 12.

In principle, heterogeneity with regard to EH/MIH prevalence is expected within a certain range. However, the documented extent of the range of results is surprising and appears to be difficult to explain in view of the points mentioned above. Therefore, some methodological considerations seem appropriate. First, the meaning of the selected indices should be discussed, as the registration of EH/MIH has been subject to methodological changes in recent decades. It should be emphasized at this point that the EAPD criteria for the detection and diagnosis of demarcated opacities, enamel breakdowns, and atypical restorations [3, 7, 13–15] have become established worldwide due to their simplicity, clarity, and potentially standardized clinical examinations. This dominance in epidemiological studies can be seen in Tables 1–6. The criteria enable an exact description of the clinical entity and have, therefore, been found to be increasingly accepted for clinical diagnostics in recent years, which in turn should have increased the comparability of studies. It might be of clinical – and less epidemiological – importance to note that the EAPD criteria do not distinguish between pre-eruptive defects and post-eruptive enamel breakdowns, do not differentiate between breakdowns restricted to enamel or dentine, and do not consider the marginal integrity or other characteristics of atypical restorations. Alternative indices, e.g., the MIH-TNI or MIH-SSS, have been developed. The DDE/mDDE index [10–12] is currently used only sporadically. However, more recently published diagnostic systems, such as the MIH-TNI or MIH-SSS, have been used only rarely in epidemiological trials so far. Another aspect to be discussed is the diagnosis of MIH using index teeth. According to the definition of the EAPD, the diagnosis can be made only if signs of EH are found in at least one first permanent molar [3, 7]. The use of index teeth is not entirely unproblematic, as this procedure deviates from standard caries epidemiological practice. Here, individuals affected by caries are always identified independently of index teeth. In addition, the determination of the various phenotypes, e.g., DMH, HSPM, hypomineralisation on other permanent teeth, MIH, or M + IH, is considered challenging even for experienced epidemiologists, as this requires the complete documentation of EH in the entire dentition during clinical examination to analyze the respective index teeth and their findings later during statistical data exploration. Sometimes, for the sake of simplicity, only the index teeth are assessed in the surveys, which prevents further analyses. In some cases, the MIH prevalence was determined only by a yes/no decision in the course of the clinical examination. However, these methodological aspects should not lead to any serious deviations in prevalence.

Furthermore, the terminology potentially makes it difficult to precisely determine MIH in studies. This can be illustrated simply by the term "molar incisor hypomineralisation," as this suggests that EH must be present in both permanent molars and incisors. In fact, however, MIH is diagnosed only if at least one first permanent molar is affected [3, 7]. Nevertheless, M + IH has been reported in a few studies (Tables 1, 4, and 5) and is a subset of the MIH group. If the group of individuals with at least one EH in the permanent dentition – independent of index teeth – is determined (EH ≥ 1), this group size is usually substantially larger – sometimes by a factor of 2 – than the MIH group size [8, 9, 165]. Based on the documented approaches and phenotypes for recording EH/MIH prevalence in permanent dentition, e.g., EH ≥1, MIH, and M + IH, it appears to be clear what influence the correct application of the index teeth has on the determination of MIH prevalence. Therefore, at this point, the clinical appearance of EH should be detected using the EAPD criteria, and the prevalence of MIH should be determined using the phenotypes EH ≥1, MIH, and M + IH with the above-described index teeth.

At this point, the importance of careful differential diagnosis should also be emphasized, as this method is sometimes not always clinically easy when differentiating between caries and EH. This applies in particular to permanent molars and enamel breakdown. To avoid distortions in the results, both entities must be strictly separated from each other in epidemiological studies. Ideally, the study design should allow caries and EH to be recorded separately using the established standard criteria. This approach ultimately also enables valid comparisons between the joint occurrence of both diseases.

This scoping review has several limitations. With respect to limited resources, we systematically searched only one database and did not include a second independent researcher to countercheck the identified publications. Furthermore, we did not assess the quality, including the risk of bias, for each included report, and we were unable to perform a meta-analysis. This could be a crucial weakness of this study.

Conclusions

According to this scoping review, it can be concluded that MIH is a prevalent condition in children and adolescents worldwide. While the majority of epidemiological surveys documented prevalence rates between ~10 and ~20%, several author groups published significantly greater proportions. With the aim of standardizing and generating comparable examination data in epidemiological studies, the use of the established EAPD criteria for the detection of EH appears to be valuable. Since the determination of MIH prevalence depends on the correct use of the index teeth, their application according to the definitions must be meticulously observed. It is also recommended that possible MIH phenotypes (EH ≥1, MIH, and M + IH) should be reported in future epidemiological studies.

Statement of Ethics

For this type of study, no ethical approval and no informed consent were needed.

Conflict of Interest Statement

The authors declare that they have no conflicts of interest.

Funding Sources

The study received no funding.

Author Contributions

Jan Kühnisch: conceptualization and study design; Karl-Ferdinand Fresen: search of the literature; Karl-Ferdinand Fresen: data management; Jan Kühnisch and Karl-Ferdinand Fresen: writing – original draft; Jan Kühnisch and Karl-Ferdinand Fresen: writing – review and editing.

References

1 Crombie F, Manton D, Kilpatrick N. Aetiology of molar-incisor hypomineralization: a critical review. Int J Paediatr Dent. 2009;19:73–83.
2 Alaluusua S. Aetiology of molar-incisor hypomineralisation: a systematic review. Eur Arch Paediatr Dent. 2010; 11:53–8.
3 Lygidakis NA, Wong F, Jälevik B, Vierrou AM, Alaluusua S, Espelid I. Best clinical practice guidance for clinicians dealing with children presenting with molar-incisor-hypomineralisation (MIH): an EAPD policy document. Eur Arch Paediatr Dent. 2010;11:75–81.
4 Silva MJ, Scurrah KJ, Craig JM, Manton DJ, Kilpatrick N. Etiology of molar incisor hypomineralization – a systematic review. Community Dent Oral Epidemiol. 2016;44:342–53.
5 Fatturi AL, Wambier LM, Chibinski AC, Assunção L, Brancher JA, Reis A, et al. A systematic review and meta-analysis of systemic exposure associated with molar incisor hypomineralization. Community Dent Oral Epidemiol. 2019;47:407–15.
6 Vieira AR, Manton DJ. On the variable clinical presentation of molar-incisor hypomineralization. Caries Res. 2019; 53:482–8.
7 Lygidakis NA, Garot E, Somani C, Taylor GD, Rouas P, Wong FSL. Best clinical practice guidance for clinicians dealing with children presenting with molar-incisor-hypomineralisation (MIH): an updated European Academy of Paediatric Dentistry policy document. Eur Arch Paediatr Dent. 2022;23:3–21.
8 Kühnisch J, Heitmüller D, Thiering E, Brockow I, Hoffmann U, Neumann C, et al: Proportion and extent of manifestation of molar-incisor-hypomineralizations according to different phenotypes. J Public Health Dent. 2014;74:42–9.
9 Kühnisch J, Kabary L, Malyk Y, Rothmaier K, Metz I, Hickel R, et al. Relationship between caries experience and demarcated hypomineralised lesions (including MIH) in the permanent dentition of 15-year-olds. Clin Oral Investig. 2018;22:2013–9.
10 An epidemiological index of developmental defects of dental enamel (DDE Index). Commission on Oral Health, Research and Epidemiology. Int Dent J. 1982;32:159–67.
11 Clarkson J, O'Mullane D. A modified DDE Index for use in epidemiological studies of enamel defects. J Dent Res. 1989;68:445–50.
12 A review of the developmental defects of enamel index (DDE Index). Commission on Oral Health, Research & Epidemiology. Report of an FDI Working Group. Int Dent J. 1992;42:411–26.
13 Weerheijm KL, Jälevik B, Alaluusua S. Molar-incisor hypomineralisation. Caries Res. 2001;35:390–1.
14 Weerheijm KL, Duggal M, Mejàre I, Papagiannoulis L, Koch G, Martens LC, et al. Judgement criteria for molar incisor hypomineralisation (MIH) in epidemiologic studies: a summary of the European meeting on MIH held in Athens, 2003. Eur J Paediatr Dent. 2003;4:110–3.
15 Weerheijm KL, Mejàre I. Molar incisor hypomineralization: a questionnaire inventory of its occurrence in member countries of the European Academy of Paediatric Dentistry (EAPD). Int J Paediatr Dent. 2003;13:411–6.
16 Ghanim A, Elfrink M, Weerheijm K, Mariño R, Manton D. A practical method for use in epidemiological studies on enamel hypomineralisation. Eur Arch Paediatr Dent. 2015;16:235–46.
17 Steffen R, Krämer N, Bekes K. The Würzburg MIH concept: the MIH treatment need index (MIH TNI): a new index to assess and plan treatment in patients with molar incisor hypomineralisation (MIH). Eur Arch Paediatr Dent. 2017;18:355–61.
18 Bekes K, Steffen R, Krämer N. Update of the molar incisor hypomineralization: Würzburg concept. Eur Arch Paediatr Dent. 2023;24:807–13.
19 Elfrink ME, Veerkamp JS, Aartman IH, Moll HA, Ten Cate JM. Validity of scoring caries and primary molar hypomineralization (DMH) on intraoral photographs. Eur Arch Paediatr Dent. 2009; 10(suppl 1):5–10.
20 Elfrink ME, ten Cate JM, Jaddoe VW, Hofman A, Moll HA, Veerkamp JS. Deciduous molar hypomineralization and molar incisor hypomineralization. J Dent Res. 2012;91:551–5.
21 Elfrink ME, Schuller AA, Weerheijm KL, Veerkamp JS. Hypomineralized second primary molars: prevalence data in Dutch 5-year-olds. Caries Res. 2008; 42:282–5.
22 Ghanim A, Manton D, Mariño R, Morgan M, Bailey D. Prevalence of demarcated hypomineralisation defects in second primary molars in Iraqi children. Int J Paediatr Dent. 2013;23:48–55.
23 Cabral RN, Nyvad B, Soviero VLVM, Freitas E, Leal SC. Reliability and validity of a new classification of MIH based on severity. Clin Oral Investig. 2020 Feb;24(2):727–34.
24 Kevrekidou A, Kosma I, Kotsanos I, Arapostathis KN, Kotsanos N. Enamel opacities in all other than Molar Incisor Hypomineralisation index teeth of adolescents. Int J Paediatr Dent. 2021 Mar;31(2):270–7.
25 Tricco, AC, Lillie, E, Zarin, W, O'Brien, KK, Colquhoun, H, Levac, D, et al. PRISMA extension for scoping reviews (PRISMA-ScR): checklist and explanation. Ann Intern Med. 2018;169(7):467–73.
26 Jälevik B. Prevalence and diagnosis of molar-incisor- hypomineralisation (MIH): a systematic review. Eur Arch Paediatr Dent. 2010 Apr;11(2):59–64.
27 Wogelius P, Haubek D, Nechifor A, Norgaard M, Tvedebrink T, Poulsen S. Association between use of asthma drugs and prevalence of demarcated opacities in permanent first molars in 6-to-8-year-old Danish children. Community Dent Oral Epidemiol. 2010;38:145–51.
28 Martinez Gomez TP, Guinot Jimeno F, Bellet Dalmau LJ, Tarrida LG. Prevalence of molar-incisor hypomineralisation observed using transillumination in a group of children from Barcelona (Spain). Int J Paediatr Dent. 2012;22: 100–9.
29 Condo R, Perugia C, Maturo P, Docimo R. MIH: epidemiologic clinic study in paediatric patient. Oral Implantol. 2012;5:58–69.
30 Balmer R, Toumba J, Godson J, Duggal M. The prevalence of molar incisor hypomineralisation in Northern England and its relationship to socioeconomic status and water fluoridation. Int J Paediatr Dent. 2012;22:250–7.
31 Heitmüller D, Thiering E, Hoffmann U, Heinrich J, Manton D, Kühnisch J, et al. Is there a positive relationship between molar incisor hypomineralisations and the presence of dental caries? Int J Paediatr Dent. 2013;23:116–24.

32 Robles MJ, Ruiz M, Bravo-Perez M, Gonzalez E, Penalver MA. Prevalence of enamel defects in primary and permanent teeth in a group of schoolchildren from Granada (Spain). Med Oral Patol Oral Cir Bucal. 2013;18:e187–93.
33 Groselj M, Jan J. Molar incisor hypomineralisation and dental caries among children in Slovenia. Eur J Paediatr Dent. 2013;14:241–5.
34 Jankovic S, Ivanovic M, Davidovic B, Lecic J. Distribution and characteristics of molar-incisor hypomineralization. Vojnosanit Pregl. 2014;71:730–4.
35 Garcia-Margarit M, Catala-Pizarro M, Montiel-Company JM, Almerich-Silla JM: Epidemiologic study of molar-incisor hypomineralization in 8-year-old Spanish children. Int J Paediatr Dent. 2014;24:14–22.
36 Petrou MA, Giraki M, Bissar AR, Basner R, Wempe C, Altarabulsi MB, et al. Prevalence of Molar-Incisor-Hypomineralisation among school children in four German cities. Int J Paediatr Dent. 2014;24:434–40.
37 Wuollet E, Laisi S, Salmela E, Ess A, Alaluusua S. Background factors of molar-incisor hypomineralization in a group of Finnish children. Acta Odontol Scand. 2014;72:963–9.
38 Kevrekidou A, Kosma I, Arapostathis K, Kotsanos N. Molar incisor hypomineralization of eight- and 14-year-old children: prevalence, severity, and defect characteristics. Pediatr Dent. 2015;37: 455–61.
39 Opydo-Szymaczek J, Gerreth K. Developmental enamel defects of the permanent first molars and incisors and their association with dental caries in the region of Wielkopolska, Western Poland. Oral Health Prev Dent. 2015;13:461–9.
40 Schmalfuss A, Stenhagen KR, Tveit AB, Crossner CG, Espelid I. Canines are affected in 16-year-olds with molar-incisor hypomineralisation (MIH): an epidemiological study based on the Tromso study: "Fit Futures". Eur Arch Paediatr Dent. 2016;17:107–13.
41 Wuollet E, Laisi S, Salmela E, Ess A, Alaluusua S. Molar-incisor hypomineralization and the association with childhood illnesses and antibiotics in a group of Finnish children. Acta Odontol Scand. 2016;74:416–22.
42 Hysi D, Kuscu OO, Droboniku E, Toti C, Xhemnica L, Caglar E. Prevalence and aetiology of Molar-Incisor Hypomineralisation among children aged 8–10 years in Tirana, Albania. Eur J Paediatr Dent. 2016;17:75–9.
43 Mulic A, Cehajic E, Tveit AB, Stenhagen KR. How serious is Molar Incisor Hypomineralisation (MIH) among 8- and 9-year-old children in Bosnia-Herzegovina? A clinical study. Eur J Paediatr Dent. 2017;18:153–7.
44 Buchgraber B, Kqiku L, Ebeleseder KA. Molar incisor hypomineralization: proportion and severity in primary public school children in Graz, Austria. Clin Oral Investig. 2018;22:757–62.
45 Hernandez M, Boj JR, Espasa E, Peretz B. First permanent molars and permanent incisors teeth by tooth prevalence of molar-incisor-hypomineralisation in a group of Spanish schoolchildren. Acta Stomatol Croat 2018;52:4–11.
46 Negre-Barber A, Montiel-Company JM, Catala-Pizarro M, Almerich-Silla JM. Degree of severity of molar incisor hypomineralization and its relation to dental caries. Sci Rep. 2018;8:1248.
47 Wuollet E, Laisi S, Alaluusua S, Waltimo-Siren J. The association between molar-incisor hypomineralization and dental caries with socioeconomic status as an explanatory variable in a group of Finnish children. Int J Environ Res Public Health. 2018;15:1324.
48 Glodkowska N, Emerich K. Molar Incisor Hypomineralization: prevalence and severity among children from Nothern Poland. Eur J Paediatr Dent. 2019;20: 59–66.
49 Arslanagic-Muratbegovic A, Markovic N, Zukanovic A, Tiro A, Dzemidzic V. Molar Incisor Hypomineralization: prevalence and severity in six to nine-year-old Sarajevo children. Eur J Paediatr Dent. 2020;21:243–7.
50 Amend S, Nossol C, Bausback-Schomakers S, Wleklinski C, Scheibelhut C, Pons-Kuhnemann J, et al: Prevalence of molar-incisor-hypomineralisation (MIH) among 6–12-year-old children in Central Hesse (Germany). Clin Oral Investig. 2021;25:2093–100.
51 Glodkowska N, Emerich K. The impact of environmental air pollution on the prevalence of molar incisor hypomineralization in schoolchildren: a cross-sectional study. Adv Clin Exp Med. 2020; 29:1469–77.
52 Abdelaziz M, Krejci I, Banon J. Prevalence of molar incisor hypomineralization in over 30,000 schoolchildren in Switzerland. J Clin Pediatr Dent. 2022; 46:1–5.
53 Wogelius P, Viuff JH, Haubek D. Use of asthma drugs and prevalence of molar incisor hypomineralization. Int J Paediatr Dent. 2020;30:734–40.
54 Jurlina D, Uzarevic Z, Ivanisevic Z, Matijevic N, Matijevic M. Prevalence of molar-incisor hypomineralization and caries in eight-year-old children in Croatia. Int J Environ Res Public Health. 2020;17:6358.
55 Nisii F, Mazur M, De Nuccio C, Martucci C, Spuntarelli M, Labozzetta S, et al. Prevalence of molar incisor hypomineralization among school children in Rome, Italy. Sci Rep. 2022;12:7343.
56 Grieshaber A, Waltimo T, Haschemi AA, Erb J, Steffen R, Bornstein MM, et al. Prevalence of and factors associated with molar-incisor hypomineralisation in schoolchildren in the canton of Basel-Landschaft, Switzerland. Clin Oral Investig. 2023;27:871–7.
57 Vanhee T, Poncelet J, Cheikh-Ali S, Bottenberg P. Prevalence, caries, dental anxiety and quality of life in children with MIH in Brussels, Belgium. J Clin Med. 2022;11:3065.
58 Ilczuk-Rypula D, Zalewska M, Pietraszewska D, Dybek A, Nitecka-Buchta A, Postek-Stefanska L. Prevalence and possible etiological factors of molar-incisor hypomineralization (MIH) in population of Silesian children in Poland: a pilot retrospective cohort study. Int J Environ Res Public Health. 2022;19: 8697.
59 Haque Afzal S, Wigen TI, Skaare AB, Brusevold IJ. Molar-incisor hypomineralisation in Norwegian children: prevalence and associated factors. Eur J Oral Sci. 2023;131:e12930.
60 Stoica SN, Nimigean V, Moraru SA, Sirbu I, Nimigean VR. A clinical and statistical study on enamel hypomineralization of the first permanent molar in the period of mixed dentition. Rom J Morphol Embryol. 2023;64:241–9.
61 Estivals J, Fahd C, Baillet J, Rouas P, Manton DJ, Garot E. The prevalence and characteristics of and the association between MIH and HSPM in South-Western France. Int J Paediatr Dent. 2023;33:298–304.

62 Olczak-Kowalczyk D, Krämer N, Gozdowski D, Turska-Szybka A. Developmental enamel defects and their relationship with caries in adolescents aged 18 years. Sci Rep. 2023;13:4932.
63 Ciocan B, Sandulescu M, Luca R. Real-world evidence on the prevalence of molar incisor hypomineralization in school children from Bucharest, Romania. Children (Basel). 2023;10:1563.
64 Ghanim A, Morgan M, Marino R, Bailey D, Manton D. Molar-incisor hypomineralisation: prevalence and defect characteristics in Iraqi children. Int J Paediatr Dent. 2011;21:413–21.
65 Zawaideh FI, Al-Jundi SH, Al-Jaljoli MH. Molar incisor hypomineralisation: prevalence in Jordanian children and clinical characteristics. Eur Arch Paediatr Dent. 2011;12:31–36.
66 Ghanim AM, Manton DJ, Morgan MV, Marino RJ, Bailey DL. Trends of oral health care and dental treatment needs in relation to molar incisor hypomineralisation defects: a study amongst a group of Iraqi schoolchildren. Eur Arch Paediatr Dent. 2012;13:171–8.
67 Parikh DR, Ganesh M, Bhaskar V. Prevalence and characteristics of Molar Incisor Hypomineralisation (MIH) in the child population residing in Gandhinagar, Gujarat, India. Eur Arch Paediatr Dent. 2012;13:21–6.
68 Ahmadi R, Ramazani N, Nourinasab R. Molar incisor hypomineralization: a study of prevalence and etiology in a group of Iranian children. Iran J Pediatr. 2012;22:245–51.
69 Ghanim A, Bagheri R, Golkari A, Manton D. Molar-incisor hypomineralisation: a prevalence study amongst primary schoolchildren of Shiraz, Iran. Eur Arch Paediatr Dent. 2014;15:75–82.
70 Mittal NP, Goyal A, Gauba K, Kapur A: Molar incisor hypomineralisation: prevalence and clinical presentation in school children of the northern region of India. Eur Arch Paediatr Dent. 2014;15:11–8.
71 Sönmez H, Yildirim G, Bezgin T. Putative factors associated with molar incisor hypomineralisation: an epidemiological study. Eur Arch Paediatr Dent. 2013;14:375–80.
72 Pitiphat W, Savisit R, Chansamak N, Subarnbhesaj A. Molar incisor hypomineralization and dental caries in six- to seven-year-old Thai children. Pediatr Dent. 2014;36:478–82.
73 Shrestha R, Upadhaya S, Bajracharya M. Prevalence of molar incisor hypomineralisation among school children in Kavre. Kathmandu Univ Med J (KUMJ). 2014;12:38–42.
74 Pitiphat W, Luangchaichaweng S, Pungchanchaikul P, Angwaravong O, Chansamak N. Factors associated with molar incisor hypomineralization in Thai children. Eur J Oral Sci. 2014;122:265–70.
75 Allazzam SM, Alaki SM, El Meligy OA. Molar incisor hypomineralization, prevalence, and etiology. Int J Dent. 2014;2014:234508.
76 Ng JJ, Eu OC, Nair R, Hong CH. Prevalence of molar incisor hypomineralization (MIH) in Singaporean children. Int J Paediatr Dent. 2015;25:73–8.
77 Mittal N, Sharma BB. Hypomineralised second primary molars: prevalence, defect characteristics and possible association with molar incisor hypomineralisation in Indian children. Eur Arch Paediatr Dent. 2015;16:441–7.
78 Krishnan R, Ramesh M, Chalakkal P. Prevalence and characteristics of MIH in school children residing in an endemic fluorosis area of India: an epidemiological study. Eur Arch Paediatr Dent. 2015;16:455–60.
79 Hussein AS, Faisal M, Haron M, Ghanim AM, Abu-Hassan MI. Distribution of molar incisor hypomineralization in Malaysian children attending university dental clinic. J Clin Pediatr Dent. 2015;39:219–23.
80 Kirthiga M, Poornima P, Praveen R, Gayathri P, Manju M, Priya M. Prevalence and severity of molar incisor hypomineralization in children aged 11–16 years of a city in Karnataka, Davangere. J Indian Soc Pedod Prev Dent. 2015;33:213–7.
81 Mittal R, Chandak S, Chandwani M, Singh P, Pimpale J. Assessment of association between molar incisor hypomineralization and hypomineralized second primary molar. J Int Soc Prev Community Dent. 2016;6:34–9.
82 Yannam SD, Amarlal D, Rekha CV. Prevalence of molar incisor hypomineralization in school children aged 8–12 years in Chennai. J Indian Soc Pedod Prev Dent. 2016;34:134–8.
83 Ravindran R, Saji AM. Prevalence of the developmental defects of the enamel in children aged 12–15 years in Kollam district. J Int Soc Prev Community Dent. 2016;6:28–33.
84 Mishra A, Pandey RK. Molar incisor hypomineralization: an epidemiological study with prevalence and etiological factors in Indian pediatric population. Int J Clin Pediatr Dent. 2016;9:167–71.
85 Subramaniam P, Gupta T, Sharma A. Prevalence of molar incisor hypomineralization in 7–9-year-old children of Bengaluru City, India. Contemp Clin Dent. 2016;7:11–5.
86 Mittal N. Phenotypes of enamel hypomineralization and molar incisor hypomineralization in permanent dentition: identification, quantification and proposal for classification. J Clin Pediatr Dent. 2016;40:367–74.
87 Salem K, Aziz D, Asadi M. Prevalence and predictors of Molar Incisor Hypomineralization (MIH) among rural children in Northern Iran. Iran J Public Health. 2016;45:1528–30.
88 Hussain G, Al-Halabi M, Kowash M, Hassan A. The prevalence and severity of molar incisor hypomineralization and molar hypomineralization in Dubai, UAE. J Dent Child (Chic). 2018;85:102–7.
89 Rai A, Singh A, Menon I, Singh J, Rai V, Aswal GS. Molar incisor hypomineralization: prevalence and risk factors among 7–9 years old school children in Muradnagar, Ghaziabad. Open Dent J. 2018;12:714–22.
90 Saitoh M, Nakamura Y, Hanasaki M, Saitoh I, Murai Y, Kurashige Y, et al. Prevalence of molar incisor hypomineralization and regional differences throughout Japan. Environ Health Prev Med. 2018;23:55.
91 Koruyucu M, Ozel S, Tuna EB. Prevalence and etiology of molar-incisor hypomineralization (MIH) in the city of Istanbul. J Dent Sci. 2018;13:318–28.
92 Padavala S, Sukumaran G. Molar incisor hypomineralization and its prevalence. Contemp Clin Dent. 2018;9:S246–50.
93 Ahmad SH, Petrou MA, Alhumrani A, Hashim R, Splieth C. Prevalence of molar-incisor hypomineralisation in an emerging community, and a possible correlation with caries, fluorosis and socioeconomic status. Oral Health Prev Dent. 2019;17:323–7.
94 Goswami M, Bhushan U, Pandiyan R, Sharma S. Molar incisor hypomineralization-an emerging burden: a short study on prevalence and clinical characteristics in Central Delhi, India. Int J Clin Pediatr Dent. 2019;12:211–4.

95 Rai PM, Jain J, Raju AS, Nair RA, Shashidhar K, Dsouza S. Prevalence of molar incisor hypomineralization among school children aged 9 to 12 years in Virajpet, Karnataka, India. Open Access Maced J Med Sci. 2019;7: 1042–6.

96 Kilinc G, Cetin M, Kose B, Ellidokuz H. Prevalence, aetiology, and treatment of molar incisor hypomineralization in children living in Izmir City (Turkey). Int J Paediatr Dent. 2019;29:775–82.

97 Owlia F, Akhavan-Karbassi MH, Rahimi R. Could molar-incisor hypomineralization (MIH) existence be predictor of short stature? Int J Prev Med. 2020;11:101.

98 Yi X, Chen W, Liu M, Zhang H, Hou W, Wang Y. Prevalence of MIH in children aged 12 to 15 years in Beijing, China. Clin Oral Investig. 2021;25:355–61.

99 Elzein R, Chouery E, Abdel-Sater F, Bacho R, Ayoub F. Molar incisor hypomineralisation in Lebanon: prevalence and clinical characteristics. Eur Arch Paediatr Dent. 2020;21:609–16.

100 Emmatty TB, Eby A, Joseph MJ, Bijimole J, Kavita K, Asif I. The prevalence of molar incisor hypomineralization of school children in and around Muvattupuzha, Kerala. J Indian Soc Pedod Prev Dent. 2020;38:14–9.

101 Thakur H, Kaur A, Singh N, Singh R, Kumar S. Prevalence and clinical characteristics of molar-incisor hypomineralization in 8–16-year-old children in industrial town of Solan District of Himachal Pradesh. Int J Clin Pediatr Dent. 2020;13:230–4.

102 Almuallem Z, Alsuhaim A, Alqudayri A, Aljarid S, Mousa Alotaibi M, Alkraida R, et al. Prevalence and possible aetiological factors of molar incisor hypomineralisation in Saudi children: a cross-sectional study. Saudi Dent J. 2022;34:36–44.

103 Mariam S, Goyal A, Dhareula A, Gauba K, Bhatia SK, Kapur A. A case-controlled investigation of risk factors associated with molar incisor hypomineralization (MIH) in 8–12 year-old children living in Chandigarh, India. Eur Arch Paediatr Dent. 2022;23:97–107.

104 Tarannum, Ravichandra KS, Muppa R, Srikanth K, Kantipudi MJ, Ram KC. Molar incisor hypomineralization prevalence in the schoolchildren of Gannavaram Mandal, Krishna District, Andhra Pradesh, India: a cross-sectional study. Int J Clin Pediatr Dent. 2021;14:737–40.

105 Alhowaish L, Baidas L, Aldhubaiban M, Bello LL, Al-Hammad N. Etiology of molar-incisor hypomineralization (MIH): a cross-sectional study of Saudi children. Children (Basel). 2021;8:466.

106 Elzein R, Chouery E, Abdel-Sater F, Bacho R, Ayoub F. Relation between molar-incisor hypomineralization (MIH) occurrence and war pollutants in bombarded regions: epidemiological pilot study in Lebanon. Niger J Clin Pract. 2021;24:1808–13.

107 Khanmohammadi R, Seraj B, Salari A, Alipour F. Etiological factors involved in molar-incisor hypomineralization in 7 to 12-year-old children in Tehran. Front Dent. 2022;19:16.

108 Khan A, Garg N, Mayall SS, Pathivada L, Kaur H, Yeluri R. Prevalence, pattern, and severity of molar incisor hypomineralization in 8–12-year-old schoolchildren of Moradabad City. Int J Clin Pediatr Dent. 2022;15:168–74.

109 Verma S, Dhinsa K, Tripathi AM, Saha S, Yadav G, Arora D. Molar incisor hypomineralization: prevalence, associated risk factors, its relation with dental caries and various enamel surface defects in 8–16-year-old schoolchildren of Lucknow District. Int J Clin Pediatr Dent. 2022;15:1–8.

110 Berenstein Ajzman G, Dagon N, Iraqi R, Blumer S, Fadela S. The prevalence of developmental enamel defects in Israeli children and its association with perinatal conditions: a cross-sectional study. Children (Basel). 2023;10:903.

111 Al-Nerabieah Z, AlKhouli M, Dashash M. Prevalence and clinical characteristics of molar-incisor hypomineralization in Syrian children: a cross-sectional study. Sci Rep. 2023;13:8582.

112 Shah VU, Dave BH, Chari DN, Shah KA: Prevalence, severity and associated risk indicators of molar incisor hypomineralization amongst 8–13-year-old children of Vadodara District Gujarat: a cross-sectional study. Int J Clin Pediatr Dent. 2023;16: 280–6.

113 Brejawi MS, Venkiteswaran A, Ergieg SM, Sabri B. Prevalence and severity of Molar-Incisor Hypomineralisation in children in Fujairah, United Arab Emirates. Eur J Paediatr Dent. 2023; 24:139–43.

114 da Costa-Silva CM, Jeremias F, de Souza JF, Cordeiro Rde C, Santos-Pinto L, Zuanon AC. Molar incisor hypomineralization: prevalence, severity and clinical consequences in Brazilian children. Int J Paediatr Dent. 2010;20: 426–34.

115 Biondi AM, Cortese SG, Martinez K, Ortolani AM, Sebelli PM, Ienco M, et al. Prevalence of molar incisor hypomineralization in the city of Buenos Aires. Acta Odontol Latinoam. 2011; 24:81–5.

116 Biondi AM, Lopez Jordi Mdel C, Cortese SG, Alvarez L, Salveraglio I, Ortolani AM. Prevalence of molar-incisor hypomineralization (MIH) in children seeking dental care at the Schools of Dentistry of the University of Buenos Aires (Argentina) and University of la Republica (Uruguay). Acta Odontol Latinoam. 2012;25:224–30.

117 Souza JF, Costa-Silva CM, Jeremias F, Santos-Pinto L, Zuanon AC, Cordeiro RC. Molar incisor hypomineralisation: possible aetiological factors in children from urban and rural areas. Eur Arch Paediatr Dent. 2012;13:164–70.

118 Souza JF, Jeremias F, Costa-Silva CM, Santos-Pinto L, Zuanon AC, Cordeiro RC. Aetiology of molar-incisor hypomineralisation (MIH) in Brazilian children. Eur Arch Paediatr Dent. 2013; 14:233–8.

119 Jeremias F, de Souza JF, Silva CM, Cordeiro Rde C, Zuanon AC, Santos-Pinto L. Dental caries experience and Molar-Incisor Hypomineralization. Acta Odontol Scand. 2013;71:870–6.

120 de Lima Mde D, Andrade MJ, Dantas-Neta NB, Andrade NS, Teixeira RJ, de Moura MS, et al. Epidemiologic study of molar-incisor hypomineralization in schoolchildren in North-eastern Brazil. Pediatr Dent. 2015;37:513–9.

121 Dantas-Neta NB, Moura LF, Cruz PF, Moura MS, Paiva SM, Martins CC, et al. Impact of molar-incisor hypomineralization on oral health-related quality of life in schoolchildren. Braz Oral Res. 2016;30:e117.

122 Tourino LF, Correa-Faria P, Ferreira RC, Bendo CB, Zarzar PM, Vale MP. Association between molar incisor hypomineralization in schoolchildren and both prenatal and postnatal factors: a population-based study. PLoS One. 2016;11:e0156332.

123 da Silva Figueiredo Se MJ, Ribeiro APD, dos Santos-Pinto LAM, de Cassia Loiola Cordeiro R, Cabral RN, Leal SC. Are hypomineralized primary molars and canines associated with molar-incisor hypomineralization? Pediatr Dent. 2017;39:217–21.

124 Reyes MRT, Fatturi AL, Menezes J, Fraiz FC, Assuncao L, Souza JF. Demarcated opacity in primary teeth increases the prevalence of molar incisor hypomineralization. Braz Oral Res. 2019;33:e048.

125 Raposo F, de Carvalho Rodrigues AC, Lia EN, Leal SC. Prevalence of hypersensitivity in teeth affected by molar-incisor hypomineralization (MIH). Caries Res. 2019;53:424–30.

126 Portella PD, Menoncin BLV, de Souza JF, de Menezes J, Fraiz FC, Assuncao L. Impact of molar incisor hypomineralization on quality of life in children with early mixed dentition: a hierarchical approach. Int J Paediatr Dent. 2019;29:496–506.

127 Mejia JD, Restrepo M, Gonzalez S, Alvarez LG, Santos-Pinto L, Escobar A. Molar incisor hypomineralization in Colombia: prevalence, severity and associated risk factors. J Clin Pediatr Dent. 2019;43:185–9.

128 Gambetta-Tessini K, Marino R, Ghanim A, Calache H, Manton DJ. The impact of MIH/HSPM on the carious lesion severity of schoolchildren from Talca, Chile. Eur Arch Paediatr Dent. 2019;20:417–23.

129 Fatturi AL, Menoncin BL, Reyes MT, Meger M, Scariot R, Brancher JA, et al. The relationship between molar incisor hypomineralization, dental caries, socioeconomic factors, and polymorphisms in the vitamin D receptor gene: a population-based study. Clin Oral Investig. 2020;24:3971–80.

130 Laureano ICC, Farias L, Fernandes LHF, Alencar CRB, Forte FDS, Honorio DR, et al. Dental fear in children: association with dental caries and molar incisor hypomineralization. Braz Dent J. 2020;31:673–9.

131 Argote Quispe DM, de Priego GPM, Leon Manco RA, Portaro CP. Molar incisor hypomineralization: prevalence and severity in schoolchildren of Puno, Peru. J Indian Soc Pedod Prev Dent. 2021;39:246–50.

132 Bonzanini LIL, Arduim ADS, Lenzi TL, Hugo FN, Hilgert JB, Casagrande L. Molar-incisor hypomineralization and dental caries: a hierarchical approach in a populational-based study. Braz Dent J. 2021;32:74–82.

133 Rodriguez-Rodriguez M, Carrasco-Colmenares W, Ghanim A, Natera A, Acosta-Camargo MG. Prevalence and distribution of molar incisor hypomineralization in children receiving dental care in Caracas Metropolitan Area, Venezuela. Acta Odontol Latinoam. 2021;34:104–12.

134 Dourado DG, Lima CCB, Silva RNC, Tajra FS, Moura MS, Lopes TSP, et al. Molar-incisor hypomineralization in quilombola children and adolescents: a study of prevalence and associated factors. J Public Health Dent. 2021;81: 178–87.

135 Saldarriaga A, Rojas-Gualdron D, Restrepo M, Santos-Pinto L, Jeremias F. Dental fluorosis severity in children 8–12 years old and associated factors. Acta Odontol Latinoam. 2021;34:156–65.

136 Farias L, Laureano ICC, Fernandes LHF, Forte FDS, Vargas-Ferreira F, Alencar CRB, et al. Presence of molar-incisor hypomineralization is associated with dental caries in Brazilian schoolchildren. Braz Oral Res. 2021; 35:e013.

137 Freitas Fernandes LH, Laureano ICC, Farias L, Andrade NM, Soares Forte FD, Barros Alencar CR, et al. Incisor molar hypomineralization and quality of life: a population-based study with Brazilian schoolchildren. Int J Dent. 2021;2021:6655771.

138 Reis PPG, Jorge RC, Americano GCA, Thiago Pontes NS, Peres A, Silva Oliveira AGE, et al. Prevalence and severity of molar incisor hypomineralization in Brazilian children. Pediatr Dent. 2021;43:270–5.

139 Fernandes IC, Forte FDS, Sampaio FC. Molar-incisor hypomineralization (MIH), dental fluorosis, and caries in rural areas with different fluoride levels in the drinking water. Int J Paediatr Dent. 2021;31:475–82.

140 Duarte MBS, Carvalho VR, Hilgert LA, Ribeiro APD, Leal SC, Takeshita EM. Is there an association between dental caries, fluorosis, and molar-incisor hypomineralization? J Appl Oral Sci. 2021;29:e20200890.

141 Damares Lago J, Restrepo M, Girotto Bussaneli D, Patricia Cavalheiro J, Feltrin de Souza J, Santos-Pinto L, et al: Molar-incisor hypomineralization: prevalence comparative study in 6 years of interval. Sci World J. 2022; 2022:4743252.

142 Quintero Y, Restrepo M, Rojas-Gualdron DF, Farias AL, Santos-Pinto L. Association between hypomineralization of deciduous and molar incisor hypomineralization and dental caries. Braz Dent J. 2022;33:113–9.

143 Oreano MD, Santos PS, Borgatto AF, Bolan M, Cardoso M: Association between dental caries and molar-incisor hypomineralisation in first permanent molars: a hierarchical model. Community Dent Oral Epidemiol. 2023;51: 436–42.

144 de Barros LVC, Vale MP, Tourino L, Bittencourt JM, Bendo CB: Determination of dental caries, molar-incisor hypomineralization, and oral health-related quality of life in schoolchildren: a structural equation modeling approach. Int J Paediatr Dent. 2023; 33:289–97.

145 Vicioni-Marques F, Carvalho MR, Raposo F, de Paula-Silva FWG, de Queiroz AM, Leal SC, et al. Association of dental hypersensitivity and anxiety in children with molar-incisor hypomineralisation (MIH). Eur Arch Paediatr Dent. 2023;24:313–9.

146 Harz D, Catalan Gamonal B, Matute Garcia S, Jeremias F, Martin J, Fresno MC. Prevalence and severity of molar-incisor hypomineralization, is there an association with socioeconomic status? A cross-sectional study in Chilean schoolchildren. Eur Arch Paediatr Dent. 2023;24:577–84.

147 Gurrusquieta BJ, Nunez VM, Lopez ML. Prevalence of molar incisor hypomineralization in Mexican children. J Clin Pediatr Dent. 2017;41:18–21.

148 Villanueva-Gutierrez T, Barrera-Ortega CC, Garcia-Perez A, Gonzalez-Aragon Pineda AE. Relationship between Molar Incisor Hypomineralization (MIH) severity and cavitated carious lesions in schoolchildren. Acta Odontol Latinoam. 2019;32:133–40.

149 Gutierrez TV, Ortega CCB, Perez NP, Perez AG. Impact of molar incisor hypomineralization on oral health-related quality of life in Mexican schoolchildren. J Clin Pediatr Dent. 2019;43:324–30.
150 Davenport M, Welles AD, Angelopoulou MV, Gonzalez C, Okunseri C, Barbeau L, et al. Prevalence of molar-incisor hypomineralization in Milwaukee, Wisconsin, USA: a pilot study. Clin Cosmet Investig Dent. 2019;11:109–17.
151 Villanueva-Gutierrez T, Irigoyen-Camacho ME, Castano-Seiquier A, Zepeda-Zepeda MA, Sanchez-Perez L, Frechero NM. Prevalence and severity of molar-incisor hypomineralization, maternal education, and dental caries: a cross-sectional study of Mexican schoolchildren with low socioeconomic status. J Int Soc Prev Community Dent. 2019;9:513–21.
152 Irigoyen-Camacho ME, Villanueva-Gutierrez T, Castano-Seiquer A, Molina-Frechero N, Zepeda-Zepeda M, Sanchez-Perez L. Evaluating the changes in molar incisor hypomineralization prevalence: a comparison of two cross-sectional studies in two elementary schools in Mexico City between 2008 and 2017. Clin Exp Dent Res. 2020;6:82–9.
153 Sidhu N, Wang Y, Barrett E, Casas M. Prevalence and presentation patterns of enamel hypomineralisation (MIH and HSPM) among paediatric hospital dental patients in Toronto, Canada: a cross-sectional study. Eur Arch Paediatr Dent. 2020;21:263–70.
154 Sosa-Soto J, Padron-Covarrubias AI, Marquez-Preciado R, Ruiz-Rodriguez S, Pozos-Guillen A, Pedroza-Uribe IM, et al. Molar incisor hypomineralization (MIH): prevalence and degree of severity in a Mexican pediatric population living in an endemic fluorosis area. J Public Health Dent. 2022;82:3–10.
155 Garcia-Perez A, Gonzalez-Aragon Pineda AE, Villanueva Gutierrez T, Perez Perez NG, Gomez-Clavel JF. Impact of diseases of the hard tissues of teeth on oral health-related quality of life of schoolchildren in area with a high concentration of fluoride in drinking water. Community Dent Health. 2022;39:240–6.
156 Temilola OD, Folayan MO, Oyedele T. The prevalence and pattern of deciduous molar hypomineralization and molar-incisor hypomineralization in children from a suburban population in Nigeria. BMC Oral Health. 2015;15:73.
157 Oyedele TA, Folayan MO, Adekoya-Sofowora CA, Oziegbe EO, Esan TA. Prevalence, pattern and severity of molar incisor hypomineralisation in 8- to 10-year-old school children in Ile-Ife, Nigeria. Eur Arch Paediatr Dent. 2015;16:277–82.
158 Saber F, Waly N, Moheb D. Prevalence of molar incisor hypomineralisation in a group of Egyptian children using the short form: a cross-sectional study. Eur Arch Paediatr Dent. 2018;19:337–45.
159 Folayan MO, Chukwumah NM, Popoola BO, Temilola DO, Onyejaka NK, Oyedele TA, et al. Developmental defects of the enamel and its impact on the oral health quality of life of children resident in Southwest Nigeria. BMC Oral Health. 2018;18:160.
160 Abdalla HE, Abuaffan AH, Kemoli AM. Molar incisor hypomineralization, prevalence, pattern and distribution in Sudanese children. BMC Oral Health. 2021;21:9.
161 Arheiam A, Abbas S, Ballo L, Borowis E, Rashwan S, El Tantawi M. Prevalence, distribution, characteristics and associated factors of molar-incisor hypo-mineralisation among Libyan schoolchildren: a cross-sectional survey. Eur Arch Paediatr Dent. 2021;22:595–601.
162 Mahoney EK, Morrison DG. Further examination of the prevalence of MIH in the Wellington region. N Z Dent J. 2011;107:79–84.
163 Gambetta-Tessini K, Marino R, Ghanim A, Calache H, Manton DJ. Carious lesion severity and demarcated hypomineralized lesions of tooth enamel in schoolchildren from Melbourne, Australia. Aust Dent J. 2018;63:365–73.
164 Schwendicke F, Elhennawy K, Reda S, Bekes K, Manton DJ, Krois J. Global burden of molar incisor hypomineralization. J Dent. 2018;68:10–8.
165 Jordan RA, Micheelis W. Fünfte deutsche Mundgesundheitsstudie. Köln: Deutscher Zahnärzteverlag (DÄV); 2016.

Jan Kühnisch
Klinikum der Ludwig-Maximilians-Universität München
Poliklinik für Zahnerhaltung und Parodontologie
Goethestraße 70, DE–80336 Munich (Germany)
jan.kuehnisch@med.uni-muenchen.de

Published online: July 1, 2024
Rios D, Santos-Pinto L (eds): Molar Incisor Hypomineralisation: New Perceptions. Monogr Oral Sci. Basel, Karger, 2024, vol 32, pp 117–139 (DOI: 10.1159/000538874)

Systemic and Environmental Risk Factors Associated with Molar Incisor Hypomineralisation

Juliana Feltrin-Souza[a] Gabriela Fonseca-Souza[a] Emanuella Pinheiro[b] Fabian Calixto Fraiz[a] Paulo Sérgio Cerri[c]

[a]Department of Stomatology, Federal University of Paraná, Curitiba, Brazil; [b]Department of Pediatric Dentistry, School of Dentistry, University of São Paulo, São Paulo, Brazil; [c]Laboratory of Histology and Embryology, Department of Morphology, Genetics, Orthodontics and Pediatric Dentistry, Dental School, São Paulo State University (Unesp), Araraquara, Brazil

Abstract

The etiology of molar incisor hypomineralisation (MIH) has been attributed to systemic and environmental factors since 2001. The identification of MIH etiology is fundamental to better understand this condition, for differential diagnosis, and to identify the patient group at risk of MIH. Although the etiology of MIH is still unclear, it is stated as a multifactorial origin, with an overlap of systemic and genetic risk factors. The aim of this chapter was to discuss the systemic and environmental factors associated with MIH according to scientific evidence in the literature, relating it to the basic knowledge of amelogenesis and tooth development chronology. In this chapter, amelogenesis is described and illustrated in detail. Some characteristics of the amelogenesis process could explain some clinical features of the developmental defect of enamel, especially MIH. The chronology of tooth development was also referred to as a characteristic for the occurrence of MIH. Finally, the literature about systemic and environmental risk factors was revised, and the prenatal, perinatal, and postnatal factors associated with MIH were discussed. During the prenatal period, maternal health status, including illnesses during pregnancy and maternal smoking, are the main investigated factors associated with MIH. Prematurity (<37 weeks), low birth weight, and cesarean delivery are the factors associated with MIH during the perinatal period. Moreover, postnatal factors, such as common childhood illnesses, respiratory disease, infections, and antibiotic use, have been associated with MIH. New longitudinal studies that consider the synergy between exposure to environmental factors and biological susceptibility are likely to provide a new understanding of the etiology of MIH.

Introduction

The etiology of molar incisor hypomineralisation (MIH) has been widely discussed since the term “molar incisor hypomineralisation” was proposed in 2001 [1]. In this article, MIH was defined as a developmental defect of enamel (DDE) of systemic origin, since it affects first permanent molars and incisors, teeth with coincident developmental chronology.

In the literature, there are several retrospective studies investigating the systemic and environmental factors associated with this defect [2–8]. Systemic factors include general health problems or conditions that can affect an individual's health [9]. Environmental factors are all factors that are external to the human body, including physical, chemical, and biological exposures [10]. Currently, MIH pathogenesis has been investigated with an increasing number of genetic studies on this subject [11] and it is already known that it has a complex or multifactorial origin, with systemic, environmental, and genetic factors acting synergistically [12]. Thus, according to our understanding, despite the systemic or environmental triggers, the occurrence of MIH may be influenced by genetic variability [13].

An understanding of the risk factors of MIH is important for the basic scientific point of view, highlighting the factors able to disrupt amelogenesis. And, for the clinical interest, this knowledge is helpful in the differential diagnosis of DDE. Besides, it allows clinicians to identify patient groups at risk of MIH, improving the care provided to these patients, given the unfavorable clinical consequences and treatments needed related to this condition. Since some risk factors can be modified and avoided, this information may also contribute to the prevention of MIH.

DDEs result from insults in the amelogenesis process. Once enamel is formed, it is not able to be remodeled; therefore, such insults are permanently registered as biomarkers in the mineral structure [14]. For the investigation of MIH or DDE etiology, it is fundamental to analyze the clinical characteristics of DDE that will direct to the amelogenesis phase that was affected. Thus, for a better understanding of the etiopathogenesis of MIH, this chapter will discuss the phases of amelogenesis, the chronology of tooth development, and the systemic and environmental risk factors associated with MIH.

Fig. 1. a, b Photomicrographs of a frontal section of a rat head showing dental germ in the advanced bell stage, consisting of enamel organ (EO) and dental papilla (DP). The EO, derived from the ectoderm, contains four distinct layers of cells: preameloblasts (PAMs) or inner enamel epithelium (IE), stratum intermedium (SI), stellate reticulum (SR), and outer epithelium (OtE). Note that the future cusp tip region of the EO exhibits a continuous layer of cylindrical cells (PAMs), while in the more cervical portion, the epithelium is cuboidal (IE). The DP is situated in the concavity of the EO. In the cusp tip region, the peripheral cells of DP underlying the PAMs are cylindrical, forming the pre-odontoblasts (POd). Note that in the more cervical portion of the dental germ, ectomesenchymal cells (arrows) show similar features to the other cells in the DP, indicating that they are not yet differentiated. The dental follicle (DF) is represented by ectomesenchymal cells that surround the dental germ. AP, developing alveolar process; DL, dental lamina; OE, oral epithelium. Hematoxylin & Eosin. **b** Higher magnification of a portion of the future cusp of dental germ of **a**, showing the distinct layers of cells in the EO: (1) PAMs forming a single layer of cylindrical cells, (2) SI composed of 2–3 layers of squamous cells, (3) SR containing irregular cells with extensions connecting to each other and to the cells of the SI and the OtE, and (4) the OtE of the EO represented by a layer of cuboidal and/or squamous cells. At the periphery of the dental papilla, differentiating ectomesenchymal cells appear cylindrical and polarized, forming a single layer of cells; these differentiating cells are called PODs. Between the layer of PAMs and the layer of PODs, there is a thin layer of acidophilic matrix (stained pink), which constitutes the mantle dentin (asterisk). **c** Photomicrograph of a portion of section of a dental germ in the phase of crown formation. PAMs form a single layer of cylindrical cells juxtaposed to the layer of unmineralised mantle dentin (predentine [Pd]); PODs are arranged in a single layer of polarized cylindrical cells beneath the Pd layer. Hematoxylin & Eosin. **d, e** Electron micrographs showing the onset of dentin formation. **d** Portions of PAMs are in close contact with the surface of the newly synthesized organic matrix of mantle dentin (Pd) by PODs. Small and electron-dense globules of mineralisation (white arrows) are dispersed in the Pd. P, odontoblast processes in the Pd. **e** High magnification of a portion of **d**, note that distal portion of PAMs exhibits short projections (thick arrows) extending between the components of the organic matrix of Pd. The Pd adjacent to the PAMs displays electron-dense areas (white arrows) representing the onset of dentin mineralisation. Bars, 140 μm (**a**), 25 μm (**b**), 10 μm (**c**), and 0.5 μm (**d** and **e**).

(For figure see next page.)

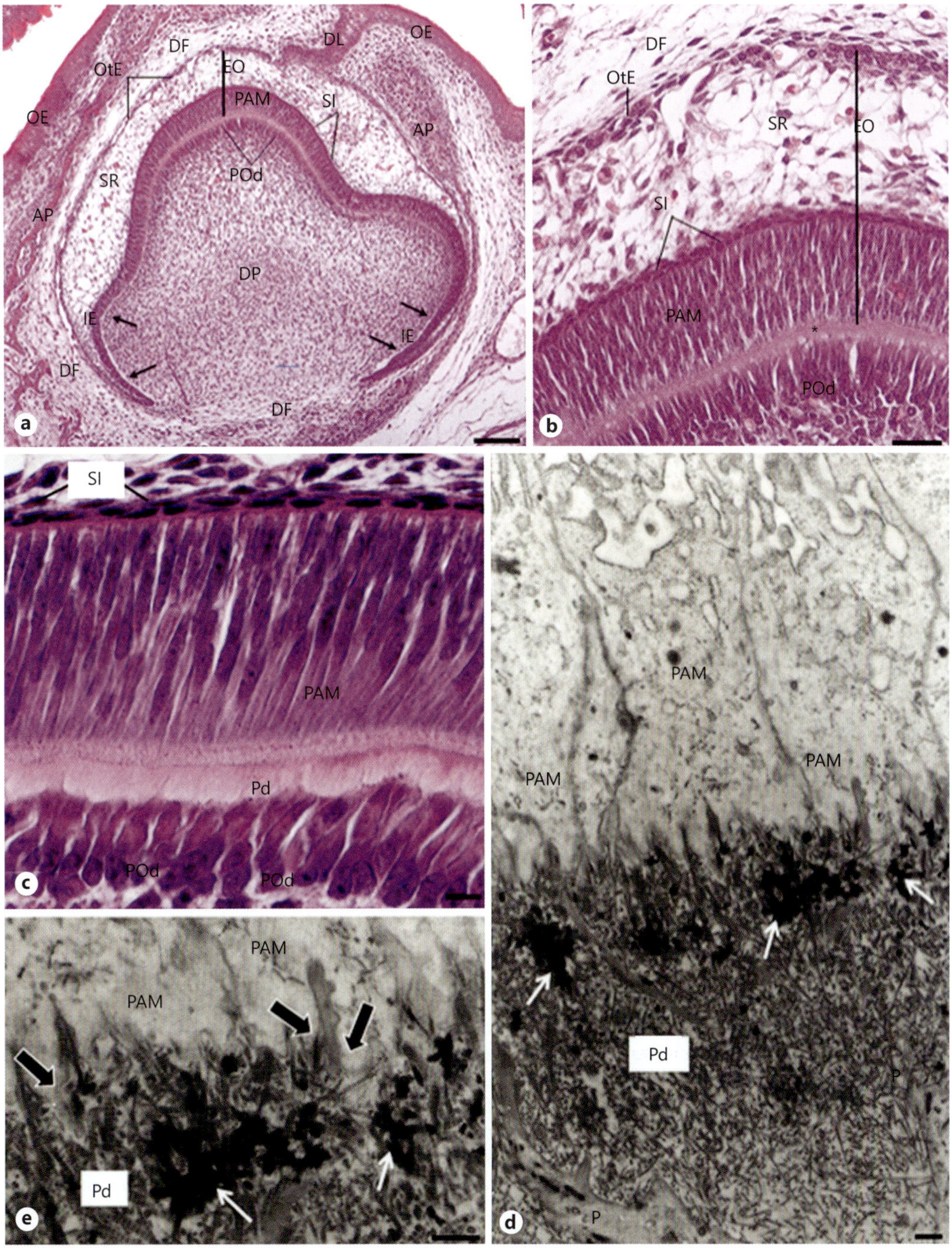

1

Considerations about Amelogenesis

Odontogenesis is a coordinated and genetically controlled process, involving the signaling of over 300 genes [15]. The enamel formation process, known as amelogenesis, initiates during the advanced bell stage, phase characterized by the histodifferentiation of the dental germ [16]. During this phase, the dental germ is characterized by the presence of the enamel organ derived from ectoderm, a structure responsible for enamel formation. The enamel organ extends laterally, partially surrounding the dental papilla, an ectomesenchymal-derived structure responsible for dentin and dental pulp formation. The dental germ (enamel organ and dental papilla) is surrounded by ectomesenchymal cells, forming the dental follicle, which gives rise to the supporting periodontal tissues [16, 17] (shown in Fig. 1a).

During the advanced bell stage, the enamel organ displays distinctive morphological features, with the presence of four morphologically well-defined layers of cells, named from the innermost boundary (closest to the dental papilla) to the outer boundary: (1) inner epithelium, (2) stratum intermedium, (3) stellate reticulum, and (4) outer epithelium (shown in Fig. 1a, b). In the inner epithelium layer, mitotic activity in these cells ceases at specific areas, contributing significantly to the establishment of crown morphogenesis for the future tooth [16, 17].

In general, mitosis ceases in the inner epithelium layer in regions corresponding to the tips of future cusps or incisal edges, while on the lateral edges, mitosis in the inner epithelium cells continues, promoting the growth of the future tooth crown [18]. As the mitosis is interrupted in the inner epithelium cells in the areas of future cusp tips, conspicuous morphological changes are observed in the inner epithelium cells as well as in the peripheral cells of the dental papilla, adjacent to the inner enamel organ. Initially, a noticeable increase in the height of the inner epithelium cells is observed in histological sections, causing these epithelial cells to become columnar. This change in cell shape is accompanied by the development and reorganization of their organelles, particularly those associated with protein synthesis. One important morphological change observed in this layer is the inversion of polarity, where the nucleus of the inner epithelium, initially positioned close to the dental papilla, gradually shifts and positions itself in the portion of the ameloblast near the stratum intermedium. The Golgi complex develops next to the nucleus, facing the distal portion of the cytoplasm (toward the dental papilla) of the columnar cell [16, 19]. At this point, the differentiating inner epithelium is referred as preameloblast (shown in Fig. 1b, c).

During the differentiation of the inner epithelium, preameloblasts secrete various growth factors, including transforming growth factor-β, which induces the differentiation of ectomesenchymal cells located on the periphery of the dental papilla into preodontoblasts (odontoblasts in differentiation). Preodontoblasts quickly organize

Fig. 2. a, **b** Photomicrographs showing a frontal section of rat molar tooth germ in the crown formation phase. Note that dentin (De) and enamel (E) formation is evident in the portions corresponding to the future cusps of the molar. Adjacent to the organic matrix of enamel (E), the layer of ameloblasts (AMs) is observed, while odontoblasts (Ods) are at the periphery of the dental papilla (DP), adjacent to the forming dentin (De). AP, alveolar process; OE, oral epithelium; SR, stellate reticulum; OtE, outer epithelium of the enamel organ. Hematoxylin & Eosin. **b** Higher magnification of a lateral portion of the forming molar of **a**. AMs exhibiting nuclei located near the stratum intermedium (arrows) are juxtaposed to the organic matrix of enamel surface (E). Note that the dentin layer (De) is thicker compared to enamel (E) due to its formation preceding enamel formation. Between the dentin layer (De) and Ods, there is a weakly stained dentin matrix layer, the pre-dentin (Pd), representing the unmineralised dentin organic matrix. Hematoxylin & Eosin. **c** Electron micrograph showing fine mineral crystals (arrows) in the enamel (E) newly synthesized by AMs. The partially mineralised enamel matrix (E) is continuous with the strongly electron-dense mineralised dentin layer (De). Bars, 80 μm (**a**), 20 μm (**b**), and 400 nm (**c**).

(For figure see next page.)

themselves into a single layer of juxtaposed columnar cells aligned perpendicularly to the basement membrane [18] (shown in Fig. 1c). Complex junctions, including the tight junction, responsible for compartmentalizing the dentin matrix, are established between the preodontoblasts, ensuring that the dentin matrix is produced by odontoblasts without the involvement of other dental pa-

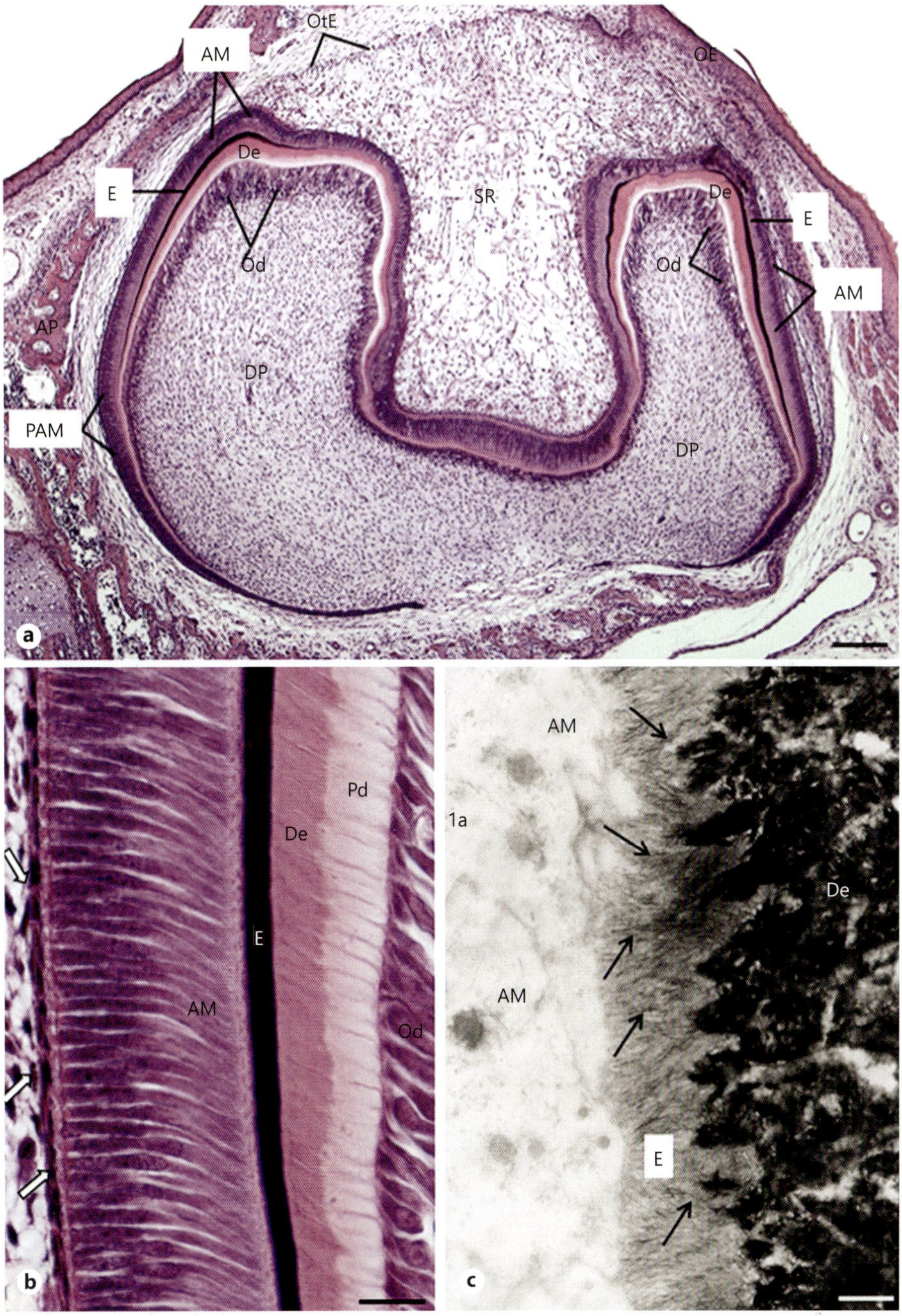

2

pilla cells [20]. Likewise, the layer of preameloblasts also organizes, and junctional complexes are established on the lateral sides, maintaining cell-to-cell adhesion. As soon as the first layer of predentin in the mantle layer is secreted by the preodontoblasts (shown in Fig. 1c–e), the enamel proteins are packaged into secretory granules and transported to the distal portion of the preameloblasts [16, 19]. Secretory granules containing enamel proteins rapidly reach the membrane of the preameloblast at its distal portion (adjacent to the future amelodentinal junction), fusing with the cell membrane and consequently releasing the granule content onto the unmineralised mantle dentin layer (shown in Fig. 3a–c). Concurrently with the formation of the first enamel layer, ameloblasts move away from the dental papilla, thus distancing themselves from the dentin surface (shown in Fig. 2a, b). At the distal portion of the ameloblast, a protrusion named Tomes' process is formed and, this thin cytoplasmic projection is observed involved by enamel matrix [17, 21, 22] (shown in Fig. 3a). Although enamel protein secretion occurs throughout the surface of the Tomes' process, it is more pronounced in its secretory region, while the nonsecretory side has a lower and slower rate of secretion. The presence of the Tomes' process and its differential secretion, along with changes in ameloblast movement during enamel formation, results in the arrangement of the basic enamel unit, known as the enamel prism (shown in Fig. 3b).

Unlike dentin, enamel is almost immediately mineralised upon secretion by ameloblasts. However, at this stage, enamel is only partially mineralised, with inorganic components accounting for only 20% of its total content. Enamel mineralisation will be completed only after the formation of the enamel matrix has finished when ameloblasts are almost in contact with the outer enamel organ. At this stage, ameloblasts decrease in size, and their distal portion, the Tomes' process, disappears (shown in Fig. 3b). Although the entire thickness of the enamel has been deposited and is partially mineralised, ameloblasts still play an active role in enamel maturation. The membrane of their distal portion, adjacent to the enamel surface, undergoes cyclic modulation, alternating between a nearly smooth distal surface (shown in Fig. 3b–d) and ruffled distal border (ruffle-ended ameloblasts). The smooth edge of the ameloblast is associated with the degradation of enamel matrix proteins. During this phase, ameloblasts release various enzymes, such as enamelysin (MMP-20), a serine protease, which degrade organic components of the enamel matrix. Therefore, the degradation of enamel proteins primarily occurs due to the release of enzymes by ameloblasts in the extracellular environment. The degradation of some enamel proteins and the removal of water from the matrix are necessary for the addition of inorganic components to the enamel, allowing the addition of hydroxyapatite crystals and the growth of existing crystals that were nucleated during initial mineralisation (shown in Fig. 3c, d).

Ion transport to the enamel occurs intracellularly (through ameloblasts), which release these ions through the ruffled border. In this maturation cycle, various vesicles, lysosomes, and calcium-adenosine triphosphatases are observed in close association with the ruffle-ended membrane of the ameloblast, indicating their involvement in pumping calcium from the ameloblast into the maturing enamel matrix. In addition to ameloblasts exhibiting strong calcium-dependent ATPase activity and alkaline phosphatase, the crenated membrane contains calcium channels. These conditions create an alkaline microenvironment that promotes the nucleation of new hydroxyapatite crystals as well as the growth of pre-existing ones. The supersaturation of hydroxyapatite crystals leads to a new cycle of the ameloblast's distal edge, which becomes smooth and active in releasing enzymes into the mineralising enamel matrix, promoting a new cycle of protein degradation and "freeing" space for the addition of inorganic components for the formation and growth of hydroxyapatite crystals [16].

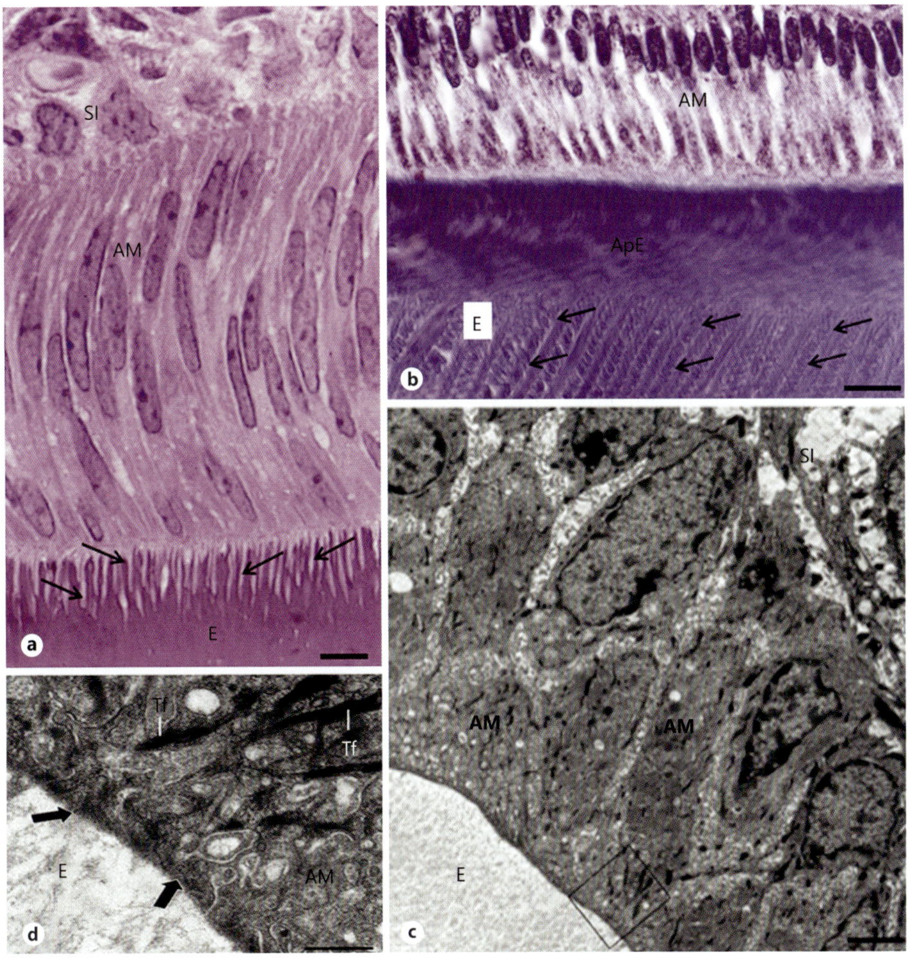

Fig. 3. a, **b** Photomicrographs showing a portion of a tooth germ in the crown formation phase. Ameloblasts (AMs) exhibit in their distal portion the Tomes' process (arrows) that occupy recesses in the surface of the enamel matrix (E). SI, stratum intermedium. Hematoxylin & Eosin. **b** AMs apposed to aprismatic enamel matrix layer (ApE); note that Tomes' process is not observed in the distal portion of AMs. In the underlying enamel (E), enamel prisms are visible (arrows). Masson's trichrome. **c**, **d** Electron micrographs of an ultrathin section of a rat molar germ in the crown formation phase, showing the interface between AMs and the maturing enamel matrix (E) surface. Note in **d**, outlined area in **c**, that the AMs exhibit a smooth membrane (thick arrows) in their distal portion in contact with the surface of the enamel matrix (E). At this stage, AMs release enzymes to degrade the enamel proteins to allow, in a subsequent phase, the addition and growth of hydroxyapatite crystals. TF, tonofilament. Bars, 7 µm (**a**), 20 µm (**b**), 2.5 µm (**c**), and 0.5 µm (**d**).

These cycles continue until the enamel reaches maturity, where inorganic components make up about 94–96% of the enamel content. The mineralisation phase is the longest, comprising about two-thirds of amelogenesis, resulting in a mineralised enamel with a mineral content of around 96%. After enamel mineralisation, ameloblasts involute into cuboidal epithelial cells that remain adjacent to the enamel. This epithelium forms a single continuous layer of cells that serve to protect the enamel, because it in direct contact with ectomesenchyme would stimulate the migration of clastic cells, which would promote the enamel resorption [16]. The cuboidal inner epithelium, associated with the cells of the stratum intermedium, the stellate reticulum cells that remain after the involuted enamel organ, along with the outer epithelium, form about four layers of cells that make up the reduced enamel epithelium [17, 23]. The reduced enamel epithelium covers the enamel along its entire length and, during the eruptive phase when it penetrates the mucosa, this epithelium fuses with the oral epithelium, creating an epithelial tunnel through which the tooth moves toward the occlusal plane. Thus, the reduced enamel epithelium constitutes the primordium of the junctional epithelium [17, 24].

From the considerations above, it becomes evident that dentinogenesis and amelogenesis initiate in the regions of the future dental cusp tips and incisal edges and extend toward the cervical loop [16]. Thus, the formation of the dental crown occurs gradually and depends on a complex cascade of cellular and molecular events that establish a chronological development [16]. In this manner, systemic changes, local factors, and mechanical traumas during this process can lead to DDE. Insults or disturbances in the secretory phase result in enamel hypoplasia, which is a quantitative defect of dental enamel, represented by a reduction of enamel thickness [25]. Insults during the mineralisation and maturation phases will result in hypomineralisation or hypomaturation, which cannot be clinically differentiated. Hypomineralisation is defined as qualitative defects of enamel, since there is no change in thickness but rather in quality, and they are detectable by alterations in enamel translucency, appearing as opacities. These opacities can be diffuse or demarcated, and their severity can vary depending on the etiological factor involved [25].

An important aspect when attempting to relate a DDE to potential etiological factors is the observation of the dental development chronology [14]. As mentioned, the formation of dental structures follows a pattern characterized by a temporal sequence of development that occurs simultaneously in the various dental groups, each at its specific stage (shown in Fig. 5). It is noteworthy that dental development begins in the fourth month of gestation. The deciduous dentition is almost entirely formed during the gestational period up to the first year of life. The last teeth to form are the second deciduous molars at around twelve months of age [26].

In the permanent dentition, the first tooth to form is the first permanent molar, which initiates mineralisation at birth and completes crown formation around the age of three. This period coincides with the development of permanent incisors and canine cusps [26]. Shown in Figure 4, the chronological development of the permanent dentition is observed, along with the framework or pattern of development in thirds of the dental crown. Thus, it can be noted that there is a chronological overlap between the development periods of regions involving the first molars, incisors, and permanent canines, as well as the deciduous second molars. This overlap is also observed in some clinical cases of children with demarcated hypomineralisation in deciduous second molars and deciduous canines (shown in Fig. 5) [27], the same chronological pattern of occurrence of opacities, which justifies MIH having a systemic or environmental component in its etiology.

Given the above, with knowledge of amelogenesis and dental development chronology, it is possible for the clinician, through the analysis of DDE signs, to estimate the period in which the triggering event occurred. Generally, factors related to the etiology of DDEs can be genetic, systemic, environmental, and local [9].

In clinical practice, it is not easy to identify the etiological factors, especially because the diagnosis of DDEs occurs a long time after the triggering

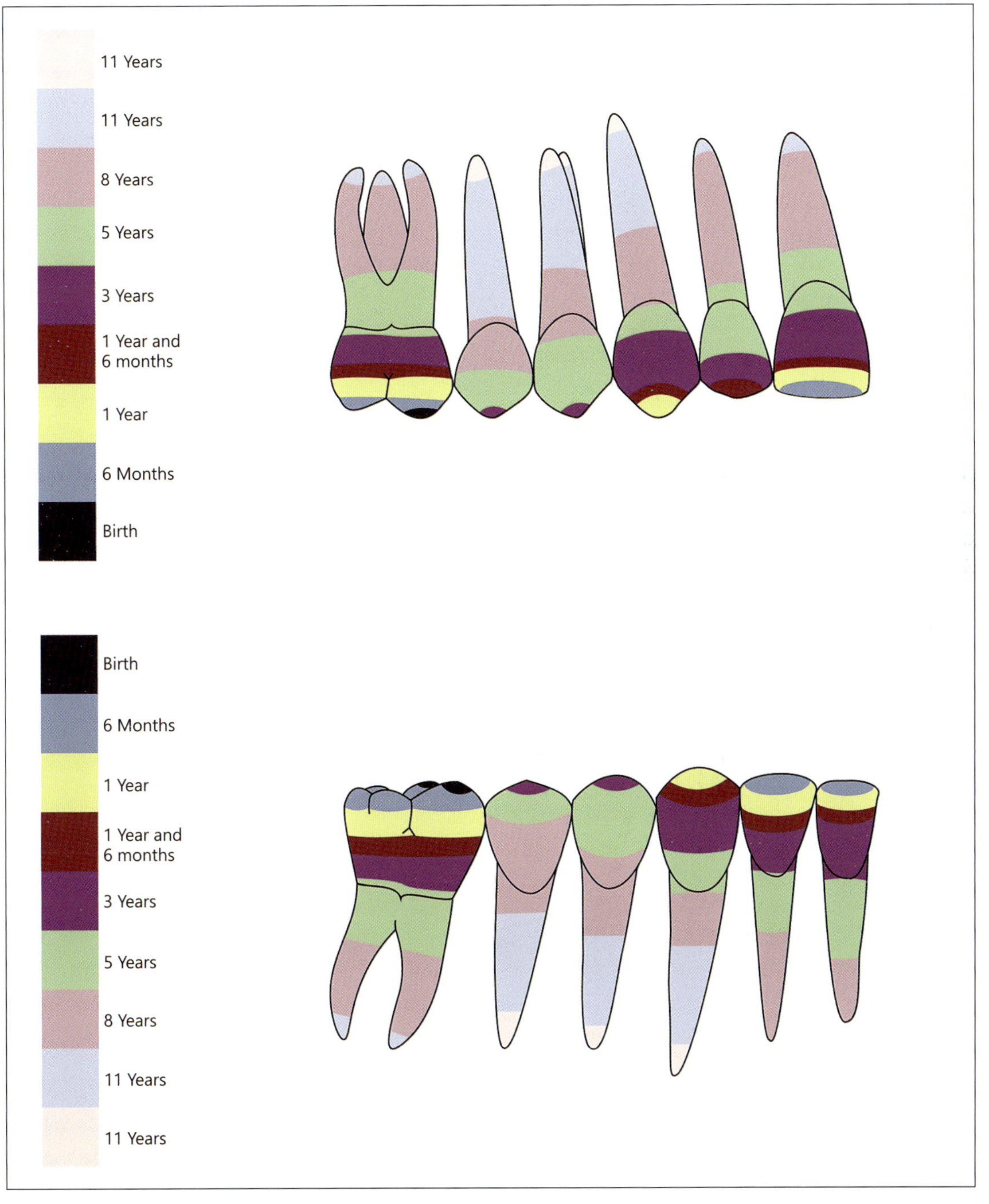

Fig. 4. Chronology of formation of permanent teeth. Adapted from McCall and Wald (1940) [73].

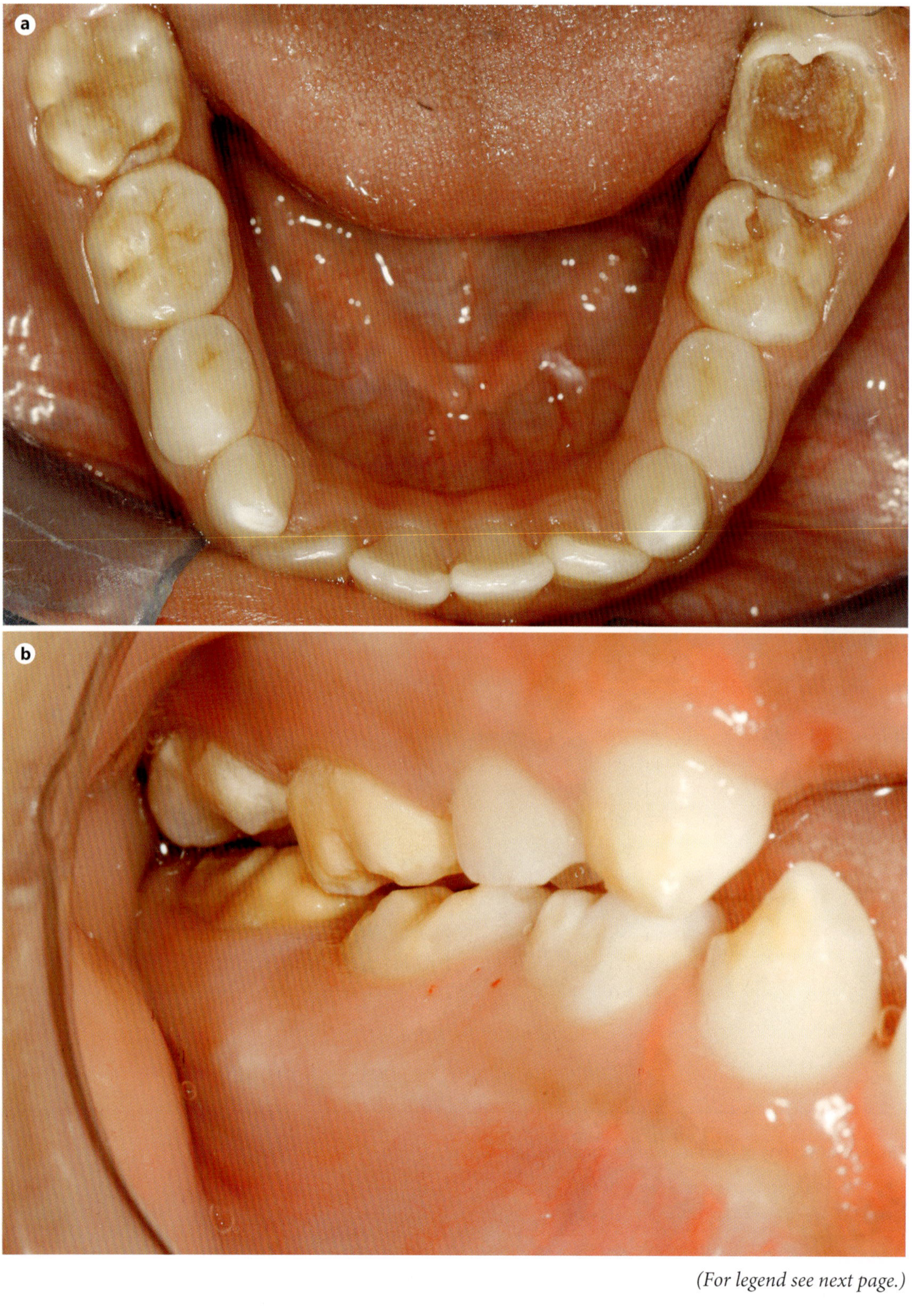

5

(For legend see next page.)

events. Therefore, the information is retrospective and, consequently, has many observation and memory biases, making it challenging to establish causality. However, according to the clinical characteristics, and medical or family history, it is possible to form hypotheses about the etiology, based on biological plausibility.

Systemic Factors Associated with MIH

The association between MIH and several systemic factors in the pre-, peri-, and postnatal periods has been investigated (Table 1), but it is still unclear. Systemic exposures refer to general health problems or conditions that can affect an individual's health [9]. Most studies on the etiology of MIH are cross-sectional and do not have the ideal design to investigate causality; retrospective data collection can introduce important biases, reducing the quality of evidence, especially considering the complexity of MIH etiology when factors can overlap and have an additive effect [9, 12, 28]. Furthermore, recent literature emphasizes the role of epigenetics in mediating environmental influences on gene expression, suggesting a link between systemic and genetic factors in MIH [28]. Longitudinal studies are scarce, more well-designed prospective cohort studies are needed, ideally with follow-up from prenatal care until the complete eruption of first permanent molar.

When cross-sectional studies are considered with a statistical approach such as meta-analysis carried out in some systematic reviews, it is possible to estimate the effects of findings from many studies more precisely, considering the quality of each study and summarizing the results [29]. The standardization of the MIH definition [1] allowed this type of analysis, which seeks to answer research questions with a greater volume of information by combining data from several studies. It is important to highlight that many primary studies have methodological flaws that compromise the quality of the findings; therefore, they should be viewed with caution [9].

Few studies have found associations between prenatal factors and MIH; however, peri- and postnatal factors seem to be more associated [28, 30] due to the chronology of mineralisation of teeth affected by MIH, which some authors claim begins close to birth [31]. Table 1 summarizes the main findings of the cohort and case-control studies.

Prenatal Factors

Some health conditions and maternal habits during pregnancy are cited in many studies as a risk factor for MIH in the offspring. Cohort or case-control studies mainly point to maternal illnesses during pregnancy, anemia, maternal infection, psychological stress, vitamin D insufficiency, use of antibiotics, and maternal smoking [30, 32–38].

Maternal illnesses during pregnancy, which may be associated with fever, can interfere with the activity of ameloblasts, altering the developing dental enamel of their children [9, 30]. The most cited conditions are pre-eclampsia, gestational diabetes, gestational hypertension, kidney disease, and maternal infections [28], but the role of each of these conditions is not entirely clear in the literature [9]. Two systematic reviews found an association between maternal diseases and MIH through their respective meta-analyses; however, they highlight that many studies do not specify which diseases were evaluated, making it difficult to identify the mechanism associated with MIH, considering that clinical manifestations can be different between the exhibitions [9, 28].

Fig. 5. a Patient with MIH and HSPM. **b** Patient with MIH, presenting opacities in their first permanent molar, second primary molar, and primary canine. HSPM, hypomineralised second primary molar.

Table 1. Characteristics of the studies included in this literature review and main findings involving the systemic factors associated with MIH, based on prenatal, perinatal, and postnatal periods

Study	Country	Sample			Study design	Associated factors
		age, years	number of participants included	children with MIH, *N* (%)		
Prenatal						
Lygidakis et al., 2008 [30]	Greece	5–12	720	360	Case control	Medical problems
Whatling and Fearne, 2008 [32]	England	6–13	109	57 (52.3%)	Case control	Maternal problems during pregnancy
Ghanim et al., 2013 [33]	Iraqi	7–9	823	153 (18.6%)	Case control	Illness in the 3rd trimester, psychological stress, hypotension-related anemia, more than 3 ultrasound scans in the 3rd trimester
Costa-Silva et al., 2013 [74]	Brazil	4–6	134	21 (15.7%)	Cohort	No significant association
Kühnisch et al., 2014 [42]	Germany	10	692	102 (14.7%)	Cohort	No significant association
Rodrigues et al., 2015 [75]	Brazil	7–14	28	14	Case control	No significant association
Giuca et al., 2018 [36]	Italy	6–13	120	60	Case control	Antibiotics used during pregnancy
Van der Tas et al., 2018 [43]	The Netherlands	6	1,780	146 (8.2%)	Cohort	No significant association
Lee et al., 2020 [38]	South Korea	6–13	1,191	607	Case control	Maternal smoking, intake of health supplements
Elzein et al., 2021 [76]	Lebanon	7–9	659	176	Case control	Pollutants
Noor Mohamed et al., 2021 [37]	Saudi Arabia	3–4 7–8	577	207 (35.9%)	Case control	Maternal infection
Børsting et al., 2022 [21]	Norway	7–9	176	55 (32%)	Cohort	Vitamin D insufficiency 2nd trimester
Lim et al., 2022 [77]	England	7–10	5,536	297 (5.4%)	Case control	No significant association
Mariam et al., 2022 [35]	India	8–12	315	104	Case control	Maternal anemia, intrauterine growth retardation
Bagattoni et al., 2022 [47]	Italy	5–17	140	78	Case control	No significant association
Perinatal						
Lygidakis et al., 2008 [30]	Greece	5–12	720	360	Case control	Medical problems

Table 1 (continued)

Study	Country	Sample			Study design	Associated factors
		age, years	number of participants included	children with MIH, *N* (%)		
Brogårdh-Roth et al., 2011 [49]	Sweden	10–12	164	44 31 (70.5%) SG 13 (29.5%) CG	Case control	Gestational age, birth weight
Ghanim et al., 2013 [33]	Iraqi	7–9	823	153 (18.6%)	Case control	Low birth weight, hypoxia with incubation, respiratory distress, hypocalcemia
Costa-Silva et al., 2013 [74]	Brazil	4–6	134	21 (15.7%)	Cohort	No significant association
Rodrigues et al., 2015 [75]	Brazil	7–14	38	14	Case control	No significant association
Garot et al., 2016 [51]	France	6–28	128	75	Case control	Hypoxia, cesarean
Sidaly et al., 2016 [78]	Norway	8–10	224	n.r. (25.4%) CG n.r. (23.5%) SG	Case control	No significant association
Andrade et al., 2017 [52]	Brazil	7–15	99	31 15 (45.5%) SG 16 (24.2%) CG	Case control	Incubator
Giuca et al., 2018 [36]	Italy	6–13	120	60	Case control	No significant association
Van der Tas et al., 2018 [43]	The Netherlands	6	1,780	146 (8.2%)	Cohort	No significant association
Portella et al., 2018 [53]	Brazil	5–15	93	31	Case control	Prematurity, prolonged delivery
Noor Mohamed et al., 2021 [37]	Saudi Arabia	3–4 7–8	577	207 (35.9%)	Case control	Prematurity and low birth weight
Ilczuk-Rypuł et al., 2022 [50]	Poland	M = 9.1 SD ±1.9	613	38 (6.2%)	Cohort	Prematurity
Mariam et al., 2022 [35]	India	8–12	315	104	Case control	Prematurity, low birth weight, neonatal jaundice, and neonatal problems
Bagattoni et al., 2022 [47]	Italy	5–17	140	78	Case control	No significant association
Postnatal						
Beentjes et al., 2002 [58]	Holland	M = 9.9 SD ±2.02	45	24	Case control	Otitis media, pneumonia, and high fever

Table 1 (continued)

Study	Country	Sample			Study design	Associated factors
		age, years	number of participants included	children with MIH, *N* (%)		
Muratbegovic et al., 2007 [79]	Bosnia and Herzegovina	12	138	69	Case control	No significant association
Lygidakis et al., 2008 [30]	Greece	5–12	720	360	Case control	Medical problems
Whatling and Fearne, 2008 [32]	England	6–13	109	57 (52.3%)	Case control	Chickenpox between 3 and 3.99 years, amoxicillin
Laisi et al., 2008 [65]	Finland	7–10	167	24 (14.4%)	Cohort	No significant association
Durmus et al., 2009 [34]	Turkey	7–14	228	54 (24%)	Case control	Asthma until 3 years old, constant medicament consumption
Fagrell et al., 2011 [64]	Sweden	9–11	477	224	Case control	Breastfeeding for more than 6 months, late introduction of gruel, late introduction of infant formula
Ghanim et al., 2013 [33]	Iraqi	7–9	823	153 (18.6%)	Case control	Pneumonia, chest infections (CIs), tonsillitis, high fever (HF), severe diarrhea & vomiting and UTI, HF & CI, & ear infection, breastfeeding less than 12 months, antibiotics in the 1st year
Kühnisch et al., 2015 [42]	Germany	10	692	102 (14.7%)	Cohort	Respiratory diseases
Peker et al., 2014 [80]	Turkey	M = 9.9 SD ±1.4 M = 10.2 SD ±4.8	60	13	Case control	No significant association
Kühnisch et al., 2015 [42]	Germany	10	1,048	143 (13.6%)	Cohort	Elevated serum 25(OH) vitamin D
Loli et al., 2015 [81]	Italy	6–13	182	91	Case control	Aerosol therapy
Rodrigues et al., 2015 [75]	Brazil	7–14	38	14	Case control	No significant association
Wuollet et al., 2016 [59]	Finland	7–12	287	33 (11.5%)	Cohort	Amoxicillin and macrolide until 3 years old, penicillin in the 1st year, acute otitis media
Andrade et al., 2017 [52]	Brazil	7–15	99	31 15 (45.5%) SG 16 (24.2%) CG	Case control	Protease inhibitors

Table 1 (continued)

Study	Country	Sample			Study design	Associated factors
		age, years	number of participants included	children with MIH, *N* (%)		
Giuca et al., 2018 [36]	Italy	6–13	120	60	Case control	Ear, nose, throat disorders
Van der Tas et al., 2018 [43]	The Netherlands	6	1,780	146 (8.2%)	Cohort	No significant association
Portella et al., 2018 [53]	Brazil	5–15	93	31	Case control	Recurrent fevers
Lee et al., 2020 [38]	South Korea	6–13	1,191	607	Case control	Respiratory infection until 3 years old
Flexeder et al., 2020 [82]	Germany	10–15	730	101 (13.8%)	Case control	Asthma at age 15
Elzein et al., 2021 [76]	Lebanon	7–9	659	176	Case control	Pollutants
Noor Mohamed et al., 2021 [37]	Saudi Arabia	3–4 7–8	577	207 (35.9%)	Case control	Childhood infection
Doğusal et al., 2021 [83]	Turkey	6–18	455	33 (7.3%)	Case control	No significant association
Khazaei et al., 2021 [84]	Germany	10	1,070	n.r. (13.7%)	Cohort	No significant association
Ilczuk-Rypuł et al., 2022 [50]	Poland	M = 9.1 SD ±1.9	613	38 (6.2%)	Cohort	Otitis and atopic dermatitis until 3 years old
Mariam et al., 2022 [35]	India	8–12	315	104	Case control	Frequent episodes of fever, tonsillitis, bronchitis, and gastroenteritis in the first 3 years of life, early childhood illnesses, amoxycillin + clavulanic acid, hospitalization, breastfeeding duration <12 months, initiation of top feed at <12 months
Bagattoni et al., 2022 [47]	Italy	5–17	140	78	Case control	No significant association

CG, control group; M, mean; SD, standard deviation; SG, study group.

Two case-control studies found an association between maternal anemia during pregnancy and MIH in their children [9, 35]. According to the authors, this relationship may be related to the decrease in the general oxygen transport capacity of mothers with anemia; in addition, maternal anemia during pregnancy may be a risk factor for premature birth [9, 39].

Vitamin D participates in the absorption process of calcium and phosphate [40]; these minerals play an important role in the mineralisation of enamel [41], which is why their relationship with MIH has been investigated. The association between vitamin D deficiency or insufficiency during pregnancy and MIH remains controversial. In a retrospective German study, lower vitamin D levels at 10 years of age were associated with an increased prevalence of MIH [42]. In a Dutch birth cohort, the association between vitamin D status and MIH was not evidenced; serum vitamin D concentrations were measured in the second gestational trimester, at birth, and at the child's sixth birthday, when dental examination was also performed [43]. The authors also emphasize that most children (62.5%) did not have their first permanent molars erupted [43]. In another retrospective cohort study, vitamin D status was measured in the second and third trimester of pregnancy but was also not associated with the prevalence of MIH in children aged 7–9 years. However, a greater number of teeth affected by MIH were associated with vitamin D insufficiency in the second trimester [21].

Intrauterine growth restriction (IUGR) has been associated with MIH [35]. The authors emphasize that IUGR is related to placental insufficiency, when there is a reduction in the supply of nutrients and oxygen to the fetus [44]. Therefore, the underlying mechanism of IUGR would have the potential to interfere with amelogenesis [35].

The relationship between ultrasound exams during pregnancy and MIH is controversial; one study observed a positive association with multiple exposures in the third trimester [33]. In another investigation, the relationship between the number of prenatal ultrasound scans and MIH was not evidenced [32]. However, it is still unknown whether ultrasound waves have any negative effect on the fetus; in addition, there may be a confusion between a greater need for ultrasound scans due to a maternal comorbidity that could have the potential to cause MIH [33].

One study showed an association between the use of antibiotics during pregnancy and MIH; however, the type of medication and the period used are not reported [36]. However, according to a systematic review and meta-analysis, MIH was not associated with the use of medications during pregnancy, including antibiotics, medication for diabetes, and hypertension. Due to the diversity reported, some studies group this prenatal exposure, and therefore, the authors were unable to evaluate it individually [9].

Maternal smoking during pregnancy is investigated as a possible risk factor for MIH; animal studies have shown that exposure to nicotine affected the function of ameloblasts, altering enamel mineralisation [45, 46]. In a case-control study, this association was demonstrated, and mothers who smoked during pregnancy had children with 2.37 more chances of having MIH compared to mothers who did not smoke [38]; on the other hand, in a design study similarly, this exposure could not be confirmed due to low precision of the estimate [47]. This association was also not found by two systematic reviews [9, 48]; the authors point out a difficulty in analysis due to the lack of standardization in data collection in relation to the number of cigarettes and at what point the habit persisted during pregnancy [9].

Ghanim et al. [33] found an increased likelihood of MIH and maternal stress. The authors mention that Iraq, the country where the study was carried out, was in a situation of war for a long period and that this circumstance has a negative impact on people's health and can result in stress-related malnutrition that is indirectly related to MIH [33]. These results were estimated by two meta-analyses that added a second study, and maternal stress remained associated with MIH [9, 28].

Perinatal Factors

Events occurring during childbirth or close to it can interfere with the mineralisation of the first permanent molars [12, 31]. Factors such as prematurity, low birth weight, hypocalcemia, hypoxia, respiratory distress, cesarean, prolonged delivery, and need for an incubator are cited as potential risk factors for MIH [33, 35, 37, 49–53]. These findings were evidenced in meta-analyses that also evaluated the association between perinatal factors and MIH, except for hypoxia, hypocalcemia, and respiratory distress [9, 28, 54].

The association between prematurity (<37 weeks) and low birth weight (<2,500 g) with MIH may be related to systemic conditions pertinent to these perinatal conditions, such as the immaturity of the respiratory system, which can compromise oxygen supply and inadequacies of calcium and phosphorus due to the lower capacity of the gastrointestinal tract to absorb minerals [22, 33, 35, 37, 49, 55]. Additionally, physiological immaturity in premature babies is associated with gastrointestinal and respiratory changes (hypoxia) and infections [55]. Hypocalcemia and hypoxia can affect the normal function of ameloblasts, resulting in defects in enamel development [12, 30, 35, 49].

Cesarean delivery can be elective or emergency when there is an associated complication; this differentiation is essential to control confounders [9]. Some questions regarding cesarean section may explain the association with MIH, such as the type of anesthesia used or due to complications associated with the type of delivery that can alter the oxygen supply [51]. Spinal anesthesia can produce hypotension and generate hypoxia for the baby [56]. In a cohort study, babies born by elective cesarean section at 37–39 weeks were two- to four-fold increased risk of respiratory morbidity compared to children born vaginally [57]; these facts could infer in an overlap between prenatal, perinatal, and postnatal factors in relation to MIH.

Postnatal Factors

After birth, postnatal factors such as common childhood illnesses in early childhood have been linked to MIH, especially when there are episodes of fever [9, 28]. The use of some medications and the need for hospital care have also been reported [9, 28]. Some studies indicate that children with MIH become ill more frequently when compared to children without this condition [30, 33, 58, 59].

The most investigated childhood diseases associated with MIH are otitis media, pneumonia, chickenpox, asthma, bronchitis, tonsillitis, chest infections, throat diseases, infections, severe diarrhea, and vomiting, gastroenteritis, and atopic dermatitis [32–38, 42, 50, 58, 59, 82].

Respiratory diseases have been repeatedly associated with MIH due to hypoventilation that alters oxygen saturation [9, 28, 60]. Respiratory acidosis caused by variations in oxygen supply can change the pH of the enamel matrix [61]. These changes are capable of inhibiting proteolytic enzymes and impacting the growth of hydroxyapatite crystals [30, 60].

Several classes of antibiotics have been investigated, and amoxicillin appears to be most associated with MIH [35]. In an animal study, amoxicillin was able to disrupt amelogenesis [62]. There is discussion in the literature about the difficulty of distinguishing the causal factor of MIH between the childhood illnesses, fever, and the use of antibiotics, considering that they may overlap in time [9, 28]. However, in some primary studies and one meta-analysis, antibiotic use was associated with MIH [3, 32, 35, 59]. On the other hand, a systematic review that investigated the use of medications implicated in MIH did not show this association [63].

Some infectious diseases, such as otitis media, urinary tract infection, tonsillitis, and gastroenteritis, have been associated with MIH in primary studies [32, 33, 35–37, 50, 58, 59]; however, the result is controversial in the meta-analyses carried out [9, 28], remaining associated with just one of them [28]. Another important point is related to the heterogeneity of reports of childhood diseases and infections; many studies group exposures together, preventing them from being assessed in isolation [9]. Therefore, the relevance of prospective data collection and/or from medical records filled with established criteria for the diagnosis of each health problem, hospitalizations, and medication prescription, as well as statistical planning that allows confounding variables to be controlled, is highlighted [9, 28].

A case-control investigation using data from a large prospective medical and social population study from birth found a positive association between MIH and breastfeeding more than 6 months, late introduction to gruel and infant formula [64]. However, the role of environmental pollutants has not been investigated, and the authors suggest that differences in nutrition in the first months may be related to MIH, as in cases of premature children, but this relationship has not been explored [64]. Ghanim et al. reported that breastfeeding for up to 6 or 12 months was associated with more cases of MIH. These data should be viewed with caution as subsequent reasons were not investigated, and breastfeeding for more than 2 years had a protective role against the occurrence of MIH [33]. On the other hand, the association between breastfeeding and MIH was not found by other prospective cohort studies [42, 65].

Environmental Factors Associated with MIH

Environmental factors are all that are external to the human body, being divided into physical, chemical, and biological [10]. Some examples of these factors include dioxins, heavy metals, air pollutants, biphenyls, and pesticides.

Dioxins are a group of persistent environmental pollutants (persistent organic pollutants) reported to be associated with MIH. These compounds are generated from products of industrial processes and can be found in some soils, sediments, and foods [66]. One of the first studies that hypothesized this association found a positive correlation between MIH and the exposure to a dioxin called polychlorinated dibenzo-p, present in the breastfeeding milk in a Finland population [67]. Over the years, it was observed that the levels of dioxins in mother's milk decreased in Finland; thus, the same research group conducted a new study and found no association between MIH and the exposure to dioxins [65]. Therefore, the authors assumed that this lack of association was a result of the reduced levels of dioxins in Finland and reduced time of breastfeeding, which may suggest a dose-response association.

In a population of Lebanese children, association between MIH and the exposition to heavy metals used in wars was found [3]. It is known that heavy metals present negative effects on health, leading to acute and toxic effects. The main sources of contamination include water, air, and food [68]. Besides that, a correlation between higher levels of air pollutants and MIH was observed in Poland [5].

A more recent study [2] investigated the association between MIH and polychlorinated biphenyls, organochlorine pesticides, and perfluorinated alkyl substances. The exposition to two of the organochlorine pesticides studied was associated with a reduced risk of MIH, while polychlorinated biphenyls and perfluorinated alkyl substances were not associated with MIH or seemed to be sex specific, once boys presented a higher risk of MIH.

An animal study found association between MIH and bisphenol A [69]. This compound is an endocrine-disrupting chemical used in the production of polycarbonate plastics and epoxy resins, which can be found in food contact materials [66]. Jedeon et al. [69] observed a disruption in the protein removal from the enamel matrix in the teeth of rats exposed to bisphenol A, resulting in a hypomineralised enamel.

The exact mechanisms of how these environmental factors act on amelogenesis are still not understood. It is possible that environmental and systemic factors are overlapped, since the exposition to some environmental factors may cause systemic diseases associated with MIH, such as otitis media and respiratory problems [9]. Furthermore, certain environmental factors can present epigenetic influence, interacting with genes, and consequently causing the expression of the MIH phenotype [70, 71]. The interaction between these factors reinforces the understanding of MIH as a complex condition since it includes more than one factor acting in synergism.

Final Considerations

Risk factors are markers aimed at predicting future events; in the case discussed in this book: the occurrence of MIH. This chapter reinforces the need to understand MIH from a systemic perspective, which will expand the possibility of identifying risk factors. Understanding the probability of MIH occurrence and its risk factors will undoubtedly enable preventive measures that have a real impact on reducing its prevalence. The evidence presented in this chapter indicates that the occurrence of MIH cannot be explained by a random distribution model. As research begins to incorporate the temporal assessment of the cause-effect relationship, the hypothesis that identifiable risk factors exist for this condition begins to solidify, and therefore, the temporal anticipation and predictability of its occurrence become possible. However, it is essential to understand that since risk is a finding relative to the aggregate dimension (to a particular group of people or population), the identified risk factors for population groups may not be entirely applicable to the individual dimension [72].

This is even more challenging in the case of MIH, where the etiology is complex and acknowledged to be multifactorial. At the current stage of research on MIH, it is especially difficult to distinguish whether a specific event is a determining factor or merely predisposes to or contributes to its occurrence. Additionally, studies that do not account for temporality may erroneously label as risk factors those that are only incidentally associated. Therefore, although scientific production on this topic has been prolific in recent years, new longitudinal studies that consider the synergy between exposure to environmental factors and biological susceptibility are likely to provide a new understanding of the etiology of MIH.

Lastly, the aspects raised in this chapter clearly indicate that the prevention of MIH will never be achieved solely through individual actions. It will be necessary for all health care professionals to collaborate in expanding actions aimed at improving living conditions during pregnancy and the early years of life.

Acknowledgment

We thank the Federal University of Paraná for their support and resources that have greatly contributed to the success of this manuscript. Additionally, we extend our acknowledgment to Laboratory of Histology and Embryology, Department of Morphology, Genetics, Orthodontics and Pediatric Dentistry, Dental School, São Paulo State University (Unesp) for providing valuable images and technical assistance, which enriched the content of this manuscript.

Statement of Ethics

We state that the pictures of patients were obtained by patient's written informed consent for publication of the images. The intraoral photographs were obtained during clinical research, which was previously approved by the Ethics Committee from the Federal University of Paraná (protocol number: 4.095.306).

Conflict of Interest Statement

The authors have no conflicts of interest to declare.

Funding Sources

The authors declare no funding sources for this work.

Author Contributions

Juliana Feltrin-Souza participated in the manuscript design, selection of the content and conceptions, and elaborated the pictures, and wrote and revised the manuscript. Gabriela Fonseca-Souza revised the literature about the environmental factors related to MIH, wrote this content, organized the references, and revised the manuscript. Emanuella Pinheiro revised the literature about the systemic factors related to MIH, wrote this content, and revised the manuscript. Fabian Calixto Fraiz participated in the manuscript design, selection of the content and conceptions, and wrote the final considerations, and revised the manuscript. Paulo Sérgio Cerri revised the literature and wrote about the amelogenesis, elaborated the pictures of amelogenesis and described it, and revised the manuscript.

References

1 Weerheijm KL, Jälevik B, Alaluusua S. Molar-incisor hypomineralisation. Caries Res. 2001;35(5):390–1.

2 Boyer E, Monfort C, Lainé F, Gaudreau É, Tillaut H, Bonnaure-Mallet M, et al. Prenatal exposure to persistent organic pollutants and molar-incisor hypomineralization among 12-year-old children in the French mother-child cohort PELAGIE. Environ Res. 2023;231(Pt 3): 116230.

3 Elzein R, Chouery E, Abdel-Sater F, Bacho R, Ayoub F. Relation between molar-incisor hypomineralization (MIH) occurrence and war pollutants in bombarded regions: epidemiological pilot study in Lebanon. Niger J Clin Pract. 2021;24(12):1808–13.

4 Fonseca-Souza G, Fatturi AL, Fraiz FC, Assunção LRdS, Feltrin-Souza J. What are the systemic factors associated with the molar-incisor hypomineralization etiology? Pesqui Bras Odontopediatria Clín Integr. 2021;21:e0041.

5 Głódkowska N, Emerich K. The impact of environmental air pollution on the prevalence of molar incisor hypomineralization in schoolchildren: a cross-sectional study. Adv Clin Exp Med. 2020; 29(12):1469–77.

6 Elfrink ME, Moll HA, Kiefte-de Jong JC, Jaddoe VW, Hofman A, ten Cate JM, et al. Pre- and postnatal determinants of deciduous molar hypomineralisation in 6-year-old children. The Generation R Study. PLoS One. 2014;9(7):e91057.

7 Souza JF, Costa-Silva CM, Jeremias F, Santos-Pinto L, Zuanon AC, Cordeiro RC. Molar incisor hypomineralisation: possible aetiological factors in children from urban and rural areas. Eur Arch Paediatr Dent. 2012;13(4):164–70.

8 Souza JF, Jeremias F, Costa-Silva CM, Santos-Pinto L, Zuanon AC, Cordeiro RC. Aetiology of molar-incisor hypomineralisation (MIH) in Brazilian children. Eur Arch Paediatr Dent. 2013;14: 233–8.

9 Fatturi AL, Wambier LM, Chibinski AC, Assunção L, Brancher JA, Reis A, et al. A systematic review and meta-analysis of systemic exposure associated with molar incisor hypomineralization. Community Dent Oral Epidemiol. 2019;47(5):407–15.

10 Prüss-Üstün A, Corvalán C. Preventing Disease Through Healthy Environments: Towards an Estimate of the Environmental Burden of Disease. Geneva: World Health Organization; 2006.

11 Manton DJ, Crombie FA, Silva MJ. The pathogenesis and aetiology of MIH: more questions than answers. In: Bekes K, editor. Molar Incisor Hypomineralization – A Clinical Guide to Diagnosis and Treatment. Austria: Springer; 2020. p. 33–44.

12 Alaluusua S. Aetiology of molar-incisor hypomineralisation: a systematic review. Eur Arch Paediatr Dent. 2010; 11(2):53–8.

13 Vieira AR, Kup E. On the etiology of molar-incisor hypomineralization. Caries Res. 2016;50(2):166–9.

14 Collignon AM, Vergnes JN, Germa A, Azogui S, Breinig S, Hollande C, et al. Factors and mechanisms involved in acquired developmental defects of enamel: a scoping review. Front Pediatr. 2022;10:836708.

15 Thesleff I. The genetic basis of tooth development and dental defects. Am J Med Genet A. 2006;140(23):2530–5.

16 Nanci A. Desenvolvimento do Dente e de seus Tecidos de Suporte. In: Nanci A, editor. Ten Cate – Histologia Oral. 9th ed. São Paulo: Grupo GEN; 2019. p. 117–54.

17 Garant PR. Early tooth development. In: Garant PR, editor. Oral Cells and Tissues. 35. Chicago: Quintessence Publishing Company; 2003. p. 1–80.

18 Lungová V, Radlanski RJ, Tucker AS, Renz H, Míšek I, Matalová E. Tooth-bone morphogenesis during postnatal stages of mouse first molar development. J Anat. 2011;218(6):699–716.

19 Katchburian E, Holt SJ. Studies on the development of ameloblasts. I. Fine structure. J Cell Sci. 1972;11(2):415–47.

20 Arana-Chavez VE, Massa LF. Odontoblasts: the cells forming and maintaining dentine. Int J Biochem Cell Biol. 2004;36(8):1367–73.

21 Børsting T, Schuller A, van Dommelen P, Stafne SN, Skeie MS, Skaare AB, et al. Maternal vitamin D status in pregnancy and molar incisor hypomineralisation and hypomineralised second primary molars in the offspring at 7–9 years of age: a longitudinal study. Eur Arch Paediatr Dent. 2022;23(4):557–66.
22 Jain A, Agarwal R, Sankar MJ, Deorari A, Paul VK. Hypocalcemia in the newborn. Indian J Pediatr. 2010;77(10): 1123–8.
23 Cerri PS, de Faria FP, Villa RG, Katchburian E. Light microscopy and computer three-dimensional reconstruction of the blood capillaries of the enamel organ of rat molar tooth germs. J Anat. 2004;204(pt 3):191–5.
24 de Pizzol Júnior JP, Sasso-Cerri E, Cerri PS. Apoptosis and reduced microvascular density of the lamina propria during tooth eruption in rats. J Anat. 2015; 227(4):487–96.
25 FDI World Dental Federation. A review of the developmental defects of enamel index (DDE Index). Commission on Oral Health, Research & Epidemiology. Report of an FDI Working Group. Int Dent J. 1992;42(6):411–26.
26 Dean MC, Humphrey L, Groom A, Hassett B. Variation in the timing of enamel formation in modern human deciduous canines. Arch Oral Biol. 2020;114: 104719.
27 da Silva Figueira R, Mustafa Gomes Muniz FW, Costa LC, Silva de Moura M, Moura L, Mello de Oliveira B, et al. Association between genetic factors and molar-incisor hypomineralisation or hypomineralised second primary molar: a systematic review. Arch Oral Biol. 2023;152:105716.
28 Garot E, Rouas P, Somani C, Taylor GD, Wong F, Lygidakis NA. An update of the aetiological factors involved in molar incisor hypomineralisation (MIH): a systematic review and meta-analysis. Eur Arch Paediatr Dent. 2022;23(1):23–38.
29 Glass GV. Primary, secondary, and meta-analysis of research. Educ Res. 1976; 5(10):3–8.
30 Lygidakis NA, Dimou G, Marinou D. Molar-incisor-hypomineralisation (MIH). A retrospective clinical study in Greek children. II. Possible medical aetiological factors. Eur Arch Paediatr Dent. 2008;9(4):207–17.
31 Reid DJ, Dean MC. Variation in modern human enamel formation times. J Hum Evol. 2006;50(3):329–46.
32 Whatling R, Fearne JM. Molar incisor hypomineralization: a study of aetiological factors in a group of UK children. Int J Paediatr Dent. 2008;18(3):155–62.
33 Ghanim A, Manton D, Bailey D, Mariño R, Morgan M. Risk factors in the occurrence of molar-incisor hypomineralization amongst a group of Iraqi children. Int J Paediatr Dent. 2013;23(3):197–206.
34 Durmus B, Abbasoglu Z, Peker S, Kargul BJASC. Possible medical aetiological factors and characteristics of molar incisor hypomineralisation in a group of Turkish children/Moguci medicinski etioloski cimbenici i znacajke molarno incizivne hipomineralizacije u skupini turske djece. Acta Stomatol Croat. 2013;47(4):297–306.
35 Mariam S, Goyal A, Dhareula A, Gauba K, Bhatia SK, Kapur A. A case-controlled investigation of risk factors associated with molar incisor hypomineralization (MIH) in 8–12 year-old children living in Chandigarh, India. Eur Arch Paediatr Dent. 2022;23(1):97–107.
36 Giuca MR, Cappè M, Carli E, Lardani L, Pasini M. Investigation of clinical characteristics and etiological factors in children with molar incisor hypomineralization. Int J Dent. 2018;2018:7584736.
37 Noor Mohamed R, Basha S, Virupaxi SG, Idawara Eregowda N, Parameshwarappa P. Hypomineralized primary teeth in preterm low birth weight children and its association with molar incisor hypomineralization-a 3-year-prospective study. Children (Basel). 2021;8(12):1111.
38 Lee DW, Kim YJ, Oh Kim S, Choi SC, Kim J, Lee JH, et al. Factors associated with molar-incisor hypomineralization: a population-based case-control study. Pediatr Dent. 2020;42(2):134–40.
39 Rahmati S, Azami M, Badfar G, Parizad N, Sayehmiri K. The relationship between maternal anemia during pregnancy with preterm birth: a systematic review and meta-analysis. J Matern Fetal Neonatal Med. 2020;33(15):2679–89.
40 DeLuca HF. Overview of general physiologic features and functions of vitamin D. Am J Clin Nutr. 2004;80(6 suppl):1689s–96s.
41 Lacruz RS, Habelitz S, Wright JT, Paine ML. Dental enamel formation and implications for oral health and disease. Physiol Rev. 2017;97(3):939–93.
42 Kühnisch J, Thiering E, Kratzsch J, Heinrich-Weltzien R, Hickel R, Heinrich J. Elevated serum 25(OH)-vitamin D levels are negatively correlated with molar-incisor hypomineralization. J Dent Res. 2015;94(2):381–7.
43 van der Tas JT, Elfrink MEC, Heijboer AC, Rivadeneira F, Jaddoe VWV, Tiemeier H, et al. Foetal, neonatal and child vitamin D status and enamel hypomineralization. Community Dent Oral Epidemiol. 2018;46(4):343–51.
44 Bruin C, Damhuis S, Gordijn S, Ganzevoort W. Evaluation and management of suspected fetal growth restriction. Obstet Gynecol Clin North Am. 2021; 48(2):371–85.
45 Chowdhury IG, Bromage TG. Effects of fetal exposure to nicotine on dental development of the laboratory rat. Anat Rec. 2000;258(4):397–405.
46 Dong Q, Wu H, Dong G, Lou B, Yang L, Zhang L. The morphology and mineralization of dental hard tissue in the offspring of passive smoking rats. Arch Oral Biol. 2011;56(10):1005–13.
47 Bagattoni S, Carli E, Gatto MR, Gasperoni I, Piana G, Lardani L. Predisposing factors involved in the aetiology of molar incisor hypomineralization: a case-control study. Eur J Paediatr Dent. 2022; 23(2):116–20.
48 Silva MJ, Scurrah KJ, Craig JM, Manton DJ, Kilpatrick N. Etiology of molar incisor hypomineralization – A systematic review. Community Dent Oral Epidemiol. 2016;44(4):342–53.
49 Brogårdh-Roth S, Matsson L, Klingberg G. Molar-incisor hypomineralization and oral hygiene in 10- to-12-yr-old Swedish children born preterm. Eur J Oral Sci. 2011;119(1):33–9.
50 Ilczuk-Rypuła D, Zalewska M, Pietraszewska D, Dybek A, Nitecka-Buchta A, Postek-Stefańska L. Prevalence and possible etiological factors of molar-incisor hypomineralization (MIH) in population of Silesian children in Poland: a pilot retrospective cohort study. Int J Environ Res Public Health. 2022; 19(14):8697.
51 Garot E, Manton D, Rouas P. Peripartum events and molar-incisor hypomineralisation (MIH) amongst young patients in southwest France. Eur Arch Paediatr Dent. 2016;17(4):245–50.

52 Andrade NS, Pontes AS, Paz HES, de Moura MS, Moura LF, Lima MD. Molar incisor hypomineralization in HIV-infected children and adolescents. Spec Care Dentist. 2017;37(1):28–37.
53 Portella PD, Fraiz FC, Soares RC, Nagata AG, de Oliveira Tomaz C, da Silva Assunção LR. Molar-incisor hypomineralization and associated factors: a case-control study. Pesqui Bras Odontopediatria Clín Integr. 2018;18(1): 4320.
54 Wu X, Wang J, Li YH, Yang ZY, Zhou Z. Association of molar incisor hypomineralization with premature birth or low birth weight: systematic review and meta-analysis. J Matern Fetal Neonatal Med. 2020;33(10):1700–8.
55 Saigal S, Doyle LW. An overview of mortality and sequelae of preterm birth from infancy to adulthood. Lancet. 2008;371(9608):261–9.
56 Cyna AM, Andrew M, Emmett RS, Middleton P, Simmons SW. Techniques for preventing hypotension during spinal anaesthesia for caesarean section. Cochrane Database Syst Rev. 2006;(4): CD002251.
57 Hansen AK, Wisborg K, Uldbjerg N, Henriksen TB. Risk of respiratory morbidity in term infants delivered by elective caesarean section: cohort study. BMJ. 2008;336(7635):85–7.
58 Beentjes VE, Weerheijm KL, Groen HJ. Factors involved in the aetiology of molar-incisor hypomineralisation (MIH). Eur J Paediatr Dent. 2002;3(1):9–13.
59 Wuollet E, Laisi S, Salmela E, Ess A, Alaluusua S. Molar-incisor hypomineralization and the association with childhood illnesses and antibiotics in a group of Finnish children. Acta Odontol Scand. 2016;74(5):416–22.
60 Né YGS, Frazão DR, Lopes GO, Fagundes NCF, Souza-Rodrigues RD, Paula-Silva FWG, et al. Association between respiratory diseases and molar-incisor hypomineralization: a systematic review and meta-analysis. Front Med (Lausanne). 2022;9:990421.
61 Whitford GM, Angmar-Månsson B. Fluorosis-like effects of acidosis, but not NH+4, on rat incisor enamel. Caries Res. 1995;29(1):20–5.
62 Sahlberg C, Pavlic A, Ess A, Lukinmaa PL, Salmela E, Alaluusua S. Combined effect of amoxicillin and sodium fluoride on the structure of developing mouse enamel in vitro. Arch Oral Biol. 2013;58(9):1155–64.
63 Serna C, Vicente A, Finke C, Ortiz AJ. Drugs related to the etiology of molar incisor hypomineralization: a systematic review. J Am Dent Assoc. 2016;147(2): 120–30.
64 Fagrell TG, Ludvigsson J, Ullbro C, Lundin SA, Koch G. Aetiology of severe demarcated enamel opacities—an evaluation based on prospective medical and social data from 17,000 children. Swed Dent J. 2011;35(2):57–67.
65 Laisi S, Kiviranta H, Lukinmaa PL, Vartiainen T, Alaluusua S. Molar-incisor-hypomineralisation and dioxins: new findings. Eur Arch Paediatr Dent. 2008;9(4):224–7.
66 World Health Organization. Dioxins and their effects on human health 2016 [cited 2023 Sep 15]. Available from: https://www.who.int/news-room/fact-sheets/detail/dioxins-and-their-effects-on-human-health.
67 Alaluusua S, Lukinmaa PL, Vartiainen T, Partanen M, Torppa J, Tuomisto J. Polychlorinated dibenzo-p-dioxins and dibenzofurans via mother's milk may cause developmental defects in the child's teeth. Environ Toxicol Pharmacol. 1996;1(3):193–7.
68 Balali-Mood M, Naseri K, Tahergorabi Z, Khazdair MR, Sadeghi M. Toxic mechanisms of five heavy metals: mercury, lead, chromium, cadmium, and arsenic. Front Pharmacol. 2021;12: 643972.
69 Jedeon K, De la Dure-Molla M, Brookes SJ, Loiodice S, Marciano C, Kirkham J, et al. Enamel defects reflect perinatal exposure to bisphenol A. Am J Pathol. 2013;183(1):108–18.
70 Lygidakis NA, Garot E, Somani C, Taylor GD, Rouas P, Wong FSL. Best clinical practice guidance for clinicians dealing with children presenting with molar-incisor-hypomineralisation (MIH): an updated European Academy of Paediatric Dentistry policy document. Eur Arch Paediatr Dent. 2022;23(1):3–21.
71 da Silva FMF, de Carvalho FM, Franco A, Soares TRC, Fonseca-Gonçalves A, Vieira AR, et al. Association between molar hypomineralization, genes involved in enamel development, and medication in early childhood: a preliminary study. Int J Paediatr Dent. 2024 May;34(3):211–8.
72 Filho NA, Castiel LD, Ayresbe JR. Risco: Conceito básico da epidemiologia. In: Filho NdA, Barreto ML, editors. Epidemiologia & Saúde – Fundamentos, Métodos e Aplicações. Rio de Janeiro: Grupo GEN; 2011.
73 McCall J, Wald S. Roentgenologia Clínica Dentária. Rio de Janeiro: Atheneu; 1959.
74 Costa-Silva CM, Paula JSD, Ambrosano GMB, Mialhe FL. Influence of deciduous molar hypomineralization on the development of molar-incisor hypomineralizarion. Braz J Oral Sci. 2013;12:335–8.
75 Rodrigues FCN, Ribeiro PHB, Thomaz ÉBAF, Lima GQT, Neves PAM, Ribeiro CCC. Molar-incisor hypomineralization in Schoolchildren of São Luis, Brazil Maranhão: prevalence and associated factors. Pesqui Bras Odontopediatria Clín Integr. 2015;15(1):271–8.
76 Elzein R, Chouery E, Abdel-Sater F, Bacho R, Ayoub F. Molar-incisor hypomineralisation in Lebanon: association with prenatal, natal and postnatal factors. Eur Arch Paediatr Dent. 2021; 22(2):283–90.
77 Lim QY, Taylor K, Dudding T. The effects of modifiable maternal pregnancy exposures on offspring molar-incisor hypomineralisation: a negative control study. Community Dent Health. 2022; 39(4):231–9.
78 Sidaly R, Schmalfuss A, Skaare AB, Sehic A, Stiris T, Espelid I. Five-minute Apgar score ≤ 5 and molar incisor hypomineralisation (MIH) – a case control study. BMC Oral Health. 2016;17(1):25.
79 Muratbegovic A, Markovic N, Ganibegovic Selimovic M. Molar incisor hypomineralisation in Bosnia and Herzegovina: aetiology and clinical consequences in medium caries activity population. Eur Arch Paediatr Dent. 2007;8(4):189–94.
80 Peker S, Mete S, Gokdemir Y, Karadag B, Kargul B. Related factors of dental caries and molar incisor hypomineralisation in a group of children with cystic fibrosis. Eur Arch Paediatr Dent. 2014; 15(4):275–80.
81 Loli D, Costacurta M, Maturo P, Docimo R. Correlation between aerosol therapy in early childhood and molar incisor hypomineralisation. Eur J Paediatr Dent. 2015;16(1):73–7.

82 Flexeder C, Kabary Hassan L, Standl M, Schulz H, Kühnisch J. Is there an association between asthma and dental caries and molar incisor hypomineralisation? Caries Res. 2020;54(1):87–95.

83 Doğusal G, Sönmez I, Ünüvar T. Evaluation of serum 25(OH)D levels in obese and normal-weight children with carious and hypomineralized teeth. J Clin Pediatr Dent. 2021;45(1):35–40.

84 Khazaei Y, Harris CP, Heinrich J, Standl M, Kühnisch J. Association study on nutrition in the first year of life and molar-incisor hypomineralization (MIH)-results from the GINIplus and LISA birth cohort studies. Int J Environ Res Public Health. 2021;18(21):11411.

Juliana Feltrin-Souza
Department of Stomatology, Federal University of Paraná
Rua Pref. Lothário Meissner, 632
Curitiba, Paraná 80210-170 (Brazil)
julianafeltrin@ufpr.br

Published online: July 1, 2024
Rios D, Santos-Pinto L (eds): Molar Incisor Hypomineralisation: New Perceptions. Monogr Oral Sci. Basel, Karger, 2024, vol 32, pp 140–146 (DOI: 10.1159/000538875)

Genetic *Theory* behind the Molar Incisor Hypomineralisation

Alexandre R. Vieira
East Carolina University School of Dental Medicine, Greenville, NC, USA

Abstract
Much effort has been spent in the identification of an environmental factor that explains the occurrence of molar incisor hypomineralisation (MIH). The best explanation, however, is accepting that MIH has a complex or multifactorial mode of inheritance. This chapter provides an analysis of how multifactorial inheritance operates in determining MIH, an explanation that accommodates the variation seen in the phenotype and the frequency of the problem around the world.

Introduction

The editors proposed the title of this chapter, and when I accepted to write it, I decided that I would not change their original title proposal (I only added the italics font to the word theory). The word *theory* in everyday use often means an untested hunch or a guess without supporting evidence. But, for us scientists, a *theory* has nearly the opposite meaning. A theory is a well-substantiated explanation of an aspect of the natural world that can incorporate laws, hypothesis, and facts [1].

Molar incisor hypomineralisation (MIH) was originally described as an idiopathic condition likely related to an environmental factor [2]; however, it has all the characteristics of a trait that has a complex mode of inheritance, such as height, weight, intelligence, sexual orientation, or most diseases and conditions, such as cardiovascular risks, cancer, obesity, arthritis, dementia, premature birth, many structural birth defects among many. The goal of this chapter is presenting the evidence that excludes an environmental factor as the sole cause of MIH.

The Name "Molar Incisor Hypomineralisation"

The reason for writing this book relates to an event that dates back to the fifth European Academy of Paediatric Dentistry congress held in Bergen, Norway, between June 7 and 11, 2000. Dur-

Table 1. Characteristics of multifactorial or complex modes of inheritance [5]

	Characteristics
1	Reliability of estimates: Accurate estimates of population frequency are difficult to obtain because of variation in reliability of reporting
2	Sex ratio: It is very common to see differences in frequency with one sex being more commonly affected than the other
3	Side of the defect: Very commonly bilateral structures are not affected at the same degree
4	Environmental factors: No striking associations are often seen in conditions with multifactorial modes of inheritance
5	Variation between populations: It is common to see differences of frequency estimates. It is difficult to know how much of the variation represents differences in geographic origin, location variation in teratogenic factors, or differences in reporting
6	Variation in geographic origin: The greatest contribution to variation in population frequency is likely that associated with their origins
7	Relationship between population frequency and frequency in relatives: Using the threshold model and reasonable assumptions, it is possible to derive fixed relationships between the frequency of the condition in relatives and the frequency in the general population
8	Rapid decrease in frequency with decreasing degree of relationship: For a trait determined by a single gene, the frequency in near relatives will decrease by 50% with each degree of relationship removed from the proband. For multifactorial conditions, their distribution in the population approaches a normal distribution, and the proportions of affected relatives are represented for the area under the curve beyond the threshold in the respective distribution. Since the tail of the curve becomes progressively flatter, the drop in frequency between first- and second-degree relatives should be greater than that between second- and third-degree relatives
9	Risks for relatives versus population incidence: In groups where the frequency of the condition is increased, the risk for relatives should also be increased, though not proportionally
10	Twins: In any condition determined in part by genetic factors, the concordance rate is expected to be higher in monozygotic than in dizygotic pairs
11	Risk of recurrence after 2 affected: Unaffected parents who have had an affected child have declared themselves to carry more than the average number of genes contributing to the condition. If a second affected child is born, the parents can be assumed to carry still more predisposing genes and to be still closer to the threshold
12	Effect of affected near relative on recurrence risk: If the existence of an affected first-degree relative increases the recurrence risk, it is reasonable to suppose that the same will be true for affected relatives of more distant degree, though the increase would be smaller
13	Recurrence risk varies with sex of proband: In traits that occur more frequently in one sex than the other, it must be assumed that the threshold is nearer the tail of its distribution in the sex less often affected
14	Recurrence risk varies with severity of defect in the proband: According to the threshold model, a severely affected case would lie nearer the tail of the distribution and would be expected to be more genetically predisposed than a mild case
15	Syndromes: It is not uncommon that a phenotype can be part of a syndrome. After removal of cases accounted for by mutant genes, chromosomal aberrations, or environmental insults, there remains a great majority of cases that can be reasonably attributed to the interaction of several genes and several environmental factors – the multifactorial group
16	Microforms: Any developmental deviation that suggests the person had been near the developmental threshold of the phenotype. Microforms may be difficult to detect and affect prevalence estimates

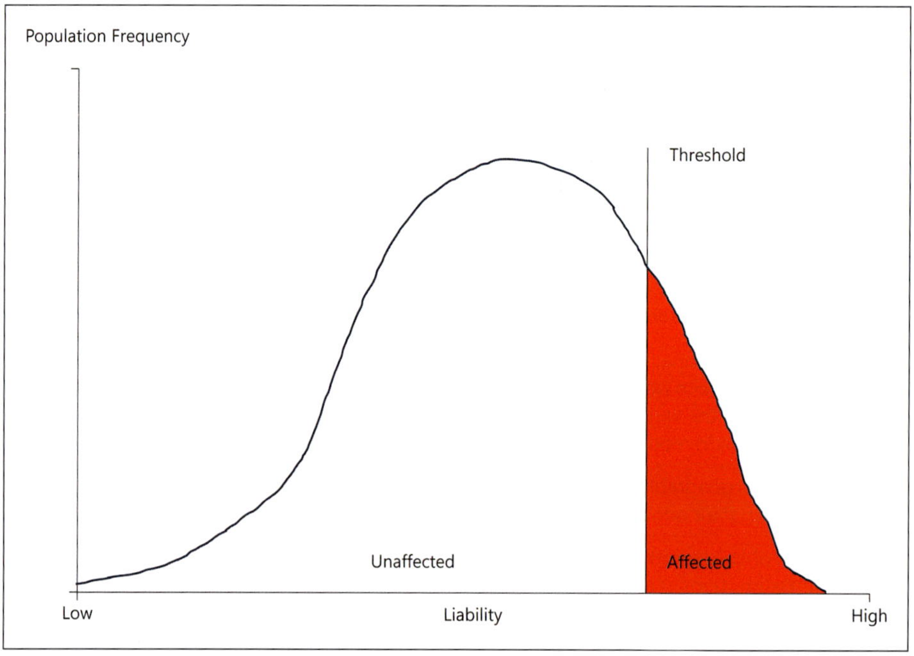

Fig. 1. The multifactorial threshold model. This model assumes that there are a number of different risk factors that contribute in an additive way to an unmeasured, continuously distributed variable called the *liability*. The *y*-axis is the number of individuals in a population; the *x*-axis is the unmeasured contributing factor.

ing the congress, four papers on permanent first molars with enamel developmental defects were presented [3]. Those similar cases were called originally by their authors "hypomineralised permanent first molars," "idiopathic enamel hypomineralisation in the permanent molars," "non-fluoride hypomineralisation in first permanent molars," and "cheese molars." Enamel developmental defects in permanent molars were a phenotype that other Bergen congress participants described seeing before. Also, the author remembers similar cases during his training in dental school back in the late 80s. In fact, MIH could be seen in medieval times [4].

Following the congress in Bergen, a proposal of creating the name MIH was published, and that document also suggested that multiple environmental factors were responsible for these fairly uniform defects [3]. The consequence of this initial report went beyond creating a unified name; it steered almost two decades of research away from one of the contributing factors leading to MIH.

Complex Mode of Inheritance

MIH, similar to the vast majority of more common adult diseases and several structural birth defects in isolation, is the result of contributions of more than one gene and can be also influenced by the environment. There are some characteristics that suggest a condition has a multifactorial or complex mode of inheritance (Table 1).

MIH fits well a threshold model, which provides a quantitative genetic framework for it. In this model (Fig. 1), we can assume that MIH is caused by variation in an unobservable but normally distributed contributing factor or liability [6].

Many items listed in Table 1 are yet to be defined for MIH. Ascertaining MIH in older relatives is difficult due to the possibility of lost teeth, extensive restorations on teeth that are commonly affected by caries lesions, and individuals not remembering or knowing the treatments they received when they were younger.

There is some variation on population estimates of the frequency of MIH, and that has been globally estimated at 13.5%. America appears to be the continent with the highest prevalence, 15.3%, and Asia the one with the lowest at 10.7% [7]. There is also some evidence that the frequency decreases in Europe from North to South [8]. There appears also to be no difference in the frequency of MIH between females and males [7, 9–12] or Blacks and Whites [12].

As expected, there is greater concordance in MIH in monozygotic twins when compared to dizygotic [13]. There is also some evidence that frequency of affected molars may be different between left and right molars [14].

There is a possibility that close to subclinical forms of MIH exist which are not easily identified. This would affect population estimates and estimates by subgroups. MIH environmental factors and association with cleft lip and palate will be discussed next.

The Environment

The original description of MIH defined its name and also established a research agenda with emphasis on identifying an environmental factor that explained the occurrence of MIH [3]. Several studies followed testing if pre- and perinatal factors and early childhood experiences were linked to MIH [15]. It comes with no surprise that none of them demonstrated an obvious relationship. When a condition has a multifactorial or complex mode of inheritance, environmental contributions happen in the background of typically several genetic variants with small individual effects. Statistical evidence of associations has arisen when gene-environmental models have been tested. Transforming growth factor beta 1 receptor (*TGFBR1*) was associated with MIH in the presence of childhood pneumonia [10]. Also, interferon regulatory factor 6 (*IRF6*) and transforming growth factor alpha (*TGFA*) were associated with MIH in the presence of medication intake up to 3 years of age [11]. Similarly, variants in enamelin (*ENAM*), ameloblastin (*AMBN*), and kallikrein 4 (*KLK4*) were associated with MIH in the presence of medication intake before 4 years of age [12]. Medication intake early in life is a proxy of infection.

Cleft Lip and Palate

Isolated forms of cleft lip and palate have a complex or multifactorial mode of inheritance and 90% heritability [16]. Heritability is a statistic used to estimate the degree of variation in a phenotype in a population that is due to genetic variation between individuals in that population. The only calculation of heritability for MIH suggested it to be 20% [17]. The data used [13] had 124 monozygotic twins and 112 dizygotic pairs. However, only 34 pairs of monozygotic twins had both children affected by MIH, whereas 11 dizygotic twins had both members of the pair affected by the condition. That means that several pairs in both groups were discordant. One has to assume that their discordance may be due to different environmental exposures, despite living at the same household with the same parents. The authors did not measure infective episodes of the children or their medication intake, and there may be differences between the individual members of the twin pairs. Further, very mild changes in dental enamel may have gone undetected in the children considered unaffected. The other possibility is that discordant twins may be discordant for certain genetic variants.

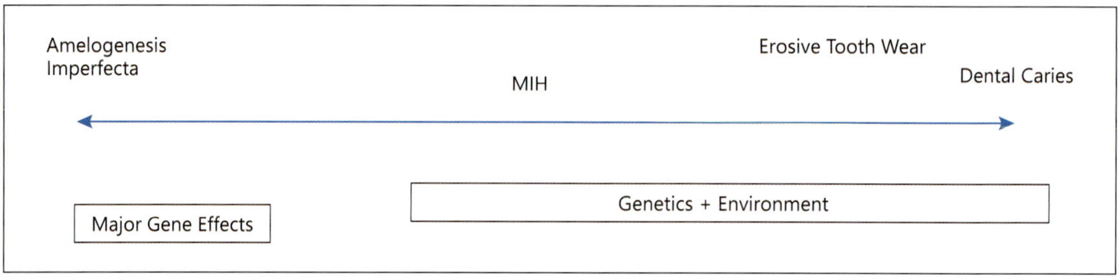

Fig. 2. Molar incisor hypomineralisation is part of a spectrum of genetic consequences that ranges from amelogenesis imperfecta to dental caries and erosive tooth wear.

Virtually all children born with cleft lip and palate have developmental dental alterations [18]. This finding has led us to suggest that isolated forms of clefts are in fact craniofacial syndromes that include dental changes [19]. A large number of these changes affect the dental enamel [20]. MIH was reported in individuals born with cleft lip and palate [21]. When compared to the general population, the frequency of MIH is 4 times higher among individuals born with cleft lip and palate [22]. One can argue that the higher frequency of MIH among individuals born with cleft lip and palate is the result of the higher frequency of infections children born with clefts experience. However, when compared to the general population, the increase in the number of infections is 2-fold [23], and infection alone probably does not explain the frequency with which MIH affects individuals born with cleft lip and palate. This is likely the strongest evidence that multiple interacting genes contribute to MIH. Further, when children born with a smaller cleft lip and palate and who therefore underwent primary bone grafting were compared to children born with a larger cleft lip and palate and who therefore underwent secondary bone grafting, children who were treated with a primary bone grafting were more likely to have incisors affected [24]. These data suggested that severity of MIH can depend on whether primary or secondary alveolar grafting was done [25]. These data provide definitive evidence that a complex genetic component is the reason certain individuals have MIH.

Genes

Finally, a brief word on genes that might contribute to MIH. The first hypothesis generated was that genes involved in dental enamel formation contributed to MIH [9]. Genes involved in immune response have also been suggested as contributing to MIH [10, 26, 27]. Developmental genes previously associated with cleft lip and palate [11] or supernumerary teeth [19] have also been tested for association with MIH. Results are inconsistent but likely some studies' sample sizes were too small to allow for detecting associations [26, 27], since we believe many contributing genes have relatively small effect sizes.

Mutations in enamel formation genes, such as amelogenin (*AMELX*) and metalloproteinase 20 (*MMP20*), cause forms of amelogenesis imperfecta [28]. These same genes have been associated with dental caries, erosive tooth wear, and MIH [29, 30]. For additional genes related to amelogenesis or other gene pathways, such as immune response, xenobiotic detoxication, and ion transport, the reader can consult the study by Figueira et al. [31]. Following the concept of complex or multifactorial inheritance, MIH is a relatively common microform (Table 1) of amelogenesis imperfecta and is part of a spectrum that includes susceptibility to dental caries (Fig. 2).

In conclusion, MIH has a complex or multifactorial mode of inheritance, with contributions from several genes with relatively small individual effects and the presence of infection early in life. This is the process *theory* for MIH or the best system of ideas that explain how MIH changes and develops.

Acknowledgment

The author thanks all the scientists that currently work and have worked on the topic of MIH and for having had the open mind to concede that MIH is the result of a multifactorial mode of inheritance. Using the multifactorial mode of inheritance premise in future study designs will only benefit the children who suffer from this developmental disturbance and save valuable resources, research dollars, and time.

Conflict of Interest Statement

The author has no conflict of interest to declare.

Funding Sources

None.

References

1 American Museum of Natural History. What is a theory? Available from: https://www.amnh.org/exhibitions/darwin/evolution-today/what-is-a-theory (accessed July 15, 2023).
2 Weerheijm KL. Molar incisor hypomineralisation (MIH). Eur J Paediatr Dent. 2003 Sep;4(3):114–20.
3 Weerheijm KL, Jälevik B, Alaluusa S. Molar-incisor hypomineralisation. Caries Res. 2001 Sep-Oct;35(5):390–1.
4 Curzon ME, Ogden AR, Williams-Ward M, Cleaton-Jones PE. Case report: a medieval case of molar-incisor-hypomineralization. Br Dent J. 2015 Dec;219(12):583–7.
5 Fraser FC. The genetics of cleft lip and cleft palate. Am J Hum Genet. 1970 May;22(3):336–52.
6 Wright S. An analysis of variability in number of digits in an inbred strain of guinea pigs. Genetics. 1934 Nov;19(6):506–36.
7 Lopes LB, Machado V, Mascarenhas P, Mendes JJ, Botelho J. The prevalence of molar-incisor hypomineralization: a systematic review and meta-analysis. Sci Rep. 2021 Nov;11(1):22405.
8 Vieira AR. Prevalence of molar incisor hypomineralisation has a North-South gradient between Europe and North Africa. Eur J Paediatr Dent. 2019 Oct;20(5):501–2.
9 Jeremias F, Koruyucu M, Küchler EC, Bayram M, Tuna EB, Deeley K, et al. Genes expressed in dental enamel development are associated with molar-incisor hypomineralization. Arch Oral Biol. 2013 Oct;58(10):1434–42.
10 Bussaneli DG, Restrepo M, Fragelli CMB, Santos-Pinto L, Jeremias F, Cordeiro RCL, et al. Genes regulating immune response and amelogenesis interact in increasing the susceptibility to molar-incisor hypomineralization. Caries Res. 2019;53(2):217–27.
11 Bezamat M, Souza JF, Silva FMF, Corrêa EG, Fatturi AL, Brancher JA, et al. Gene-environment interaction in molar-incisor hypomineralization. PLoS One. 2021 Jan;16(1):e0241898.
12 Silva FMF, Carvalho FM, Franco ALMM, Soares TRC, Gonçalves AF, Vieira AR, et al. Association between molar hypomineralization, genes involved in enamel development, and medication in early childhood: a preliminary study. Int J Paediatr Dent. 2024;34(3):211–8.
13 Teixeira RJPB, Andrade NS, Queiroz LCC, Mendes FM, Moura MS, Moura LFAD, et al. Exploring the association between genetic and environmental factors and molar incisor hypomineralization: evidence from a twin study. Int J Paediatr Dent. 2018 Mar;28(2):198–206.
14 Vieira AR, Manton DJ. On the variable clinical presentation of molar-incisor hypomineralization. Caries Res. 2019;53(4):482–8.
15 Silva MJ, Scurrah KJ, Craig JM, Manton DJ, Kilpatrick N. Etiology of molar incisor hypomineralization—a systematic review. Community Dent Oral Epidemiol. 2016 Aug;44(4):342–53.
16 Rosen D, Bille C, Petersen I, Skytthe A, von Bornemann Hjelmborg J, Pedersen JK, et al. Risk of oral clefts in twins. Epidemiology. 2011 May;22(3):313–9.
17 Vieira AR. On the genetic contribution to molar incisor hypomineralisation. Int J Paediatr Dent. 2019 Jan;29(1):2–3.
18 Lacerda RHW, Vieira AR. Dental anomalies and genetic polymorphisms as predictors of maxillofacial growth in individuals born with cleft lip and palate. J Dent Res. 2023 Aug;102(9):979–87.
19 Koruyucu M, Kasimoğlu Y, Seymen F, Bayram M, Patir A, Ergöz N, et al. Rethinking isolated cleft lip and palate as a syndrome. Oral Surg Oral Med Oral Pathol Oral Radiol. 2018 Apr;125(4):307–12.
20 Lavôr JR, Lacerda RHW, Modesto A, Vieira AR. Maxillary incisor enamel defects in individuals born with cleft lip/palate. PLoS One. 2020 Dec;15(12):e0244506.

21 Hartsock LA, Burnheimer J, Modesto A, Vieira AR. A snapshot of the prevalence of molar incisor hypomineralization and fluorosis in Pittsburgh, Pennsylvania, USA. Pediatr Dent. 2020 Jan;42(1):36–40.
22 Lacerda RHW, Filgueiras VM, Mendonça AC, Vieira AR. Molar-incisor hypomineralization in a cohort of individuals born with cleft lip and palate. Orthod Craniofac Res. 2024 Jun;27(Suppl 1): 21–6.
23 Sato Y, Yoshioka E, Saijo Y, Miyamoto T, Azuma H, Tanahashi Y, et al. Lower respiratory tract infections and orofacial clefts: a prospective cohort study from the Japan Environment and Children's Study. J Epidemiol. 2022 Jun;32(6):270–6.
24 Allam E, Ghoneima A, Tholpady SS, Kula K. Enamel hypomineralization in children with clefts and the relationship to treatment: a cross-sectional retrospective study. Ann Plast Surg. 2018 Nov;81(5):544–7.
25 Vieira AR. Molar-incisor hypomineralization and cleft lip and palate. Ann Plast Surg. 2019 Feb;82(2):252.
26 Hočevar L, Kovač J, Podkrajšek KT, Batelino S, Pavlič A. The possible influence of genetic aetiological factors on molar-incisor hypomineralisation. Arch Oral Biol. 2020 Oct;118:104848.
27 Georgina-Pérez L, Ribas-Pérez D, Dehesa-Santos A, Mendoza-Mendoza A. Relationship between the TGFBR1 gene and molar incisor hypomineralization. J Pers Med. 2023 May;13(5):777.
28 Vieira AR. Beyond amelogenesis imperfecta mutations: hypomorphic forms. Monogr Oral Sci. 2021;30:20–35.
29 Vieira AR. Genetic basis of enamel and dentin defects. In: Vieira AR, editor. Genetic Basis of Oral Health Conditions. 1st ed. Cham: Springer; 2019. p. 9–21.
30 Vieira AR, Modesto A. Amelogenesis imperfecta enamel changes, amelogenin, and dental caries susceptibility. Front Dent Med. 2020 Nov;1:613851.
31 Figueira RS, Muniz FWMG, Costa LC, Moura MS, Moura LFAD, Oliveira BM, et al. Association between genetic factors and molar-incisor hypomineralization or hypomineralized second primary molar: a systematic review. Arch Oral Biol. 2023 Aug;152:105716.

Alexandre R. Vieira
Department of Foundational Sciences
School of Dental Medicine, East Carolina University
4216 Ross Hall, Greenville, NC 27858 (USA)
vieiraa23@ecu.edu

Published online: July 1, 2024
Rios D, Santos-Pinto L (eds): Molar Incisor Hypomineralisation: New Perceptions. Monogr Oral Sci. Basel, Karger, 2024, vol 32, pp 147–156 (DOI: 10.1159/000538884)

Deciduous Teeth Hypomineralisation and Perinatal Risk Factors

Kasandra Yupanqui[a] Diego Girotto Bussaneli[a] Aline Leite de Farias[b] Manuel Restrepo[b] Lourdes Santos-Pinto[a]

[a]Department of Morphology and Pediatric Dentistry, Araraquara School of Dentistry, São Paulo State University (Unesp), Araraquara, Brazil; [b]School of Dentistry, CES University, Medellin, Colombia

Abstract

Hypomineralisation defects with demarcated opacities are also observed in the deciduous dentition and have been found to be a predictive factor for hypomineralisation defects in the permanent dentition. Deciduous molar hypomineralisation (DMH) represents a qualitative enamel defect primarily afflicting deciduous second molars, albeit its presence is not limited solely to deciduous second molars, as it can manifest in deciduous canines and first molars. Thus, the presence of demarcated hypomineralisation defects in deciduous teeth could be called as deciduous teeth hypomineralisation. Clinically, these defects are characterized by demarcated opacities, post-eruptive enamel breakdown, atypical caries lesions, and atypical restorations. The accurate diagnosis of DMH continues to present a clinical challenge, and the reported prevalence of this defect exhibits notable variability across different countries. Its precise etiology remains elusive; however, there is a prevailing suspicion that events occurring during the prenatal, perinatal, or early postnatal periods, particularly those unfolding during the perinatal phase, are intricately linked to DMH development. Factors such as delivery complications, neonatal complications, prematurity, and low birth weight have been associated with DMH. Notably, there exists a possibility that, the more health-related events occur during this critical period, the greater the likelihood of a child presenting with this enamel defect. Nevertheless, the establishment of these associations warrants further investigation through prospective studies. Acquiring knowledge regarding the factors associated with this defect holds paramount importance for effective diagnosis, guidance for families with affected children, and the formulation of strategies to mitigate the incidence of these contributory factors.

Introduction

Developmental defects of enamel are structural alterations in tooth enamel resulting from factors that impact ameloblasts during the enamel formation process [1]. These defects can be of the hypoplastic or hypomineralised type. Among hypomineralisations, a particular category of de-

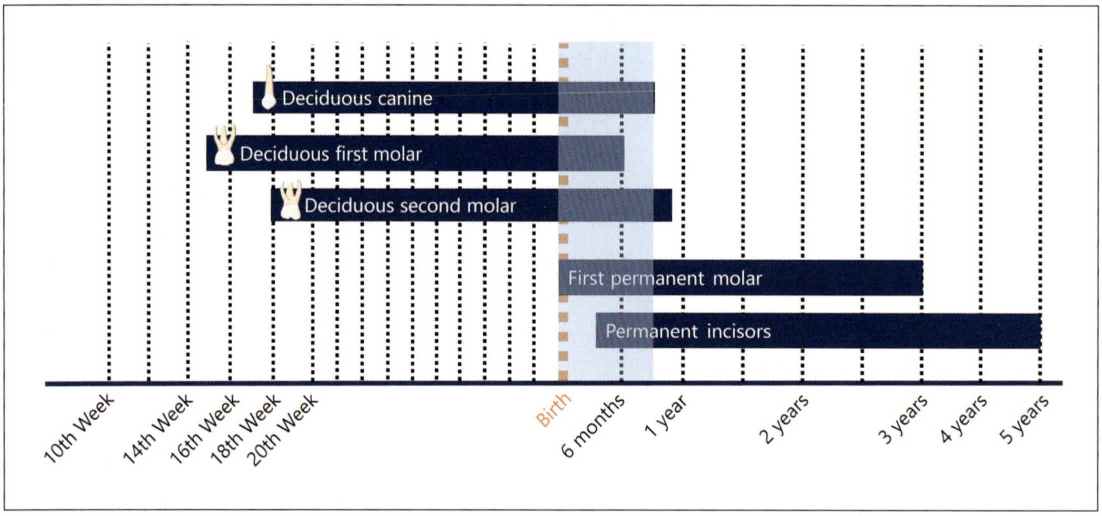

Fig. 1. Crown mineralisation period of deciduous and permanent teeth. Note also the coincident period of formation between them. Own elaboration based on McDonald and Avery; Santos-Pinto et al. [26, 43].

fects, known as molar incisor hypomineralisation (MIH), has garnered significant attention from both clinicians and researchers.

MIH was formally defined in 2001 by Weerheijm et al. [2] and is a qualitative defect that affects at least one first permanent molar and can affect permanent incisors [3]. Clinically, it is characterized by demarcated opacities, posteruptive enamel breakdown, atypical caries lesions, atypical restorations, or even the loss of the affected tooth [4–6]. Subsequently, numerous studies have been conducted to investigate its prevalence, etiology, and therapeutic approaches. Additionally, these investigations have raised the possibility of detecting hypomineralisation defects similar to MIH in other types of teeth, including deciduous second molars, second permanent molars, and the cusps of permanent canines [4]. Thus, defects in deciduous second molars were defined as deciduous molar hypomineralisation (DMH) and, more recently, defects in other permanent teeth were called hypomineralisation of other permanent teeth [7–9].

Research focused on elucidating the characteristics and prevalence of DMH has been published since 2008 [7]. Although in the deciduous dentition the defect is more prevalent in second molars, it can also be present in canines and first molars, but there are few studies that provide data on the prevalence and factors associated with these teeth [10–13].

The evidence that DMH and MIH may be associated has made DMH a predictive factor for MIH [14]. The presence of the defect in both dentitions could be explained by the coincidence of the formation period of the deciduous second molars with the permanent first molars and incisors (as shown in Fig. 1).

Much like MIH, the etiology of these defects in deciduous molars remains unknown. Extensive inquiry has been directed toward events occurring during pregnancy, childbirth, and early childhood, with particular emphasis on perinatal risk factors, which appear to be most frequently associated with these conditions, followed by prenatal factors [15].

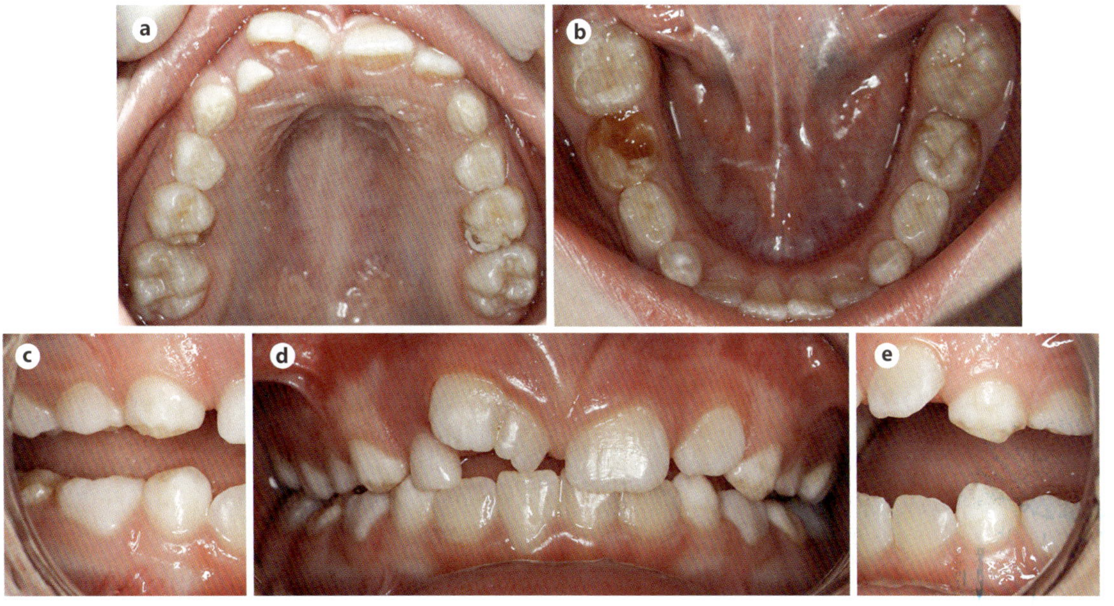

Fig. 2. Patient aged 7 years and 1 month in the mixed dentition stage, showing deciduous teeth hypomineralisation. **a** Maxillary arch, showing posteruptive enamel breakdown defects in teeth 55, 53, 63 and atypical restoration in tooth 65. **b** Mandibular arch, showing atypical restoration defects in tooth 75 and extensive posteruptive enamel breakdown in tooth 85. **c–e** The detail of hypomineralisation defects in deciduous canines, in teeth 53, 63, 73, and 83.

The literature points out that the risk factors frequently associated with DMH occur in the perinatal period, considering this period to be the days before labor or shortly after, both in the mother and in the newborn [15]. Thus, perinatal factors would be those occurring from labor until 28 days of life [15]. However, according to the World Health Organization, the perinatal period is the time between week 22 of pregnancy and 7 days after birth and the neonatal period is the time between birth and 28 days [16]. For this review, and for didactic reasons, we chose to consider the perinatal period as reported in research on DMH, which is the time from birth to 28 days of life.

The aim of this review is to present information on demarcated hypomineralisation defects in the deciduous dentition and the risk factors that occur in the perinatal period.

Deciduous Teeth Hypomineralisation

DMH, also referred to as hypomineralised second primary molars (HSPMs), constitutes an enamel developmental anomaly that shares analogous characteristics with MIH. It is defined as a hypomineralisation defect observed in one to four deciduous second molars [7]. This nomenclature stems from the observation that the deciduous second molar is the tooth most afflicted by this condition. Nevertheless, similar defects have also been documented in deciduous canines and first molars [10–13] (as shown in Fig. 2). Thus, to use a broader term, since the defect can be present in deciduous molars and canines, it could be called deciduous teeth hypomineralisation.

A recent systematic review reports the global prevalence of DMH to be 6.8%, albeit with a substantial variability in reported rates, ranging from 0 to 41% [17]. It is unclear whether these differences actually occur or result from difficulties in defect recognition, characteristics of the studied population, and methodological variations across the conducted studies. Furthermore, data on the prevalence of other affected deciduous teeth are scarce. The prevalence of affected canines ranges from 2.22% to 11.11% [10–13], and the prevalence of deciduous first molars has not been clearly determined at the child level, since in the studies found, assessments of these teeth were generally carried out on children who already had DMH and not on the total sample assessed [11, 12]. Consequently, like with MIH research, there is a pronounced need for standardized investigations, assessment of the entire deciduous dentition, featuring meticulously trained evaluators employing established criteria and indices for defect diagnosis. Such standardization is crucial both for clinical recordkeeping and epidemiological research [6, 18, 19].

The demarcated hypomineralisation defect, as seen in both MIH and DMH, is characterized by demarcated opacities, spanning a spectrum of colors from white to brown. These opacities signify a more porous and mechanically compromised enamel, rendering it susceptible to fractures in the affected region, often occurring shortly after eruption due to masticatory forces [4]. The porosity and posteruptive enamel breakdown areas create a conducive environment for dental plaque accumulation and subsequently foster the development of carious lesions. These lesions on the affected teeth are called atypical carious lesions because their location, extent, and rapid progression do not correspond to the pattern of biofilm accumulation and a usual carious lesion. Likewise, when these teeth are restored, it is called an atypical restoration. Thus, hypomineralised enamel may contribute to an elevated prevalence of carious lesions in deciduous second molars [20]. Children with DMH, for instance, are at up to three times higher risk of experiencing caries compared to their unaffected counterparts [21].

Additionally, patients with MIH and DMH may frequently report sensitivity, whether in response to air exposure or commonplace mechanical stimuli like tooth brushing. This heightened sensitivity can also pose challenges in maintaining proper oral hygiene for the affected teeth [4, 22].

Furthermore, DMH is regarded as a predictive factor for MIH, as children with DMH exhibit up to a 5-fold higher likelihood of subsequently developing MIH [14, 23], particularly in cases of mild DMH [23]. It has recently been observed that demarcated canine hypomineralisations have also been associated with MIH [10]. Hence, diligent monitoring of children presenting with any of these defects is crucial until the eruption of permanent molars and incisors. It is known that the presence of the defect in both dentitions is due to the overlapping period of formation between them, and that the occurrence of some risk factor in the mineralisation period would result in a hypomineralisation defect. Thus, knowledge of the common etiological factors would also make it possible to recognize patients at risk of MIH.

Perinatal Risk Factors

Although the etiological factors associated with DMH remain incompletely elucidated, several risk factors occurring during the prenatal, perinatal, and early postnatal periods in the first year of life are under suspicion [24]. This suspicion arises from the fact that the development of the deciduous second molar begins during intrauterine life and extends throughout the initial year after birth [15, 25, 26]. Considering that perinatal events, those encompassing the period from birth to 28 days thereafter, appear to be most strongly correlated with DMH [15], a systematic and comprehensive search was carried out on perinatal factors and DMH. The databases used were PubMed/MEDLINE, Scopus, and Web of Science. All studies evaluating risk factors in the perinatal period associated with DMH were included and analyzed.

Data concerning potential etiological factors of DMH are primarily derived from comprehensive health questionnaires, indicating that children with DMH tend to have a higher incidence of medical conditions, with a substantial proportion occurring during the perinatal period (45.3%) [15, 27]. Emphasizing the importance of investigating perinatal events is founded on the finding that the formation and mineralisation of deciduous second molars occur during this critical period. Observations by Kraus and Jordan underscore that the initiation of deciduous second molar development occurs around the 12th and 13th weeks of intrauterine life, with calcification possibly commencing as early as the 18th week [26]. However, at birth, only a portion of the occlusal surface exhibits mineralisation [26]. Similarly, the crowns of deciduous first molars and deciduous canines begin to calcify around weeks 15 and 17, respectively, and continue to mineralise a few months after birth [26] (as shown in Fig. 1). Given that the mineralisation process remains underway at birth, the presence of disturbing factors during this time frame holds the potential to influence the subsequent, inadequate mineralisation of the enamel.

The risk factors present in the perinatal period include prematurity [15, 28, 29], low birth weight [15, 27–31], mode of delivery (cesarean) [15, 29, 31], delivery complications, pre-eclampsia [15, 27, 28], neonatal complications, such as hospitalization within the first week of life and respiratory distress [15, 27, 29], incubator usage [28, 29], Apgar score [27], vitamin D levels [30, 31], and twin pregnancies [28]. Of these factors, delivery complications [15, 28], neonatal complications [15], low birth weight [15, 28], prematurity [29], and high vitamin D levels at birth [31] showed a significant association with DMH, which will be reported below.

Delivery Complications and Neonatal Complications

In some studies, delivery complications [15, 28], pre-eclampsia [27], and the mode of delivery (caesarean) [15, 29, 31] were considered risk factors. Of these, delivery complications were significantly associated with DMH [15, 32]. These delivery complications encompass conditions, such as retained placenta, bleeding, maternal hypoxia, and prolonged labor, with the latter being implicated in hypoxic episodes in the neonate [32]. Furthermore, additional events related with oxygen deprivation could be those occurring in neonatal complications [15] that result in hospitalization within the first week of life [27], episodes of hypoxia, respiratory difficulties [29], and the utilization of incubators [28, 29]. Consequently, events linked to oxygen deficiency may be the result of complications during childbirth and the neonate's health status, and this potentially exerts an influence on the activity of ameloblasts.

Assessment of hypoxia episodes stemming from potential birth asphyxia were conducted using the Apgar score. However, no statistically significant association between Apgar scores and DMH was discerned [27, 32]. It is imperative to underscore that the Apgar score serves as a descriptor of the neonate's overall condition at the first and fifth minutes after birth. The signs assessed are heart rate, breathing, muscle tone, reflex irritability, and skin color, using a score of 0–2 for each item. The sum of the scores ranges from 0 to 10, with values of 7–10 being considered normal, and a value of less than 7 being considered low, indicating the need for special medical attention or even resuscitation [33].

However, the Apgar score alone does not suffice to establish a definitive diagnosis of birth asphyxia, as such a diagnosis necessitates complementary physical and laboratory assessments [33]. While a direct link between low Apgar scores and hypoxia remains undetermined, it is conceivable that low Apgar scores may serve as an indicator of the neonate's initial compromised health status and challenges encountered during the transition from the intrauterine to the external environment. Such disruptions could potentially precipitate alterations in ameloblastic activity.

Low Birth Weight and Prematurity

In investigations concerning perinatal factors associated with DMH, a notable association has been observed between low birth weight [15, 27] and prematurity [29]. This association was further substantiated through a comprehensive systematic review with meta-analysis, revealing that children born with low birth weight exhibit a 1.5-fold elevated likelihood of presenting DMH, while this likelihood escalates to nearly twice as high in prematurely born children [32].

It is well documented that children born with low birth weight face heightened susceptibility to various diseases and infections [34]. Premature infants, in addition to enduring potential episodes of oxygen deprivation, are also susceptible to a spectrum of diseases and metabolic disorders owing to the disruption of normal fetal development [29]. Consequently, this augmented vulnerability to diseases and infections may have an impact on the developmental process of enamel, which is still undergoing mineralisation. Nonetheless, the precise mechanisms through which both factors may be intricately linked to the manifestation of DMH remain incompletely elucidated.

One proposed hypothesis posits that the perturbation of overall intrauterine development may influence the activity of ameloblasts during the enamel formation and mineralisation phase [29]. This alteration in ameloblastic function could potentially stem from the oxygen deficiency that may occur as a consequence of neonatal complications in premature infants [32]. Furthermore, it is plausible that the inadequate incorporation of essential chemical elements, such as calcium (Ca), phosphorus (P), carbon (C), and oxygen (O), plays a contributory role. Calcium deposition, a critical facet of enamel development, is intricately regulated by factors, including magnesium, acid-base equilibrium, parathyroid hormone, and vitamin D. It is noteworthy that the culmination of calcium accumulation in the body predominantly transpires during the final trimester of gestation [35, 36].

Additionally, low birth weight may be intricately linked to maternal health-related factors [27], potentially setting in motion a cascade of events encompassing premature deliveries and complications both during childbirth and in the neonatal period. A significant revelation emerged, indicating that children who experienced neonatal illnesses and whose mothers encountered complications during pregnancy and childbirth were six times more likely to manifest DMH in comparison to those solely experiencing childbirth complications [15]. Consequently, the cumulative occurrence of health-related events appears to intensify the likelihood of DMH occurrence [15]. This multifaceted interplay of health events during the perinatal period renders it challenging to pinpoint a singular risk factor, as many of these events are interconnected and often occur concurrently [29].

Vitamin D and Other Factors

Vitamin D levels have been assessed to both MIH [30, 37] and DMH [30, 31] at the prenatal, perinatal, and postnatal periods. Regrettably, none of the conducted studies have succeeded in establishing a definitive association with DMH. Notably, vitamin D plays a pivotal role in bone calcification, dental mineralisation, and the maintenance of plasma calcium concentrations [30]. Consequently, it is postulated that a deficiency in vitamin D during tooth development might impede the mineralisation process [37], potentially contributing to the presence of weakened or even hypomineralised enamel [30].

In the studies carried out on vitamin D, a patient is considered to have a vitamin D deficiency when they have concentrations of 25-hydroxyvitamin D of less than 50 nmol/L and a severe deficiency with values of less than 25/30 nmol/L [30, 38]. The greatest amount of vitamin D is obtained from exposure to the sun, through the action of UVB rays, so this deficiency could be due to reduced exposure to UVB rays, a nutritional deficiency, or a deficiency in the absorption of the vitamin in the body [38]. However, more studies need to be carried out to establish its relationship with DMH.

Investigations into twin pregnancies have been undertaken to explore potential genetic interrelationships with DMH. However, no statistically significant association has emerged [31]. It is crucial to acknowledge that twin pregnancies may also be linked to childbirth and neonatal complications, variables that warrant consideration in future research endeavors.

As previously delineated, perinatal factors appear to be the most prevalent in association with DMH [15]. Nonetheless, evidence suggests a correlation between certain prenatal and postnatal factors as well. A systematic review conducted by Lima et al. [32] revealed, in conjunction with perinatal factors, an association between DMH and maternal tobacco use during pregnancy, maternal hypertension, the absence of breastfeeding, antibiotic utilization, fever, and childhood asthma. However, another systematic review scrutinizing medication use during pregnancy and the initial year of life yielded inconclusive evidence regarding this association [39].

Given the potential exposure of children to diverse causal agents and the intricacies of isolating a single contributory factor associated with the defect, the etiology of DMH is increasingly regarded as multifactorial. Genetic factors may intertwine with environmental variables, influencing the development of these defects [40]. A recent systematic review addressed the genetic aspects of MIH and DMH, albeit characterized by very low-quality evidence, unveiled an association between hypomineralised deciduous second molars and a gene correlated with hypoxia, as well as methylation in genes linked to amelogenesis [41]. The identification of genes associated with these defects holds the potential to shed light on the mechanisms by which enamel formation becomes disrupted, leading to hypomineralisation [41].

Conclusion

The recognition and diagnosis of DMH bear substantial clinical implications for health care professionals engaged in the care of children. To facilitate the diagnosis of this enamel defect, the age of 5 years has been recommended, considering that at this age, a child can collaborate in oral assessments [18]. Nevertheless, whenever feasible, clinical diagnosis should be conducted upon the emergence of the deciduous second molar in the oral cavity, particularly among populations at a high risk of dental caries. This approach is essential due to the potential for more severe defects or extensive carious lesions emerging at later stages, rendering accurate defect visualization challenging. Timely diagnosis would enable the implementation of preventive measures, treatment, and follow-up protocols for children afflicted by DMH [10].

Intraoral assessments should include the comprehensive evaluation of the entire deciduous dentition to ascertain whether the patient exhibits defects in other deciduous teeth aside from the second molar. Analogous defects have been documented in deciduous canines and first molars [10–13], with the presence of canine defects also being correlated with MIH [10]. Additionally, it has been established that DMH serves as a predictive factor for MIH [14, 42] and that the absence of defects in deciduous teeth does not indicate a lack of risk of MIH. Consequently, in clinical practice, it is prudent to inform parents of the necessity for regular follow-ups until the eruption of permanent teeth.

With regard to the etiological factors of DMH, this review sought to present the most recent evidence on risk factors occurring in the perinatal period. Thus, of the perinatal factors found in the literature, those that showed a significant association with DMH were delivery complications [15, 28], neonatal complications [15], low birth weight [15, 27], and prematurity [29]. Other factors such as vitamin D and the Apgar score still require further research to verify their possible association with the defect. It is worth noting that research endeavors dedicated to unraveling the etiology of DMH are comparatively scarce in comparison to MIH. Therefore, there is a compelling demand for an expanded body of studies in this domain, particularly prospective investigations [15, 24, 28, 39] that encompass comprehensive analyses adjusted for potential confounding factors [24].

The acquisition of knowledge pertaining to factors associated with DMH holds substantial clinical significance, primarily for the early monitoring and diagnosis of children exposed to risk factors. Furthermore, given the pivotal role of research in decision-making in public health, further investigation into the etiological factors of DMH is imperative. Such endeavors would enable us to know the risk factors involved in the development of this defect and thereby facilitate the establishment of preventive measures aimed at mitigating or avoid exposure to these risk factors.

Statement of Ethics

Written informed consent was obtained from the parents for publication of the images.

Conflict of Interest Statement

The authors have no conflicts of interest to declare.

Funding Sources

This study was financed in part by the Coordenação de Aperfeiçoamento de Pessoal de Nível Superior – Brasil (CAPES) – Finance Code 001.

Author Contributions

K.Y.: conceptualization, wrote the original draft and review; D.G.B.: conceptualization, wrote the original draft and review; A.L.F.: conceptualization, writing review; M.R.: conceptualization, writing review; L.S.-P.: conceptualization, wrote the original draft and review.

References

1 Seow WK. Developmental defects of enamel and dentine: challenges for basic science research and clinical management. Aust Dent J. 2014;59(suppl 1): 143–54.

2 Weerheijm KL, Jälevik B, Alaluusua S. Molar-incisor hypomineralisation. Caries Res. 2001;35(5):390–1.

3 Bussaneli DG, Vieira AR, Santos-Pinto L, Restrepo M. Molar-incisor hypomineralisation: an updated view for aetiology 20 years later. Eur Arch Paediatr Dent. 2022;23(1):193–8.

4 Weerheijm KL, Duggal M, Mejàre I, Papagiannoulis L, Koch G, Martens LC, et al. Judgement criteria for molar incisor hypomineralisation (MIH) in epidemiologic studies: a summary of the European meeting on MIH held in Athens, 2003. Eur J Paediatr Dent. 2003;4(3): 110–3.

5 Lygidakis NA, Wong F, Jälevik B, Vierrou AM, Alaluusua S, Espelid I. Best Clinical Practice Guidance for clinicians dealing with children presenting with molar-incisor-hypomineralisation (MIH): an EAPD policy document. Eur Arch Paediatr Dent. 2010;11(2):75–81.

6 Lygidakis NA, Garot E, Somani C, Taylor GD, Rouas P, Wong FSL. Best clinical practice guidance for clinicians dealing with children presenting with molar-incisor-hypomineralisation (MIH): an updated European Academy of Paediatric Dentistry policy document. Eur Arch Paediatr Dent. 2022;23(1):3–21.

7 Elfrink MEC, Schuller AA, Weerheijm KL, Veerkamp JSJ. Hypomineralized second primary molars: Prevalence data in Dutch 5-year-olds. Caries Res. 2008; 42(4):282–5.

8 Elfrink MEC, Veerkamp JSJ, Aartman IHA, Moll HA, Cate JM Ten. Validity of scoring caries and primary molar hypomineralization (DMH) on intraoral photographs. Eur Arch Paediatr Dent. 2009; 10(suppl 1):5–10.
9 Kevrekidou A, Kosma I, Kotsanos I, Arapostathis KN, Kotsanos N. Enamel opacities in all other than molar incisor hypomineralisation index teeth of adolescents. Int J Paediatr Dent. 2021;31(2): 270–7.
10 Da Silva Figueiredo Sé MJ, Ribeiro APD, Dos Santos-Pinto LAM, De Cassia Loiola Cordeiro R, Cabral RN, Leal SC. Are hypomineralized primary molars and canines associated with molar-incisor hypomineralization? Pediatr Dent. 2017; 39(7):445–9.
11 Vlachou C, Arhakis A, Kotsanos N. Distribution and morphology of enamel hypomineralisation defects in second primary molars. Eur Arch Paediatr Dent. 2021;22(2):241–6.
12 Goyal A, Dhareula A, Gauba K, Bhatia SK. Prevalence, defect characteristics and distribution of other phenotypes in 3- to 6-year-old children affected with Hypomineralised Second Primary Molars. Eur Arch Paediatr Dent. 2019; 20(6):585–93.
13 Borrego-Martí N, Peris-Corominas R, Maura-Solivellas I, Ferrés-Padró E, Ferrés-Amat E. Hypomineralisation of second primary molars and primary canines: prevalence and description of lesions in a population of 153 patients visited at a hospital paediatric dentistry service. Eur J Paediatr Dent. 2021;22(3): 237–42.
14 Garot E, Denis A, Delbos Y, Manton D, Silva M, Rouas P. Are hypomineralised lesions on second primary molars (HSPM) a predictive sign of molar incisor hypomineralisation (MIH)? A systematic review and a meta-analysis. J Dent. 2018;72:8–13.
15 Ghanim AM, Morgan MV, Mariño RJ, Bailey DL, Manton DJ. Risk factors of hypomineralised second primary molars in a group of Iraqi schoolchildren. Eur Arch Paediatr Dent. 2012;13(3):111–8.
16 World Health Organization (WHO). WHO mortality database [Internet]. Available from: https://platform.who.int/mortality/themes/theme-details/topics/topic-details/MDB/perinatal-conditions.
17 McCarra C, Olegário IC, O'Connell AC, Leith R. Prevalence of hypomineralised second primary molars (HSPM): a systematic review and meta-analysis. Int J Paediatr Dent. 2022;32(3):367–82.
18 Elfrink MECC, Ghanim A, Manton DJ, Weerheijm KL. Standardised studies on molar incisor hypomineralisation (MIH) and hypomineralised second primary molars (HSPM): a need. Eur Arch Paediatr Dent. 2015 Jun;16(3):247–55.
19 Ghanim A, Silva MJ, Elfrink MEC, Lygidakis NA, Mariño RJ, Weerheijm KL, et al. Molar incisor hypomineralisation (MIH) training manual for clinical field surveys and practice. Eur Arch Paediatr Dent. 2017;18(4):225–42.
20 Elfrink MECC, Schuller AA, Veerkamp JSJJ, Poorterman JHGG, Moll HA, ten Cate BJMM. Factors increasing the caries risk of second primary molars in 5-year-old Dutch children. Int J Paediatr Dent. 2010;20(2):151–7.
21 Costa FS, Silveira ER, Pinto GS, Nascimento GG, Thomson WM, Demarco FF. Developmental defects of enamel and dental caries in the primary dentition: a systematic review and meta-analysis. J Dent. 2017;60(March):1–7.
22 Americano GCA, Jacobsen PE, Soviero VM, Haubek D. A systematic review on the association between molar incisor hypomineralization and dental caries. Int J Paediatr Dent. 2017;27(1):11–21.
23 Elfrink MECC, Ten Cate JM, Jaddoe VWV, Hofman A, Moll HA, Veerkamp JSJJ. Deciduous molar hypomineralization and molar incisor hypomineralization. J Dent Res. 2012;91(6):551–5.
24 Silva MJ, Scurrah KJ, Craig JM, Manton DJ, Kilpatrick N. Etiology of molar incisor hypomineralization – a systematic review. Community Dent Oral Epidemiol. 2016;44(4):342–53.
25 Elfrink MECC, Moll HA, Kiefte-De Jong JC, El Marroun H, Jaddoe VWV, Hofman A, et al. Is maternal use of medicines during pregnancy associated with deciduous molar hypomineralisation in the offspring? A prospective, population-based study. Drug Saf. 2013;36(8): 627–33.
26 McDonald RE, Avery DR. Development and morphology of the primary teeth. In: McDonald RE, Avery DR. Dentistry for the Child and Adolescent. 9th ed. Mosby Elsevier; 2011. p. 41–6.
27 Elfrink MECC, Moll HA, Kiefte-de Jong JC, Jaddoe VWV, Hofman A, Ten Cate JM, et al. Pre- and postnatal determinants of deciduous molar hypomineralisation in 6-year-old children. The generation R study. PLoS One. 2014;9(7): 1–8.
28 Lopes-Fatturi AA, Nogara Borges Menezes JV, Fraiz FC, da Silva Assuncao LR, de Souza JF, Menezes JVNB, et al. Systemic exposures associated with hypomineralized primary second molars. Pediatr Dent. 2019;41(5):364–70.
29 Lima LRS, Pereira AS, de Moura MS, Lima CCB, Paiva SM, Moura LFAD, et al. Pre-term birth and asthma is associated with hypomineralized second primary molars in pre-schoolers: a population-based study. Int J Paediatr Dent. 2020;30(2):193–201.
30 van der Tas JT, Elfrink MEC, Heijboer AC, Rivadeneira F, Jaddoe VWV, Tiemeier H, et al. Foetal, neonatal and child vitamin D status and enamel hypomineralization. Community Dent Oral Epidemiol. 2018;46(4):343–51.
31 Silva MJ, Kilpatrick NM, Craig JM, Manton DJ, Leong P, Burgner D, et al. Etiology of hypomineralized second primary molars: a prospective twin study. J Dent Res. 2019;98(1):77–83.
32 Lima LJS, Ramos-Jorge ML, Soares MEC. Prenatal, perinatal and postnatal events associated with hypomineralized second primary molar: a systematic review with meta-analysis. Clin Oral Investig. 2021;25(12):6501–16.
33 American Academy of Pediatrics Committee on Fetus and Newborn; American College of Obstetricians and Gynecologists Committee on Obstetric Practice. The Apgar score. Pediatrics. 2015;136(4):819–22.
34 Corrêa-Faria P, Martins-Júnior PA, Vieira-Andrade RG, Oliveira-Ferreira F, Marques LS, Ramos-Jorge ML. Developmental defects of enamel in primary teeth: prevalence and associated factors. Int J Paediatr Dent. 2013;23(3):173–9.
35 Tsang RC, Donovan EF, Steichen JJ. Calcium physiology and pathology in the neonate. Pediatr Clin North Am. 1976; 23(4):611–26.
36 Habelitz S, DenBesten PK, Marshall SJ, Marshall GW, Li W. Amelogenin control over apatite crystal growth is affected by the pH and degree of ionic saturation. Orthod Craniofacial Res. 2005;8(4):232–8.

37 Kühnisch J, Thiering E, Kratzsch J, Heinrich-Weltzien R, Hickel R, Heinrich J. Elevated serum 25(OH)-vitamin D levels are negatively correlated with molar-incisor hypomineralization. J Dent Res. 2015;94(2):381–7.
38 Cashman KD. Vitamin D deficiency: defining, prevalence, causes, and strategies of addressing. Calcif Tissue Int. 2020;106(1):14–29.
39 Serna Muñoz C, Ortiz Ruiz AJ, Pérez Silva A, Bravo-González LA, Vicente AA, Serna Munoz C, et al. Second primary molar hypomineralisation and drugs used during pregnancy and infancy. A systematic review. Clin Oral Investig. 2020;24(3):1287–97.
40 Vieira AR, Kup E. On the etiology of molar-incisor hypomineralization. Caries Res. 2016;50(2):166–9.
41 da Silva Figueira R, Mustafa Gomes Muniz FW, Costa LC, Silva de Moura M, Moura L de FA de D, Mello de Oliveira B, et al. Association between genetic factors and molar-incisor hypomineralisation or hypomineralised second primary molar: a systematic review. Arch Oral Biol. 2023;152:105716.
42 Negre-Barber A, Montiel-Company JM, Boronat-Catalá M, Catalá-Pizarro M, Almerich-Silla JM. Hypomineralized second primary molars as predictor of molar incisor hypomineralization. Sci Rep. 2016;6(May):1–6.
43 Santos-Pinto L, Fragelli C, Bussaneli DG, Ary SP. Hipomineralização de Molares Decíduos. In: Hipomineralização de Molares e Incisivos. Nova Odessa, SP: Napoleão-Quintessence Publishing Brazil; 2020. p. 216.

Lourdes Santos-Pinto
Department of Morphology and Pediatric Dentistry
Araraquara School of Dentistry, São Paulo State University (Unesp)
Rua Humaitá 1680, Araraquara, SP 14801-385 (Brazil)
lourdes.santos-pinto@unesp.br

Published online: July 1, 2024
Rios D, Santos-Pinto L (eds): Molar Incisor Hypomineralisation: New Perceptions. Monogr Oral Sci. Basel, Karger, 2024, vol 32, pp 157–165 (DOI: 10.1159/000538886)

Factors Associated with Hypersensitivity, Management, and Treatment Options for Teeth with Molar Incisor Hypomineralisation

Marco Aurélio Benini Paschoal[a] Fabrício Kitazono de Carvalho[b]
Marina Deus Moura Lima[c] Soraya Coelho Leal[d]

[a]Department of Pediatric Dentistry, School of Dentistry, Federal University of Minas Gerais, Belo Horizonte, Brazil; [b]Department of Pediatric Dentistry, Ribeirão Preto School of Dentistry, University of São Paulo, Ribeirao Preto, Brazil; [c]Department of Pathology and Oral Health, Federal University of Piauí, Teresina, Brazil; [d]Department of Dentistry, Faculty of Health Science, University of Brasília, Brasília, Brazil

Abstract

Tooth hypersensitivity is a common symptom in molar incisor hypomineralisation (MIH) patients and can affect children's quality of life. During daily routine, children with MIH often report sensitivity to various thermal and mechanical stimuli, and difficulty in achieving effective analgesia is a common issue becoming a challenge for dentists. Research has focused on the possible pathophysiological mechanisms behind this phenomenon, which, in turn, have not been determined. Even with the apparently intact enamel of MIH-teeth, the porosity of the hypomineralised enamel acts as an open door for the invasion of oral microorganisms, which reach the dentinal tubules, and stimulate subclinical inflammatory reactions in the pulp. Tissue inflammation may, in turn, lead to morphological and cytochemical changes within sensory neurons, resulting in sensitization of these nerve fibers. This phenomenon is complex, and the treatment modalities focus on inflammation management followed by tubule obliteration by using different materials and technologies. In conclusion, this chapter reviews the concept and etiology of hypersensitivity in teeth with MIH and summarizes the clinical management according to the best evidence available.

Hypersensitivity in Molar Incisor Hypomineralisation

Molar incisor hypomineralisation (MIH), as defined and characterized in previous chapters, has proven to be a very challenging condition for various reasons, such as children and parents are often unfamiliar with the problem. To date, MIH etiology is not fully understood; first permanent molars are the most affected teeth; mechanical and chemical properties of MIH-teeth are reduced in comparison to nonaffected ones, which may lead to a posteruptive breakdown (PEB). In

Table 1. The prevalence of hypersensitivity reported by studies conducted in different countries

Study	Country	Measurement	Prevalence
Haidary [33], 2014	Dubai	Self-report[a]	98.3
Oyedele et al. [34], 2015	Nigeria	Self-report[a]	15
Petrou et al. [35], 2015	Germany	Self-report[a]	38.3
Raposo et al. [2], 2019	Brazil	Air blast and tactile examination	34.7
de Castro et al. [6], 2021	Brazil	Air blast	28
Linner et al. [36], 2021	Germany	SCASS[b] and self-report	3.8–13.3

[a]VAS, visual analogue scale. [b]The Schiff Cold Air Sensitive Scale.

these MIH-PEB cases, a progression in severity is inevitable. Currently, available dental technology and/or knowledge do not provide materials/techniques/procedures to prevent enamel breakdown where affected molars are more prone to develop an aggressive pattern of caries lesions in comparison to molars without this enamel defect. Yet, opacities might be located at cusp slopes and cusp tips, which, in case of enamel breakdown, lead to the formation of atypical cavities, making the restorative procedure more complex, and increasing the odds of presenting hypersensitivity. Consequently, difficulty in achieving proper analgesia may be observed. All the factors mentioned above, when analyzed together, may make the patient less compliant with the dental treatment. Therefore, the professional needs to focus on the aspects he/she can control to offer the child a non-traumatic experience. And indeed, one of these aspects is the management of dental hypersensitivity (DH).

Although most of the papers that have been published about MIH refer to the high prevalence of hypersensitivity in affected teeth, a worldwide prevalence rate is unknown, as just a few studies aimed to investigate this aspect (Table 1). This might be explained, in part, by the difficulties in expressing quantitatively a subjective perception that varies from individual to individual and is influenced by many different factors such as population screened and diagnostic criteria [1]. In terms of MIH, a complicating factor to gathering reliable information refers to the age of the patients affected, as its diagnostic is usually performed when the first permanent molars are recently erupted, i.e., young children. The use of different scales to measure pain is recommended due to its subjective aspect. However, in children, this strategy may present some limitations regarding the immaturity of subjects [2].

Thus, this chapter aims to present what is known up to this moment of the mechanisms involved with MIH hypersensitivity, management, and the current treatment options available.

Mechanisms/Etiology of MIH-DH

Defining MIH-teeth hypersensitivity is a quite hard task since the current mechanism and tissues involved in the source of pain are not very clear and discussed properly. So, the etiology of MIH-DH is multifactorial, and the neurosensory mechanisms underlying this symptom remain unclear. Due to this statement, describing this clinical symptom as a DH (including symptoms of the dentine and inflamed pulp tissues) may be more reasonable rather than the term dentine hypersensitivity.

Hypomineralised enamel exhibits certain characteristics compared to normal enamel that could contribute to the occurrence of DH [2–6] as lower mineral content and reduced hardness values, higher density of pulp innervation, a greater number of immune cells, and increased interprismatic gaps [7–10]. The porous hypomineralised enamel not only facilitates bacterial penetration but also inadequately shields the dentin layer against various stimuli such as cold. Consequently, it fails to sufficiently protect the underlying pulp tissue from thermal, physical, and chemical stimuli within the oral cavity. Hence, individuals with MIH present odds to more frequently chronic pulp inflammation.

Accordingly, the pain clinical feature phenomena occurring in MIH-teeth could be defined by the dentin acute pain in combination with the chronic pain feature from pulp inflammation. Thus, an adapted version of the classical definition of dentin hypersensitivity might be used to define the tooth hypersensitivity of MIH-teeth as follows: "MIH-hypersensitivity is an acute, short, sharp pain that arises from porous enamel or PEB, allowing dentin to respond to thermal, tactile, osmotic, chemical, or evaporative stimuli." This sensitivity cannot be attributed to any other form of dentin exposure or pathology [3]. Additionally, there is a chronic inflammatory state in the pulp associated with MIH.

Hypomineralised teeth with PEB show a higher prevalence of DH, but PEB is not a necessary condition for the occurrence of DH [6]. The color of the opacity is a predictor of DH where teeth with yellow-brownish opacities show DH more frequently than those with white-creamy [11]. Accordingly, the darker opacities present a lower percentual of mineral content and increased interprismatic gaps, which favor the spread of stimuli to the dentin, so they are predisposed to PEB and bacterial invasion as well [11, 12].

Factors Involving Symptomatology and Its Impact on Oral Health and Daily/Routine Life

The morphological and chemical characteristics of teeth affected by MIH, previously discussed, make them more prone to break and more painful worsening the general and oral health subjects' quality of life. In the enamel dynamics under various oral conditions (e.g., chewing forces, temperature fluctuations, pH changes, among others), an MIH severely affected tooth can be part of a vicious cycle of destruction, through PEB and/or caries. The first permanent molars, considered the most affected teeth, are particularly exposed to this dynamic, especially because they are in areas that are more difficult to access for proper oral hygiene and are more exposed to chewing impacts. A mildly affected first permanent molar by MIH (exhibiting a large yellow/brownish demarcated opacity, for instance, on the occlusal surface) due to its higher porosity characteristics can experience increased DH, leading to insufficient dental hygiene, thus raising the odds of caries risk of this tooth.

Other factors may contribute to the establishment of this cycle. Since the affected tooth surface is more porous, it may be more susceptible to the adhesion of cariogenic biofilm [13]. This fact in conjunction with a cariogenic diet may prone a more aggressive pattern of caries in MIH-affected teeth. In this context, another issue is the presence of bacteria inside dentinal tubules of teeth with MIH, even in teeth with an intact surface [8]. Thus, although still not extensively studied, there is evidence that children with MIH face greater difficulty in cleaning the more severely affected teeth [14]. These same authors also found that children with severe MIH have a higher occurrence of dietary restrictions (i.e., problems with the intake of food), particularly solid food and/or hot/cold foods. This could be associated with the child adopting a diet that is softer and more cariogenic, further perpetuating the vicious cycle.

Furthermore, since MIH commonly presents in an asymmetric and heterogeneous manner, often more severe on one side of the child's oral cavity, it can lead the child to avoid chewing on that side, which may result in alterations in their masticatory muscles [15]. All these factors, combined with the DH present in MIH, can impact their oral health-related quality of life [16].

In addition, child's characteristics at the age of over 6 years when they are in the process of developing autonomy often perform their oral hygiene without parental supervision in most cases. Many parents still mistake the first permanent molar for a primary tooth since its eruption is not associated with any exfoliation of a primary tooth. As a result, there is a high likelihood of delayed detection of the problem, and often the tooth already exhibits more severe clinical consequences, such as PEB exposing dentin or even an extensive carious lesion. Here, it is crucial to emphasize the significant importance of oral health education for all stakeholders involved with children in this age group, including teachers, educators, parents, pediatricians, and other health care professionals, as well as the children themselves.

On the other hand, considering all these factors associated with severe MIH, along with the increased need for repeated dental treatments in these cases, one could argue that this condition might be associated with higher levels of anxiety and dental fear in these children. However, current evidence shows no such association [16, 17]. Anxiety and dental fear might be established in a multifactorial manner, with previous experiences playing a more significant role than factors related solely to a specific dental element. Thus, the perceived challenges in treating MIH-affected teeth are primarily related to difficulties in achieving adequate anesthesia and managing DH rather than being driven by fear of dental care.

Therefore, from a clinical perspective, when examining children with MIH-DH, it is necessary to routinely inquire about difficulties or pain during oral hygiene; dietary restrictions related to cold/hot and/or solid foods; alterations or symptoms in masticatory muscles, and any other possible disruptions in the child's routine (Fig. 1).

Management of Patients and Teeth with MIH-DH-Related Discomfort

The studies focusing on MIH-DH-related discomfort are limited. The subjectivity of the symptom can explain this fact, the limited cases of high-intensity DH, and the asymmetric and heterogeneous manner of this condition, making the "ideal" study design a challenging task for investigators. Thus, many strategies to face MIH-DH-related discomfort are driven mainly by case reports, literature reviews, and clinical experience.

Fundamental steps are needed to manage MIH cases including identification of risk, prompt diagnosis, desensitization, preventing the occurrence of PEB and dental caries, restoration of affected teeth or extraction if beyond possible repair, and follow-up and maintenance [18].

When dealing with patients with MIH-DH-related discomfort, it is necessary to identify pain by thermic (i.e., cold stimulus), physical (i.e., air blast by triple syringe), and/or mechanical (i.e., tactile stimulus), and supported by subjective methods (i.e., scales) aiming to measurement of this clinical symptom. Usually, the use of face scales to measure pain in children is a common strategy but shows limitations [2]. Therefore, other methodologies, such as the use of the Visual Analog Scale (VAS) using a numerical reference, are better recommended [2]. In addition, the Schiff Cold Air Sensitivity Scale (SCASS) shows higher sensitivity and specificity to reduce subjective bias in the assessment of this challenging symptom [19]. Using the SCASS, the examiner assesses the reaction of the individual to the stimulus. If the subject responds to the stimulus and moves, DH diagnosis is confirmed [8, 20]. This can be quite useful when the clinician wants to determine how effective a procedure to control hypersensitivity is (before and after).

During the investigation, a hand mirror can guide both the patient and professional in showing the tooth/teeth presenting MIH-DH-related discomfort. After this step, with the support of the

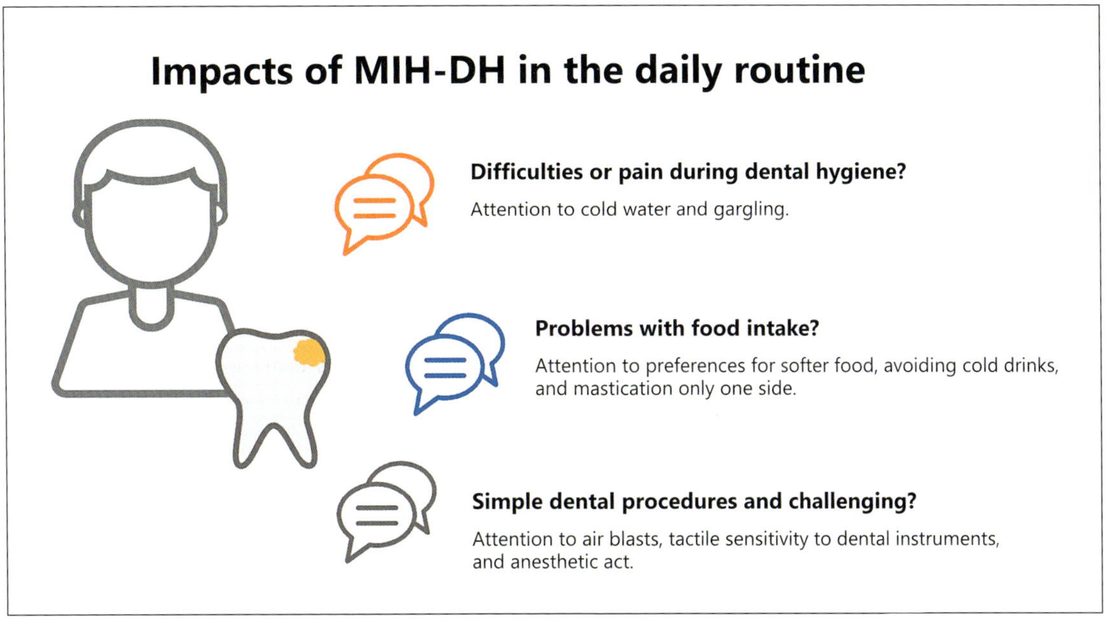

Fig. 1. Impacts in the daily routine related to individual with MIH and hypersensitivity.

stimulus cited, the patient is asked to fulfill the scales (e.g., Face Scale, VAS) or professionally analyze by SCASS.

The evaluation of the pain intensity by VAS can provide the need for immediate care (values higher than 8) or postponement (values lower than 3). In this way, after the different treatments have been applied, and evaluated for a period, the values can guide the proper management [21] (Fig. 2).

Main Modalities for Treatment of MIH-DH-Related Discomfort

Since there is a specific chapter for the management of MIH with PEB (see Chapter 19), this topic will focus only on MIH-DH opacities. As stated previously, teeth with MIH-DH-related discomfort present chronic pulp inflammation due to its unique characteristics. So, the clinical management of those teeth is, didactically, first focused on the treatment of inflammation (1st phase, known as the neural phase) followed by the obliterative phase (2nd phase) (Table 2).

In the 1st phase, the following are the main goals:

- To block the nervous impulse;
- To modify the sodium pump mechanism;
- To alter temporarily the end of the sensory axons;

These objectives can be driven using toothpaste containing potassium nitrate 5% (at-home therapy) and the use of laser technology using photobiomodulation therapy (known as *laser therapy*) (in-office therapy) in doses higher than 10 J distributed in strategic points in the MIH-affected teeth including cervical and root regions and the number of appointments depends on the host's response [22]. However, a reduction of VAS values ranging from 3 to 5 is an optimal signal to follow to the next approaching phase.

In the 2nd phase, the following are the main goals:

Table 2. A comprehensive review of treatment approaches to DH-MIH

Phase	Objectives	Treatment approaches
1st Phase	To modulate neural sensitivity and impulse transmission mechanisms	- Toothpaste containing potassium nitrate 5% (at-home therapy) - Photobiomodulation therapy with infrared laser (in-office therapy)
2nd Phase	To create a protective barrier and close dentinal tubules	- Toothpaste containing arginine or casein phosphopeptide amorphous calcium phosphate (CPP-ACP) and fluoride varnish - Resin infiltrant - Silicon-rich fluoride-enriched enamel - Tetrasodium pyrophosphate/silica ions - Cyanocrilate physical barrier

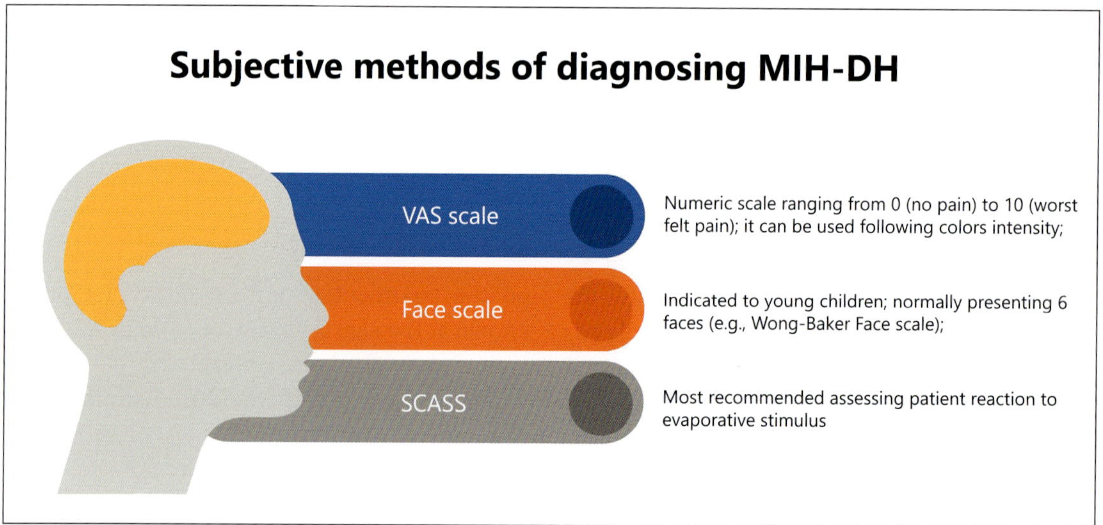

Fig. 2. Main subjective methods for measuring MIH teeth with hypersensitivity.

- To close dentinal tubules;
- To form a mechanical barrier;
- To precipitate ions/minerals into the enamel prisms;

In the case of using both approaches, the evidence points out a faster remission of MIH-DH discomfort [23]. However, there is no robust evidence supporting the need to follow this sequence for approaching hypersensitivity of MIH-teeth [24]. We can hypothesize that with the establishment of an effective and prolonged mechanical barrier, the cause of inflammation aggression may cease, leading to the disappearance of symptoms. However, it is possible to apply directly in the second phase; this process might take longer to occur. So, the use of toothpaste solely containing arginine [25, 26], casein phosphopeptide amorphous calcium phosphate, and fluoride varnish has been pointed out as feasible clinical options [27]. Some new approaches that fill the un-

Table 3. Main treatments of in vivo interventions for DH-MIH

Study	Study type	Groups of treatment	Follow-up, months	Types of treatment	Conclusion
Paschoal et al. [22], 2021	Case report	None	1	- Combination of four sessions of infrared L (48 h of interval) followed by four sessions of CPP-ACP FV (interval of 1 week)	- Improvement of quality of life and reduction of hypersensitivity
Bekes et al. [25], 2017	NRCT	1	2	- Toothpaste and rinse of 8% arginine and calcium carbonate	- Reduction of hypersensitivity
Muniz et al. [23], 2020	RCT	Group 1: L Group 2: FV Group 3: L + FV	1	- Infrared L was applied two sessions (48 h of interval); sodium fluoride FV was applied in four sessions (interval of 1 week); two sessions of infrared L (48 h of interval) + four sessions of sodium fluoride FV (interval of 1 week)	- L application promoted an immediate remission of pain, whereas FV alone a late effect; however, no difference of pain was verified between G1 and G3
Nogueira et al. [28], 2021	RCT	Group 1: FV Group 2: FV + 37% acid etching Group 3: RI	18	- FV was applied four sessions (interval of 1 week); four sessions of 30 s of 37% acid etching followed by sodium fluoride FV (interval of 1 week); RI was applied once	- RI positively influenced the integrity of MIH-affected teeth, might being a promising strategy for reducing DH-MIH

L, laser therapy; FV, fluoride varnish; NRCT, nonrandomized clinical trial; RCT, randomized clinical trial; RI, resin infiltration.

derneath enamel (e.g., resin infiltrant) [28], form an enriched enamel with fluoride silicon-rich, tetrasodium pyrophosphate/silica ions [29], and cyanocrilate physical barrier [30] might be promising approaches that deserve more clinical investigations. In cases of immediate care when there is no time to postpone any treatment, restorative procedures with/without lidocaine 2% with the support of anti-inflammatory drugs are the clinical priority [31, 32] (Table 3).

Conclusion

Managing hypersensitive MIH-teeth is one of the outmost challenges in pediatric dentistry. The presence of this symptom can affect many aspects of a child's daily life, including eating habits and chewing. Correctly diagnosing MIH DH with different scales and knowing how and when to use different materials and technologies is critical to achieving optimal results when dealing with this dental condition.

Statement of Ethics

Children's parents gave their consent for the publication of their children's teeth photographs for educational purposes.

Conflict of Interest Statement

The authors have no conflict of interest to declare.

Funding Sources

There are no funding sources associated with this manuscript.

Author Contributions

Marco A.B. Paschoal, Fabricio K. de Carvalho, Marina D.M. Lima, and Soraya C. Leal drafted, critically revised the manuscript, and gave approval to the final version. Also, all authors contributed to original illustrations and tables.

References

1 Favaro LZ, Soares PV, Cunha-Cruz J. Prevalence of dentin hypersensitivity: systematic review and meta-analysis. J Dent. 2019;81:1–6.

2 Raposo F, de Carvalho Rodrigues AC, Lia ÉN, Leal SC. Prevalence of hypersensitivity in teeth affected by molar-incisor hypomineralization. Caries Res. 2019; 53(4):424–30.

3 Canadian Advisory Board on Dentin Hypersensitivity. Consensus-based recommendations for the diagnosis and management of dentin hypersensitivity. J Can Dent Assoc. 2003 Apr;69(4):221–6.

4 Brannstrom M. Dentin sensitivity. Arsb Goteb Tandlak Sallsk. 1964:15–35.

5 Liu XX, Tenenbaum HC, Wilder RS, Quock R, Hewlett ER, Ren YF. Pathogenesis, diagnosis and management of dentin hypersensitivity: an evidence-based overview for dental practitioners. BMC Oral Health. 2020 Aug 6;20(1):220.

6 de Castro CRN, Lima CCB, Costa LC, Silva RNC, Pascotto RC, Moura MS, et al. Hypomineralization teeth have higher frequency of dental hypersensitivity. Ped Dent. 2021;43(3):218–22.

7 Rodd HD, Boissonade FM, Day PF. Pulpal status of hypomineralized permanent molars. Pediatr Dent. 2007;29(6):514–20.

8 Fagrell TG, Lingström P, Olsson S, Steiniger F, Norén JG. Bacterial invasion of dentinal tubules beneath apparently intact but hypomineralized enamel in molar teeth with molar incisor hypomineralization. Int J Paediatr Dent. 2008;18(5):333–40.

9 Fagrell TG, Dietz W, Jälevik B, Norén JG. Chemical, mechanical and morphological properties of hypomineralized enamel of permanent first molars. Acta Odontol Scand. 2010;68(4):215–22.

10 Elhennawy K, Manton DJ, Crombie F, Zaslansky P, Radlanski RJ, Jost-Brinkmann PG, et al. Structural, mechanical and chemical evaluation of molar-incisor hypomineralization-affected enamel: a systematic review. Arch Oral Biol. 2017;83:272–81.

11 Neves AB, Americano GCA, Soares DV, Soviero VM. Breakdown of demarcated opacities related to molar-incisor hypomineralization: a longitudinal study. Clin Oral Investig. 2019;23(2):611–5.

12 Jorge RC, Dos Papoula GorniReis P, Marañón-Vásquez GA, Masterson D, Cople Maia L, Mendes Soviero V. Are yellow-brownish opacities in hypomineralized teeth more prone to breakage than white-creamy ones? A systematic review. Clin Oral Investig. 2022;26(9):5795–808.

13 Hernández M, Planells P, Martínez E, Mira A, Carda-Diéguez M. Microbiology of molar-incisor hypomineralization lesions. A pilot study. J Oral Microbiol. 2020 May 20;12(1):1766166.

14 Ebel M, Bekes K, Klode C, Hirsch C. The severity and degree of hypomineralisation in teeth and its influence on oral hygiene and caries prevalence in children. Int J Paediatr Dent. 2018 Nov;28(6):648–57.

15 Carvalho MR, Regalo SCH, Siéssere S, Gonçalves LMN, Paula-Silva FWG, Vicioni-Marques F, et al. Electromyographic analysis of the stomatognathic system of children with molar-incisor hypomineralization. PLoS One. 2023 Feb 24;18(2):e0277030.

16 Jälevik B, Sabel N, Robertson A. Can molar incisor hypomineralization cause dental fear and anxiety or influence the oral health-related quality of life in children and adolescents? A systematic review. Eur Arch Paediatr Dent. 2022 Feb;23(1):65–78.

17 Reis PPG, Jorge RC, Ferreira DMTP, Marañón-Vásquez GA, Maia LC, Soviero VM. Do patients with molar incisor hypomineralization have more dental anxiety and behavior management problems? A systematic review with meta-analysis. Braz Oral Res. 2023 Jul 10;37:e069.

18 William V, Messer LB, Burrow MF. Molar incisor hypomineralization: review and recommendations for clinical management. Pediatr Dent. 2006 May-Jun;28(3):224–32.

19 Rocha MOC, Cruz AACF, Santos DO, Douglas-DE-Oliveira DW, Flecha OD, Gonçalves PF. Sensitivity and specificity of assessment scales of dentin hypersensitivity: an accuracy study. Braz Oral Res. 2020;34:e043.

20 Özgül BM, Saat S, Sönmez H, Öz FT. Clinical evaluation of desensitizing treatment for incisor teeth affected by molar incisor hypomineralization. J Clin Pediatr Dent. 2013;38(2):101–5.

21 Myles PS, Myles DB, Galagher W, Boyd D, Chew C, MacDonald N, et al. Measuring acute postoperative pain using the visual analog scale: the minimal clinically important difference and patient acceptable symptom state. Br J Anaesth. 2017 Mar;118(3):424–9.

22 Paschoal MAB, Costa HE, Santos-Pinto L, Ferreira MC. Photobiomodulation therapy for hypersensitivity associated with molar-incisor hypomineralization: a case report. Gen Dent. 2021 Nov-Dec;69(6):50–3.

23 Muniz RSC, Carvalho CN, Aranha ACC, Dias F, Ferreira MC. Efficacy of low-level laser therapy associated with fluoride therapy for the desensitisation of molar-incisor hypomineralisation: randomised clinical trial. Int J Paediatr Dent. 2020; 30(3):323–33.

24 Gevert MV, Soares R, Wambier LM, Ribeiro AE, Avais LS, de Souza JF, et al. How is the quality of the available evidence on molar-incisor hypomineralization treatment? An overview of systematic reviews. Clin Oral Investig. 2022 Oct;26(10):5989–6002.

25 Bekes K, Heinzelmann K, Lettner S, Schaller HG. Efficacy of desensitizing products containing 8% arginine and calcium carbonate for hypersensitivity relief in MIH-affected molars: an 8-week clinical study. Clin Oral Investig. 2017; 21(7):2311–7.

26 da Cunha Coelho ASE, Mata PCM, Lino CA, Macho VMP, Areias CMFGP, Norton APMAP, et al. Dental hypomineralization treatment: a systematic review. J Esthet Restor Dent. 2019 Jan;31(1):26–39.

27 Ritto FP, Tiwana KR, Schmitz TA, Dacus ZL, Borges MAP, Canellas JV. A qualitative analysis of treatment patterns for mild and severe molar hypomineralization in permanent teeth: a systematic review. Pediatr Dent. 2023 Jul 15;45(4):281–91.

28 Nogueira VKC, Mendes Soares IP, Fragelli CMB, Boldieri T, Manton DJ, Bussaneli DG, et al. Structural integrity of MIH-affected teeth after treatment with fluoride varnish or resin infiltration: an 18-month randomized clinical trial. J Dent. 2021 Feb;105:103570.

29 Vilhena FV, de Oliveira SML, Matochek MHM, Tomaz PLS, Oliveira TS, D'Alpino PHP. Biomimetic mechanism of action of fluoridated toothpaste containing proprietary REFIX technology on the remineralization and repair of demineralized dental tissues: an in vitro study. Eur J Dent. 2021 May;15(2):236–41.

30 Torres ADS, Martins OBL, Otoni RP, Henrique Soares K, Torres MG, Firoozi P, et al. Effectiveness of cyanoacrylate in the treatment of dentin hypersensitivity: a systematic review. Int J Dent. 2023 Aug 23;2023:1465957.

31 Vicioni-Marques F, Paula-Silva FWG, Carvalho MR, Queiroz AM, Freitas O, Duarte MPF, et al. Preemptive analgesia with ibuprofen increases anesthetic efficacy in children with severe molar: a triple-blind randomized clinical trial. J Appl Oral Sci. 2022 Apr 20;30: e20210538.

32 Haidar M, Raslan N. Comparative study of articaine 4% versus lidocaine 2% in the local anesthesia of permanent mandibular first molars affected by MIH: a randomized controlled trial. Eur Arch Paediatr Dent. 2023 Oct;24(5):621–30.

33 Haidary S. Comparison of the prevalence of molar incisor hypomineralization in Dubai/United Arab Emirates and Greifswald/Germany. 2014. Available from: https://epub.ub.uni-greifs-wald.de/frontdoor/deliver/index/docId/1495/file/Diss_Haidary_Somayeh.pdf.

34 Oyedele TA, Folayan MO, Adekoya-Sofowora CA, Oziegbe EO. Co-morbidities associated with molar-incisor hypomineralisation in 8 to 16 year old pupils in Ile-Ife, Nigeria. BMC Oral Health. 2015 Mar 13;15:37.

35 Petrou MA, Giraki M, Bissar A-R, Wempe C, Schäfer M, Schiffner U, et al. Severity of MIH findings at tooth surface level among German school children. Eur Arch Paed Dent. 2015;16(3):271–6.

36 Linner T, Khazaei Y, Bücher K, Pfisterer J, Hickel R, Kühnisch J. Hypersensitivity in teeth affected by molar-incisor hypomineralization (MIH). Sci Rep. 2021 Sep 9;11(1):17922.

Marco Aurélio Benini Paschoal
Department of Pediatric Dentistry, Federal University of Minas Gerais
R. Prof. Moacir Gomes de Freitas, 688
Belo Horizonte 31270-901 (Brazil)
marcoabp@ufmg.br

Chapter 14

Published online: July 1, 2024

Rios D, Santos-Pinto L (eds): Molar Incisor Hypomineralisation: New Perceptions. Monogr Oral Sci. Basel, Karger, 2024, vol 32, pp 166–172 (DOI: 10.1159/000538885)

Molar Incisor Hypomineralisation as a Dental Caries Risk Factor – Is It True?

Elsa Garot[a] Alexandre R. Vieira[b] David John Manton[c, d]

[a]Université de Bordeaux, UFR des Sciences Odontologiques, Center for Rare Oral and Dental Diseases, CCMR O-Rares, C.H.U. de Bordeaux, Bordeaux, France; [b]School of Dental Medicine, East Carolina University, Greenville, NC, USA; [c]Department of Cariology, Centre for Dentistry and Oral Hygiene, University of Groningen, University Medical Centre Groningen, Groningen, The Netherlands; [d]Department of Paediatric Dentistry, Academic Center for Dentistry Amsterdam (ACTA), University of Amsterdam and Vrije Universiteit, Amsterdam, The Netherlands

Abstract

The development of the human dentition is susceptible to disruption owing to its intricate and delicate nature, encompassing variations in tooth number, anatomical configuration, and the characteristics of enamel, dentine, and cementum. This chapter will specifically address the prevalent defect of molar incisor hypomineralisation (MIH), which can impose a significant treatment burden on individuals. MIH is linked to deleterious alterations in the properties of affected enamel, which can lead to rapid enamel breakdown and carious lesion formation in those at a heightened caries risk. In addition, MIH is associated with tooth sensitivity, dental anxiety, difficulty eating, aesthetic concerns, and negative influence during the child's psychological growth, especially when the MIH is severe. Regarding dental caries, it is essential to note that MIH does not directly increase the risk of caries. However, MIH can alter the way the caries process manifests by creating niches where biofilm can accumulate, complicating oral cleaning efforts. Additionally, MIH adversely modifies the physicochemical properties of enamel, influencing how this "hardest of tissues" responds to cariogenic challenges.

Introduction

This chapter will focus on molar incisor hypomineralisation (MIH) and how these qualitative defects influence caries risk and outcomes. MIH is a developmental defect of dental enamel, the hardest and outermost layer of the tooth, and it serves as a protective barrier against mechanical and chemical damage and as a functioning masticatory surface. Amelogenesis is the process of tooth enamel formation, and disruptions or genetic mutations in the amelogenesis process can lead to enamel defects or disorders, such as enamel hypoplasia (a quantitative defect) or enamel hypomineralisation (a qualitative defect), which can result in weakened or discolored teeth. The presence of MIH itself does not increase caries risk as this relates mainly to frequent consumption of sugars and less than ideal oral hygiene, but MIH may influence the manifestation of the carious lesion in the context of a dysbiotic cariogenic biofilm in the presence of cariogenic substrates.

Amelogenesis and MIH

Amelogenesis is a highly complex genetically moderated process, and therefore, disruption may occur, even with minor systemic or local insults or (epi)genetic influences on the processes [1]. It is a complex biological process that occurs in several stages:

Initiation. Amelogenesis begins during tooth development in the embryonic and fetal stages. Dental enamel is derived from ectoderm-derived ameloblasts, which are specialized epithelial cells that develop from the inner enamel epithelium of the tooth germ. The ameloblasts play a crucial role in enamel formation [2].

Secretory Stage. This is the first major stage of amelogenesis. During this phase, ameloblasts actively secrete proteins and minerals that make up the initial enamel template/matrix. The primary protein secreted is amelogenin, which acts as a scaffold for enamel crystal formation. As the ameloblasts deposit minerals (primarily impure hydroxyapatite crystals), the enamel matrix begins to harden and develop its characteristic structure and morphology [2].

Transitional Stage. This phase marks the transition from the secretory stage to the maturation stage. During this stage, there is a decrease in protein secretion and an increase in mineral deposition, and apoptosis of the ameloblasts begins. The enamel matrix continues to increase in mineral density, and the enamel rods (also known as enamel prisms) begin to form [3].

Maturation Stage. In this stage, ameloblasts continue to promote mineralisation and help the enamel reach its final hardness. The enamel crystals grow larger and more tightly packed, making the enamel increasingly resistant to wear, fracture, and dissolution [2].

Apoptosis Stage. This is the final stage of amelogenesis. During this stage, the ameloblasts, which have been actively involved in enamel formation, become inactive and are ultimately removed via apoptosis. The enamel layer is now fully developed and serves as a protective covering for the underlying dentine and pulp of the tooth [2].

Throughout amelogenesis, the enamel undergoes significant changes in its composition and structure, becoming highly mineralised and resilient, and this process is susceptible to insult. Once amelogenesis is complete, the enamel cannot regenerate or repair itself, so maintaining good oral hygiene practices is essential to protect the enamel from damage and decay.

The etiology of MIH is not entirely understood, but it is believed to have a multifactorial mode of inheritance with a combination of genetic, environmental, and systemic factors playing a role [4, 5]. MIH is a qualitative anomaly of the enamel (decreased mineral density) affecting at the least one permanent first molar and often the incisors [6]. These asymmetrical defects manifest themselves as demarcated white, cream, or yellow-brown opacities with possible posteruptive breakdown (PEB) of enamel [7]. The clinical forms of MIH can vary: white-cream opacities indicate a milder expression (shown in Fig. 1) of MIH, while yellow-brown opacities reflect a more severe defect [8] (shown in Fig. 2). MIH is due to a pre-eruptive disruption of mineralisation putatively due to an overabundance of albumin, which interferes with the mineralisation process. Analyses of the microstructure of sound enamel and hypomineralised enamel showed two modifications in the microstructure of the region affected by MIH: a structure of less dense enamel prisms

1

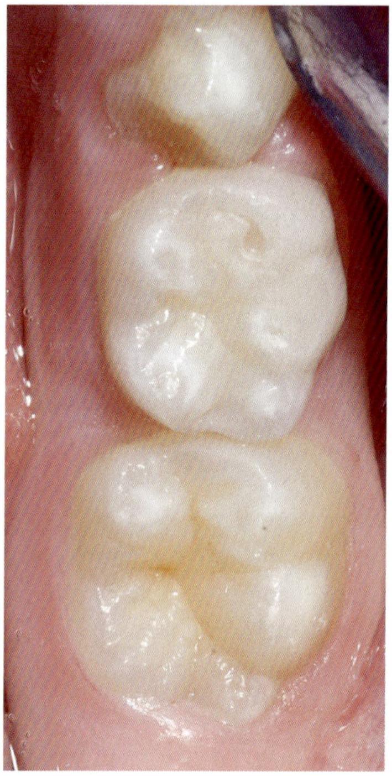

2

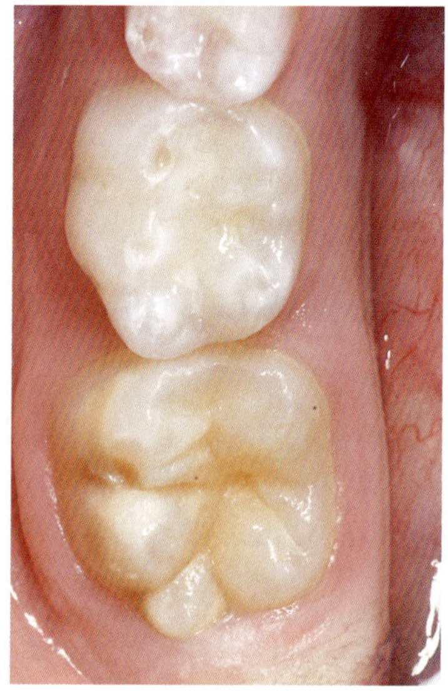

Fig. 1. White demarcated opacity on tooth 46 in a patient with MIH.
Fig. 2. Brown demarcated opacity with posteruptive enamel breakdown on tooth 36 in a patient with MIH.

with less dense apatite crystals and a widening of the prismatic sheath [9]. These changes most likely occur during enamel maturation and may explain the decrease in mineral density, hardness, and elastic modulus of the affected enamel [10]. Semiquantitative energy-dispersive X-ray spectroscopy and transverse microradiography analyses of teeth with MIH have shown that mineral densities in these lesions are lower, with mineral deficits greater than 50% in some lesions [11, 12]. Hypomineralised enamel has a significantly higher protein content than normal enamel (mostly serum albumin), but a concentration of residual amelogenin close to normal, differing from defects such as amelogenesis imperfecta [13, 14]. Brown enamel opacities (the most severe appearance of MIH) tend to have the lowest mineral density and the highest protein content, corresponding to a level 15–21 times higher than healthy enamel [12, 14]. The carbonate content of MIH lesions is also increased by up to 50%, indicating the stress that the ameloblast was under during amelogenesis and increasing the solubility of the already susceptible defective enamel [12]. Additionally, the ability of dental enamel to absorb deformational energy and maintain itself without fracture is attributed to the viscoelastic layers of proteins. Therefore, the variation in enamel protein content in MIH lesions could increase the risk of PEB of enamel, for example, if it is subjected to chewing forces [14].

Hypomineralised Enamel and Dental Caries

MIH does not cause increased caries risk – a cariogenic diet, especially containing sugars, and less than ideal oral hygiene are the main factors in dental caries. There is a positive association between the prevalence of dental caries and MIH, and several factors associated with MIH and how they exacerbate the effects of even mildly in-

3

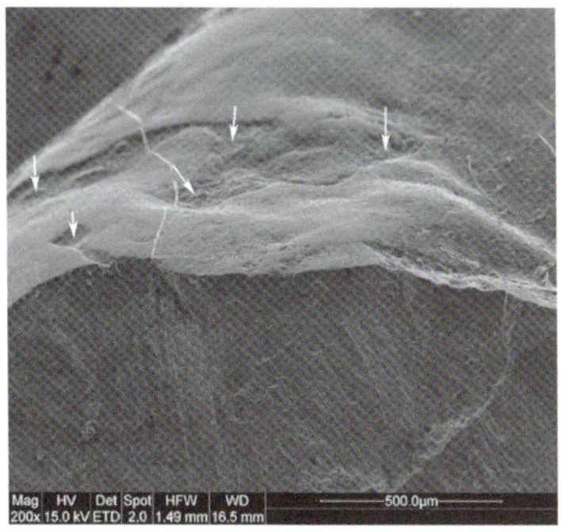

4

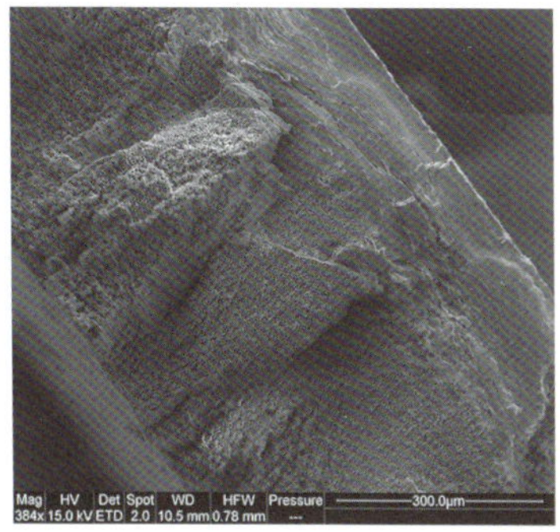

Fig. 3. Section of MIH-affected enamel (with fractured margin) illustrating surface roughness. Courtesy of Dr. Felicity Crombie, University of Melbourne.

Fig. 4. Fractured surface of MIH-affected enamel showing porosity of lesion body. Courtesy of Dr. Felicity Crombie, University of Melbourne.

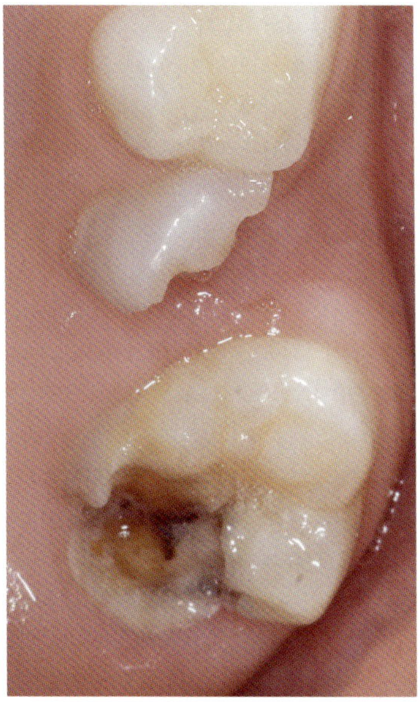

Fig. 5. Brown demarcated opacity with carious dentine lesion on tooth 26 in a patient with MIH.

creased caries risk may explain this association [15]. As an overarching statement, hypomineralised enamel is more susceptible to carious lesion development due to several physical and chemical characteristics of the lesion and their effect on the dental pulp and often the altered oral health behaviors of the affected individual.

The rough and porous and potentially broken surface enamel in MIH-affected teeth can make it challenging to maintain effective oral hygiene (shown in Fig. 3). Plaque and food particles may accumulate more easily in the rough enamel surfaces, increasing the risk of caries. The mineral density profile in MIH lesions is reversed from under the surface layer to the dentin-enamel junction compared to sound enamel, that is, mineral density is highest toward the dentin-enamel junction. Clinically, in the case of white defects, it is common for a layer of relatively sound enamel to cover this hypomineralised enamel at the surface [16]. However, in more severe lesions, this is important, especially in the situation where PEB occurs, exposing the most hypomineralised region – the body of the lesion (shown in Fig. 4), which, as stated, can have a mineral density deficit of more than 50%, porosity greater than 25%, increased carbonated apatite concentration, and increasing solubility [12, 17]. The exposed compromised enamel in the body of the lesion is therefore very susceptible to further breakdown and demineralisation in the presence of increased caries risk [18–21] (shown in Fig. 5).

Thermal, osmotic, or mechanical sensitivity in affected teeth is a prevalent clinical complaint among individuals diagnosed MIH, often prompting them to seek dental consultation [22]. As mentioned, teeth affected by MIH have enamel that is less mineralised and more porous, making them more susceptible to pain due to osmotic and thermal challenges. Tooth hypersensitivity associated with MIH may be observed in molars that have just erupted and are showing signs of breakdown [22]. Teeth affected by MIH may present hypersensitivity that prevents effective and frequent tooth brushing and increases the risk of carious lesion development in the presence of increased caries risk [7]. Added to these different issues, these teeth have a greater number of restorative failures due to reduced resin bond strengths to weakened enamel, resulting in a large number of reinterventions/retreatments increasing the anxiety of patients during care [23]. A study conducted in Brazil pointed out a significant presence of hypersensitivity in teeth affected by MIH that had undergone restoration. This heightened sensitivity could potentially be attributed to variations in the restorative techniques employed and a notable re-occurrence of additional dentine caries lesions [24]. Indeed, if all hypomineralised enamel is not removed and the restoration is not bonded to healthy enamel margins, sensitivity can persist.

Routine dental examinations, timely intervention with fluoride varnish applications (combined or not with casein phosphopeptide – amorphous calcium phosphate), and the practice of effective oral hygiene are crucial in the management and prevention of caries among individuals afflicted with MIH [8]. Any preventive measures should take into account the disease's underlying causes, the risk of cavities, the nature and extent of lesions, the level of hypersensitivity, as well as the age of the patient [25].

Discrimination between MIH lesions with PEB and MIH lesions with PEB and subsequent development of carious lesions can be challenging for the clinician and researcher alike. Limited published evidence (supported by anecdotal clinical observations) suggests that the dentine underneath MIH-like hypomineralised lesions is not "normal" and has a decrease in mineral density, just as in enamel lesions, but not as severe [26]. The authors hypothesize that this difficulty in clinically discriminating between MIH with PEB exposing dentine and the same situation with an associated carious lesion may lead to the overdiagnosis of the associated carious lesion; however, further research is required on this topic.

Conclusion

The exact cause of MIH is still unknown, but it is believed to be a combination of genetic and environmental factors. It is not related to poor oral hygiene or diet, and in itself, MIH does not "cause" an increased caries risk but can alter the outcomes. MIH can lead to increased tooth sensitivity, enamel breakdown, and an increased risk of carious lesion development in individuals at increased caries risk. In general, the approach to addressing dental caries in these patients, as in all cases, involves early detection and diagnosis (of both MIH and caries risk), reducing their susceptibility to dental caries by modifying their caries-related behaviors while also improving the physical characteristics of the defect when feasible. This process can often be intricate, especially when dealing with children, given the complexities of managing caries risk and the child's ability to handle the necessary care behaviors. Nonetheless, it is crucial to establish appropriate long-term treatment plans and management strategies in children because the enduring consequences of structural breakdown and caries can persist throughout their permanent dentition for life.

Acknowledgment

The authors acknowledge their respective universities and past and present students and colleagues for their ongoing contribution to research in the area of MIH.

Statement of Ethics

Written informed consent was obtained from subjects (or their parents) for publication of the images.

Conflict of Interest Statement

The authors declare no conflicts of interest.

Funding Sources

No funding was sourced for the writing of this chapter.

Author Contributions

Elsa Garot developed the chapter design, and both Elsa Garot, Alexandre Vieira and David Manton reviewed and edited the manuscript for critical content and approved the submitted version.

References

1 Farooq I, Ali S, Anderson P. An Illustrated Guide to Oral Histology. John Wiley & Sons; 2021. p. 194.

2 Lacruz RS, Habelitz S, Wright JT, Paine ML. Dental enamel formation and implications for oral health and disease. Physiol Rev. 2017;97(3):939–93.

3 Berkovitz BKB, Holland GR, Moxham BJ. Oral Anatomy, Histology and Embryology E-Book. Elsevier Health Sciences; 2017. p. 472.

4 Vieira AR, Manton DJ. On the variable clinical presentation of molar-incisor hypomineralization. Caries Res. 2019; 53(4):482–8.

5 Garot E, Rouas P, Somani C, Taylor GD, Wong F, Lygidakis NA. An update of the aetiological factors involved in molar incisor hypomineralisation (MIH): a systematic review and meta-analysis. Eur Arch Paediatr Dent. 2022;23(1):23–38.

6 Weerheijm KL, Jälevik B, Alaluusua S. Molar-incisor hypomineralisation. Caries Res. 2001;35(5):390–1.

7 Weerheijm KL, Duggal M, Mejàre I, Papagiannoulis L, Koch G, Martens LC, et al. Judgement criteria for molar incisor hypomineralisation (MIH) in epidemiologic studies: a summary of the European meeting on MIH held in Athens, 2003. Eur J Paediatr Dent. 2003;4(3): 110–3.

8 Lygidakis NA, Garot E, Somani C, Taylor GD, Rouas P, Wong FSL. Best clinical practice guidance for clinicians dealing with children presenting with molar-incisor-hypomineralisation (MIH): an updated European Academy of Paediatric Dentistry policy document. Eur Arch Paediatr Dent. 2022;23(1):3–21.

9 Elhennawy K, Manton DJ, Crombie F, Zaslansky P, Radlanski RJ, Jost-Brinkmann PG, et al. Structural, mechanical and chemical evaluation of molar-incisor hypomineralization-affected enamel: a systematic review. Arch Oral Biol. 2017;83:272–81.

10 Fagrell TG, Dietz W, Jälevik B, Norén JG. Chemical, mechanical and morphological properties of hypomineralized enamel of permanent first molars. Acta Odontol Scand. 2010;68(4):215–22.

11 Jälevik B, Odelius H, Dietz W, Norén J. Secondary ion mass spectrometry and X-ray microanalysis of hypomineralized enamel in human permanent first molars. Arch Oral Biol. 2001;46(3):239–47.

12 Crombie FA, Manton DJ, Palamara JEA, Zalizniak I, Cochrane NJ, Reynolds EC. Characterisation of developmentally hypomineralised human enamel. J Dent. 2013;41(7):611–8.

13 Mangum JE, Crombie FA, Kilpatrick N, Manton DJ, Hubbard MJ. Surface integrity governs the proteome of hypomineralized enamel. J Dent Res. 2010;89(10):1160–5.

14 Farah RA, Monk BC, Swain MV, Drummond BK. Protein content of molar-incisor hypomineralisation enamel. J Dent. 2010;38(7):591–6.

15 Oreano MD, Santos PS, Borgatto AF, Bolan M, Cardoso M. Association between dental caries and molar-incisor hypomineralisation in first permanent molars: a hierarchical model. Community Dent Oral Epidemiol. 2023;51(3): 436–42.

16 Garot E. Distinction entre processus pathologique de type hypominéralisation molaire-incisive et processus taphonomique par différentes méthodes de micro-analyse de l'émail dentaire [PhD]. 2017. Available from: https://www.theses.fr/2017BORD0791.

17 Baig AA, Fox JL, Young RA, Wang Z, Hsu J, Higuchi WI, et al. Relationships among carbonated apatite solubility, crystallite size, and microstrain parameters. Calcif Tissue Int. 1999;64(5):437–49.

18 Americano GCA, Jacobsen PE, Soviero VM, Haubek D. A systematic review on the association between molar incisor hypomineralization and dental caries. Int J Paediatr Dent. 2017;27(1):11–21.

19 Kosma I, Kevrekidou A, Boka V, Arapostathis K, Kotsanos N. Molar incisor hypomineralisation (MIH): correlation with dental caries and dental fear. Eur Arch Paediatr Dent. 2016;17(2):123–9.

20 Kühnisch J, Kabary L, Malyk Y, Rothmaier K, Metz I, Hickel R, et al. Relationship between caries experience and demarcated hypomineralised lesions (including MIH) in the permanent dentition of 15-year-olds. Clin Oral Investig. 2018;22(5):2013–9.

21 Farah RA, Swain MV, Drummond BK, Cook R, Atieh M. Mineral density of hypomineralised enamel. J Dent. 2010; 38(1):50–8.

22 Linner T, Khazaei Y, Bücher K, Pfisterer J, Hickel R, Kühnisch J. Hypersensitivity in teeth affected by molar-incisor hypomineralization (MIH). Sci Rep. 2021; 11(1):17922.

23 Somani C, Taylor GD, Garot E, Rouas P, Lygidakis NA, Wong FSL. An update of treatment modalities in children and adolescents with teeth affected by molar incisor hypomineralisation (MIH): a systematic review. Eur Arch Paediatr Dent. 2022;23(1):39–64.

24 Raposo F, de Carvalho Rodrigues AC, Lia ÉN, Leal SC. Prevalence of hypersensitivity in teeth affected by molar-incisor hypomineralization (MIH). Caries Res. 2019;53(4):424–30.

25 Jiménez ADP, Mora VSA, Dávila M, Montesinos-Guevara C. Dental caries prevention in pediatric patients with molar incisor hypomineralization: a scoping review. J Clin Pediatr Dent. 2023;47(4):9–15.

26 Heijs SCB, Dietz W, Norén JG, Blanksma NG, Jälevik B. Morphology and chemical composition of dentin in permanent first molars with the diagnose MIH. Swed Dent J. 2007;31(4):155–64.

David John Manton
Department of Cariology, University of Groningen, Centre for Dentistry and Oral Hygiene
University Medical Centre Groningen
A. Deusinglaan 1, NL–9700 AD Groningen (The Netherlands)
d.j.manton@umcg.nl

Published online: July 1, 2024
Rios D, Santos-Pinto L (eds): Molar Incisor Hypomineralisation: New Perceptions. Monogr Oral Sci. Basel, Karger, 2024, vol 32, pp 173–184 (DOI: 10.1159/000538887)

Is It Possible to Remineralise Hypomineralised Enamel Lesions in Patients with Molar Incisor Hypomineralisation?

Marília Afonso Rabelo Buzalaf[a] Daniela Rios[b]

[a]Department of Biological Sciences, Bauru School of Dentistry/University of São Paulo, Bauru, Brazil; [b]Department of Pediatric Dentistry, Orthodontics and Public Health, Bauru School of Dentistry/University of São Paulo, Bauru, Brazil

Abstract

Molar incisor hypomineralisation (MIH) is characterized with reduced enamel mineral quantity, especially in the calcium and phosphate content, with increases in the carbonate and protein contents. Albumin is the main protein that accumulates pre-eruptively, leading to defective initiation of mineralisation. Other oral-fluid proteins are found in cases of posteruptive enamel surface breakdown. Most of the lesions extend through the full thickness of enamel. Due to the lower mineral quantity and increased carbon and protein content, MIH teeth are more prone to fractures once exposed to mastication. In addition, susceptibility to dental caries is increased and hypersensitivity is common in MIH patients. For these reasons, MIH-affected teeth might benefit from exposure to remineralising agents that will decrease caries susceptibility and reduce sensitivity. Several in vitro, in situ, and in vivo studies have shown that improving the mineralisation of MIH teeth after eruption is possible, especially at the surface. However, complete resolution is difficult due to the depth/thickness of these lesions. In fact, the process is similar to posteruptive maturation. Thus, this nomenclature should be used instead of remineralisation. The evidence available so far indicates that among the several available remineralising agents, casein phosphopeptide-amorphous calcium phosphate (CPP-ACP) cream and fluoride (F) varnish show the best results and are equally effective in remineralising MIH-affected teeth. Fluoride varnish demands no patient adherence, while CPP-ACP cream can be applied at home. However, it is important to consider that fluoride varnish is generally more economical than CPP-ACP cream. Consequently, the choice between these agents can be tailored to the patient's specific requirements.

Introduction

Dental enamel is the hardest and most densely mineralised substance in the human body. The process of amelogenesis begins during the bell stage of tooth development. Situated in the inner enamel epithelium, ameloblasts progress through various stages of development, ultimately producing a protein-laden enamel matrix. This matrix, once released by the ameloblasts, coalesces into nanospheres, establishing a detailed three-dimensional structure that supports the organization of enamel crystals. Concurrently, a range of enzymes orchestrates the gradual breakdown of the enamel matrix, culminating in the formation of dental enamel that is predominantly composed of hydroxyapatite, accounting for about 95% of its weight [1, 2]. If any key process such as the production, secretion, organization of the matrix, formation of crystals, or resorption of the matrix is disrupted or altered, it can lead to an enamel defect. Defects that are visible on a macroscopic level and primarily arise from disruptions in the matrix secretion phase during amelogenesis are termed enamel hypoplasia. Nonetheless, qualitative defects, which stem from disturbances in the calcification or maturation phases, are identified as enamel hypomineralisation [3].

Molar incisor hypomineralisation (MIH) is a highly prevalent qualitative enamel developmental defect, with a global prevalence around 14%, ranging between 11 and 18%, depending on the region [4, 5]. At least one of the four first permanent molars is affected, with or without the involvement of the permanent incisors [6, 7]. Clinically, MIH is characterized by demarcated white/creamy or yellow/brownish opacities, larger than 1 mm, located on permanent first molars with or without the involvement of incisors. Posteruptive breakdown (PEB) may or may not occur [7, 8]. When there is no PEB, MIH is classified as mild; when PEB occurs, it is classified as severe [8]. It is important to highlight that these demarcated hypomineralisation defects might be found in the deciduous second molars and, in this case, they are predictors of MIH in the permanent dentition [9].

Despite a plethora of studies, including several systematic reviews, have explored the etiology of MIH, the exact mechanisms underlying its development are not known so far. Nevertheless, the multifactorial nature of the defect is acknowledged, where exposure to a combination of prenatal, perinatal, and postnatal factors in addition to genetic susceptibility drives its occurrence and severity [10]. Children with general illness in childhood and those whose mothers underwent illnesses during the last trimester of pregnancy might be more susceptible to MIH [11]. In addition, the asymmetry of the defect, the variability in the prevalence of MIH in distinct populations worldwide, and the fact amelogenesis is controlled genetically suggests that MIH might be a defect with multifactorial inheritance, probably influenced by more than one gene, besides suffering influence from the environment (epigenetics) [10]. There are some studies associating polymorphisms in genes that participate in the enamel formation with MIH [12–18], but additional studies are needed to better understand the influence of genetic and epigenetic factors on the development of MIH.

Since the classical report by Backer Dirks, it is known that noncavitated white spot lesions resulting from the action of bacterial acids along time can be remineralised [19]. The pattern of demineralisation seen in the white spot lesions is due to the existence of mineral phases with distinct solubilities in the dental tissues. When bacteria metabolize sugars producing acids, pH decreases in saliva and in the biofilm fluid ($4.5 < pH < 5.5$). These fluids become undersaturated with respect to carbonate hydroxyapatite (CHAP) but are still supersaturated with respect to fluorhydroxyapatite (FAP). As a consequence, CHAP dissolves from the subsurface and FAP forms in the surface layers. Due to the strong buffering capacity of saliva, together with the outward diffusion of the acids, the biofilm pH increases rapidly. When it becomes greater than 5.5, the oral fluids become supersaturated with respect to HAP again and the partially demineralised crystals suffer remineralisation. The net result of several de- and remineralisation cycles, with preponderance of the latter, leads to remineralisation. One of the most widespread agents used to potentiate the remineralisation effect of saliva is fluoride (F). Considering that $KSP_{FAP} < KSP_{CHAP}$ (KSP = solubility product constant), the presence of traces of F in the solution during the dissolution of CHAP will make the solution highly supersaturated with respect to FAP. Thus, remineralisation will occur promptly since F will adsorb to the surface of the partially demineralised crystals and attract Ca^{+2}. Low-carbonate or carbonate-free apatite will form preferentially, instead of the original CHAP, under the nucleating action of the partially dissolved minerals, since the first are less soluble. Because of the exclusion of carbonate and inclusion of F, this new coating will be less soluble than the original mineral and more resistant to future acidic challenges [20–22]. This pattern of remineralisation occurs in demineralised teeth that had their amelogenesis undisturbed. Both demineralisation and remineralisation are part of a chemical process with the aim of achieving balance. Does the same occur in teeth affected by MIH that had disturbance in the calcification or maturation phases of amelogenesis?

To answer this question, it is necessary to know the chemical, mechanical, and structural composition of enamel affected by MIH. Several studies on these topics have been conducted, and their findings were compiled in a systematic review [23]. Histologically, MIH is characterized with reduced mineral quantity, especially in the calcium and phosphate content, despite most of the studies report no significant difference regarding the Ca/P ratio in MIH-affected teeth compared to normal teeth. The reduction in mineral quantity leads to a decrease in the modulus of elasticity and enamel hardness. Enamel crystals are less densely packed, with thicker prism sheaths and inter/intraprismatic organic content.

Moreover, MIH-affected teeth exhibit an increase in the protein content (3–21-fold), especially in the yellow and brown lesions, with a more porous enamel surface compared to sound teeth [23–27]. However, the level of residual amelogenins is close to normality [28], which distinguishes MIH from dental fluorosis that contains high residual amelogenins [29]. Moreover, ameloblastin has only been found in MIH brown lesions. All major proteins identified in MIH enamel are normally associated with body fluids found intraorally (saliva, crevicular fluid, and blood). In addition, the protein composition of MIH enamel varies with surface integrity. Intact lesions contain mainly albumin, while in broken lesions, albumin is found infrequently and at lower levels [27]. Higher concentrations of alpha-1 antitrypsin, serum albumin, and antithrombin III have been reported in yellow and brown lesions than in white lesions [26, 28, 30]. These proteins might play a role in hypomineralisation, since albumin is a serum protein not typically found in mature enamel and enamel mineralisation can be inhibited by albumin, kallikrein 4, alpha-1 antitrypsin, or antithrombin III [23, 31]. Thus, MIH, as a dynamic defect, encompasses pre- and posteruptive characteristics, each with mechanistically distinct features. Pre-eruptively, there is defective initiation of mineralisation probably by accumulation of albumin, since there is near-complete removal of amelogenins. Intact lesions contain accumulated albumin but not other oral-fluid proteins with hydroxyapatite-binding ability. These are found posteruptively, in cases of PEB in severe MIH cases [28]. Considering the increase of residual proteins in MIH lesions, it has been suggested that the remineralisation of these lesions would benefit from prior removal of inhibitory proteins [32, 33]. However, this need varies remarkably, depending on the integrity of the lesion surface, since this has a direct influence on the type of protein that is accumulated [28].

Due to the lower mineral quantity, increased carbon content (up to 10% compared to 3% in normal enamel), and increased protein quantity, MIH teeth are more prone to fractures once exposed to the forces of mastication [23]. In addition, susceptibility to dental caries is increased [34] and hypersensitivity is common in MIH patients [23, 35, 36]. Most of the lesions extend through the full thickness of enamel, starting at the enamel-dentin junction and ending at the enamel surface [23]. Thus, a first insight was to treat MIH-affected teeth with therapeutic agents that could promote remineralisation. However, given the knowledge described above regarding the chemistry of de-remineralisation, and considering the origin and structure of hypomineralised enamel, it becomes apparent that remineralising MIH opacities is not feasible. In hypomineralised enamel, the crystals already exhibit chemical stability, and thus, there is no mechanism for a reaction to take place. However, if there is no mineralisation of hypomineralised enamel opacities, why are there so many studies confirming an alteration in the enamel surface? Before answering this question, an overview of the studies that evaluated the remineralisation potential of distinct active compounds for MIH-affected teeth is provided below.

"Remineralising" Agents for Hypomineralised Enamel Opacities

The first study involving the use of remineralising agents for teeth with MIH defects was published in 2011 (Table 1). The application of a mousse containing 10% casein phosphopeptide-amorphous calcium phosphate (CPP-ACP) for 20 min in a tray for 4 months in thirty 6- to 9-year-old children presenting with MIH molars improved the enamel morphology, as evaluated in vivo by replicas. Moreover, scanning electron microscopy/energy-dispersive X-ray spectroscopy analyses of enamel biopsies revealed a significant decrease in C and a significant increase in Ca and P, without significant differences in O, Mg, or Ca/P ratio [37]. The combination of hydrogen peroxide bleaching with CPP-ACP mousse has been suggested to improve aesthetics, but the evidence for this is limited to a case report [38].

Although the characteristics of enamel affected by MIH vary widely, they typically share features such as the entire enamel layer being affected, along with a thin outer layer that exhibits decreased porosity and enhanced hardness and mineral density (MD) [24]. In natural caries lesions, a similarly mineral-rich surface layer is noted, which is believed to serve as a barrier against deeper mineralisation [39, 40]. Moreover, although both caries and MIH involve enamel with lower mineralisation, MIH is characterized by an unusually high content of enamel proteins, predominantly serum proteins [26, 28]. This includes albumin, which is believed to hinder the growth of apatite crystals [31]. Therefore, removing these proteins from the affected areas could potentially enhance the effectiveness of mineralisation treatments [32]. With this in mind, the study by Crombie et al. [41] was designed to prove the concept that MIH lesions can be remineralised. The authors initially removed (by abrasion) a surface layer (50–75 μm) of enamel of MIH-affected molars. The remaining surface was submitted to deproteination by treatment with 0.95% w/v NaOCl for 2 min. Then one group was treated with 1% w/v casein phosphopeptide-amorphous calcium fluoride phosphate (CPP-ACFP) solution (pH 5.5) for 14 days. Lesions were highly variable, but treatment with the remineralising solution increased mineral content and reduced porosity. The deproteination treatment appeared to show some additional benefit. This in vitro study established proof-of-concept evidence that MIH enamel can be improved after eruption both in terms of increasing the mineral content and reducing the porosity of the lesion using gold standard techniques (transverse microradiography and polarized light microscopy). The potential to enhance the properties of MIH lesions posteruption suggests that the underlying enamel structure is essentially sound, indicating that MIH is primarily a result of a disruption in the maturation process. Achieving optimal clinical improvements in treating MIH involves the difficulty of effecting changes throughout the entire thickness of the enamel and modifying the

Table 1. Studies that evaluated the MIH-remineralising effect of distinct agents (in chronological order)

Tested products	Response variables/ condition	Main results	References
CPP-ACP mousse for 4 months	Mineralisation, morphology, and porosity (SEM, ESEM, and EDX)/in vivo	Enamel morphology improved; decrease in C and increase in Ca and P	Baroni and Marchionni (2011) [37]
CPP-ACP mousse + hydrogen peroxide gel for 5 months	Photographic evaluation/in vivo	Noticeable improvement in aesthetics	Mastroberardino et al. (2012) [38]
Surface layer removal + 0.95% NaOCl pretreatment + 1% CPP-ACFP solution for 14 days	Transverse microradiography + polarized light microscopy/in vitro	MIH enamel can be improved after eruption both in terms of increasing the mineral content and reducing the porosity of the lesion	Crombie et al. (2013) [41]
4 weekly applications of 5% NaF varnish vs. usual home care control	Quantitative light-induced fluorescence/in vivo	No significant difference between the groups	Restrepo et al. (2016) [57]
3 fortnightly applications of 5% NaF varnish, 5%NaF varnish + TCP, or CPP-ACP paste	Laser fluorescence (DIAGNOdent)/in vivo	The NaF varnish containing TCP and the NaF varnish alone was more effective for mild lesions and moderate lesions, respectively	Biondi et al. (2017) [52]
Daily application of zinc hydroxyapatite paste for 1 year[a]	Remineralisation (photo) and pain relief/in vivo	Esthetical and sensitivity improvements with treating a 4-year-old child with stage 4b MIH	Solinas et al. (2021) [50]
1 single professional application of 5% NaF varnish vs. daily applications of CPP-ACP paste for 15 days	Laser fluorescence (DIAGNOdent)/in vivo	Both products significantly remineralised the MIH lesions, without significant differences between them	Singh et al. (2021) [48]
1 single application of self-assembling peptide[b]	Laser fluorescence (DIAGNOdent)/in vivo	There was a decrease in the mean fluorescence score, indicating remineralisation	Singh et al. (2021) [49]
About 1,450 ppm fluoride toothpaste vs. CaGP paste vs. CPP-ACFP paste		There was a significant improvement in MIH lesions over time in all groups, with no differences between the groups. In lesions with laser fluorescence ≤20, the highest percentage of change was observed for CPP-ACFP, while for lesions with laser fluorescence >20, the highest percentage of change was found for the CaGP group	Sezer and Kargul (2022) [45]
CaGP paste vs. CPP-ACFP paste	Laser fluorescence (DIAGNOdent)/in vivo	No significant difference was found between the remineralisation effect of CaGP and CPP-ACFP pastes on white/creamy and yellow/brown demarcated opacities in incisors in children with MIH	Sezer et al. (2022) [46]

Table 1 (continued)

Tested products	Response variables/ condition	Main results	References
NaF varnish (single application) vs. CPP-ACP paste (daily) over 6 months	Field emission scanning microscopy and energy-dispersive spectroscopy/in situ	Both CPP-ACP cream and fluoride varnish are equally effective in achieving remineralisation of MIH affected teeth. After 6 months of application, no significant difference was found between the two groups with regard to increase in mineral content	Kumar et al. (2022) [55]
Microcrystalline HAP (30%) or 1,450 ppm fluoride toothpaste over 15 days	Microcomputed tomography/in situ	Both toothpastes remineralised the MIH lesions. The remineralisation was enhanced by the pretreatment with the acid etchant	Amaechi et al. (2022) [44]
5% NaF varnish (once/ week for 4 weeks every 6 months during the first year) vs. CPP-ACP paste vs. CPP-ACFP paste. Pastes applied twice daily. Follow-up for 24 months	ICDAS and laser fluorescence (DIAGNOdent)	All remineralisation agents increased remineralisation rates in both creamy-white and yellow-brown colored defects without presenting any statistically significant difference at the end of the follow-up period. However, the effects of fluoride varnishes were late to observe when compared to pastes containing CPP-ACP and CPP-ACFP	Olgen et al. (2022) [47]

[a]Case report. [b]Pilot study. EDX, energy-dispersive X-ray spectroscopy; ESEM, environmental scanning electron microscopy; ICDAS, International Caries Detection and Assessment System; SEM, scanning electron microscopy.

surface layer while preserving its relatively higher mineralisation. If these lesions can be "matured" to match the quality of healthy enamel, it might become feasible to manage MIH without the need for restorative intervention [41].

From then on, a plethora of studies was published, whose results have been compiled in systematic reviews [42, 43]. The most comprehensive one and up-to-date one is the systematic review by Enax et al. [42]. The authors included studies of different designs (in vitro, in situ, or in vivo – randomized clinical trials [RCTs]), with distinct response variables, such as transverse microradiography [41], microcomputed tomography [44], laser fluorescence (DIAGNOdent™) [45–52], hardness test [53], Raman microscopy [54], scanning electron microscopy [37], or energy-dispersive spectroscopy [55]. The diversity of designs and distinct techniques to evaluate the remineralising effect of the different agents on MIH teeth makes the comparison between the studies difficult. Considering the in vivo studies, the most used response variable is laser fluorescence (DIAGNOdent) [45–52] (Table 1). Among them, one evaluated the use of self-assembling peptide (SAP) to remineralise MIH lesions. However, it was a pilot study. Ten MIH lesions were first deproteinized with 5% NaOCl, then etched with 37% phosphoric acid for 30 s to open up the pores for the subsurface lesion, and then the SAP was applied for 2 min. A significant decrease was observed in the mean fluorescence score after 1 month, indicating remineralisation [49]. Despite the promising results obtained with this pilot study, future RCTs, with longer evaluation periods and larger samples sizes, should be designed to compare the effect of SAP with other remineralising agents. Moreover, the high cost of SAP makes it difficult to implement this modality of treatment, especially in low-income countries. Another publication reported a case of aesthetical and sensitivity improvements with treating a 4-year-old child with severe MIH using a cream containing 30% zinc hydroxyapatite. The cream was used at home daily for 5 min in a tray [50] (Table 1).

Several RCTs compared the performance of CPP-ACP and or CPP-ACFP versus NaF varnish to remineralise MIH lesions with distinct severities using laser fluorescence as response variable. CPP, a part of the casein protein, in the form of ACP, carries and stabilizes phosphate and calcium ions. This complex serves as a delivery system for bioavailable calcium and phosphate ions [56]. In the study by Biondi et al. [52], the MD of 92 teeth with mild or moderate MIH treated with 5% NaF varnish, 5% NaF containing tricalcium phosphate (TCP), or with CPP-ACP paste was evaluated. The remineralising agents were applied for 1 min immediately after the laser fluorescence reading at baseline and after days 15 and 30. An additional laser fluorescence reading was performed on day 45. The NaF varnish containing TCP and the NaF varnish alone were more effective for mild lesions and moderate lesions, respectively. However, the authors stated in the discussion that their results do not allow the conclusion that NaF without TCP is more effective than CPP-ACP paste. The outperformance of CPP-ACP paste when compared with the NaF varnishes might have been due to the regimen of application. In the study by Singh et al. [48], in which a single professional application of 5% NaF varnish was compared with daily application of CPP-ACP paste for 15 min, there was significant remineralisation in both groups, without difference between them. The most well-designed study was conducted by Olgen et al. [47]. In this study, 120 teeth with yellow-brown or creamy-white defects in 67 children aged 6–9 years who had MIH lesions without substance loss, caries, or restoration were randomized into 4 groups: control (oral hygiene motivation only), 5% NaF varnish, CPP-ACP paste, and CPP-ACFP paste. The varnish was applied once/week for 4 weeks every 6 months during the first year. As for the pastes, parents were advised to brush their children's teeth and then apply the paste onto the defective teeth with a cotton swab or their fingers in the morning and in the evening in the first 3 months and for another 3 months from the sixth month onward. Children were followed up for 24 months. The evaluations were based on laser fluorescence (DIAGNOdent) and on the International Caries Detection and Assessment System criteria. However, the International Caries Detection and Assessment System was designed to clinically evaluate caries lesions, not MIH opacities. All agents increased remineralisation rates in both creamy-white and yellow-brown colored defects without presenting any statistically significant difference at the end of the follow-up period. However, the effects of fluoride varnishes were late to observe when compared to the pastes, i.e., the fact that the latter resulted in a quicker increase in remineralisation compared to fluoride varnish suggests that they are superior in terms of action time. The delayed action of fluoride-containing varnishes on teeth with MIH may be related to hindered mineral transition due to high protein content [57]. A significant increase was also observed in the formation of fissure caries lesion in the fluoride varnish group, unlike the other study groups, suggesting that CPP-ACP pastes may also be more effective in preventing the formation of fissure caries lesions in teeth with white-creamy defects [47]. In addition, CPP-ACFP was found to be a faster remineralisation agent even in teeth with yellow-brown defects, providing the most protection against caries and material loss. However, along time, the difference between the groups was not detected. These findings are similar to those reported by Llena et al. [58] for the remineralisation of early carious lesions, despite CPP-ACP also provided rapid remineralisation in creamy-white lesions [47]. An in situ study was conducted to compare the effect of daily application of CPP-ACP paste with one single NaF varnish application on the remineralisation of MIH-affected teeth over 6 months. The response variables were field emission scanning microscopy and energy-dispersive spectroscopy to evaluate ultrastructure and mineral content, respectively. A significant increase in calcium and phosphorus content and a decrease in carbon content was observed within the 6 months' period, suggesting remineralisation in both the groups. On comparing the Ca:P and Ca:C ratios, a significant increase in the Ca:C ratio was evident in the two groups. No significant difference was seen in the Ca:P ratio in the CPP-ACP group at 6 months. There were no significant differences between the two groups either at baseline or at 6 months' postintervention [55] (Table 1).

Interestingly, despite fluorides are widely recommended for MIH patients [8], there are only a few studies investigating the use of fluoride-based formulations on MIH opacities. Most of these studies focus on the professional application of fluoride varnishes or daily use of fluoride toothpastes [44, 47, 48, 52, 55] (Table 1). In the first published study [52], 9- to 12-year-old children were randomly divided into two groups: (a) 4 applications of 5% NaF varnish, with one-week interval and (b) usual home care (control). At each visit, the mean change in fluorescence and area of lesion were measured by quantitative light-induced fluorescence. There was no statistically significant difference in the mean of fluorescence and area of lesion between groups over the studied time [57]. However, the lack of significant difference between the groups might be related to the response variable used. The MIH defect involves a large enamel thickness. Thus, light scattering in the lesion, which is much stronger than in sound enamel, makes the light path in the lesion much shorter. In consequence, the light absorption per volume is smaller in the lesion, and therefore, the fluorescence is weaker [59]. Some studies also compare fluoride toothpastes with CPP-ACP and/or CPP-ACFP pastes. In the study by Sezer and Kargul [45], 53 children brushed twice daily with one of the following pastes: CPP-ACFP (10% CPP-ACP + 0.2% NaF), calcium glycerophosphate (CaGP), or 1,450 ppm fluoride for 3 months. The remineralisation of MIH lesions was assessed by laser fluorescence (DIAGNOdent) at baseline and at the end of the experimental period. There was a significant improvement in MIH opacities over time in all groups, with no differences between the groups. In opacities with laser fluorescence ≤20, the highest percentage of change was observed for CPP-ACFP, while for opacities with laser fluorescence >20, the highest percentage of change was found for the CaGP group. CaGP is an organic polyphosphate that can adsorb to enamel surfaces through the PO_4 radicals. Many mechanisms have been proposed for its anticariogenic properties: direct interaction with enamel, reduction in plaque mass, plaque pH buffering, increase of plaque Ca and PO_4 levels, and changes in plaque metabolism [60]. In another RCT by the same group, no significant difference was found between the remineralisation effect of CaGP and CPP-ACFP pastes on white/creamy and yellow/brown demarcated opacities in incisors in children with MIH by using laser fluorescence [46]. Fluoride toothpastes have also been compared with HAP toothpastes. Amaechi et al. [44], in an in situ study, compared the efficacy of toothpastes based on microcrystalline HAP (30%) or 1,450 ppm fluoride, in remineralising MIH. In addition, half of the opacities had their surfaces etched with 32% phosphoric acid for 5 s. Baseline and post-treatment MD was quantified using microcomputed tomography. Both toothpastes remineralised the MIH opacities. The remineralisation was enhanced by the pretreatment with the acid-etchant (Table 1). On the other hand, etching yellow or brown MIH lesions in 6- to 12-year-old children with 37% phosphoric acid for 30 s before the application of fluoride varnish (5% NaF) had no effect on the reduction of PEB over 18 months when compared with the application of fluoride varnish alone [61]. Thus, additional studies on this topic are necessary.

Remineralisation or Posteruptive Maturation?

When a tooth is in the oral environment, it is constantly exposed to acidic challenges, whether they are of erosive or carious origin. In addition, regardless of the presence of enamel developmental defects, after eruption, enamel undergoes a modification in the degree of mineralisation of its surface, known as posteruptive maturation, characterized by the formation of less soluble apatites [62]. Saliva has a natural remineralising action, as it is supersaturated in relation to HAP at pH values above 5.5. However, there are several active ingredients that can enhance the remineralising action of saliva. Given that enamel affected by MIH contains more carbonate than healthy enamel, and assuming that carbonate exists in the form of CHAP, the deposition of more stable mineral phases like HAP and FAP during posteruptive maturation could be advantageous. This is why previous in vivo studies or studies involving the application of acids on the surface of hypomineralised enamel, followed by the application of remineralising agents, observed what was termed as "remineralisation." However, this essentially represents enamel maturation [37, 44–48, 52, 55, 57].

Another important question arises: how can we explain that there is a mineral gain when the hypomineralised enamel is deproteinized? It is straightforward, as another form of transformation takes place on the enamel surface, akin to the processes observed in erosive tooth wear [63]. Here, the enamel porosity, formerly occupied by proteins, becomes infused with minerals. However, this is not mineralisation; it is merely mineral deposition, and clinically, there is a question about how much this deposition can strengthen the enamel. Thus, there is no clinical evidence to support the claim that enamel remineralisation in the context of MIH leads to reduced posteruptive loss.

Finally, the methodologies used to evaluate enamel remineralisation, except for microradiography, which serves as the gold standard to evaluate mineral loss/gain, have many limitations. Conclusions based on these methodologies may lead to misinterpretation.

Conclusion

Several in vitro, in situ, and in vivo studies have shown that improving the mineralisation of MIH teeth after eruption is possible. However, the mineralisation is superficial and does not reach the opacities in depth or thickness. The evidence available so far indicates that among the several available remineralising agents, CPP-ACP cream and fluoride varnish are equally effective for MIH opacities. A benefit of fluoride varnish is that it demands no patient adherence, in contrast to CPP-ACP cream, which offers the convenience of at-home application, eliminating the need for dental clinic visits. Consequently, the choice between these agents can be tailored to the patient's specific requirements. It is important to consider that fluoride varnish is generally more economical than CPP-ACP cream. It should be emphasized, however, that additional clinical trials with larger sample sizes and appropriate response variables are necessary to provide adequate evidence to support the recommendations for the choice of protocols for MIH-affected teeth. In addition, evidence from in vitro and in situ studies suggests acid etching the surface with phosphoric acid to open a pathway to remineralising agents as well as removing the proteins (with NaOCl). However, the protocols for these approaches still need to be tested and validated in clinical trials.

Considering the biochemical concepts related to de-remineralisation, the term "remineralisation" for opacities in hypomineralised enamel seems inappropriate. This may give the false impression that hypomineralised enamel, in the preeruptive phase, can be improved to resemble normal enamel in the posteruptive phase. In reality, what occurs is a superficial chemical modification of enamel when exposed to the oral cavity, and in the presence of mineralising agents, it results in the formation of less soluble enamel. However, this modification does not necessarily translate into an enamel that is more resistant clinically. Therefore, we discourage researchers and clinicians from using the term "remineralisation" in cases of MIH to avoid creating misleading expectations regarding outcomes. Instead, we propose using the term "posteruptive maturation" of hypomineralised enamel opacities.

Statement of Ethics

Ethics approval was not required.

Conflict of Interest Statement

The authors have no conflicts of interest to declare.

Funding Sources

There were no funding sources.

Author Contributions

M.A.R.B. and D.R. conceived the manuscript; acquired and interpreted the data; drafted the manuscript and provided final approval for its publication.

References

1 Robinson C, Briggs HD, Atkinson PJ, Weatherell JA. Matrix and mineral changes in developing enamel. J Dent Res. 1979;58(Spec Issue B):871–82.
2 Robinson C, Kirkham J, Weatherell JA, Richards A, Josephsen K, Fejerskov O. Developmental stages in permanent porcine enamel. Acta Anat (Basel). 1987;128(1):1–10.
3 Clarkson J. Review of terminology, classifications, and indices of developmental defects of enamel. Adv Dent Res. 1989; 3(2):104–9.
4 Schwendicke F, Elhennawy K, Reda S, Bekes K, Manton DJ, Krois J. Global burden of molar incisor hypomineralization. J Dent. 2018;68:10–8.
5 Dave M, Taylor G. Global prevalence of molar incisor hypomineralisation. Evid Based Dent. 2018;19(3):78–9.
6 Almuallem Z, Busuttil-Naudi A. Molar incisor hypomineralisation (MIH) – an overview. Br Dent J. 2018;225(7):601–9.
7 Weerheijm KL, Duggal M, Mejare I, Papagiannoulis L, Koch G, Martens LC, et al. Judgement criteria for molar incisor hypomineralisation (MIH) in epidemiologic studies: a summary of the European meeting on MIH held in Athens, 2003. Eur J Paediatr Dent. 2003;4(3): 110–3.
8 Lygidakis NA, Garot E, Somani C, Taylor GD, Rouas P, Wong FSL. Best clinical practice guidance for clinicians dealing with children presenting with molar-incisor-hypomineralisation (MIH): an updated European Academy of Paediatric Dentistry policy document. Eur Arch Paediatr Dent. 2022;23(1):3–21.
9 Garot E, Denis A, Delbos Y, Manton D, Silva M, Rouas P. Are hypomineralised lesions on second primary molars (HSPM) a predictive sign of molar incisor hypomineralisation (MIH)? A systematic review and a meta-analysis. J Dent. 2018;72:8–13.
10 Bussaneli DG, Vieira AR, Santos-Pinto L, Restrepo M. Molar-incisor hypomineralisation: an updated view for aetiology 20 years later. Eur Arch Paediatr Dent. 2022;23(1):193–8.
11 Juarez-Lopez MLA, Salazar-Treto LV, Hernandez-Monjaraz B, Molina-Frechero N. Etiological factors of molar incisor hypomineralization: a systematic review and meta-analysis. Dent J (Basel). 2023; 11(5):111.
12 Jeremias F, Koruyucu M, Kuchler EC, Bayram M, Tuna EB, Deeley K, et al. Genes expressed in dental enamel development are associated with molar-incisor hypomineralization. Arch Oral Biol. 2013;58(10):1434–42.
13 Jeremias F, Pierri RA, Souza JF, Fragelli CM, Restrepo M, Finoti LS, et al. Family-based genetic association for molar-incisor hypomineralization. Caries Res. 2016;50(3):310–8.
14 Kuhnisch J, Thiering E, Heitmuller D, Tiesler CM, Grallert H, Heinrich-Weltzien R, et al. Genome-wide association study (GWAS) for molar-incisor hypomineralization (MIH). Clin Oral Investig. 2014;18(2):677–82.

15 Fatturi AL, Menoncin BL, Reyes MT, Meger M, Scariot R, Brancher JA, et al. The relationship between molar incisor hypomineralization, dental caries, socioeconomic factors, and polymorphisms in the vitamin D receptor gene: a population-based study. Clin Oral Investig. 2020;24(11):3971–80.
16 Hocevar L, Kovac J, Podkrajsek KT, Battelino S, Pavlic A. The possible influence of genetic aetiological factors on molar-incisor hypomineralisation. Arch Oral Biol. 2020;118:104848.
17 Pang L, Li X, Wang K, Tao Y, Cui T, Xu Q, et al. Interactions with the aquaporin 5 gene increase the susceptibility to molar-incisor hypomineralization. Arch Oral Biol. 2020;111:104637.
18 Silva FMF, Carvalho FM, Franco ALMM, Soares TRC, Fonseca-Gonçalves A, Vieira AR, et al. Association between molar hypomineralization, genes involved in enamel development, and medication in early childhood: a preliminary study. Int J Paediatr Dent. 2024;34(3):211–8.
19 Backer Dirks O. Posteruptive changes in dental enamel. J Dent Res. 1966;45:503–11.
20 Buzalaf MAR, Pessan JP, Honorio HM, Ten Cate JM. Mechanisms of action of fluoride for caries control. Monogr Oral Sci. 2011;22:97–114.
21 Featherstone JD. Prevention and reversal of dental caries: role of low level fluoride. Community Dent Oral Epidemiol. 1999;27(1):31–40.
22 Ten Cate JM, Buzalaf MAR. Fluoride mode of action: once there was an observant dentist. J Dent Res. 2019;98(7):725–30.
23 Elhennawy K, Manton DJ, Crombie F, Zaslansky P, Radlanski RJ, Jost-Brinkmann PG, et al. Structural, mechanical and chemical evaluation of molar-incisor hypomineralization-affected enamel: a systematic review. Arch Oral Biol. 2017;83:272–81.
24 Crombie FA, Manton DJ, Palamara JE, Zalizniak I, Cochrane NJ, Reynolds EC. Characterisation of developmentally hypomineralised human enamel. J Dent. 2013;41(7):611–8.
25 Fagrell TG, Dietz W, Jalevik B, Noren JG. Chemical, mechanical and morphological properties of hypomineralized enamel of permanent first molars. Acta Odontol Scand. 2010;68(4):215–22.
26 Farah RA, Monk BC, Swain MV, Drummond BK. Protein content of molar-incisor hypomineralisation enamel. J Dent. 2010;38(7):591–6.
27 Farah RA, Swain MV, Drummond BK, Cook R, Atieh M. Mineral density of hypomineralised enamel. J Dent. 2010;38(1):50–8.
28 Mangum JE, Crombie FA, Kilpatrick N, Manton DJ, Hubbard MJ. Surface integrity governs the proteome of hypomineralized enamel. J Dent Res. 2010;89(10):1160–5.
29 Wright JT, Chen SC, Hall KI, Yamauchi M, Bawden JW. Protein characterization of fluorosed human enamel. J Dent Res. 1996;75(12):1936–41.
30 Fraser SJ, Natarajan AK, Clark ASS, Drummond BK, Gordon KC. A Raman spectroscopic study of teeth affected with molar-incisor hypomineralisation. J Raman Spectrosc. 2015;46(2):202–10.
31 Robinson C, Kirkham J, Brookes SJ, Shore RC. The role of albumin in developing rodent dental enamel: a possible explanation for white spot hypoplasia. J Dent Res. 1992;71(6):1270–4.
32 Robinson C, Hallsworth AS, Shore RC, Kirkham J. Effect of surface zone deproteinisation on the access of mineral ions into the subsurface carious lesions of human enamel. Caries Res. 1990;24:226–30.
33 Mathu-Muju K, Wright JT. Diagnosis and treatment of molar incisor hypomineralization. Compend Contin Educ Dent. 2006;27:604–10.
34 Americano GC, Jacobsen PE, Soviero VM, Haubek D. A systematic review on the association between molar incisor hypomineralization and dental caries. Int J Paediatr Dent. 2017;27(1):11–21.
35 Linner T, Khazaei Y, Bucher K, Pfisterer J, Hickel R, Kuhnisch J. Hypersensitivity in teeth affected by molar-incisor hypomineralization (MIH). Sci Rep. 2021;11(1):17922.
36 Raposo F, de Carvalho Rodrigues AC, Lia EN, Leal SC. Prevalence of hypersensitivity in teeth affected by molar-incisor hypomineralization (MIH). Caries Res. 2019;53(4):424–30.
37 Baroni C, Marchionni S. MIH supplementation strategies: prospective clinical and laboratory trial. J Dent Res. 2011;90(3):371–6.
38 Mastroberardino S, Campus G, Strohmenger L, Villa A, Cagetti MG. An innovative approach to treat incisors hypomineralization (MIH): a combined use of casein phosphopeptide-amorphous calcium phosphate and hydrogen peroxide-a case report. Case Rep Dent. 2012;2012:379593.
39 Cochrane NJ, Anderson P, Davis GR, Adams GG, Stacey MA, Reynolds EC. An X-ray microtomographic study of natural white-spot enamel lesions. J Dent Res. 2012;91(2):185–91.
40 ten Cate JM, Arends J. Remineralization of artificial enamel lesions in vitro. II. Determination of activation energy and reaction order. Caries Res. 1978;12(4):213–22.
41 Crombie FA, Cochrane NJ, Manton DJ, Palamara JE, Reynolds EC. Mineralisation of developmentally hypomineralised human enamel in vitro. Caries Res. 2013;47(3):259–63.
42 Enax J, Amaechi BT, Farah R, Liu JA, Schulze Zur Wiesche E, Meyer F. Remineralization strategies for teeth with molar incisor hypomineralization (MIH): a literature review. Dent J (Basel). 2023;11(3):80.
43 Ritto FP, Tiwana KR, Schmitz TA, Dacus ZL, Borges MAP, Canellas JV. A qualitative analysis of treatment patterns for mild and severe molar hypomineralization in permanent teeth: a systematic review. Pediatr Dent. 2023;45(4):281–91.
44 Amaechi BT, Farah R, Liu JA, Phillips TS, Perozo BI, Kataoka Y, et al. Remineralization of molar incisor hypomineralization (MIH) with a hydroxyapatite toothpaste: an in-situ study. BDJ Open. 2022;8(1):33.
45 Sezer B, Kargul B. Effect of remineralization agents on molar-incisor hypomineralization-affected incisors: a randomized controlled clinical trial. J Clin Pediatr Dent. 2022;46(3):192–8.
46 Sezer B, Tugcu N, Caliskan C, Durmus B, Kupets T, Bekiroglu N, et al. Effect of casein phosphopeptide amorphous calcium fluoride phosphate and calcium glycerophosphate on incisors with molar-incisor hypomineralization: a cross-over, randomized clinical trial. Biomed Mater Eng. 2022;33(4):325–35.
47 Olgen IC, Sonmez H, Bezgin T. Effects of different remineralization agents on MIH defects: a randomized clinical study. Clin Oral Investig. 2022;26(3):3227–38.

48 Singh K, Goyal A, Gauba K, Rathore M. A comparative evaluation of CPP-ACP cream and fluoride varnish in remineralization of MIH-affected teeth using laser fluorescence. J South Asian Ass Pediatr Dent. 2021;4:117–21.

49 Singh K, Rathore M, Goyal A. Assesment of remineralization of hypomineralized enamel lesions using self-assembling peptide using laser fluorescence – a pilot study. Saudi J Oral Dent Res. 2021;6:498–501.

50 Solinas G, Grabesu V, Lattari M, Strinna R, Arnould N, Amodeo AA. Management of a hypomineralisation of the enamel by applying a remineraliser based on zinc hydroxyapatite (microRepair). Case Rep Dent. 2021;2021: 5291858.

51 Bakkal M, Abbasoglu Z, Kargul B. The effect of casein phosphopeptide-amorphous calcium phosphate on molar-incisor hypomineralisation: a pilot study. Oral Health Prev Dent. 2017;15(2):163–7.

52 Biondi AM, Cortese SG, Babino L, Fridman DE. Comparison of mineral density in molar incisor hypomineralization applying fluoride varnishes and casein phosphopeptide-amorphous calcium phosphate. Acta Odontol Latinoam. 2017;30:118–123.

53 Cardoso-Martins I, Arantes-Oliveira S, Coelho A, Pessanha S, P FM. Evaluation of the efficacy of CPP-ACP remineralizing mousse in MIH white and yellow opacities-in vitro vickers microhardness analysis. Dent J (Basel). 2022;10(10):186.

54 Franco S, Cardoso-Martins I, Arantes-Oliveira S, Pessanha S, Marques PF. In vitro polarized Raman analysis for the evaluation of the efficacy of CPP-ACP remineralizing mousse in tooth hypomineralization. Results Chem. 2021;3: 100232.

55 Kumar A, Goyal A, Gauba K, Kapur A, Singh SK, Mehta SK. An evaluation of remineralised MIH using CPP-ACP and fluoride varnish: an in-situ and in-vitro study. Eur Arch Paediatr Dent. 2022; 23(1):79–87.

56 Reynolds EC, Cai F, Cochrane NJ, Shen P, Walker GD, Morgan MV, et al. Fluoride and casein phosphopeptide-amorphous calcium phosphate. J Dent Res. 2008;87(4):344–8.

57 Restrepo M, Jeremias F, Santos-Pinto L, Cordeiro RC, Zuanon AC. Effect of fluoride varnish on enamel remineralization in anterior teeth with molar incisor hypomineralization. J Clin Pediatr Dent. 2016;40(3):207–10.

58 Llena C, Leyda AM, Forner L. CPP-ACP and CPP-ACFP versus fluoride varnish in remineralisation of early caries lesions. A prospective study. Eur J Paediatr Dent. 2015;16(3):181–6.

59 Angmar-Mansson B, ten Bosch JJ. Quantitative light-induced fluorescence (QLF): a method for assessment of incipient caries lesions. Dentomaxillofac Radiol. 2001;30(6):298–307.

60 Lynch RJ. Calcium glycerophosphate and caries: a review of the literature. Int Dent J. 2004;54(5 suppl 1):310–4.

61 Nogueira VKC, Soares IPM, Fragelli CMB, Boldieri T, Manton DJ, Bussanelli D, et al. Strucftural integrity of MIH-affected teeth after treatment with fluoride varnish or resin infiltration: an 18-month randomized clinical trial. J Dent. 2021;105:103570.

62 Cardoso CAB, Magalhães AC, Rios D, Lima JEO. Cross-sectional hardness of enamel from human teeth at different posteruptive ages. Caries Res. 2009;43(6):491–4.

63 Shellis RP, Featherstone JD, Lussi A. Understanding the chemistry of dental erosion. Monogr Oral Sci. 2014;25:163–79.

Marília Afonso Rabelo Buzalaf
Department of Biological Sciences
Bauru School of Dentistry/University of São Paulo
Alameda Octávio Pinheiro Brisolla, 9–75, Bauru 17012-901 (Brazil)
mbuzalaf@fob.usp.br

Published online: July 1, 2024
Rios D, Santos-Pinto L (eds): Molar Incisor Hypomineralisation: New Perceptions. Monogr Oral Sci. Basel, Karger, 2024, vol 32, pp 185–194 (DOI: 10.1159/000538888)

Fissure Sealants for Managing Hypersensitivity and Posteruptive Breakdown in MIH-Affected Molars

Katrin Bekes
Department of Paediatric Dentistry, University Clinic of Dentistry, Medical University of Vienna, Vienna, Austria

Abstract

Molar incisor hypomineralisation (MIH) is defined as hypomineralisation of systemic origin of one to four first permanent molars with or without the involvement of the permanent incisors. In addition to opacities and posteruptive breakdown, hypersensitivity may be a common problem, especially in the molars. Children then often report that hot and cold drinks and meals, toothbrushing, and even air flow cause pain. Therapy approaches to reduce and stop the hypersensitivity include the sealing of affected teeth. Fissure sealants can be placed in mildly affected molars that show no breakdowns in the occlusal surfaces. Thereby, resin-based sealants can be considered for fully erupted teeth, whereas glass ionomers are the treatment of choice in difficult clinical conditions as an interim treatment where isolation is inadequate and the molar has not fully erupted. The aim of this chapter is to describe the phenomenon of hypersensitivity in MIH-affected teeth, to discuss treatment approaches including the placement of sealants as well as the management of posteruptive breakdowns, and to present data on oral health-related quality of life in children suffering from hypersensitivity.

Introduction

Molar incisor hypomineralisation (MIH) is a significant developmental dental condition characterized by a qualitative defect of the enamel, affecting one or more permanent molars with or without the involvement of the incisors [1]. First identified in the late 1980s as idiopathic hypomineralisation, the term "molar-incisor hypomineralisation" was introduced in the dental literature in 2001 [1]. MIH has emerged as a prevalent condition that poses considerable challenges for dental practitioners worldwide. A systematic review found a worldwide prevalence of MIH of 12.9% (11.7–14.3%) [2, 3]. The etiology has not yet been clarified; however, it appears to be multifactorial, with systemic and epigenetic/genetic factors acting in a synergistic or additive manner [4]. The clinical presentation of MIH can range from mild localized defects to severe enamel loss. Depending on the severity, affected teeth can show rapid wear, enamel loss, increased susceptibility to caries, loss of fillings, and hypersensitiv-

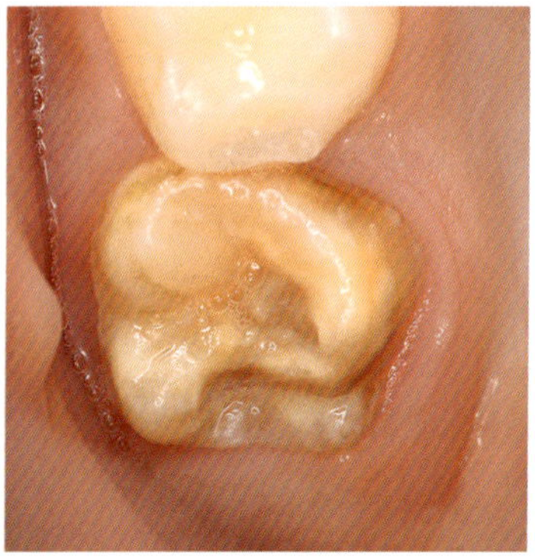

Fig. 1. Hypersensitive upper right MIH molar. In the mesial part of the fissure, breakdown of enamel and plaque can be seen. The child reported pain while eating and drinking.

ity [5]. At dental examination, behaviour management problems and even dental fear are common [5]. Therefore, early diagnosis of the condition is essential to facilitate timely intervention and mitigate potential long-term complications.

Hypersensitivity of MIH-Affected Teeth

In patients with MIH (shown in Fig. 1), hypersensitivity of affected teeth is a common symptom. In addition to opacities and posteruptive breakdowns, it can definitively be considered a key symptom [6, 7] and one of the biggest challenges in the treatment of the condition. Affected children report more or less severe chronic pain sensations starting with the beginning of eruption of the tooth (especially of the molars). While extreme stimuli can cause pain to all teeth, "hypersensitivity" is a painful response to stimuli not normally associated with pain. The occurrence of hypersensitivity does not necessarily have to be linked to the presence of an enamel breakdown.

For this reason, Bekes and Steffen [6, 7] developed an index to classify MIH teeth taking into account the presence/absence of enamel breakdowns as well as hypersensitivities. The so-called MIH treatment need index (MIH-TNI) is part of the Wuerzburg concept, which also provides a therapy plan based on the index. The MIH-TNI can be subdivided into four categories (Table 1):

Index 1: no hypersensitivity, no breakdown
Index 2: no hypersensitivity, breakdown
Index 3: hypersensitivity, no breakdown
Index 4: hypersensitivity, breakdown

Mechanism

Dentine hypersensitivity is a common condition characterized by transient tooth pain arising from exposed dentine in response to different stimuli. According to Brännström's hydrodynamic theory, it occurs due to movement of fluid within the dentin tubules in response to mechanical, osmotic, and evaporative stimuli. Cold stimuli cause an outward flow of fluid, and hot stimuli cause an inward flow [8]. In MIH teeth, the mechanism involved in hypersensitivity is not fully understood [9]. However, it is thought that the high porosity of the affected enamel facilitates the penetration of oral bacteria into the dentinal tubules, causing inflammatory reactions in the pulp, thus possibly contributing to hypersensitivity [9, 10]. This also appears to be possible in MIH teeth with an intact surface (MIH TNI 3) and means that even teeth without enamel breakdown need to be well assessed clinically and checked on a regular basis in order to avoid pulpal complications [9].

Association between Severity and Level of Hypersensitivity

Although hypersensitivity is one of the key symptoms, scientific data on the prevalence as well as on associations between tooth sensitivity and the severity of MIH are scarce. To date, only three studies have been published on this topic [11–13]. All three confirmed the existence of hypersensitivity and described a proportional increase with increasing MIH severity. Ebel et al. [12] were the first ones to show possible associations between the occurrence of hypersensitivity, its intensity, and the severity of MIH. They demonstrated that

Table 1. MIH-treatment need index as part of the Wuerzburg concept taking into account the presence or the absence of breakdowns and hypersensitivity [6, 7]

Index	Definition		
Index 1	No hypersensitivity No breakdown		
Index 2	No hypersensitivity Breakdown	2a 2b 2c	Extension of defect <1/3 Extension of defect ≥1/3 to <2/3 Extension of defect ≥2/3 and/or defect close to pulp or extraction or atypical restoration
Index 3	Hypersensitivity No breakdown		
Index 4	Hypersensitivity Breakdown	4a 4b 4c	Extension of defect <1/3 Extension of defect ≥1/3 to <2/3 Extension of defect ≥2/3 and/or defect close to pulp or extraction or atypical restoration

severely affected teeth show higher hypersensitivity than mildly affected. These results were supported by Raposo et al. [11] who also evaluated the prevalence of hypersensitivity in MIH-affected molars in 8-year-old schoolchildren. Here, all in all, teeth showed hypersensitivity in 34.7% of the cases. Thereby, sensitivity was significantly more prevalent in moderate (55%) and severe cases (51.6%) than in mild cases (29.8%). A recent study by Linner et al. [13] assessed potential associations between patient- and tooth-related variables and the intensity of hypersensitivity in permanent MIH teeth. MIH teeth with demarcated opacities, and atypical restorations had moderate sensitivity, whereas teeth with enamel breakdown were mostly linked to severe hypersensitivity. Furthermore, a significantly lower level of hypersensitivity was observed in patients aged ≥8 years.

Clinical Problems

Children with hypersensitive MIH teeth show multiple clinical problems. They often report that hot and cold or sweet drinks and meals and sometimes even air flow or breathing cause pain [1, 14, 15]. However, the response to the stimulus varies from person to person due to differences in pain tolerance, environmental factors, and emotional state [16]. Depending on the intensity of pain, problems with oral hygiene habits may also be described. This, in turn, leads to a higher susceptibility of carious lesions due to an increased plaque accumulation. The risk of caries is further increased by a cariogenic diet, especially containing sugars, and less than ideal oral hygiene. Furthermore, difficulties in achieving an effective local anesthesia may also be encountered during dental procedures [17]. This observation could be explained as follows: It is well known that preoperative pain can serve as a risk factor for inadequate local anesthesia in patients with irreversible pulpitis. A considerable help and a possible solution is to give analgesic premedication to children with hypersensitive MIH teeth before the treatment [18]. Steffen and Stratigaki [19] developed an appropriate treatment protocol for this purpose, based on the findings in treatments of patients with chronic back pain. Finally, the presence of hypersensitivity may also increase the child's anxiety and cause behavioral problems during clinical workflows [14].

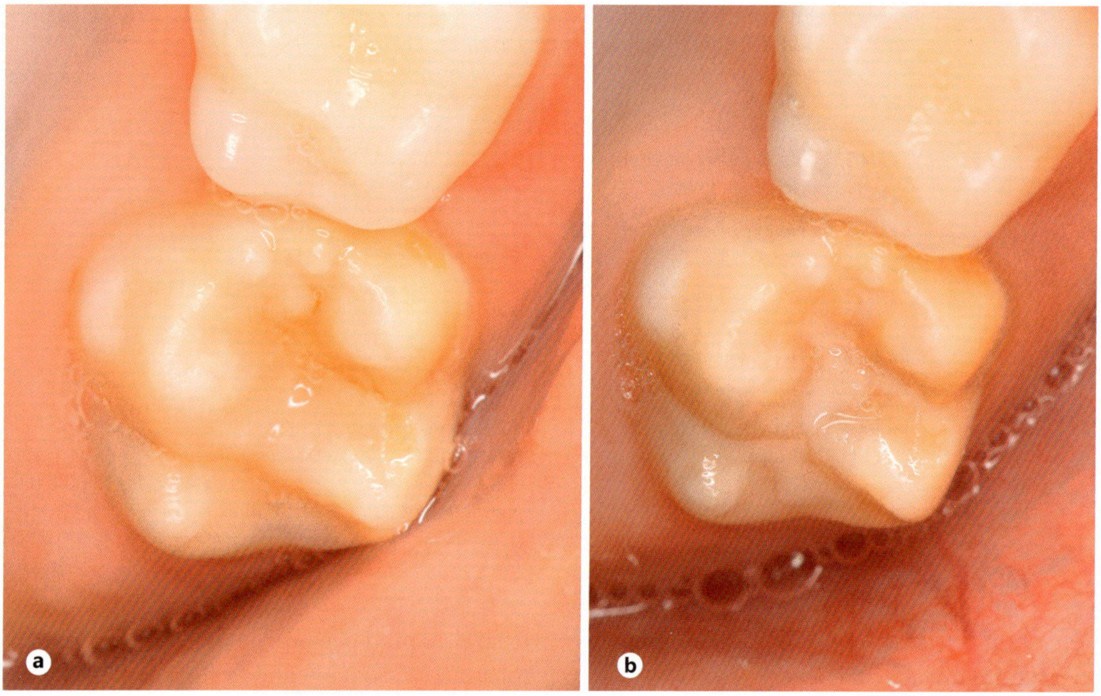

Fig. 2. Sealing of tooth 26 with a resin-based fissure sealant. A self-etch adhesive was applied before the placement of the fissure sealant. **a** Before sealing. **b** After sealing.

Fissure Sealants

Background

Fissure sealants are one of the most highly recommended and widely accepted preventive dental procedures. Their effectiveness in preventing caries lesions, particularly on the occlusal surfaces of teeth in children and adolescents, has been shown in numerous clinical studies [20]. Sealants act as a physical barrier to decay. They prevent cariogenic bacteria from gaining access to their source of fermentable nutrients [21]. However, the ability to provide this protection is determined by and directly related to the retention of the sealant on the tooth surface. For noncompromised molars, well-evaluated application protocols and material recommendations exist.

Sealing of MIH Teeth

Sealing of MIH molars was initially recommended only if the tooth showed mild defects, no sensitivity, and no posteruptive breakdowns [15, 22, 23]. However, the observation of retention losses in clinical practice first called in question the effectiveness of this treatment approach for some time. For example, Kotsanos et al. [24] observed that hypomineralised sealed molars required retreatment approximately 2 years earlier than sound teeth. Furthermore, the risk of loss of the sealant was approximately three times higher using classical treatment protocols.

Since then, sealing approaches have changed or have been adapted. First of all, altered clinical workflows have been suggested. Regarding step-by-step procedures, adhesives are now proposed before sealant application when resin-based sealants are placed as this step has clearly shown to

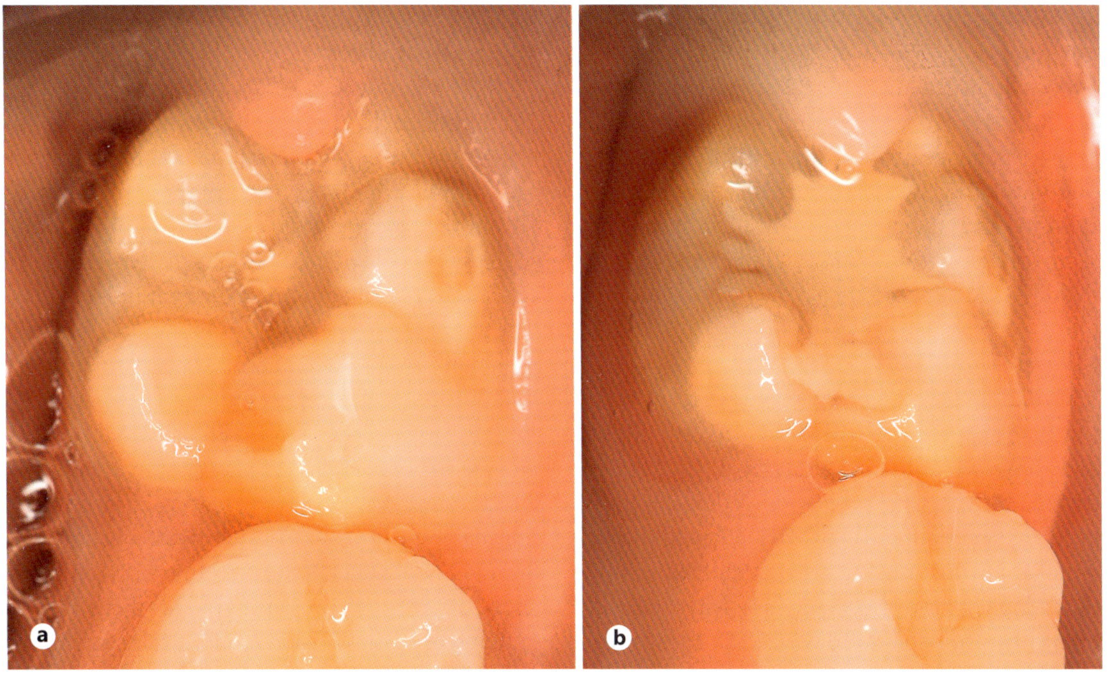

Fig. 3. Sealing of tooth 36 with a glass ionomer cement. The tooth was not fully erupted, and it was difficult to reach adequate isolation. **a** Before sealing. **b** After sealing.

increase the retention rate [25]. This is due to the fact that the hypomineralised enamel is characterized by a reduction in mineral quantity and quality, a reduced hardness and modulus of elasticity, increased porosity, and higher protein contents. In comparison to sound enamel, the retentive etch patterns of MIH-affected enamel are suboptimal [26]. Some other studies proposed additional application of 5% sodium hypochlorite (NaOCl) for 60 s after etching (deproteinisation) to enhance enamel bonding by removing excess protein content from the tooth surface [27, 28]. However, the current best clinical practice guidance of the EAPD is neither in favor nor against this additional step [29], and further studies are needed to clarify this point. Furthermore, fissure sealants are now also considered if mildly affected molars that are hypersensitive or present minimal breakdowns, which are not located on the occlusal surface [30].

Materials
Regarding materials, resin-based sealants as well as glass ionomers can be chosen (shown in Fig. 2, 3). However, existing studies on these two materials are primarily based on sound enamel. Clinical studies on MIH are generally rare at present, so the current approach is to transfer the knowledge gained from sound enamel to hypomineralised enamel and research it further.

It is largely recognized that resin-based sealants present higher retention rates compared to glass ionomer cement (GIC) sealants in sound enamel [31]. However, they need optimal conditions for placement, including excellent moisture control [32]. Therefore, they can only be an option when the tooth is fully erupted and the patient has good compliance (shown in Fig. 2). Conversely, GIC sealants can be used as an interim treatment in difficult clinical conditions where isolation is inadequate (shown in Fig. 3), as they are less technique sensitive, cure rapidly, and do not require intermediate steps such as etching. Especially in situations when an MIH molar has not fully erupted but a sealing is indicated as well as in less-cooperative and anxious children or patients suffering from hypersensitive molars, GIC sealants and their easy application procedure seem preferable and more convenient for the child [33].

Clinical Data

It should be noted, however, that current scientific data on sealing of MIH teeth are very limited, and there are also contradictory data. As mentioned above, a Greek study described an earlier need for retreatment in MIH-affected molars than in healthy molars and calculated a three times higher risk of sealant loss when classical treatment protocols were used [24]. Lygidakis et al. [25] studied molars with mild forms of MIH over 4 years in a split-mouth design after sealing with and without additional application of an etch-and-rinse adhesive system. In all molars, mechanical preparation of the superficial enamel of the fissure was performed before. When fissure sealants were placed with the adhesive, higher complete retention rates were observed (70% vs. 26%).

In contrast, a Brazilian study with 18 months of follow-up showed no significant differences in retention rates of mildly affected molars compared to sound ones (72% vs. 62%). Here, fissure sealants were placed under rubber dam using the conventional method after a previous 4-week application of fluoride (1× per week).

A recent study that was conducted in Turkey focused on the clinical success of giomer- and conventional resin-based sealants and found retention rates of 8% and 68% after 12 months, respectively [34].

Sealing as an Approach to Treat Hypersensitivities

In addition to the classic functions of caries prevention or the arrest of carious lesions without cavities [35], sealing appears to have another important effect in the treatment of MIH molars. Bekes et al. [33] demonstrated that sealing of hypersensitive teeth can also help to reduce the pain immediately. The study was carried out in children with hypersensitive molars (without enamel breakdown, MIH TNI 3) using two different sealing techniques (classical fissure sealant with additional use of a self-etching adhesive; GIC) in a split-mouth design. The effectiveness of the treatment was measured by thermal tests immediately after treatment and 1, 4, 8, and 12 weeks later. Before treatment, the children showed severe hypersensitivity of their molars (Schiff score 2 or 3, Visual Analog Scale score in the upper range of the scale ranging from 0 to 10 [>7]). Regardless of the material used, hypersensitivities decreased immediately after placement of the sealant. This decrease remained stable over the 12-week study period.

It should be added that the underlying mechanism is currently still unclear. The study included teeth that showed opacities not only on the occlusal surface. The observation that covering the occlusal surface prevents hypersensitivity, although there may still be uncovered hypomineralised areas, has not yet been conclusively explained. The same enigma also applies to MIH teeth with post-eruptive breakdowns, which do not necessarily have to be hypersensitive.

The limitations of the evidence related to this topic explicitly emphasize the need for further studies to draw stronger conclusions and establish clinical guidelines.

Despite the insights gained from the existing research mentioned, limitations of the evidence related to this topic still exist. There is an ongoing need for additional studies to address uncertainties and refine the understanding of sealing as an approach to treat hypersensitivities.

Sealing as an Approach to Cover Breakdowns

In addition to the traditional sealing process, sealants can also be chosen to cover small breakdowns on the occlusal surface. Although Lygidakis et al. [36] suggested in 2010 that application of a GIC sealant can protect MIH-affected molars, so far, however, there is only one study that has focused on this issue [37]. The working group evaluated the preventive effect of a glass ionomer sealant versus no sealant application with regard to posteruptive breakdowns and dental caries after a 12-month follow-up period. Only MIH molars presenting opacities on the occlusal surface were included. The results showed that molars that were not sealed were 77% more likely to develop dental caries compared to molars that received a sealant application. However, the placement of a glass ionomer sealant did not protect molars against posteruptive breakdown, atypical restoration, atypical caries, or extraction due to MIH. With regard to the cited study, it should be noted that by covering the occlusal surface with a sealant, only the areas that are covered by the material can theoretically be protected. However, the authors do not provide detailed information on which surface the PEB actually occurred in the sealed teeth – whether in the sealed area or elsewhere.

Furthermore, Schraverus et al. [37] observed a significant association regarding posteruptive breakdown and the color of the opacities. Teeth with yellow-brown opacities were 5 times more likely to have posteruptive breakdown, atypical restoration, atypical caries, or extraction due to MIH after a 12-month follow-up. This is probably related to yellow-brown opacities being more porous and less mineralised than white-creamy [38], which may be a risk factor for a breakdown.

In conclusion, without dismissing the significance of the existing study, it is evident that its limitations warrant further investigation to refine the understanding of sealing as an approach to cover and protect from breakdowns and establish definitive clinical guidelines.

Oral Health-Related Quality of Life

Background

Oral health is an integral component of overall well-being and plays a fundamental role in an individual's ability to perform essential functions related to eating, speaking, and expressing emotions. Beyond the traditional clinical indicators, there is a growing recognition that oral health encompasses a broader concept, which includes the impact of oral conditions on an individual's quality of life. In this context, oral health-related quality of life (OHRQoL) has emerged as a pivotal aspect of oral health research, focusing on the physical, psychological, and social dimensions of an individual's life that are influenced by the condition of their oral health [39].

The most widely used method for assessing OHRQOL is the use of multiple-item questionnaires. As oral health and health cognition are considered to be age dependent, specific issues may arise when measuring OHRQoL in younger patients due to their stage of physical, cognitive, emotional, social, and linguistic development [40, 41]. Several instruments have been specifically developed for specific age groups. For schoolchildren and adolescents, the most often used ones include the Child Perceptions Questionnaire [42, 43], the Child Oral Health Impact Profile [44], and the Child Oral Impacts on Daily Performances [45].

OHRQoL in MIH Patients with Hypersensitivity

OHRQoL is often altered in patients with MIH. This is because the pain associated with hypomineralised teeth causes noticeable and frequent discomfort. However, data on the relationship between MIH and OHRQoL are still scarce, even though MIH has been known for more than 20 years [46]. These studies all point to the same direction. Joshi et al. were able to show that the presence of MIH significantly impacted OHRQoL. MIH-affected children had a 3 times more impaired OHRQoL. Furthermore, regarding severity of

MIH, reduced OHRQoL increased with increasing severity of MIH. The impact of hypersensitivity could also be demonstrated. MIH children with hypersensitive teeth (with or without breakdown, TNI 3 and 4) [6, 7] had a worse OHRQoL compared to children with MIH teeth that were not hypersensitive (TNI 1 and 2). Most often reported problems of MIH patients in this study were "pain or sensitivity towards cold drinks and foods," "bad breath," "pain in the teeth or mouth," "needed longer time than others to eat meal because of teeth or mouth," and "been upset because of teeth or mouth" ($N = 35$, 37.23%). The item "pain in teeth or mouth" showed a seven-fold increase in MIH-affected children compared those without MIH.

To date, there is only one study that assessed OHRQoL in patients with hypersensitive MIH molars before and after treatment with a sealing [47]. Bekes et al. included MIH-affected children with two molars showing hypersensitivity (Schiff Cold Air Sensitivity Scale 2 or 3 [48]) and nonocclusal breakdowns (MIH-TNI 3) [6, 7]. Both molars were sealed using a split-mouth design: a resin-based fissure sealant in combination with the use of a self-etch adhesive, and a GIC, respectively. The validated German version of the CPQ8–10 was used to assess the OHRQoL of the child before and at different time points after treatment [49]. The questionnaire includes a total of 25 items, which can be split into four domains: oral symptoms (five questions), functional limitations (five questions), emotional well-being (five questions), and social well-being (ten questions). Questions ask about the frequency of events in the child's last four weeks.

Prior to treatment, all enrolled patients had two MIH molars with severe hypersensitivity (Schiff score 2 or 3, Visual Analog Scale score in the upper range of the scale ranging from 0 to 10 [>7]). Irrespective of the material used, hypersensitivity decreased immediately after treatment and remained constant over the 12-week study period. This was also the case in the patients' self-perception. Pretreatment quality of life limitations (particularly pain frequency and food restriction) were reduced with the sealant application. The mean CPQ-G8–10 score at baseline was 14.7 (±5.9; range = 4–31). At the one-week follow-up, the score decreased significantly, and it was reduced again after the 12-week follow-up (2.7 [±3.2; range = 0–14]), showing a large effect size. This indicates that the children noticed themselves as having a significant improvement in their overall OHRQoL. The same results were seen in all subdomains. As anticipated, the children showed high scores in the subdomain "oral symptoms" and "functional limitations." These include questions on the frequency of pain and the frequency of food intake restriction.

Conclusions

Molars with mild forms of MIH only show opacities and no occlusal breakdowns, but sensitivity can be considered for a sealing approach. The choice of material – resin-based sealers or glass ionomer – depends on the state of eruption, the possibility of moisture control, and the compliance of the patient. Immediate sealing can increase OHRQoL in these patients.

Statement of Ethics

Written informed consent was obtained from patients (or their parents/legal guardians/next-of-kin) for publication of the images.

Conflict of Interest Statement

The author has no conflicts of interest to declare.

Funding Sources

The author declares that the mentioned studies regarding sealing of hypersensitive MIH teeth were funded by 3M [33, 47].

References

1 Weerheijm KL, Jalevik B, Alaluusua S. Molar-incisor hypomineralisation. Caries Res. 2001 Sep-Oct;35(5):390–1.
2 Schwendicke F, Elhennawy K, Reda S, Bekes K, Manton DJ, Krois J. Global burden of molar incisor hypomineralization. J Dent. 2018;68:10–18.
3 Schwendicke F, Elhennawy K, Reda S, Bekes K, Manton DJ, Krois J. Corrigendum to "Global burden of molar incisor hypomineralization" [J Dent. 2018;68C:10–18]. J Dent. 2019 Jan;80:89–92.
4 Garot E, Rouas P, Somani C, Taylor GD, Wong F, Lygidakis NA. An update of the aetiological factors involved in molar incisor hypomineralisation (MIH): a systematic review and meta-analysis. Eur Arch Paediatr Dent. 2022;23(1):23–38.
5 Lygidakis NA. Treatment modalities in children with teeth affected by molar-incisor enamel hypomineralisation (MIH): a systematic review. Eur Arch Paediatr Dent. 2010 Apr;11(2):65–74.
6 Bekes K, Steffen R. The Wuerzburg MIH concept: part 1. The MIH treatment need index (MIH TNI). A new index to assess and plan the treatment in patients with molar incisior hypomineralization (MIH). Oralprophylaxe Kinderzahnheilkunde. 2016;38(4):165–70.
7 Steffen R, Kramer N, Bekes K. The Wurzburg MIH concept: the MIH treatment need index (MIH TNI): a new index to assess and plan treatment in patients with molar incisior hypomineralisation (MIH). Eur Arch Paediatr Dent. 2017 Oct;18(5):355–61.
8 Brannstrom M. The hydrodynamic theory of dentinal pain: sensation in preparations, caries, and the dentinal crack syndrome. J Endod. 1986 Oct;12(10): 453–7.
9 Fagrell TG, Lingstrom P, Olsson S, Steiniger F, Noren JG. Bacterial invasion of dentinal tubules beneath apparently intact but hypomineralized enamel in molar teeth with molar incisor hypomineralization. Int J Paediatr Dent. 2008 Sep;18(5):333–40.
10 Fagrell TG, Ludvigsson J, Ullbro C, Lundin SA, Koch G. Aetiology of severe demarcated enamel opacities – an evaluation based on prospective medical and social data from 17,000 children. Swed Dent J. 2011;35(2):57–67.
11 Raposo F, de Carvalho Rodrigues AC, Lia EN, Leal SC. Prevalence of hypersensitivity in teeth affected by molar-incisor hypomineralization (MIH). Caries Res. 2019;53(4):424–30.
12 Ebel M, Bekes K, Klode C, Hirsch C. The severity and degree of hypomineralisation in teeth and its influence on oral hygiene and caries prevalence in children. Int J Paediatr Dent. 2018;28(6): 648–57.
13 Linner T, Khazaei Y, Bucher K, Pfisterer J, Hickel R, Kuhnisch J. Hypersensitivity in teeth affected by molar-incisor hypomineralization (MIH). Sci Rep. 2021 Sep 9;11(1):17922.
14 Jalevik B, Klingberg GA. Dental treatment, dental fear and behaviour management problems in children with severe enamel hypomineralization of their permanent first molars. Int J Paediatr Dent. 2002 Jan;12(1):24–32.
15 William V, Messer LB, Burrow MF. Molar incisor hypomineralization: review and recommendations for clinical management. Pediatr Dent. 2006 May-Jun;28(3):224–32.
16 Orchardson R, Collins WJ. Clinical features of hypersensitive teeth. Br Dent J. 1987 Apr 11;162(7):253–6.
17 Rodd HD, Morgan CR, Day PF, Boissonade FM. Pulpal expression of TRPV1 in molar incisor hypomineralisation. Eur Arch Paediatr Dent. 2007 Dec;8(4):184–8.
18 Bekes K, Steffen R. Pain control. In: Bekes K, editor. Molar Incisor Hypomineralization. Berlin: Quintessence Publishing; 2022. p. 81–9.
19 Steffen R, Stratigaki E. Schmerzausschaltung bei Kindern und Jugendlichen – Grundlagen der Lokalanästhesie. Zahnmedizin Up2date. 2019;13(3):219–31.
20 Ahovuo-Saloranta A, Forss H, Walsh T, Nordblad A, Makela M, Worthington HV. Pit and fissure sealants for preventing dental decay in permanent teeth. Cochrane Database Syst Rev. 2017 Jul 31;7:CD001830.
21 American Academy of Paediatric Dentistry. Guideline on restorative dentistry. Pediatr Dent. 2016 Oct;38(6):250–62.
22 Fayle SA. Molar incisor hypomineralisation: restorative management. Eur J Paediatr Dent. 2003 Sep;4(3):121–6.
23 Mathu-Muju K, Wright JT. Diagnosis and treatment of molar incisor hypomineralization. Compend Contin Educ Dent. 2006 Nov;27(11):604–10; quiz 11.
24 Kotsanos N, Kaklamanos EG, Arapostathis K. Treatment management of first permanent molars in children with Molar-Incisor Hypomineralisation. Eur J Paediatr Dent. 2005 Dec;6(4):179–84.
25 Lygidakis NA, Dimou G, Stamataki E. Retention of fissure sealants using two different methods of application in teeth with hypomineralised molars (MIH): a 4 year clinical study. Eur Arch Paediatr Dent. 2009 Dec;10(4):223–6.
26 Elhennawy K, Manton DJ, Crombie F, Zaslansky P, Radlanski RJ, Jost-Brinkmann PG, et al. Structural, mechanical and chemical evaluation of molar-incisor hypomineralization-affected enamel: a systematic review. Arch Oral Biol. 2017 Nov;83:272–81.
27 Sonmez H, Saat S. A clinical evaluation of deproteinization and different cavity designs on resin restoration performance in MIH-affected molars: two-year results. J Clin Pediatr Dent. 2017; 41(5):336–42.
28 Ekambaram M, Anthonappa RP, Govindool SR, Yiu CKY. Comparison of deproteinization agents on bonding to developmentally hypomineralized enamel. J Dent. 2017 Dec;67:94–101.
29 Lygidakis NA, Garot E, Somani C, Taylor GD, Rouas P, Wong FSL. Best clinical practice guidance for clinicians dealing with children presenting with molar-incisor-hypomineralisation (MIH): an updated European Academy of Paediatric Dentistry policy document. Eur Arch Paediatr Dent. 2022 Feb;23(1):3–21.
30 Bekes K, Krämer N, van Waes H, Steffen R. The Wuerzburg MIH concept: part 2. The treatment plan. Oralprophylaxe Kinderzahnheilkunde. 2016;38(4):171–75.
31 Kuhnisch J, Bedir A, Lo YF, Kessler A, Lang T, Mansmann U, et al. Meta-analysis of the longevity of commonly used pit and fissure sealant materials. Dent Mater. 2020 May;36(5):e158–68.
32 Cvikl B, Moritz A, Bekes K. Pit and fissure sealants-a comprehensive review. Dent J (Basel). 2018 Jun 12;6(2):18.

33 Bekes K, Amend S, Priller J, Zamek C, Stamm T, Krämer N. Hypersensitivity relief of MIH-affected molars using two sealing techniques: a 12-week follow-up. Clin Oral Investig. 2022;26(2):1879–88.
34 Ozgur B, Kargin ST, Olmez MS. Clinical evaluation of giomer- and resin-based fissure sealants on permanent molars affected by molar-incisor hypomineralization: a randomized clinical trial. BMC Oral Health. 2022 Jul 5;22(1):275.
35 Welbury R, Raadal M, Lygidakis NA, European Academy of Paediatric D. EAPD guidelines for the use of pit and fissure sealants. Eur J Paediatr Dent. 2004 Sep;5(3):179–84.
36 Lygidakis NA, Wong F, Jalevik B, Vierrou AM, Alaluusua S, Espelid I. Best clinical practice guidance for clinicians dealing with children presenting with molar-incisor-hypomineralisation (MIH): an EAPD policy document. Eur Arch Paediatr Dent. 2010 Apr;11(2):75–81.
37 Schraverus MS, Olegario IC, Bonifacio CC, Gonzalez APR, Pedroza M, Hesse D. Glass ionomer sealants can prevent dental caries but cannot prevent posteruptive breakdown on molars affected by molar incisor hypomineralization: one-year results of a randomized clinical trial. Caries Res. 2021;55(4):301–09.
38 Jalevik B, Noren JG. Enamel hypomineralization of permanent first molars: a morphological study and survey of possible aetiological factors. Int J Paediatr Dent. 2000 Dec;10(4):278–89.
39 Sischo L, Broder HL. Oral health-related quality of life: what, why, how, and future implications. J Dent Res. 2011 Nov;90(11):1264–70.
40 Tapsoba H, Deschamps JP, Leclercq MH. Factor analytic study of two questionnaires measuring oral health-related quality of life among children and adults in New Zealand, Germany and Poland. Qual Life Res. 2000;9(5):559–69.
41 Barbosa TS, Gaviao MB. Oral health-related quality of life in children: part I. How well do children know themselves? A systematic review. Int J Dent Hyg. 2008 May;6(2):93–9.
42 Jokovic A, Locker D, Stephens M, Kenny D, Tompson B, Guyatt G. Validity and reliability of a questionnaire for measuring child oral-health-related quality of life. J Dent Res. 2002 Jul;81(7):459–63.
43 Jokovic A, Locker D, Tompson B, Guyatt G. Questionnaire for measuring oral health-related quality of life in eight- to ten-year-old children. Pediatr Dent. 2004 Nov-Dec;26(6):512–8.
44 Broder HL, Wilson-Genderson M. Reliability and convergent and discriminant validity of the Child Oral Health Impact Profile (COHIP Child's version). Community Dent Oral Epidemiol. 2007 Aug;35(suppl 1):20–31.
45 Gherunpong S, Tsakos G, Sheiham A. Developing and evaluating an oral health-related quality of life index for children; the CHILD-OIDP. Community Dent Health. 2004 Jun;21(2):161–9.
46 Joshi T, Rahman A, Rienhoff S, Rienhoff J, Stamm T, Bekes K. Impact of molar incisor hypomineralization on oral health-related quality of life in 8–10-year-old children. Clin Oral Investig. 2022;26(2):1753–9.
47 Bekes K, Amend S, Priller J, Zamek C, Stamm T, Krämer N. Changes in oral health-related quality of life after treatment of hypersensitive molar incisor hypomineralization–affected molars with a sealing. Clin Oral Investig. 2021;25(11):6449–54.
48 Schiff T, Delgado E, Zhang YP, Cummins D, DeVizio W, Mateo LR. Clinical evaluation of the efficacy of an in-office desensitizing paste containing 8% arginine and calcium carbonate in providing instant and lasting relief of dentin hypersensitivity. Am J Dent. 2009 Mar;22 Spec No A:8A–15A.
49 Bekes K, Ebel M, Omara M, Boukhobza S, Dumitrescu N, Priller J, et al. The German version of Child Perceptions Questionnaire for children aged 8 to 10 years (CPQ-G8–10): translation, reliability, and validity. Clin Oral Investig. 2021 Mar;25(3):1433–39.

Katrin Bekes
Department of Paediatric Dentistry
University Clinic of Dentistry, Medical University of Vienna
Sensengasse 2a, AT–1190 Vienna (Austria)
katrin.bekes@meduniwien.ac.at

Published online: July 1, 2024
Rios D, Santos-Pinto L (eds): Molar Incisor Hypomineralisation: New Perceptions. Monogr Oral Sci. Basel, Karger, 2024, vol 32, pp 195–211 (DOI: 10.1159/000538889)

MIH-Affected Substrate: An Overview of Adhesive Challenges to the Dental Structures

Linda Wang[a] Victor Mosquim[a] Giovanna Speranza Zabeu[a]
Juliana Feltrin-Souza[b]

[a]Department of Operative Dentistry, Endodontics and Dental Materials, Bauru School of Dentistry, University of São Paulo, Bauru, Brazil; [b]Department of Stomatology, Federal University of Paraná, Curitiba, Brazil

Abstract

Based on the current state of the art regarding molar incisor hypomineralisation (MIH)-affected enamel, bonding systems are expected to play a relevant role on the restorative procedures when required. MIH-affected enamel is often subjected to posteruptive breakdown combined or not with carious lesions, predominantly on molars, and may also affect the aesthetics of anterior teeth. As unbalanced mineral and protein contents occur, understanding these alterations is essential before selecting the most appropriate adhesive systems, while bearing in mind their limitations. In particular, when dentin is involved due to enamel breakdown, the use of functional monomer-based bonding systems present in self-etching and universal systems produce a chemical interaction that enhance the bonding. So far, the overall recommendation relies on placing the margin of the restoration on clinically sound enamel, regardless of the category of the adhesive system.

Introduction

It is known that the teeth affected by molar incisor hypomineralisation (MIH) demands more dental treatments due to enamel breakdown and caries risk in patients with cariogenic diet. Thus, when the restorative treatment is required, it should be associated with a prevention plan and patient's oral care education [1].

Previously, due to the wide clinical variability of MIH, it is essential to properly clinically diagnose the hypomineralised lesion affecting enamel, taking in consideration aspects that will further help to predict the success of the treatment, regardless of the selection of the adhesive systems and restorative materials [2, 3].

Significant efforts have been made by researchers to develop safe and conservative guidelines addressing the management of a patient with MIH that have been constantly updated over the last decades [1, 4, 5]. However, bonding to MIH-affected tissue is still a challenge, and long-term clinical trials on this subject are encouraged,

Table 1. Local and overall conditions to consider on a lesion before making a clinical decision

Local	Overall
- Color (white, yellow, or brown) - Area to be bonded (involving enamel and/or dentin) - The presence or absence of carious tissue/lesion - Report or not of sensitivity	- Occlusion characteristics - Age of the patient - Follow-up availability - Cooperation of the patient

as they will provide sufficient evidence to support the clinical practice, while also considering the constant innovation of products developed by the industry. Thus, it is important for clinicians to stay up to date.

Before deciding on the most appropriate bonding agent, it is necessary to consider both the severity of the condition and the area to be bonded. The current state-of-the-art classification for MIH ranges from demarcated opacities that do not show any compromised clinical structure to conditions with evident enamel breakdown or atypical cavity [1, 5]. In general, darker brownish opacities seem to be more severely hypomineralised, presenting higher breakdown risk than whitish/creamy ones [6–8]. Thus, while considering the appearance/color of the hypomineralised enamel, clinicians also need to simultaneously take other clinical factors into account before deciding on the most appropriate treatment (Table 1) [1, 9].

Moreover, it is relevant to state that other developmental defects might affect the enamel with similar clinical characteristics as those seen in MIH-affected teeth concurrently shown in Figure 1. These defects must be properly diagnosed and differentiated from the MIH before attempting to treat the area as they are determined by distinct etiological factors. If they are not properly identified and addressed, the treatment is likely going to fail, regardless of the bonding agent and restorative material used in the area [10–12].

Differences in the MIH-Affected Enamel

Sound enamel is considered a well-structured and homogeneous tissue mainly composed of minerals with very little organic content [13]. This aspect is a key condition that makes the bonding procedures reliable under clinical circumstances. The presence of margins on sound enamel for any dental restoration is almost synonymous of proper marginal sealing with reduced risk of bacterial infiltration; therefore, this healthy tissue should be preserved whenever possible [14].

In this perspective, once the mineral quality of enamel is affected, caution needs to be taken when considering placing a bonded restoration. Several dental malformations, posteruptive conditions, and diseases can impair the enamel and/or dentin mineral quality, such as MIH, dental caries, dental erosion, or even amelogenesis imperfecta [3, 7, 15, 16]. In particular, MIH is a qualitative developmental enamel defect, represented by demarcated opacity, affecting one or more first permanent molars and frequently permanent incisors.

MIH is associated with systemic and genetic factors occurred during the early maturation stage of enamel formation [16–18]. In sound teeth, during this stage, the organic content is normally resorbed and followed by the deposition of minerals [10, 12, 19]. In MIH pathogenesis, it is hypothesized that there is a possible setback in this maturation stage, in which the organic content is not properly resorbed, thus the mineral content cannot achieve its usual proportion [17, 18, 20]. Thus, higher protein/organic content as

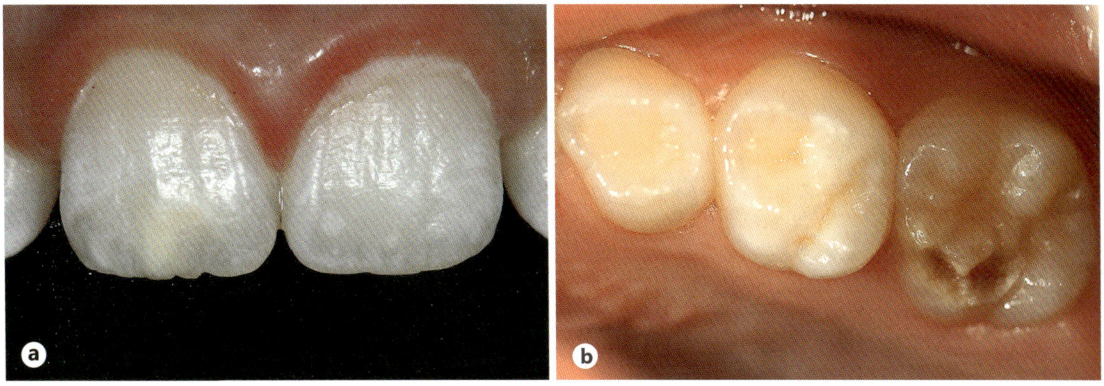

Fig. 1. Anterior teeth affected by mild fluorosis with the right central incisor also presenting a hypomineralised opacity in the incisal third (**a**). MIH lesion associated with enamel breakdown (**b**).

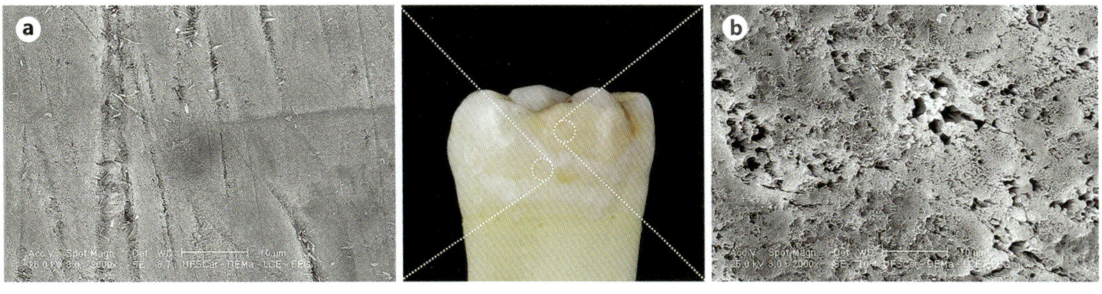

Fig. 2. Scanning electron microscopy evidencing the difference in porosity of enamel between an allegedly clinically unaffected part of the tooth (**a**) compared to the area visibly affected by MIH (**b**). The areas from which these images were taken are circled in white.

well as a higher and variable concentration of carbon and magnesium led to a lower Ca/P ratio, which hampers the growth of hydroxyapatite crystals observed for hypomineralised enamel [7, 10].

Given this overall scenario, there is a reduction in the hardness and elasticity as well as increased porosity in the affected enamel [3, 7, 16, 17]. A comparison between the area affected by the hypomineralisation and an allegedly unaffected part of the enamel in the same tooth is shown in Figure 2. As previously reported, the MIH-affected enamel is not as organized into hydroxyapatite crystals as the sound teeth, usually presenting loosely packed crystals, less-dense prismatic structure, partial loss of the prismatic pattern, less distinct prism borders, and more evident interprismatic space [1, 4, 5, 8]. These described alterations clearly result in a vulnerable substrate to be bonded.

In the case of opaque areas with no visible structural breakdown, aesthetic interventions can be requested to mask them (Fig. 3). Caution is necessary to not ignore this aspect as mere discoloration once it involves deeper enamel layers, differently from other enamel defects, such as fluorosis [11]. Considering the alterations in MIH-affected enamel, such as higher organic and lower

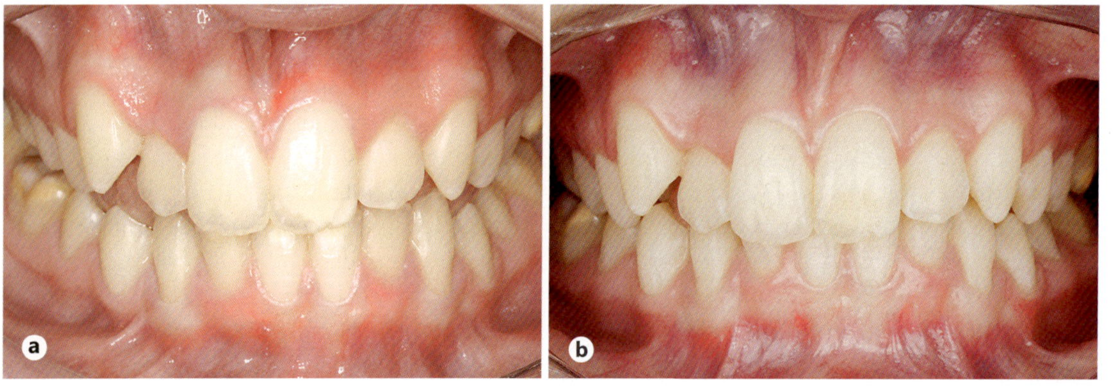

Fig. 3. White stain affecting the left upper central incisor of a patient with MIH (**a**). Final aspect 1 week after infiltration with a resin infiltrant (Icon/DMG) (**b**).

calcium content, and the relevance of this ion to promote bonding to the dental tissues [21–23], it does not seem safe to restrict the bonding treatment to this area, despite efforts being made to preserve as much dental tissue as possible.

Clinically, the sound enamel margin has been stipulated as the safe area to be involved when bonding to MIH-affected teeth [3, 14, 24–26]. This occurs because the MIH-affected enamel is known to have 8- to 21-fold higher content of proteins than sound enamel, especially albumin [7], which was shown to bind to apatite crystals and inhibit its growth [27].

Adhesion of Restorative Materials to the MIH-Affected Enamel

Some evidence indicates glass ionomer cements (GICs) as reliable options to be considered on MIH-affected enamel, despite marginal rupture or partial loss of the restoration being common [28]. For this purpose, conventional GICs and, more recently, resin-modified glass-ionomer cements (RMGICs) are available. In these situations, a weak acidic solution with high molecular weight, such as polyacrylic and/or carboxylic acid, is used to clean the surface and increase the interaction between the GIC and the dental structure. In the event an RMGIC is used, a light-curing primer is applied instead, and a mechanical interlocking mechanism can also be involved to promote adhesion to the substrate. Yet, regardless of their classifications, bonding of GICs to the enamel provides a chemical reaction with the tooth mineral content [22, 23].

This chemical bond between the material and the enamel relies basically on a result of ionic forces, in which the carboxylic groups from the material replace the phosphate (PO_4^{3-}) ions and make ionic bonds with calcium (Ca^+) ions present in the enamel's hydroxyapatite [22, 23]. As MIH-affected enamel presents a lower mineral content, it is reasonable to assume that the bond strength might be lower than it is on sound enamel. Still, this statement is purely speculative as there are scarce studies evaluating the adhesion of GICs to MIH-affected enamel compared to sound enamel. This is a particularly hard task to fulfill given that cohesive failures within the material are common in bond strength tests using GICs [29], and cohesive failures within the enamel are common in bond strength tests on MIH-affected teeth [4, 20, 30]. This basically means that the bond strength is higher than the resistance of the GIC and of the affected enamel.

Despite this lack of evidence of bond strength values for GICs on MIH-affected enamel, there is sufficient evidence that GICs are able to release fluoride, presenting an anticariogenic property and promoting remineralisation of the underlying and surrounding enamel [31, 32]. This is particularly important for patients with high risk of caries, and the GIC bonding characteristics associated with the fluoride release make this material desirable when carious lesions are associated, which is not uncommon for patients with MIH [32, 33]. Also, the adhesion of GICs to the enamel is much less susceptible to the presence of moisture than it is with resins, making it a great material to be used in those cases where proper moisture control cannot be achieved (e.g., teeth with severe sensitivity, teeth in irruptive process, and/or noncompliant children).

However, GICs do not present great mechanical properties and can be susceptible to wear and fracture, especially in stress-bearing areas [31, 32, 34, 35]. In the study of Schraverus et al. [32], GIC restorations on MIH-affected teeth were able to prevent the development of carious lesions but were not able to prevent the enamel from breaking upon chewing forces (posteruptive breakdown), which is common for MIH-affected teeth [9]. The hypothesis is that the GIC was able to promote some level of remineralisation to the point of preventing and arresting dental caries but not to the point of clinically enhancing the mechanical strength of the affected enamel [32]. Some studies suggest that this superficial mineralisation can improve bonding to MIH-affected enamel [36, 37].

Hence, it can be deduced that while glass ionomer-based materials do not offer interesting mechanical properties in load-bearing areas and are more susceptible to bonding issues with the MIH-affected enamel, it seems more reliable to be used in situations that do not involve enamel breakdown. Also, in particular conditions where carious lesions can be associated, the properties related to remineralisation and bioactive ingredients can be more relevant, making the GICs an interesting choice. In the case these materials fail mechanically prematurely, it could be repaired or even replaced by resin composite materials. Additionally, the use of sandwich-type restorations can also be an interesting alternative [4].

Mostly, the resin composite restorations have been widely used and have shown a higher survival rate when compared to other restorative materials in MIH teeth [1, 38, 39]. In the study performed by Mejàre et al. [39], only 16% of the restorations conducted with resin composites were considered unacceptable against 51% of those conducted with RMGICs. This is important because, when dental restorative procedures are necessary in stress-bearing areas, such as molars (the teeth most affected by MIH), the bonding strategies are majorly based on using composites associated with dentin bonding systems. However, regardless of the bonding agents used, MIH-affected enamel historically presents lower bond strength than sound enamel [40–42]. Representations of the characteristics of the hybrid layer created on MIH-affected and sound enamel is shown in Figure 4.

As observed by Fagrell et al. [42], after acid etching, a structureless layer with underlying prisms is seen, likely because of the higher porosity of the MIH-affected enamel (Fig. 2), which exposes the organic part of the prism sheaths due to the reduced inorganic content in the hypomineralised enamel. This generates an altered demineralisation pattern on the MIH-affected enamel, which can limit the ability of the bonding agent to penetrate within the tissue (also known as hybrid layer) and consequently jeopardize the bond strength [40, 42–44].

William et al. [45] demonstrated that, regardless of the category of adhesive systems, poorer bond strength is yielded on MIH-affected enamel. As mentioned for the GIC restoration performance, increase in cohesive failures within enamel was seen for the hypomineralised enamel. This can be interpreted as a prediction of early failures,

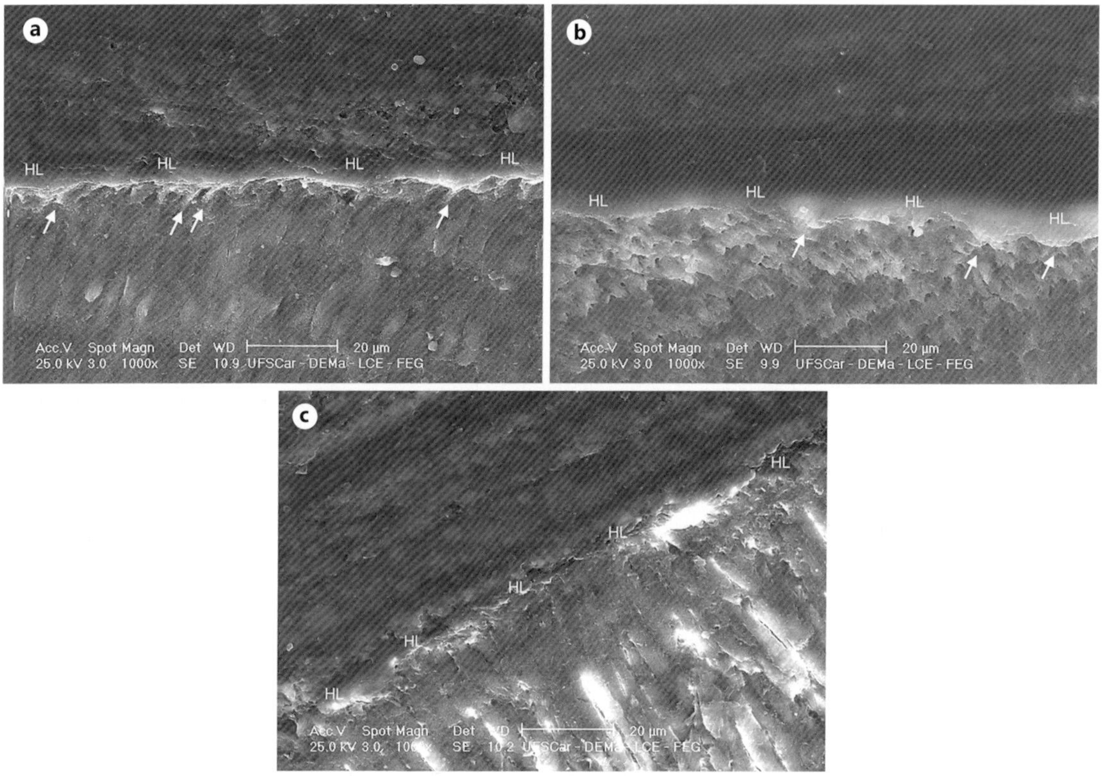

Fig. 4. Sound enamel after application of 37% phosphoric acid followed by Clearfil SE (Kuraray) self-etching adhesive system (interface analysis). Note the presence of a uniform hybrid layer (HL) with the formation of thin and homogeneous resin tags (arrows) (**a**). Enamel affected by MIH under the same protocol. It is possible to observe the lack of regularity in the HL and scarce imbrication (arrows), even with the application of phosphoric acid (**b**). Enamel affected by MIH after application of the Clearfil SE self-etching adhesive system without prior etching with 37% phosphoric acid. This approach further impaired the adhesive interface, forming an irregular HL with voids and gaps (**c**).

as it occurred during the preparation of the specimens for bonding tests [1, 41].

In order to overcome this issue with the higher organic content in the MIH enamel, some authors have suggested applying sodium hypochlorite (NaOCl) to the enamel as a deproteinization step [14, 20, 30, 40, 46]. The concentration of NaOCl and whether it was applied before or after acid etching varied between the studies, making it difficult to compare the results. Nonetheless, an improvement in the in vitro bond strength was seen for those who applied the NaOCl after acid etching and in a concentration around 5% [20, 30]. Krämer et al. [40] did not detect a significant improvement in bond strength after deproteinizing the enamel, but less premature failures (cohesive failure within the enamel) were observed.

Sönmez and Saat [14] evaluated this approach clinically for 24 months. When 5% NaOCl was applied for 1 min after acid etching, an increase in the survival rate of restorations was observed at 24 months. No differences were detected before 12 months. Nonetheless, it is worth noting that the 5% NaOCl improved the survival rate of restorations placed on clinically hard enamel. It was obtained after removing the softened carious/porous enamel with a bur until significant resistance from the hypomineralised enamel was detected. Additionally, it did not differ from the group in which the margins of the restoration were placed on sound enamel (not affected by MIH) [14]. Lagarde et al. [41] concluded in a systematic review that the application of NaOCl resulted in higher bond strength values.

Therefore, there is no consensus on the best bonding agent to be used on MIH-affected enamel since there is conflicting evidence between the studies [41]. In in vitro studies, William et al. [4] found no differences between etch-and-rinse and self-etching adhesives, whilst Krämer et al. [40] observed a significantly better performance by the etch-and-rinse system compared to the self-etching system. The universal bonding system presented intermediate bond strength values and was statistically similar to both the etch-and-rinse and the self-etching adhesives. However, attention must be paid to the type of adhesive used in the studies, as William et al. [45] used a two-step etch-and-rinse adhesive and Krämer et al. [40] used a three-step etch-and-rinse adhesive. Thus, the differences between these results could also be attributed to the presence of hydrophilic monomers, which could reduce the bond strength if in excess.

One of the most relevant clinical trials concerning these aspects is presented by de Souza et al. [26], who compared two bonding agents, a self-etching and an etch-and-rinse adhesive system. In this study, there was no significant difference between the bonding agents, but a slightly higher survival rate was found for the self-etching agent (68%) compared to the etch-and-rinse one (54%) after 18 months. Other interesting clinical trials compared the use of a universal adhesive system based on the total-etch and self-etching modes of 64 first permanent molars affected by MIH (with breakdown or atypical lesions associated or not with carious lesions). Twelve-month follow-up revealed that the use of the phosphoric acid was mandatory to a successful performance (80.8% rather than 62.3% in terms of retention). As also observed by Bekes et al. [47], both studies included reports related to dental pain and anxiety/quality of life of the patients who underwent the treatment. As the responses are positive, the successful treatment is notable beyond the retention/restoration themselves [48].

It is essential to emphasize that adhesive systems containing 10-methacryloyloxydecyl dihydrogen phosphate and/or other functional monomers promote a chemical bond with calcium from the apatite, forming a stable salt [21]. This adds a chemical bond to the micromechanical bond promoted by conventional etch-and-rinse adhesives, so this strategy could be beneficial for MIH patients. Moreover, self-etching adhesives are recognized to cause less postoperative sensitivity, which is already a prevalent clinical complaint by patients affected by MIH [49]. Rolim et al. [48] presented self-reported sensitivity by patients treated with self-etching or etch-and-rinse mode of a universal bonding system, revealing significant less postoperative sensitivity for the first mode, in particular related to early pain. According to these authors based on other similar studies, pre-etching with phosphoric acid causes additional step to the restorative protocol, as rinsing and drying, which increases the chances of postoperative sensitivity.

Adhesion of Sealant Materials to the MIH-Affected Enamel

It is also relevant to state some information regarding the use of sealants indicated for posterior teeth when no MIH enamel breakdown occurs, since their interaction to the enamel is also based on the adhesive capacity combined or not with additional adhesive systems. This category of materials is indicated for posterior teeth with mild MIH [36, 47].

No differences in the behavior of resin-based sealants on MIH-affected and sound enamel for

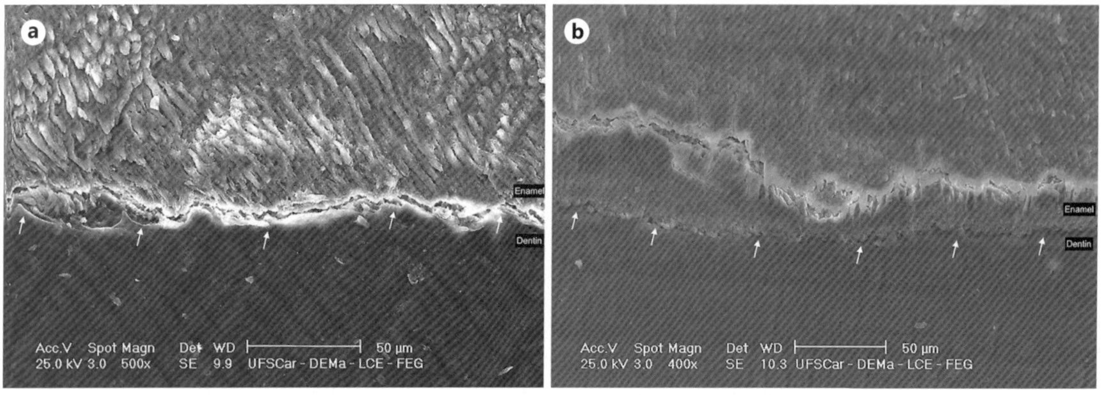

Fig. 5. Dentin-enamel junction (DEJ; arrows) of a sound tooth (**a**) and of an MIH-affected tooth (**b**). Note the presence of a crack in the enamel (**b**) due to the fragility of the affected tissue.

18 months was observed by Fragelli et al. [36]. In the comparison of retention, Bekes et al. [47] also observed similar performance after 12 months, regardless of GIC-based or resin composite-based sealants.

Based on the in vitro study performed by Gandhi et al. [46], no differences in the hybrid layer were detected when NaOCl was applied before acid etching at MIH-affected enamel, even though this step led to a significant improvement in the retention of sealants.

Usually, the viscosity of the resin-based sealants is sufficient to fill the porosities of the enamel and serve as a mechanical barrier, which can be helpful to prevent biofilm retention [32]. However, some investigations have suggested using an adhesive system before the placement of the resinous sealant [50, 51]. This premise is justified as bonding agents show lower viscosity than the sealant itself, which would improve the penetration into the tissue and somehow enhance the sealant imbrication to the affected enamel. Despite this strategy making sense and the outcomes being favorable [50, 51], it is still conflicting as there are few clinical trials to sustain it, especially because it is not common in regular indications of sealants [52]. Systematic reviews have demonstrated that in other substrates, favorable results are observed when adhesive systems are applied before the sealant. Moreover, the etch-and-rinse adhesive system results in better behavior than self-etch ones in these scenarios [52–54].

When Dentin Is Involved

Although enamel is primarily affected by hypomineralisation, studies have evidenced that the porosity seems to extend to the dentin-enamel junction [10, 42]. Thus, professionals cannot ignore the possible involvement of dentin in the area to be bonded, especially in cases associated with dental caries or even in those teeth with the presence of darker yellowish/brownish opacities at the surface, which are more susceptible to post-eruptive breakdown as shown in Figure 5. This is particularly important while considering where the margin of the restoration will be placed [9, 55].

In the last decades, major efforts have been put into developing materials and techniques to overcome the complexity of bonding to the dentin substrate [56–58]. Since sound enamel is a homogeneous and well-organized hydroxyapatite-rich tissue with low amounts of proteins and water, the constitution of a thin hybrid layer has been shown to achieve clinical long-term success [22]. Thus, until this day, placing the margin on sound enamel becomes almost synonymous with safety due to its higher impermeability/sealing [14]. When dentin is involved, a different mechanism is attributed due to the complexity of its nature. Then, dentin conditioning is no longer a necessary step since the introduction of acidic functional monomers [21, 23, 59, 60]. 10-Methacryloyloxydecyl dihydrogen phosphate is most commonly used by different brands, but it is not exclusively the only functional monomer available [21, 23, 59, 60]. By these types of monomers, it is possible to modify the smear layer enough to expose the calcium and establish a chemical reaction. This is the base of all self-etching mode systems, including the universal ones [48]. This is sufficient to preserve the minerals and allow this reliable interaction, rather than promoting dentin conditioning with strong acid (phosphoric acid) in a previous step [21, 23, 59, 60]. Also, the preservation of the minerals minimizes the exposure of collagen fibrils and the intrinsic enzymes such as the matrix metalloproteinases and the cysteine cathepsins, which can contribute to the degradation of the interface [61–63]. Despite the reason for treating dentin, in case bonding procedures are indicated, the self-etch systems are preferable due to all these benefits and the reduction of one step for the operator. The use of this strategy seems to be less technically sensitive and generates less postoperative sensitivity. Nonetheless, when dentin is involved, even when these improved systems are used, the presence of sound enamel at the margins is mandatory to assure longevity of the restorative procedure.

Therefore, the expected safety by limiting the restorations to enamel margin needs to be considered with caution when MIH-affected tissue is being restored with bonding strategies. Besides, as mentioned before, regardless of the presence of MIH or not, moisture control is a major step to achieve long-lasting bonding while placing resin composite restorations [64].

It is also interesting to report the bonding to dentin of teeth affected by MIH. In this context, Krämer et al. [40] pointed that the adhesion to dentin is not affected by the presence of MIH on the overlying enamel. In fact, the bond strength to the dentin was significantly higher than that of the enamel (regardless of the presence of MIH). This study is particularly important because it confirms that dentin adhesion in these areas is not affected by hypomineralisation in terms of bonding capacity, despite some speculations [40]. Yet, it is necessary to take into account that the tests were based on laboratory experiments.

Also, another important scenario is related to the case of MIH followed by subsequent carious lesions occurrence, as it is not uncommon to observe and cause a more extensive cavity than usual [33]. It determines atypical restorations as the caries factors act on a less mineralised and more porous tissue that facilitates its spread toward the pulp. As mentioned before, besides dental caries, this weak substrate is also susceptible to breakdown even after restoration and in the absence of carious lesions [33]. This should also be considered while choosing the restorative material to treat the lesions.

However, even after treating the lesions, dental caries and/or breakdown are still common. In the study of Jälevik and Klingberg [65], MIH-affected teeth are normally treated twice due to restoration failure, posteruptive breakdown, or recurrence of caries, whilst the control group did not need to be retreated. This further breakdown or caries development often leads to the mentioned so called "atypical cavitation." Thus, the selection of the materials and techniques should also rely on analyzing the circumstances of eruption phase, the antagonist teeth's aspect, and occlusion, as well as the level of destruction of the tooth being restored [26].

This aspect is of great relevance to be taken before considering the use of glass-ionomer or resin-based systems, since a stronger adhesion allied to the mechanical properties of the resin composite will likely lead to choosing the composite combined with a proper dentin bonding system. Nonetheless, it cannot be overemphasized that, whenever resin composite restorations are being placed, moisture control and treatment of the margins seems to be necessary, regardless of the bonding agent used. The current state of the art indicates that self-etching and/or universal systems in the self-etching mode are the most recommended bonding agents to be used due to their interaction with calcium by the functional acidic monomers [21]. Also, the lack of phosphoric acid etching on dentin reduces the postoperative sensitivity and also helps to reduce the degradation of the collagen fibrils by diminishing the exposure of them to intrinsic proteolytic enzymes, such as the matrix metalloproteinases [26, 48, 49, 66].

Moreover, some alternatives rely on the continuous development of functional monomers, in particular if they interact with the collagen fibrils rather than depending solely on minerals [59, 60]. Also, the addition of bioactive ingredients could offer benefits to strengthen the mineralised part of the tissue [60], whilst other compounds have also been tested to decrease the activity of such proteolytic enzymes and preserve the collagen matrix, thus, increasing the longevity of the adhesive bond [61–63].

Final Considerations

The correct diagnosis of MIH-affected enamel is mandatory regardless of the indication of any adhesive. Studies pointed out in Tables 2 and 3 refer to some of the references based on clinical trials or laboratory experiments cited in this chapter. It can be seen that, given the different circumstances, it is not possible to directly compare all of them, but some conclusions can be stated by now:

1. When feasible, a noninterventional approach is preferred, aligning with a more conservative approach. However, in the case of MIH-affected enamel breakdown condition, the margin placed on sound enamel seems more appropriate to establish better performance.
2. All categories of adhesives used onto MIH-affected surfaces seem to be less effective than sound substrates, regardless of the involvement of dentin. The cohesive failures indicate fragility of the MIH-affected enamel.
3. In the case of sealants used on MIH-affected surfaces, the association of a previous step with an adhesive system seems to be an interesting alternative.
4. The use of 5% NaOCl as a deproteinization strategy seems worth it for MIH-affected enamel and deserves to be more investigated.
5. GIC-based materials seem to be indicated in no stress-bearing areas with no enamel breakdown presenting less risk of fracture.

As pointed out by some authors, professionals' unawareness still is the biggest obstacle for the appropriate management [1, 3, 4]. The success of any bonding system or strategy is only possible based on proper diagnosis and following the instructions of the selected technique. The emphasis is to always be aware that any bonding strategy is performed in a modified enamel. It is important to state that, despite the recommendation being to extend the margins to clinically sound enamel, this step might not be always possible. In areas with severe MIH or even carious lesions, it is possible that extending the cavity further might make the restoration unfeasible.

Given that GICs might not bear the mechanical stress imposed by the chewing forces on molars affected by MIH, they could be used temporarily as a restorative material until better conditions are achieved (e.g., better moisture control or patient compliance), or as a final restoration, but evidence points out that they might not achieve long-lasting survival rates [41, 55]. If resin composites are the material of choice, it seems more appropriate to determine the margin on clinically sound tissue. Minimal intervention dentistry claims for the balance among maximum preservation, safe result, and perspectives of long-term longevity, but to this day, no material available can guarantee a reliable bonding exclusively on

Table 2. Comparative performance of adhesive systems to MIH-affected teeth, based on interventional in vivo studies

Authors, year	Substrate	Enamel margin condition	Adhesive system	Test/outcome	Follow-up	Highlights
Resin composite (RC) restorations						
Lygidakis et al., 2003 [38]	More than 2 surfaces on MIH-affected permanent first molars with removal of all carious tissues together with possible previous, failed amalgam restoration and enamel easily penetrated by probe	Cavities with marginal sound enamel (although sometimes discolored) were observed in the cavity surfaces	In all groups, surfaces were etched with 35% phosphoric acid 2-step etching-and-rinse system Prime & Bond/Dentsply DeTrey RC: Brilliant Synergy/Coltene *Use of rubber dam	Modified US Public Health Service (USPHS)	Up to 48 months	Mostly restorations were rated as A, and no C was coded for any assessment, revealing good performance and no need of repair or replacement
de Souza et al., 2017 [26]	Cavities (enamel and dentin) on MIH-affected permanent first molars (classified as enamel posteruptive breakdown or unsatisfactory atypical restoration), with or without carious lesions	All cavities were first treated with glass-ionomer (Ketac Molar) and partially replaced by the following described bonding protocols after 2 months. No removal of defective margins was made	Two-step self-etching system Clearfil SE Bond or etching step with 37.5% phosphoric acid Followed by 3-step etch-and-rinse system Adper Scotchbond Multi-Purpose/3M ESPE RC: Filtek Z350/3M ESPE *Before the restorative procedures, teeth underwent 4-week treatment with fluoride varnish Duraphat *Use of rubber dam	Modified USPHS (retention)	Up to 18 months	The cumulative survival rates were 68 and 54%, respectively, for self-etching and etch-and-rinse systems, which is considered successful when defective margin was maintained
Sönmez and Saat, 2017 [14]	Cavities (enamel and dentin) on MIH-affected permanent first molars vs. caries but not MIH-affected teeth	Group I – all hypomineralised tissues were removed until healthy enamel was reached Group II – carious and cheesy hypomineralised tissue was removed until a reasonable resistance was detected in the hypomineralised tissue Group III – cavities designed as group II, differently from this group deproteinization (5% NaOCl – 60 s) of the left hypomineralised tissue was performed prior to the placement of RC Group IV – control group consisting of unaffected carious first permanent molars	In all groups, cavities were etched with 37% phosphoric acid Self-etching system Futurabond NR/Voco	Modified USPHS (retention)	Up to 24 months	No differences among groups for any aspect up to 6-month evaluation Failure of the restorations, in particular marginal defects, was predominant in group II, in which the hypomineralised tissue was left surrounding the cavities Deproteinization of the hypomineralised enamel was found to enhance the retention rates of RCs

Table 2 (continued)

Authors, year	Substrate	Enamel margin condition	Adhesive system	Test/outcome	Follow-up	Highlights
Rolim et al., 2021 [48]	Cavities (enamel and dentin) on MIH-affected permanent first molars	Hypomineralised enamel removal was selective – removal of the hypomineralised enamel with an opaque appearance, which crumbles on contact with the instruments until more resistant enamel is obtained	In etch-and-rinse group, enamel surfaces were etched with 35% phosphoric acid Universal adhesive system in both modes: etch-and-rinse and self-etching modes: Ambar/FGM RC: Tetric N-Ceram bulk-fill/Ivoclar Vivadent *Use of rubber dam	Modified USPHS	Up to 12 months	The survival rates were around 80.8 and 62.3% after 12 months for etch-and-rinse and self-etching modes, respectively. No significant difference was observed between the groups. The self-etching mode seems to be less effective in this case, but both performed adequately considering the scenario
Sealants						
Lygidakis et al., 2009 [51]	Occlusal surfaces on MIH-affected permanent first molars with occlusal enamel opacities without breakdown	Mechanical cleaning of fissures using a round bur No. 1/4 in a slow handpiece was used before acid etching	In all groups, surfaces were etched with 35% phosphoric acid Two-step etching-and-rinse system One step/Bisco Sealant: Fissurit/Voco *Use of cotton rolls	Modified USPHS	Up to 48 months	The survival rates were around 70.2% and 25.5% of fully retention, respectively, for association or not with adhesive system MIH-affected surfaces respond better using adhesive system prior to sealant
Fragelli et al., 2017 [36]	Occlusal surfaces on MIH-affected permanent first molars (mild severity presenting white, yellow, and brown opacities, and that showed both mechanical and chemical alteration of the enamel, at a high risk for carious lesion or breakdown. vs. sound surfaces)	No previous mechanical removal/treatment	In all groups, surfaces were etched with 35% phosphoric acid Sealant: Fluroshield/Dentsply *Before the restorative procedures, teeth underwent 4-week treatment with fluoride varnish Duraphat *Use of rubber dam	Modified USPHS (retention)	Up to 18 months	The survival rates were around 62.6 and 72%, respectively, for sound and MIH- affected surface, determining similar clinical performance

Table 3. Comparative performance of adhesive systems to MIH-affected teeth based on interventional in vitro studies

Authors, year	Substrate	Enamel margin/surface	Adhesive system	Test/outcome	Follow-up	Highlights
Gandhi et al., 2012 [46]	Occlusal surfaces of permanent molars affected by MIH	Sealant on enamel of MIH-affected surface Group I: conditioned with 35% phosphoric acid + sealant; Group II: conditioned with 35% phosphoric acid + 5% NaOCl – 60 s + sealant; Group III: phosphoric acid + 5% NaOCl – 60 s + sealant	Delton Sealant	Sealant tag/enamel grade observations by scanning electron microscopy	–	Acid conditioning determined enhanced tags formation compared to its no use Deproteinization with NaOCl alone (without etch) was not efficient "Poor" sealant tags in MIH enamel, regardless of treatments occurs
William et al., 2016 [45]	Enamel of sound and MIH-affected permanent first molars	No previous mechanical removal/treatment	Two-step self-etching system Clearfil SE Bond or etching step with 37.5% phosphoric acid followed by 2-step etch-and-rinse system Adper Single Bond/3M ESPE RC: Filtek Restorative Universal/3M ESPE	Microshear and interface SEM observations	12 h	Bonding to MIH-affected surface is poorer compared to sound enamel, as was the quality of tags' formation The tested adhesives did not differ between them. Limited bonding to MIH-affected enamel of the all-etch single-bottle adhesive was attributed to inadequate microtag formation The use of self-etching primer adhesive-etched hypomineralised enamel was deeper than control enamel Observation of higher frequency of cohesive failures to bonding to hypomineralised enamel
Ekambaram et al., 2017 [20]	Enamel from MIH-affected permanent first molars	Enamel of sound (groups I, II, and III) or hypomineralised as creamy-white or yellow-brown opacities surfaces (groups IV, V, and VI) treated with: Group I/IV – conditioned with 32% phosphoric acid; group II/V – conditioned with 32% phosphoric acid + 5% NaOCl – 60 s); Group III/VI – conditioned with 32% phosphoric acid + Papacarie gel – 60 s)	Two-step etch-and-rinse system Adper Single Bond 2 (3M ESPE)	Microshear	24 h	Hypomineralised enamel surface produced lower bond strength compared to sound enamel Both deproteinization agents were equally effective to improve the bonding to hypomineralised enamel

Table 3 (continued)

Authors, year	Substrate	Enamel margin/surface	Adhesive system	Test/outcome	Follow-up	Highlights
Krämer et al., 2018 [40]	Enamel of sound and MIH-affected molars and incisors and respective dentin	Longitudinal cut of enamel and dentin subsequently polished to the tests	Etching step with 37.5% phosphoric acid followed by 2-step etch-and-rinse system Optibond FL/Bisco Etching step with 37.5% phosphoric acid + 5% NaOCl, followed by 2-step etch-and-rinse system Optibond FL/Bisco Etching step with 37.5% phosphoric acid followed by universal system at etch-and-rinse mode Adper Scothbond Universal (for affected surface) Etching step with 37.5% phosphoric acid + 5% NaOCl followed by universal system at etch-and-rinse mode Adper Scothbond Universal (for affected surface) Two-step self-etching system Clearfil SE Bond Two-step self-etching system Clearfil SE Bond + 5% NaOCl *There were other groups tested involving Icon, which is not the intention of this purpose RC: Filtek Restorative Universal/3M ESPE	Microtensile test, failure analysis, and micro-morphological assessment	Not mentioned	Bonding values regarding dentin were higher than enamel for all comparisons Bonding to sound enamel was superior compared to MIH-affected enamel, despite the treatment The use of etch-and-rinse system yielded enhanced bonding values compared to universal and self-etching systems on MIF-affected enamel Treatment of affected enamel specimens with NaOCl; however, it caused less pretest failures Micromorphological analyses revealed that phosphoric acid etching produced a much less pronounced etching pattern in affected enamel and a porous structure as weak link for the resin-enamel bond was identified

the MIH-affected enamel. Clinical trials and systematic reviews have not yet been extensively performed comparing the outcomes of removing or maintaining the affected enamel.

The pursuit for strategies for effective long-term adhesive materials and techniques includes those that can also serve as a vehicle to bioactive ingredients to strengthen the structure while preserving the bonding property itself in the long term. Thus, it is safe to state that the clinician should also operate with common sense. Last, no treatment will be effective if the concern regarding prevention plan and patient's oral care education are ignored, including the purpose to offer improvement of the quality of life of the patients.

Statement of Ethics

Written informed consent was obtained from patients (or their parents/legal guardians/next-of-kin) for publication of the images for this purpose or was obtained via consent of Ethical Committee (5.724.283).

Conflict of Interest Statement

The authors have no conflicts of interest to declare.

Author Contributions

All authors have made equal contributions to the conception or design of the work; drafting the work and reviewing it critically for important intellectual content; final approval of the version to be published; agreement to be accountable for all aspects of the work in ensuring that questions related to the accuracy or integrity of any part of the work are appropriately investigated and resolved.

References

1 Lygidakis NA, Garot E, Somani C, Taylor GD, Rouas P, Wong FSL. Best clinical practice guidance for clinicians dealing with children presenting with molar-incisor-hypomineralisation (MIH): an updated European Academy of Paediatric Dentistry policy document. Eur Arch Paediatr Dent. 2022 Feb;23(1):3–21.

2 Perdigão J. Dentin bonding-variables related to the clinical situation and the substrate treatment. Dent Mater. 2010 Feb;26(2):e24–37.

3 Bastos-Bitencourt NA, Mosquim V, Zabeu GS, Rios D, Ishikiriama SK, Wang L. MIH-affected teeth: clinical challenges from diagnosis to restorative management. Int J Periodontics Restorative Dent. 2022 Mar-Apr;42(2):225–31.

4 William V, Messer LB, Burrow MF. Molar incisor hypomineralization: review and recommendations for clinical management. Pediatr Dent. 2006 May-Jun;28(3):224–32.

5 Steffen R, Krämer N, Bekes K. The Würzburg MIH concept: the MIH treatment need index (MIH TNI): a new index to assess and plan treatment in patients with molar incisior hypomineralisation (MIH). Eur Arch Paediatr Dent. 2017 Oct;18(5):355–61.

6 Chawla N, Messer LB, Silva M. Clinical studies on molar-incisor-hypomineralisation part 2:development of a severity index. Eur Arch Paediatr Dent. 2008 Dec;9(4):191–9.

7 Farah RA, Monk BC, Swain MV, Drummond BK. Protein content of molar-incisor hypomineralisation enamel. J Dent. 2010 Jul;38(7):591–6.

8 Neves AB, Americano GCA, Soares DV, Soviero VM. Breakdown of demarcated opacities related to molar-incisor hypomineralization: a longitudinal study. Clin Oral Investig. 2019 Feb;23(2):611–5.

9 Costa-Silva CM, Ambrosano GM, Jeremias F, Souza JF, Mialhe FL. Increase in severity of molar-incisor hypomineralization and its relationship with the colour of enamel opacity: a prospective cohort study. Int J Paediatr Dent. 2011; 21(5):333–41.

10 Jälevik B, Odelius H, Dietz W, Norén J. Secondary ion mass spectrometry and X-ray microanalysis of hypomineralized enamel in human permanent first molars. Arch Oral Biol. 2001 Mar;46(3): 239–47.

11 Duarte MBS, Carvalho VR, Hilgert LA, Ribeiro APD, Leal SC, Takeshita EM. Is there an association between dental caries, fluorosis, and molar-incisor hypomineralization? J Appl Oral Sci. 2021 Jul 16;29:e20200890.

12 Dulla JA, Meyer-Lueckel H. Molar-incisor hypomineralisation: narrative review on etiology, epidemiology, diagnostics and treatment decision. Swiss Dent J. 2021 Mar 25;131(11):886–95.

13 He LH, Swain MV. Understanding the mechanical behaviour of human enamel from its structural and compositional characteristics. J Mech Behav Biomed Mater. 2008 Jan;1(1):18–29.
14 Sönmez H, Saat S. A clinical evaluation of deproteinization and different cavity designs on resin restoration performance in MIH-affected molars: two-year results. J Clin Pediatr Dent. 2017; 41(5):336–42.
15 Jacobsen PE, Haubek D, Henriksen TB, Østergaard JR, Poulsen S. Developmental enamel defects in children born preterm: a systematic review. Eur J Oral Sci. 2014 Feb;122(1):7–14.
16 Elhennawy K, Manton DJ, Crombie F, Zaslansky P, Radlanski RJ, Jost-Brinkmann PG, et al. Structural, mechanical and chemical evaluation of molar-incisor hypomineralization-affected enamel: a systematic review. Arch Oral Biol. 2017 Nov;83:272–81.
17 Jälevik B. Enamel hypomineralization in permanent first molars. A clinical, histomorphological and biochemical study. Swed Dent J Suppl. 2001;149:1–86.
18 Weerheijm KL, Jälevik B, Alaluusua S. Molar-incisor hypomineralisation. Caries Res. 2001 Sep-Oct;35(5):390–1.
19 Butera A, Maiorani C, Morandini A, Simonini M, Morittu S, Barbieri S, et al. Assessment of genetical, pre, peri and post natal risk factors of deciduous molar hypomineralization (DMH), hypomineralized second primary molar (HSPM) and molar incisor hypomineralization (MIH): a narrative review. Children (Basel). 2021 May 21;8(6):432.
20 Ekambaram M, Anthonappa RP, Govindool SR, Yiu CKY. Comparison of deproteinization agents on bonding to developmentally hypomineralized enamel. J Dent. 2017 Dec;67:94–101.
21 Yoshida Y, Nagakane K, Fukuda R, Nakayama Y, Okazaki M, Shintani H, et al. Comparative study on adhesive performance of functional monomers. J Dent Res. 2004 Jun;83(6):454–8.
22 Fukuda R, Yoshida Y, Nakayama Y, Okazaki M, Inoue S, Sano H, et al. Bonding efficacy of polyalkenoic acids to hydroxyapatite, enamel and dentin. Biomaterials. 2003 May;24(11):1861–7.
23 Yoshida Y, Van Meerbeek B, Nakayama Y, Snauwaert J, Hellemans L, Lambrechts P, et al. Evidence of chemical bonding at biomaterial-hard tissue interfaces. J Dent Res. 2000 Feb;79(2): 709–14.
24 Fayle SA. Molar incisor hypomineralisation: restorative management. Eur J Paediatr Dent. 2003 Sep;4(3):121–6.
25 Pashley DH, Tay FR, Breschi L, Tjäderhane L, Carvalho RM, Carrilho M, et al. State of the art etch-and-rinse adhesives. Dent Mater. 2011 Jan;27(1):1–16.
26 de Souza JF, Fragelli CB, Jeremias F, Paschoal MAB, Santos-Pinto L, Cordeiro RCL. Eighteen-month clinical performance of composite resin restorations with two different adhesive systems for molars affected by molar incisor hypomineralization. Clin Oral Investig. 2017 Jun;21(5):1725–33.
27 Garnett J, Dieppe P. The effects of serum and human albumin on calcium hydroxyapatite crystal growth. Biochem J. 1990 Mar 15;266(3):863–8.
28 Vieira A, Emerenciano NG, Moda MD, Silva Ú, Fagundes TC, Danelon M, et al. Treatment of molar-incisor hypomineralization: a case report of 11-year clinical follow-up. Oper Dent. 2023 Mar 1;48(2):121–9.
29 Powis DR, Follerås T, Merson SA, Wilson AD. Improved adhesion of a glass ionomer cement to dentin and enamel. J Dent Res. 1982 Dec;61(12):1416–22.
30 Chay PL, Manton DJ, Palamara JE. The effect of resin infiltration and oxidative pre-treatment on microshear bond strength of resin composite to hypomineralised enamel. Int J Paediatr Dent. 2014 Jul;24(4):252–67.
31 Bueno LS, Silva RM, Magalhães APR, Navarro MFL, Pascotto RC, Buzalaf MAR, et al. Positive correlation between fluoride release and acid erosion of restorative glass-ionomer cements. Dent Mater. 2019 Jan;35(1):135–43.
32 Schraverus MS, Olegário IC, Bonifácio CC, González APR, Pedroza M, Hesse D. Glass ionomer sealants can prevent dental caries but cannot prevent posteruptive breakdown on molars affected by molar incisor hypomineralization: one-year results of a randomized clinical trial. Caries Res. 2021;55(4):301–9.
33 Fragelli CM, Souza JF, Jeremias F, Cordeiro Rde C, Santos-Pinto L. Molar incisor hypomineralization (MIH): conservative treatment management to restore affected teeth. Braz Oral Res. 2015;29: S1806-83242015000100271.
34 Menezes-Silva R, Oliveira BMB, Magalhães APR, Bueno LS, Borges AFS, Baesso ML, et al. Correlation between mechanical properties and stabilization time of chemical bonds in glass-ionomer cements. Braz Oral Res. 2020 Jun 5;34: e053.
35 de Lima Navarro MF, Pascotto RC, Borges AFS, Soares CJ, Raggio DP, Rios D, et al. Consensus on glass-ionomer cement thresholds for restorative indications. J Dent. 2021 Apr;107:103609.
36 Fragelli CMB, Souza JF, Bussaneli DG, Jeremias F, Santos-Pinto LD, Cordeiro RCL. Survival of sealants in molars affected by molar-incisor hypomineralization: 18-month follow-up. Braz Oral Res. 2017 Apr;31:e30.
37 de Souza JF, Gramasco M, Jeremias F, Santos-Pinto L, Giovanini AF, Cerri PS, et al. Amoxicillin diminishes the thickness of the enamel matrix that is deposited during the secretory stage in rats. Int J Paediatr Dent. 2016 May;26(3): 199–210.
38 Lygidakis NA, Chaliasou A, Siounas G. Evaluation of composite restorations in hypomineralised permanent molars: a four year clinical study. Eur J Paediatr Dent. 2003 Sep;4(3):143–8.
39 Mejàre I, Bergman E, Grindefjord M. Hypomineralized molars and incisors of unknown origin: treatment outcome at age 18 years. Int J Paediatr Dent. 2005 Jan;15(1):20–8.
40 Krämer N, Bui Khac NN, Lücker S, Stachniss V, Frankenberger R. Bonding strategies for MIH-affected enamel and dentin. Dent Mater. 2018 Feb;34(2): 331–40.
41 Lagarde M, Vennat E, Attal JP, Dursun E. Strategies to optimize bonding of adhesive materials to molar-incisor hypomineralization-affected enamel: a systematic review. Int J Paediatr Dent. 2020 Jul;30(4):405–20.
42 Fagrell TG, Dietz W, Jälevik B, Norén JG. Chemical, mechanical and morphological properties of hypomineralized enamel of permanent first molars. Acta Odontol Scand. 2010 Jul;68(4):215–22.
43 Jälevik B, Dietz W, Norén JG. Scanning electron micrograph analysis of hypomineralized enamel in permanent first molars. Int J Paediatr Dent. 2005 Jul; 15(4):233–40.

44 Bozal CB, Kaplan A, Ortolani A, Cortese SG, Biondi AM. Ultrastructure of the surface of dental enamel with molar incisor hypomineralization (MIH) with and without acid etching. Acta Odontol Latinoam. 2015;28(2):192–8.
45 William V, Burrow MF, Palamara JE, Messer LB. Microshear bond strength of resin composite to teeth affected by molar hypomineralization using 2 adhesive systems. Pediatr Dent. 2006 May-Jun; 28(3):233–41.
46 Gandhi S, Crawford P, Shellis P. The use of a 'bleach-etch-seal' deproteinization technique on MIH affected enamel. Int J Paediatr Dent. 2012 Nov;22(6):427–34.
47 Bekes K, Amend S, Priller J, Zamek C, Stamm T, Krämer N. Hypersensitivity relief of MIH-affected molars using two sealing techniques: a 12-week follow-up. Clin Oral Investig. 2022 Feb;26(2):1879–88.
48 Rolim TZC, da Costa TRF, Wambier LM, Chibinski AC, Wambier DS, da Silva Assunção LR, et al. Adhesive restoration of molars affected by molar incisor hypomineralization: a randomized clinical trial. Clin Oral Investig. 2021 Mar;25(3):1513–24.
49 Raposo F, de Carvalho Rodrigues AC, Lia ÉN, Leal SC. Prevalence of hypersensitivity in teeth affected by molar-incisor hypomineralization (MIH). Caries Res. 2019;53(4):424–30.
50 Bandeira Lopes L, Machado V, Botelho J, Haubek D. Molar-incisor hypomineralization: an umbrella review. Acta Odontol Scand. 2021 Jul;79(5):359–69.
51 Lygidakis NA, Dimou G, Stamataki E. Retention of fissure sealants using two different methods of application in teeth with hypomineralised molars (MIH): a 4 year clinical study. Eur Arch Paediatr Dent. 2009 Dec;10(4):223–6.
52 Botton G, Morgental CS, Scherer MM, Lenzi TL, Montagner AF, Rocha RO. Are self-etch adhesive systems effective in the retention of occlusal sealants? A systematic review and meta-analysis. Int J Paediatr Dent. 2016 Nov;26(6):402–11.
53 Bagherian A, Sarraf Shirazi A. Preparation before acid etching in fissure sealant therapy: yes or no?: A systematic review and meta-analysis. J Am Dent Assoc. 2016 Dec;147(12):943–51.
54 Martignon S, Zarta OL. The use of adhesive systems under fissure sealants improves their retention, with etch-and-rinse performing better than self-etching adhesive systems. J Evid Based Dent Pract. 2017 Mar;17(1):56–8.
55 Linner T, Khazaei Y, Bücher K, Pfisterer J, Hickel R, Kühnisch J. Comparison of four different treatment strategies in teeth with molar-incisor hypomineralization-related enamel breakdown – A retrospective cohort study. Int J Paediatr Dent. 2020 Sep;30(5):597–606.
56 Marshall GW Jr, Marshall SJ, Kinney JH, Balooch M. The dentin substrate: structure and properties related to bonding. J Dent. 1997 Nov;25(6):441–58.
57 Oliveira SS, Pugach MK, Hilton JF, Watanabe LG, Marshall SJ, Marshall GW Jr. The influence of the dentin smear layer on adhesion: a self-etching primer vs. a total-etch system. Dent Mater. 2003 Dec;19(8):758–67.
58 Schulze KA, Oliveira SA, Wilson RS, Gansky SA, Marshall GW, Marshall SJ. Effect of hydration variability on hybrid layer properties of a self-etching versus an acid-etching system. Biomaterials. 2005 Mar;26(9):1011–8.
59 Ikemura K, Tay FR, Nishiyama N, Pashley DH, Endo T. Design of new phosphonic acid monomers for dental adhesives – synthesis of (meth) acryloxyalkyl 3-phosphonopropionates and evaluation of their adhesion-promoting functions. Dent Mater J. 2006 Sep;25(3):566–75.
60 Ikemura K, Endo T. A review of our development of dental adhesives – effects of radical polymerization initiators and adhesive monomers on adhesion. Dent Mater J. 2010 Mar;29(2):109–21.
61 Giacomini MC, Candia Scaffa PM, Gonçalves RS, Jacomine JC, Zabeu GS, Carrilho MRO, et al. Performance of MDP-based system in eroded and carious dentin associated with proteolytic inhibitors: 18-month exploratory study. J Mech Behav Biomed Mater. 2021 Feb; 114:104177.
62 Speranza Zabeu G, Candia Scaffa PM, Ciccone Giacomini M, de Mattos Pimenta Vidal C, Tjäderhane L, Wang L. Gelatinolytic activity after dentin pretreatment with dimethyl sulfoxide (DMSO) combined to dental bonding systems: perspectives for biological responses. J Mech Behav Biomed Mater. 2022 Jun;130:105188.
63 Zabeu GS, Giacomini MC, Scaffa PMC, Tjäderhane L, Mosquim V, Wang L. Solvation role of dimethyl sulfoxide on the interaction with dentin bonding systems after 30 months. Dent Mater. 2023 May;39(5):478–84.
64 Knight GT, Berry TG, Barghi N, Burns TR. Effects of two methods of moisture control on marginal microleakage between resin composite and etched enamel: a clinical study. Int J Prosthodont. 1993 Sep-Oct;6(5):475–9.
65 Jälevik B, Klingberg GA. Dental treatment, dental fear and behaviour management problems in children with severe enamel hypomineralization of their permanent first molars. Int J Paediatr Dent. 2002 Jan;12(1):24–32.
66 Mukhtar U, Goyal A, Luthra-Guptasarma M, Gauba K, Kapur A, Thakur AK. Label-free quantitative proteomics reveals molecular correlates of altered biomechanical properties in molar incisor hypomineralization (MIH): an in vitro study. Eur Arch Paediatr Dent. 2022 Feb;23(1):179–91.

Linda Wang
Department of Operative Dentistry, Endodontics and Dental Materials
Bauru School of Dentistry, University of São Paulo
Dr. Octávio Pinheiro Brisolla, 9, Bauru 17012-901 (Brazil)
wang.linda@usp.br

Published online: July 1, 2024
Rios D, Santos-Pinto L (eds): Molar Incisor Hypomineralisation: New Perceptions. Monogr Oral Sci. Basel, Karger, 2024, vol 32, pp 212–235 (DOI: 10.1159/000539638)

Re-Establishing the Esthetics of Incisors in Patients with Molar Incisor Hypomineralisation

Jefferson Pires Silva Júnior[a] Rafael Pinto Mendonça[b] Rafael Santos Rocha[b] Daniela Rios[c] Eduardo Bresciani[b]

[a]Department of Dentistry, Nilton Lins University, Manaus, Brazil; [b]Department of Restorative Dentistry, Institute of Science and Technology of São José dos Campos, São Paulo State University (Unesp), São José dos Campos, Brazil; [c]Department of Pediatric Dentistry, Orthodontics, and Collective Health, Bauru Dental School, University of São Paulo, Bauru, Brazil

Abstract

The awareness of molar incisor hypomineralisation (MIH) has led to its increased clinical detection, consequently drawing more attention to its associated complications. This text offers an overview of the esthetic management of anterior teeth affected by MIH, a condition characterized by enamel defects that present significant cosmetic challenges. The focus is on the clinical presentation of MIH characteristics, considering the depth of lesions and the clinical aspects, and the treatment protocols available, despite a lack of extensive scientific evidence. To the best of the current scientific knowledge, the text evaluates the potential of minimally invasive procedures, as well as the use of traditional composite resin techniques and their possible combinations, highlighting the critical role of esthetic considerations for the impacted anterior teeth. The chapter is augmented with five illustrative clinical cases that display the practical application of these treatment approaches. These examples articulate the clinical decision-making process and personalized restorative strategies, aiming to balance function with enhanced esthetic results. The described cases act as a roadmap for clinicians tackling the complexities of MIH treatment in the context of limited empirical evidence, providing insights into achieving both satisfactory and esthetically pleasing outcomes for patients suffering from this condition.

Introduction

The etiology, prevalence, and clinical signs of molar incisor hypomineralisation (MIH) have been previously reported, with the most prevalent form affecting both molars and incisors. In contrast, a less frequently observed variant, idiopathic incisive hypomineralisation, with an occurrence rate approximately one-third as common, exclusively impacts incisors [1]. This disorder originates from a perturbation in enamel development, leading to localized defects in incisors [2]. These defects, unlike other forms of white opacities, emanate from the amelodentinal junction and progress toward the enamel surface [3]. As such, mild to moderate lesions are confined within the enamel matrix, predominantly within the innermost third, whereas severe and more conspicuous lesions might be exposed to the external surface of the enamel [4]. The implications of these specific characteristics are particularly pertinent in the context of esthetic considerations for anterior teeth and the formulation of treatment protocols, as well as in evaluating the efficacy of these interventions.

Patients more frequently require resolution of issues stemming from MIH in posterior teeth, which range from sensitivity, pain, and friable enamel to the association with caries lesions following enamel breakdown [4]. This therapeutic need is estimated to affect about 30% of individuals with MIH [5, 6]. Clinically, patients with MIH typically require dental treatment for their first permanent molars 4–10 times more often than those without MIH due to tissue fragility [7, 8]. These conditions and potential therapeutic protocols have been discussed and presented previously. Following the resolution of problems related to posterior teeth, patients may experience greater dissatisfaction with anterior teeth [9, 10], primarily concerning esthetic alterations, which often present in a moderate form [4]. Therefore, this text provides scientific information on the clinical conditions of anterior teeth in MIH scenarios, the clinical characteristics associated with the depth of the lesion, and the potential clinical treatment protocols based on the available scientific literature.

Clinical Features of Incisors with MIH

In the context of MIH, anterior teeth exhibit a lower prevalence of involvement compared to posterior teeth. Approximately 50% of MIH cases do not exhibit visible changes in anterior teeth [10]. Anterior teeth, when affected, tend to retain more intact enamel in terms of friability. This is supported by the high prevalence of mild and moderate lesions (91%) [10], which consequently maintain a covering of healthy enamel with superior mechanical properties (shown in Fig. 1). This resilience may also be attributed to the different forces exerted on these teeth compared to their posterior counterparts. For anterior teeth with MIH, esthetic concerns are more pronounced, with creamy or brownish discolorations being typical. Sensitivity in anterior teeth is rarely reported in the literature, possibly due to the lower incidence of this condition in patients.

Clinically, incisors with MIH typically present with localized color changes due to weakened enamel from defects in the mineral matrix [8]. The pigmentation is more pronounced in the lesion's central area, reflecting a yellowish hue variation and direct visualization of this zone. Defined edges often have milkier halos, demarcating the boundary of the defective region [11]. The pigmentation intensity suggests the potential severity of lesions, appearing darker when the affected area is thicker and milkier when it is thinner [12, 13]. Darkened lesions, which cause esthetic concerns, as well as those exhibiting enamel breakdown with or without dental caries, are classified as severe [14]. Severe lesions on anterior teeth often appear dark. Such lesions typically involve the full thickness of the enamel, extending to the dental surface [3] (shown in Fig. 1). Mild and moderate lesions, appearing creamy or whitish [14], are located in the inner third of the enamel, near the amelodentinal junction [4], but have sound enamel covering the alteration [3] (shown in Fig. 1). Severe lesions on incisors have a prevalence between 5% and 9% [4, 10]. When molars exhibit severe conditions, approximately 70% of incisors also display signs of MIH, usually mild or moderate.

In addition to considering the severity, thickness, and color of MIH lesions, the edges of the lesions must be observed as they can influence the effectiveness of the therapeutic protocol. A study [15] found that creamy and matte edges in white

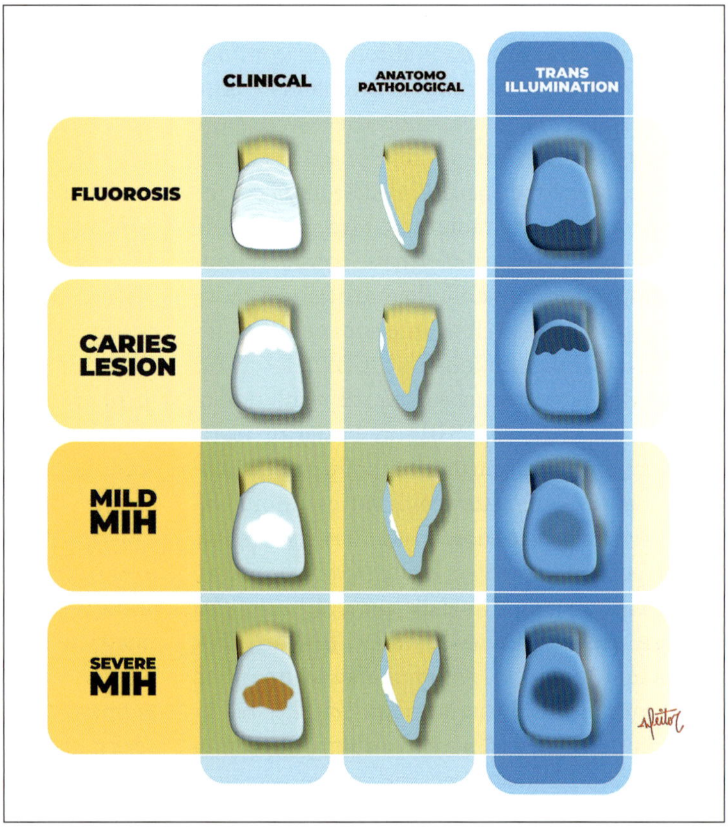

Fig. 1. Schematic illustration of the various types of enamel opacities. *Fluorosis*: Clinically, it is characterized by horizontal, more or less convergent white lines, which may be accompanied by cloudy and chalky areas that give the tooth a parchment-like appearance. Anatomopathological characteristics show that the demineralised zone extends below the surface at an obtuse angle and affects only the external part of the enamel thickness. On transillumination, the borders are defined, and the image is dark. *Caries lesion*: Clinically, caries lesions appear as chalky-white, matte, opaque spots with variable shape and size and outlines that are more or less well defined in areas where dental plaque preferentially accumulates. Anatomopathological characteristics in a transverse cross-section show that the lesion extends from the surface of the tooth to the demineralisation front at an obtuse angle. The white spot hypomineralisation remains subsurface without altering the volume of enamel. On transillumination, the borders are defined, and the image is dark. *Mild MIH*: Clinically, it is characterized by well-defined opaque white-creamy areas. Anatomopathological characteristics in a transverse cross-section show that the hypomineralised enamel is located in the inner third along the dentinoenamel junction, forming an obtuse angle with the enamel surface. A layer of normal enamel covers the hypomineralised enamel. The less severe the MIH, the deeper the localization of the hypomineralised enamel. On transillumination, there is a spot with diffuse edges, and the closer it is to the surface, the darker it appears. *Severe MIH*: Clinically, it is characterized by well-defined opaque yellow-brown areas. Anatomopathological characteristics in a transverse cross-section show that the entire depth of the enamel is affected by hypomineralisation.

spot lesions indicate a deep lesion covered by sound enamel. For minimally invasive or invasive treatment, this margin should be reduced or removed to allow the treatment to act effectively on the affected area. The same group of researchers [11] also observed that lesions with diffuse edges, as seen during transillumination, suggest that the lesion is covered by sound enamel (shown in

Fig. 1), which can hinder the effectiveness of the resin infiltration protocol. In this context, transillumination may assist in identifying and removing the sound enamel covering the MIH lesion, thereby enhancing the infiltration process [11]. After the removal of the superficial sound enamel, diffuse edges become less apparent under transillumination. At this stage, the lesions appear more uniform, and their edges are more clearly demarcated, making them more amenable to infiltration [11]. This leads to a more favorable clinical outcome. Based on our experience, the degree of darkness of the lesion under transillumination is a challenging clinical parameter to use as an indicator of potential clinical success and esthetic improvement.

Furthermore, localized defects can disrupt the harmony of a smile. Surface alterations change the "smile pattern," leading to psychosocial dissatisfaction [16, 17]. The presence of such alterations complicates esthetics and conveys a sense of fragility in the affected area, detracting from the patient's perception of an "ideal smile" [18]. The pursuit of the "ideal smile" resonates deeply with the public, as it aligns with the World Health Organization's definition of health, which includes physical, chemical, and social well-being [19].

Considerations for Treating Esthetics of Anterior Teeth with MIH

Reports have highlighted the implications on the quality of life for individuals with anterior teeth affected by MIH. Among these observations, it has been noted that the presence of an incisor with MIH impacts dental health, primarily regarding the perception of tooth color and alignment, which in turn indirectly affects the individuals' quality of life [10]. It is crucial to acknowledge that this condition is frequently diagnosed in young ages and that parental influence can significantly affect the patients' quality of life. Studies have shown that both parents and the affected individuals experience changes in their quality of life, particularly in social and psychological aspects, emphasizing the importance of addressing this issue [9]. Esthetic treatments should be carried out to satisfy the affected individuals rather than their parents.

In addition to the psychological and quality of life issues that affect MIH sufferers, especially those with anterior teeth, there have been reports of improvements in these aspects following minimally invasive [20], invasive, or combined treatments. These findings reinforce the justification for the therapeutic treatment of this condition.

Treatment Options for Incisors Affected by MIH

There are currently no randomized controlled clinical trials that evaluate and contrast potential protocols addressing the resolution of the issue at hand, with particular focus on clinical efficacy, treatment durability, and cost-effectiveness analysis. Additionally, the heterogeneity of lesion characteristics, including variations in size, pigmentation, extent of involvement, and anatomical distribution, complicates the formulation of a universally applicable standard protocol to be preferred over alternative approaches.

Among the esthetic resolution options for MIH, there are minimally invasive protocols, invasive methods, and combinations thereof. Minimally invasive protocols include tooth bleaching, microabrasion, resin infiltration, and potential combinations of these treatments. These treatments should be preferred considering the large pulp chamber, prominent pulp horns, and immature gingiva in these pediatric/adolescent patients [14]. Furthermore, a minimally invasive approach preserves tooth structure, maintaining options for future restorative interventions.

In general, there is a consensus [20] that masking with the use of minimally invasive procedures improves the quality of life of individuals. This fact reinforces the use of these techniques, which at times might be undervalued in favor of traditional restorative procedures.

There are opposing views that minimally invasive treatments should not be used for mild or moderate lesions, given that these are located in the inner third of the enamel and covered by sound enamel [4]. Therefore, a substantial layer of healthy enamel would need to be removed to access the lesion and execute the protocol, which in this case would no longer be minimally invasive.

For instance, in a study utilizing resin infiltration on teeth with mild or moderate MIH, a resolution rate of 57% for treated lesions was achieved after a full 30-min application [9]. A significant improvement in masking ability began to be observed at the 15th minute [9]. It is noteworthy that the erosive step of the treatment, performed with hydrochloric acid, was repeated three times under pressure, presumably to reach the lesion within the enamel [9]. The authors emphasize that the effectiveness of the protocol depends on the characteristics of the treated enamel, such as thickness, depth of the lesion, and the histological organization of the subsurface, especially concerning its mineralisation [9]. Additionally, the results of this study indicate the need for an infiltration time of at least 15 min. However, this recommendation will only have a scientific basis when a clinical study compares the effect of the standard application time (3 min + 1 min) with an extended application time (15 min + 1 min).

In an attempt to address these issues of lesion depth and the quality of the enamel layer covering it, a proposed approach involves deep infiltration to access the hypomineralisation [21]. This involves removing a superficial layer of enamel, between 100 and 500 μm, using an aluminum oxide jet or diamond burs. The confirmation of adequate removal is done by applying ethanol from the infiltrating resin kit, and a masking effect is observed. Ethanol masks the lesion, often not completely, due to its high refractive index. In general, regardless of the method used to remove the superficial layer over the hypomineralised enamel of mild and moderate lesions, there seems to be unanimous agreement on the necessity of removing this layer, whether through microabrasion, aluminum oxide jet, diamond burs, or hydrochloric acid (erosive agent).

The effectiveness of resin infiltration was also identified in another study that compared the resolution of white spots of different etiologies [22]. Both fluorosis and mild or moderate MIH showed high resolution rates, with minimal incidences of clinically unsatisfactory scores. However, opacities caused by trauma did not exhibit the same performance. This is justified by the fact that the margins of these lesions were not adequately masked, possibly due to the coverage of sound enamel over the lesions which, when viewed incisally, presented an acute angle with the external surface [4, 22]. It is important to note that the application of the erosive agent was also repeated three times in that study. The authors suggest the combination with teeth whitening to try and resolve issues that were not effectively addressed by resin infiltration alone.

Comparing cases 1 and 2 presented in this report, one can observe different resolution scenarios. These differences may be attributed to the varying depths of the lesions, which were somewhat discernible through transillumination [11], as described in the captions accompanying the related figures.

Resin infiltration may not address the esthetic issues associated with MIH; therefore, the costs of this treatment should be clearly outlined and discussed with patients beforehand. Currently, there is a lack of cost-effectiveness studies regarding this treatment option. Based on our experience, the cost of supplies for resin infiltration per tooth is approximately $15.00. It is important to present a combination of treatments and their associated costs to patients, aiming to avoid more invasive and traditional approaches initially.

Among the indications for microabrasion, the use of an association with remineralising agents, such as casein phosphopeptide-amorphous calcium phosphate paste, seems to optimize the outcome after a period of 6 months [23]. This is because the remineralising agent has facilitated access to the body of the lesion that was exposed after the microabrasion procedure. The isolated treatment of microabrasion in this study did not result in improvements to the esthetic appearance of the lesion even after 6 months of follow-up.

Dental bleaching can also be indicated for the treatment of MIH opacities, but these indications should be made for severe lesions with the presence of brownish discolorations [4]. This protocol can be used in conjunction with erosive/abrasive agents that will expose the body of the lesion for the whitening agent to act. The rationale for this approach is likely due to the fact that severe MIH lesions with brown discolorations are often more resistant to conventional treatments. The combination of bleaching with preparatory erosion or abrasion can reveal the deeper lesion body, allowing the whitening agents to have better access and potentially provide a more effective esthetic resolution. This method, however, should be used cautiously considering the potential for increased tooth sensitivity.

The long-term follow-up of a report [24] emphasizes the importance of a tailored approach, considering the evolution of the patient's condition and the impact of age on treatment options. The eventual inclusion of bleaching procedures, which were initially unsuitable, showcases the dynamic nature of managing MIH. The combination of microabrasion and composite resin has been shown to be a viable option for maintaining esthetics and tooth integrity over an extended period, with the flexibility to adapt to changes such as those caused by bleaching treatment [25–27]. There are other approaches that also suggest that employing whitening in conjunction with direct resin restorations can be an effective strategy, although careful planning and patient monitoring are imperative to ensure successful outcomes.

Among invasive treatments, direct adhesive restorations with composite resin are primarily used. Managing patients with MIH is reported in the literature as complicated due to uncertainties about adhesion to dental structures and the longevity of restorations [27, 28].

Laboratory studies on adhesion to these structures assist in guiding the clinical decision making. There is evidence that enamel affected by MIH negatively influences the bond strength and that adhesive protocols with a prior step of acid etching of the enamel are beneficial for adhesive outcomes [29]. Despite these results, there is also laboratory evidence that the use of resin infiltration brings benefits when used with a preceding oxidizing agent [30], contrary to the first study reported in this paragraph [31]. This information and other available literature highlight the need for bonding to healthy enamel or dentin for the longevity of an adhesive restoration. Here, as it concerns an esthetic problem, the need to remove enamel affected by MIH is generally necessary considering the esthetic results required to complete the restorative treatment. This aspect becomes somewhat different in posterior teeth where the friability of the enamel might be the most important factor for the removal of affected structure before the adhesive restorative procedure.

In comparing adhesive restorations performed on posterior teeth, statistically similar results are observed in clinical settings when using adhesive protocols with total etching or selective etching [31]. It is important to note that the evaluations were over a short period, and the enamel affected by MIH had been removed.

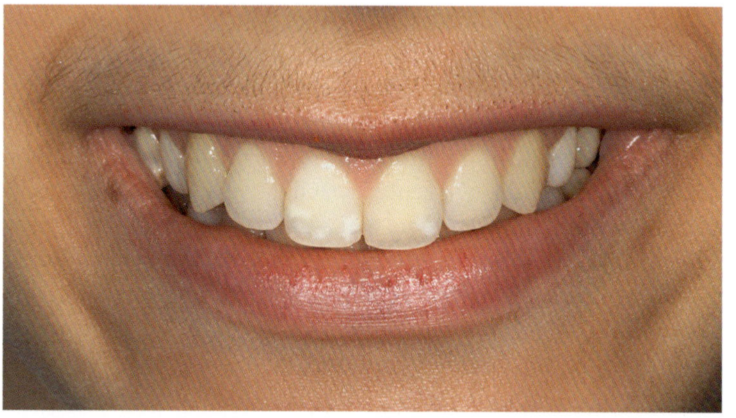

Fig. 2. Clinical aspect of smile of the patient with MIH lesion on the central incisors in case scenario 1.

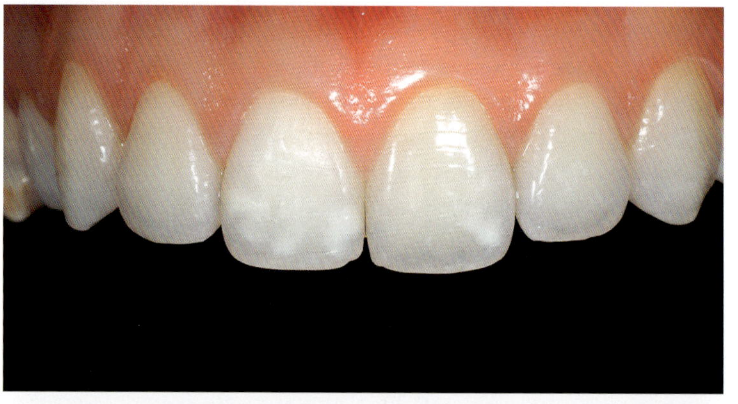

Fig. 3. Clinical intraoral aspect of MIH lesion on the central incisors in case scenario 1.

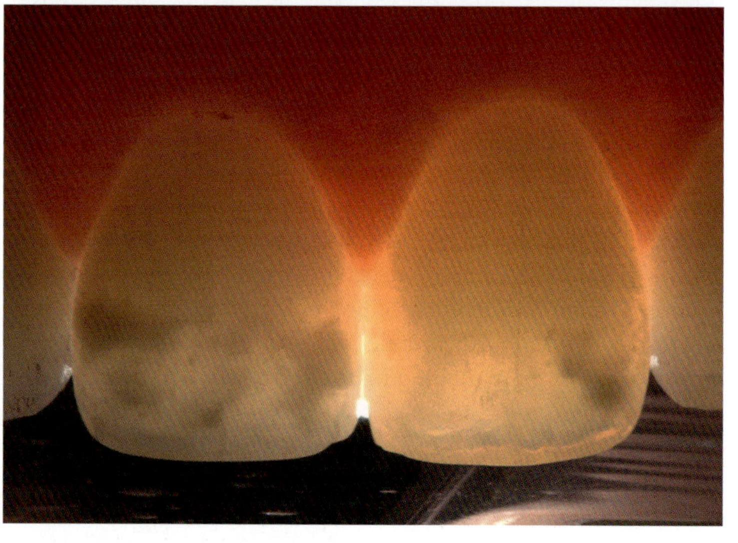

Fig. 4. MIH lesion transilluminated (Valo Grand associated with the Translume lens, Ultradent, Brazil). According to the scientific literature [11], darker lesions are deep and more difficult to mask. There is no clinical protocol currently described that adequately guides clinicians on the likelihood of achieving satisfactory results.

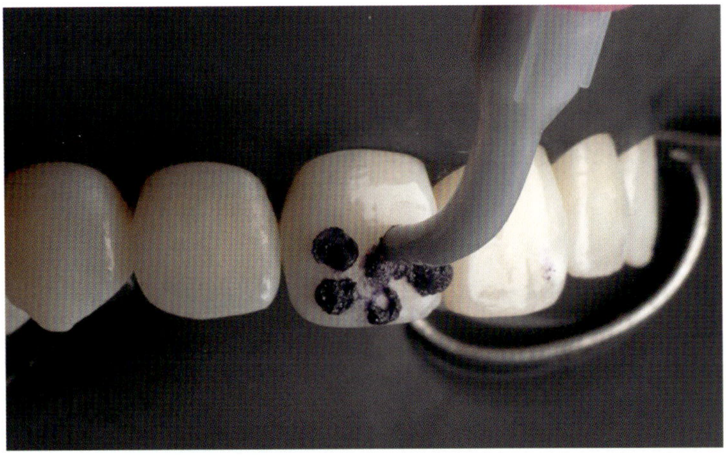

Fig. 5. Microabrasion with Opalustre being performed. Six applications of 10 s each were performed using rubber cups.

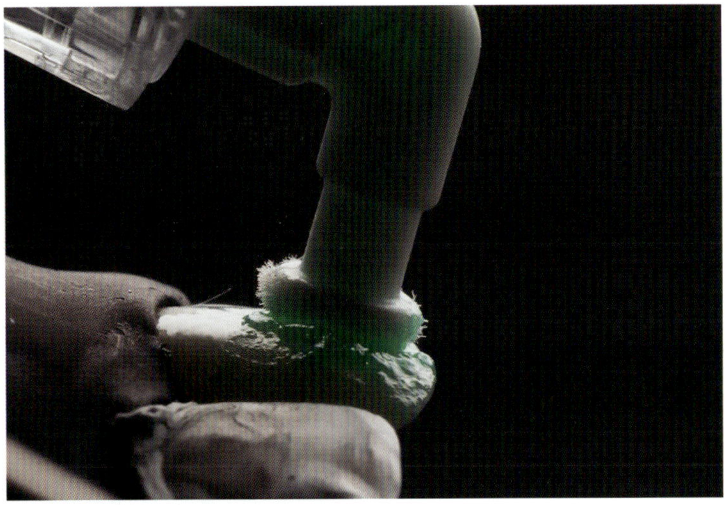

Fig. 6. Hydrochloric acid being applied for 2 min. The application was performed once, considering that the superficial layer of the enamel had been previously removed using the microabrasion protocol.

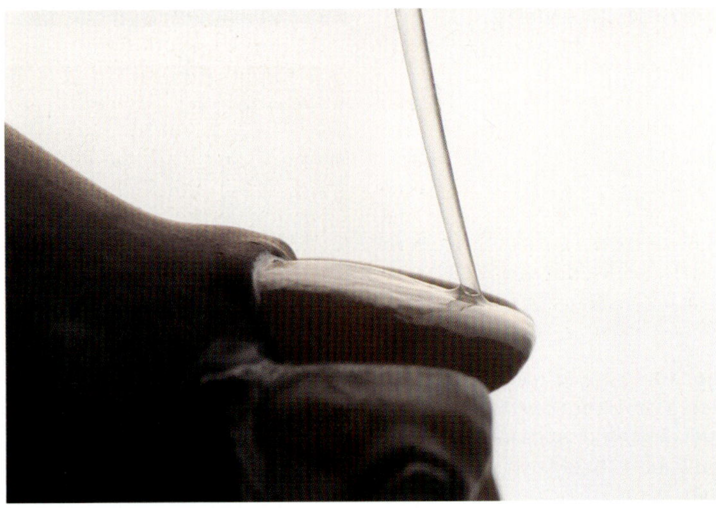

Fig. 7. Icon dry being applied for 30 s.

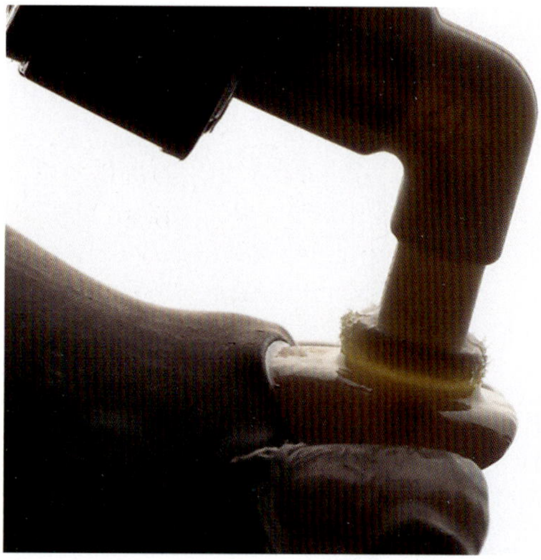

Fig. 8. Resin infiltration being applied and let sit for 3 min prior to excess removal and 40 s light activation. Second resin infiltration application for 1 min, excess removal and light curing for 40 s.

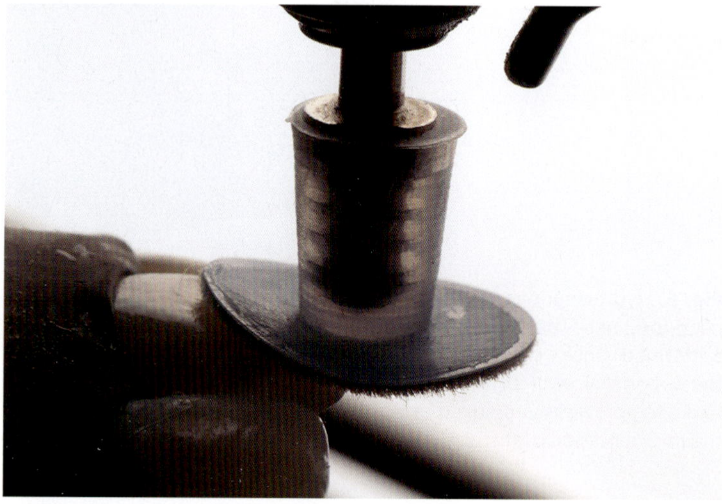

Fig. 9. Surface polishing of the resin infiltrated the surface, performed with felt discs and polishing paste (Ultradent Polishing Mint, Ultradent) using a dental handpiece.

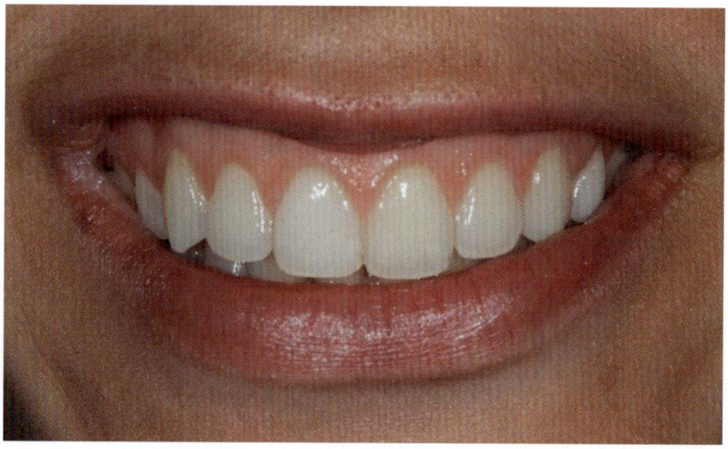

Fig. 10. Result of the resin infiltration. It can be noticed that the white spot lesions disappeared. The patient was very pleased with the results.

Case Reports

Case Scenario 1

Resolution of Mild MIH with Associated Microabrasion and Resin Infiltration

A 20-year-old female patient presented with mild white MIH lesions on the upper central incisors. After being informed about the possible protocols and their limitations, the chosen therapy was the association of an erosive/abrasive protocol (Opalustre, Ultradent, Indaiatuba, SP, Brazil) to remove the superficial layer of enamel and resin infiltration (Icon, DMG, Germany) to mask the lesions, as shown in Figures 2–10.

Case Scenario 2

Resolution of Mild MIH with Associated Microabrasion and Resin

A 22-year-old male patient presented to the dental clinic with mild white MIH lesions on the maxillary central incisors, a condition similar to the previous scenario (case 1). After being informed of the possible protocols and their limitations, the therapy of choice was the association of an erosive/abrasive protocol (Opalustre, Ultradent, Indaiatuba, SP, Brazil), for the removal of the superficial layer of enamel, and resin infiltration (Icon, DMG, Germany) for masking the lesions, as shown in Figures 11–21.

Case Scenario 3

Resolution of Severe MIH with the Association of Microabrasion, Local Bleaching, Resin Infiltration, and Restoration with Composite Resin

A 16-year-old female patient came to the dental clinic accompanied by her parents. In this scenario, she presented a severe white MIH lesion on the right maxillary central incisor. After guidance on the possible protocols and their limitations, the therapy of choice was the association of erosive/abrasive protocol (Opalustre, Ultradent, Indaiatuba, SP, Brazil), for the removal of the superficial layer of enamel, dental bleaching (Whiteness HP 35%, FGM, Joinville, SC, Brazil), and resin infiltration (Icon, DMG, Germany) for masking the lesions. After the completion of the protocol, the patient was satisfied with the esthetic results; however, a restoration with composite resin (Vitra #A2, FGM, Joinville, SC, Brazil) was made to recover the contour of the tooth surface, as shown in Figures 22–36. The patient and parents were aware that the situation could require dental restoration due to the severity of the case but agreed to try the minimally invasive protocols initially. It is worth noting that resin infiltration has its costs and may not respond as expected, requiring new interventions and additional treatment costs. A discussion on that financial issue was previously addressed.

The case in question underwent all the minimally invasive protocols that were discussed. Despite the use of transillumination and considering the clinical expertise of the clinicians, it was not possible to accurately predict the necessity for restorative treatment, the need for removal of excess enamel, the risk of inadvertently removing enamel, or the potential for sensitivity issues. This scenario highlights the unpredictable prognosis of treatments for MIH with respect to esthetic outcomes.

Case Scenario 4

MIH Treatment with Restorative Procedures on Severe Lesion

An 8-year-old male patient presented at the dental clinic with mild white MIH lesions on the maxillary central incisors and the left lateral incisor. In addition, a severe MIH lesion with a brownish appearance and loss of incisal structure was observed on the right maxillary central incisor. The parent reported that the child was complaining about comments from friends about their teeth, using terms such as “rotten,” “decayed,” and so on. After counseling on the possible protocols and their limitations, the course of action chosen was to restore the lost portion of the referred tooth. The other white lesions were

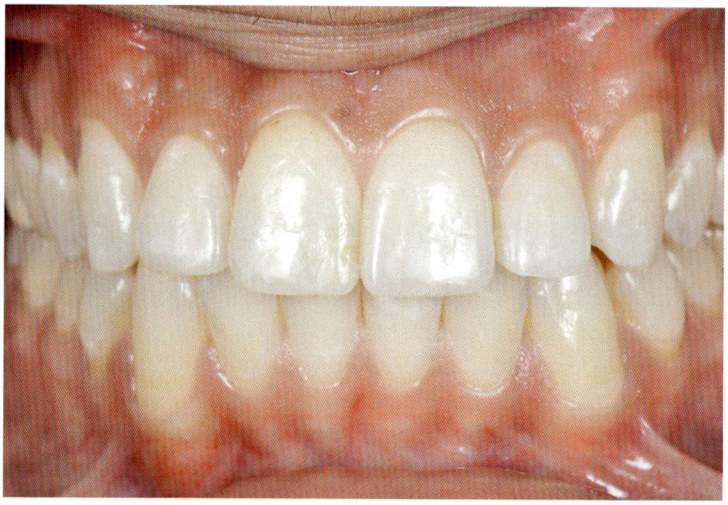

Fig. 11. Clinical aspect of the MIH lesions on the central incisors in case scenario 2.

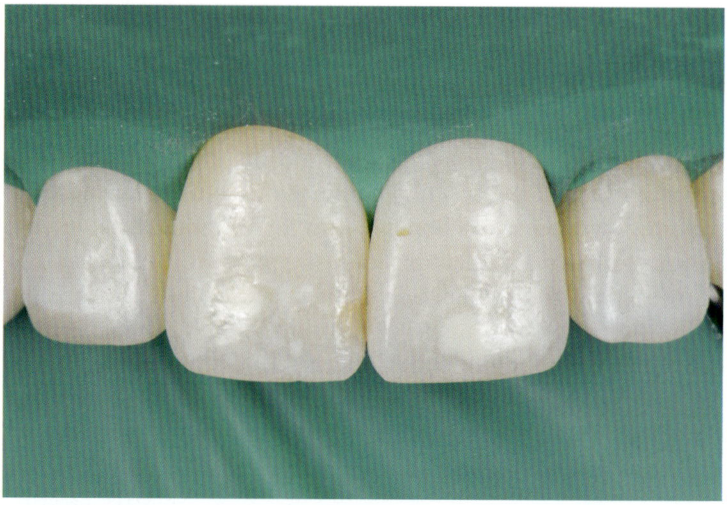

Fig. 12. Aspect evidenced after rubber dam isolation.

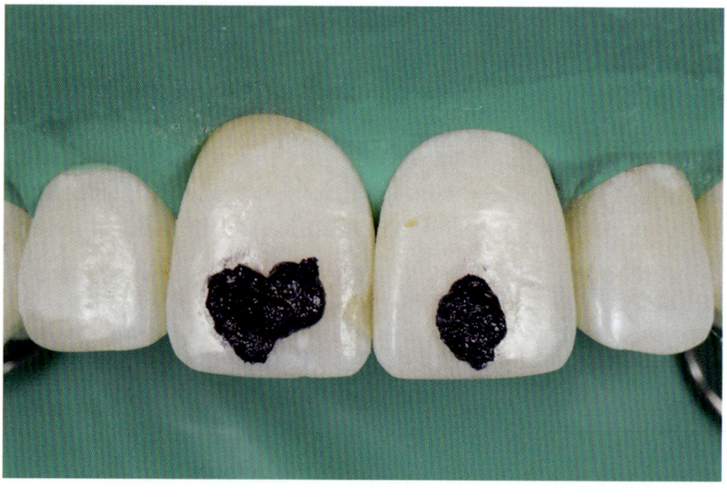

Fig. 13. Microabrasion with Opalustre being performed. Six applications of 10 s each were performed using rubber cups.

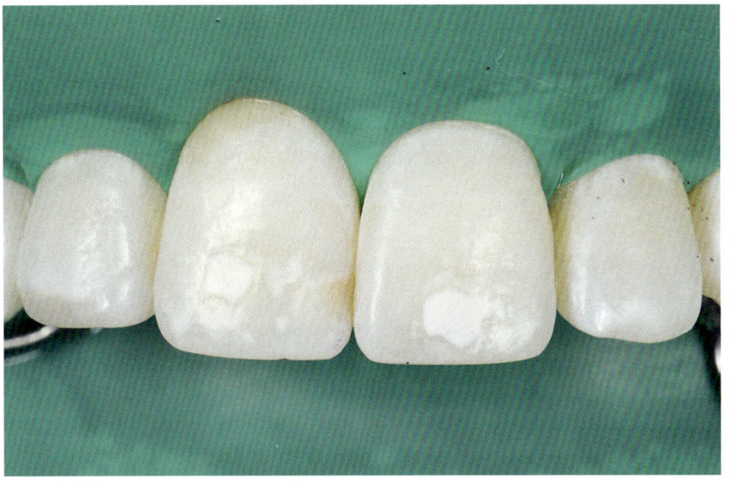

Fig. 14. Enamel surface characteristics after the microabrasion was performed. The opaque aspect of the lesions was evidenced, suggesting the sound enamel covering them was probably removed.

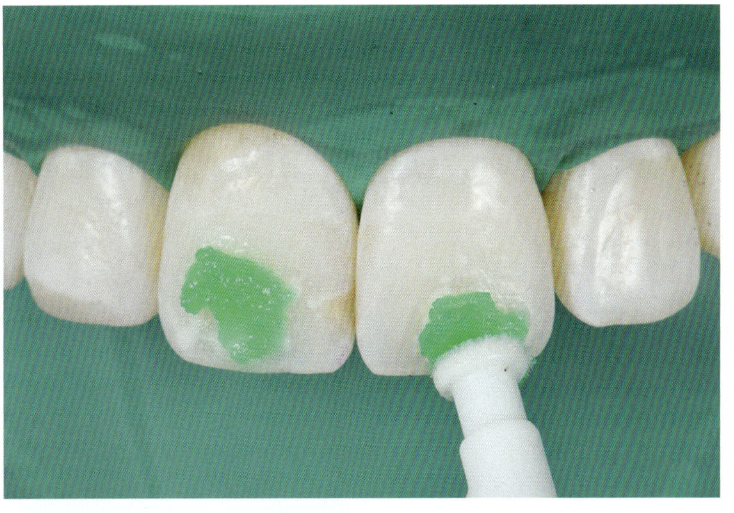

Fig. 15. Hydrochloric acid being applied for 2 min. The erosive protocol (icon etch using hydrochloric acid) was performed two times.

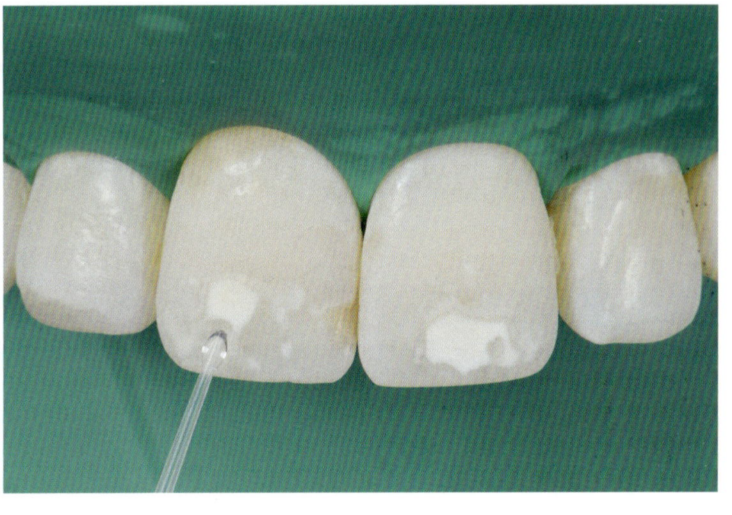

Fig. 16. Icon dry being applied for 30 s after each cycle of the icon etch.

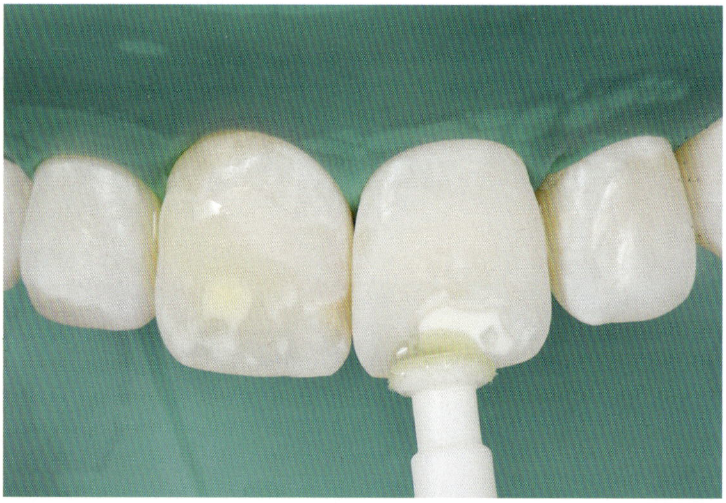

Fig. 17. Resin infiltration being applied and let sit for 3 min prior to excess removal and 40 s light activation. Second resin infiltration application for 1 min, excess removal and light curing for 40 s.

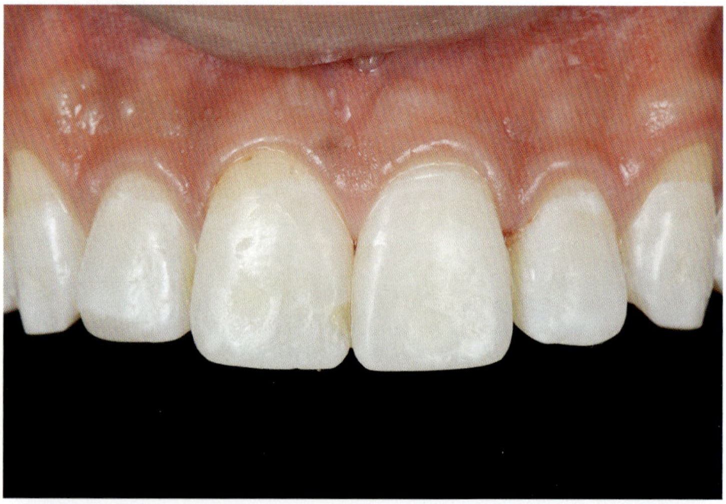

Fig. 18. Clinical aspect after resin infiltration.

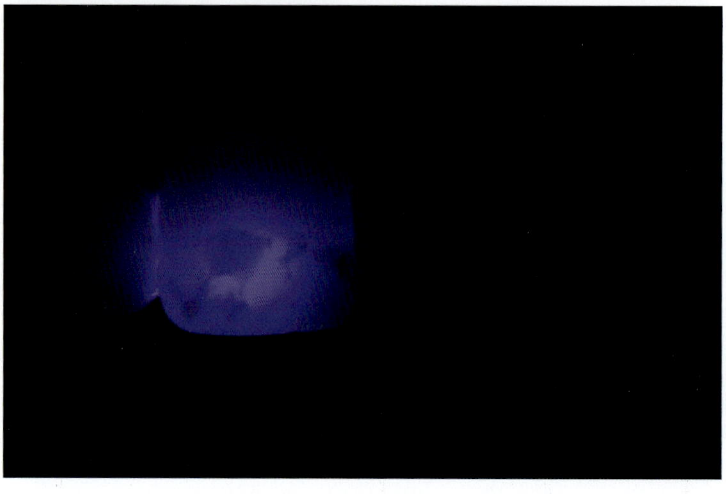

Fig. 19. MIH infiltrated lesion being transilluminated with the light of a light curing unit (Grand Valo, Ultradent) from the lingual aspect of the right central incisor. Dark images indicate that the lesion is deep, suggesting that the prognosis for successfully masking it through treatment might not be favorable.

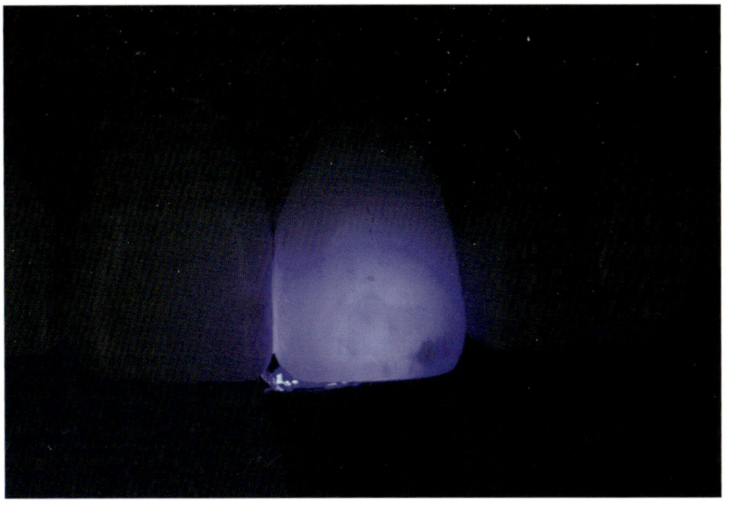

Fig. 20. MIH infiltrated lesion being transilluminated with the light of a light curing unit (Grand Valo, Ultradent) from the lingual aspect of the left central incisor.

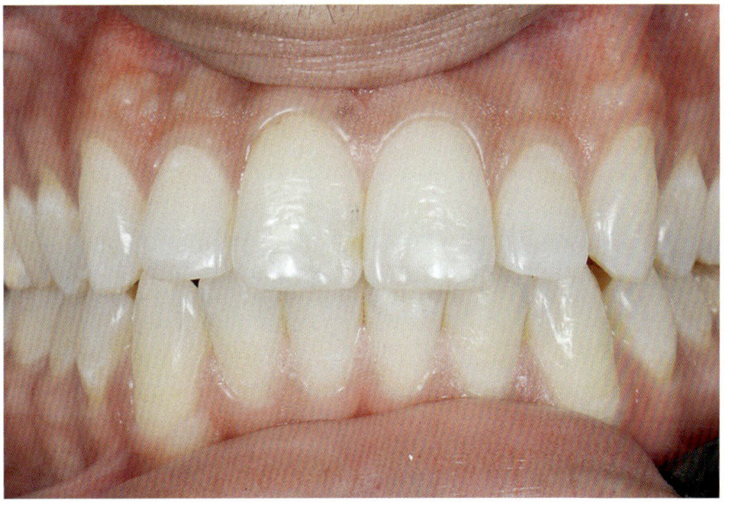

Fig. 21. Result of the resin infiltration after tooth hydration. It can be noticed that the white spot lesions are still present but in a milder manner. The patient was pleased with the results, but he still wanted to perform further protocols for complete removal of lesions.

not treated at this stage at the patient's request. If she chooses to treat the white lesions associated with the other teeth, she may be subjected to minimally invasive protocols, as shown in Figures 37–40.

Case Scenario 5

Resolution of Mild and Severe MIH Lesions with Restorative Procedures

A 15-year-old female patient presented to the dental clinic with a mild white MIH lesion on maxillary left central incisor. On the other hand, the right central incisor had a severe MIH lesion with a brown appearance and loss of tooth structure on the incisal edge and vestibular face. She reported real discomfort when smiling during social life and especially at school. After being informed about the possible protocols and their limitations, it was decided to restore the lost portion of the central incisor and the white lesion of the left incisor after selective wear of the surface with diamond tips, as shown in Figures 41 and 42.

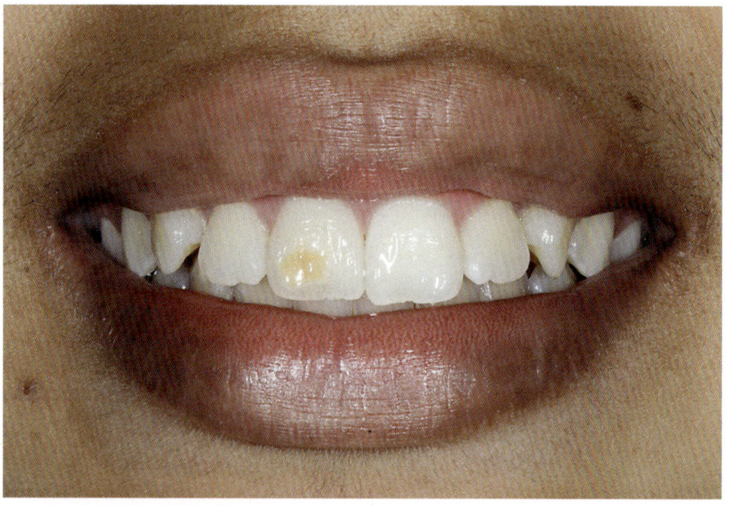

Fig. 22. Clinical aspect of the patient's smile for case scenario 3.

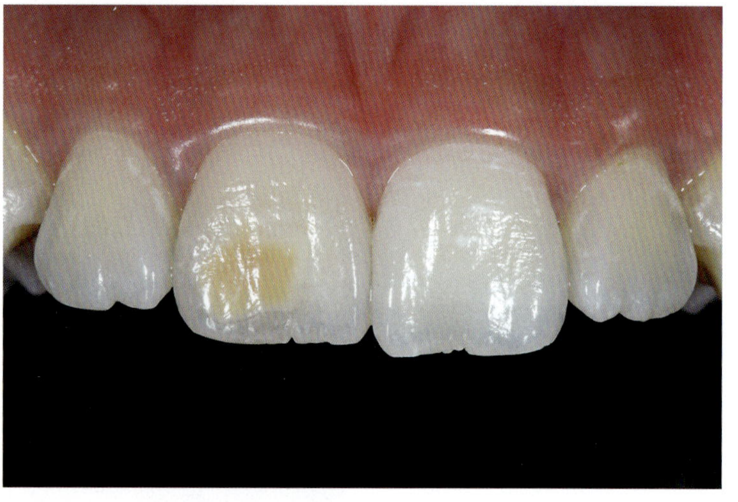

Fig. 23. Clinical aspect of an intraoral view.

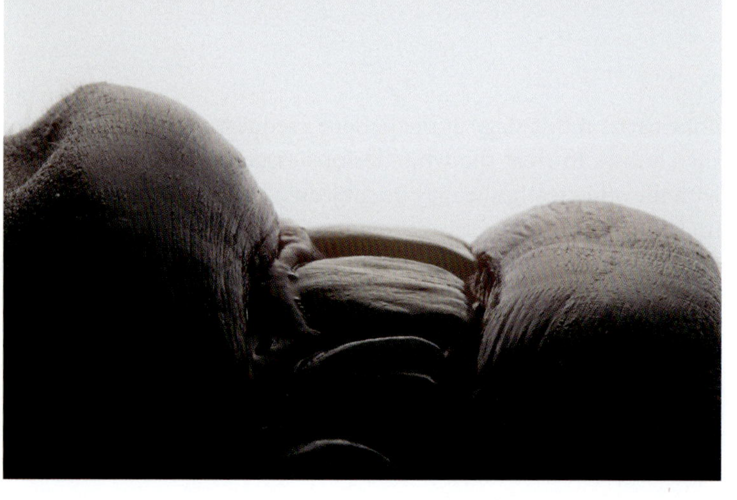

Fig. 24. Clinical aspect of the surface texture of the right central incisor in comparison to the neighboring teeth.

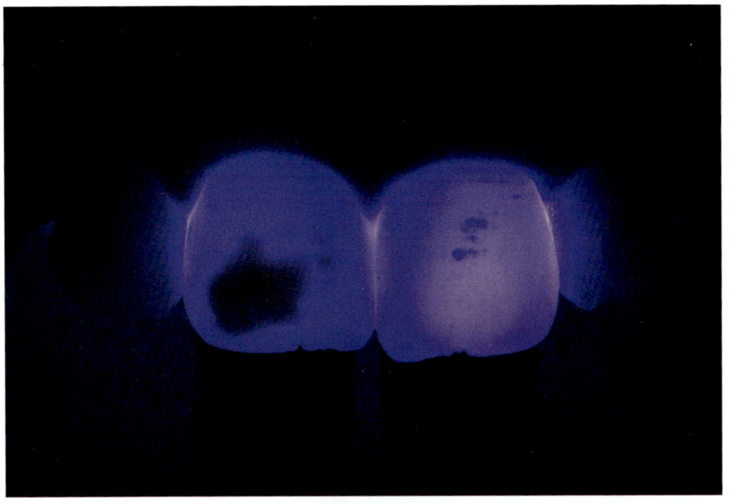

Fig. 25. Lesion transilluminated with the light of a light curing unit (Grand Valo, Ultradent) from the lingual aspect of the tooth. It can be noted as a well-defined and dark lesion, indicating that its thickness is considerable.

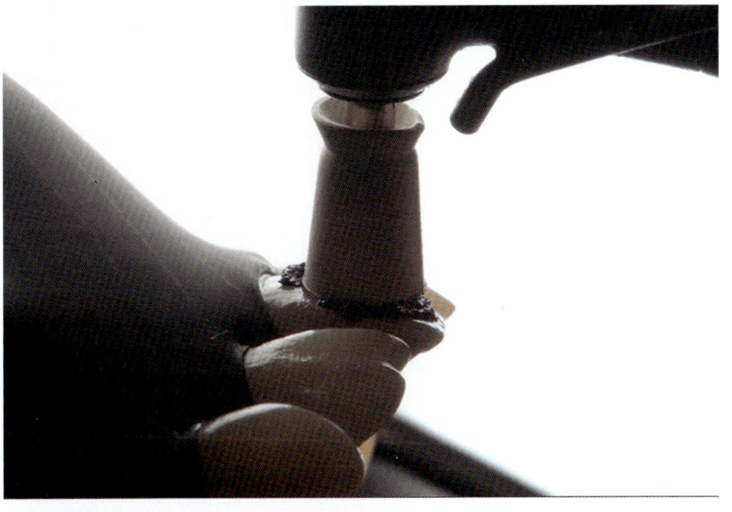

Fig. 26. Six 10-s applications of Opalustre (Ultradent, Brazil) were performed using rubber cups.

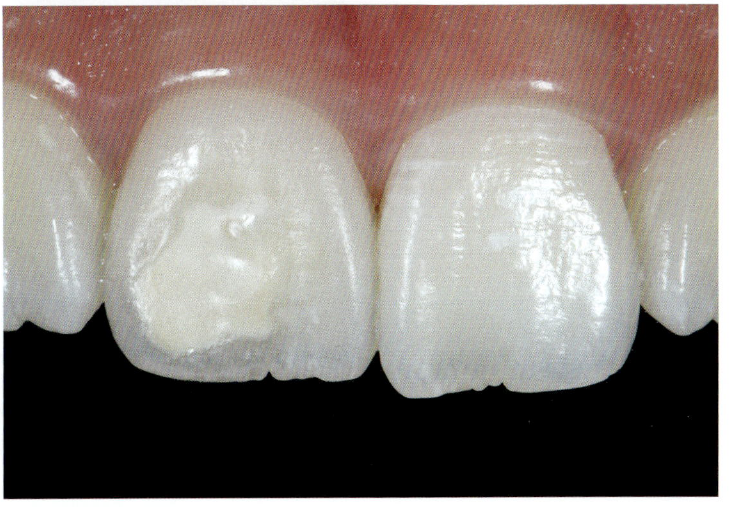

Fig. 27. Aspect after microabrasion. A removal of tooth structure can be observed, differently from the previous reported cases. Moreover, a brownish lesion can still be noticed.

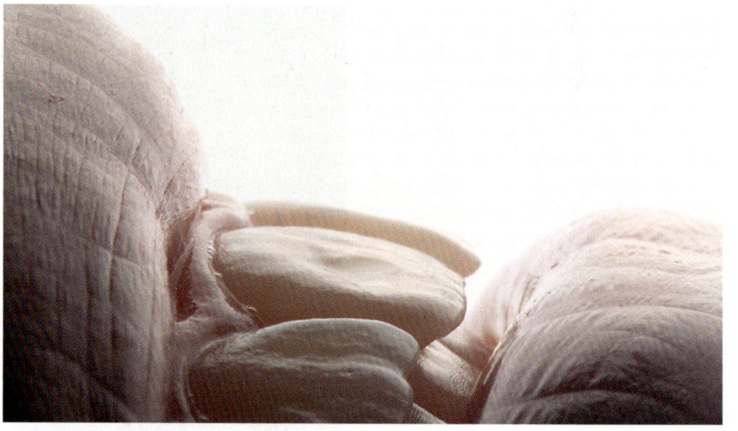

Fig. 28. The amount of tooth structure removal can be noticed in a lateral view.

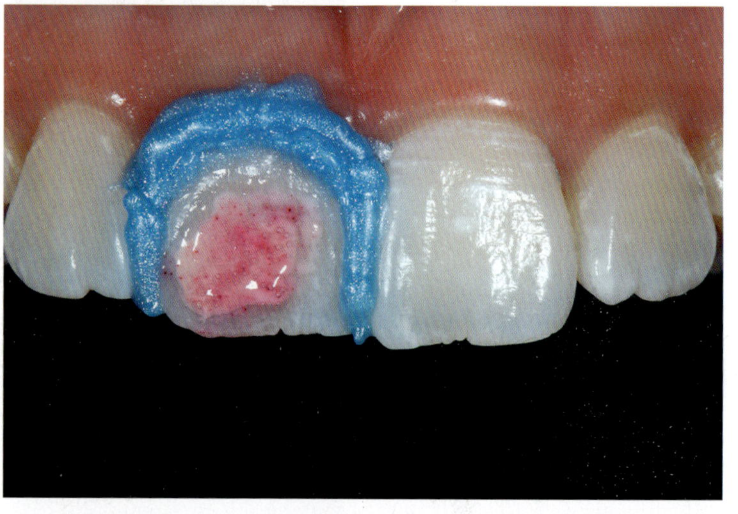

Fig. 29. An in-office session of dental bleaching was performed after 7 days in order to try to reduce the coloration of the lesion, still with brownish characteristics.

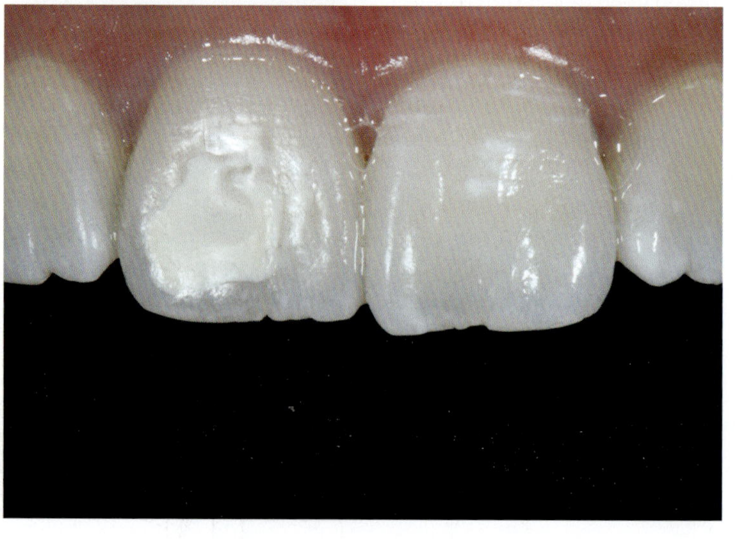

Fig. 30. A reduction in the brown hue is observed.

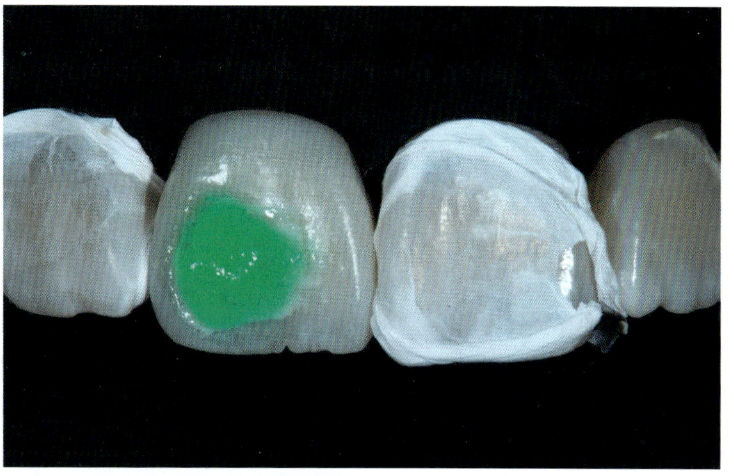

Fig. 31. Hydrochloric acid being applied for 2 min. The erosive protocol (icon etch using hydrochloric acid) was performed two times.

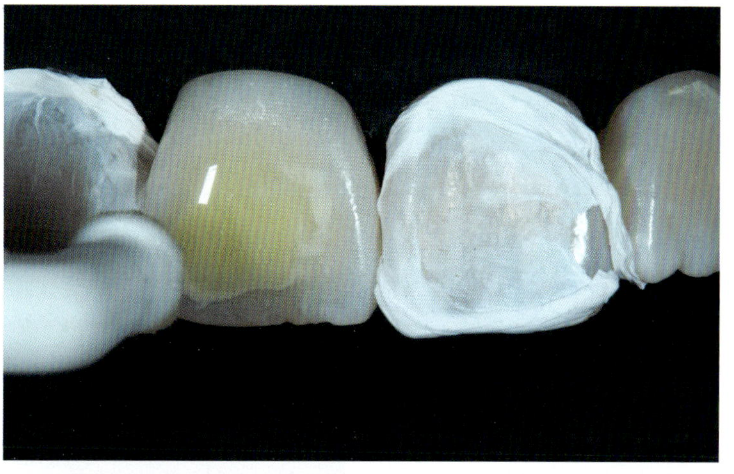

Fig. 32. Resin infiltration being applied and let sit for 3 min prior to excess removal and 40 s light activation. Second resin infiltration application for 1 min, excess removal and light curing for 40 s.

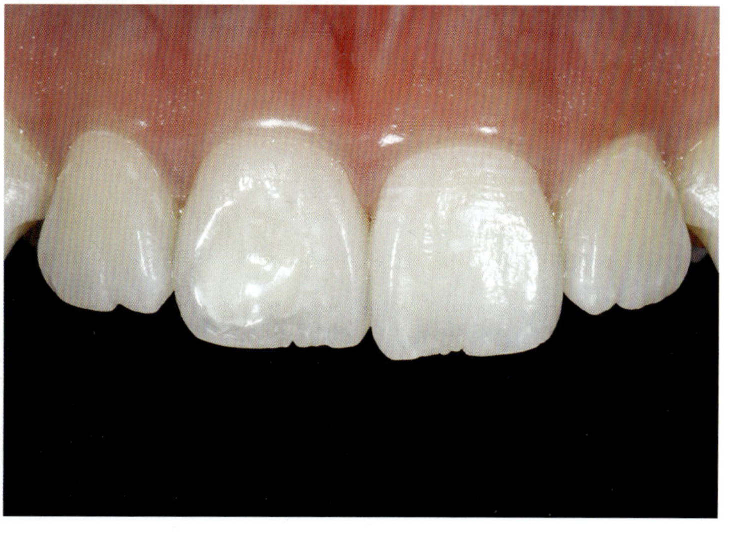

Fig. 33. Clinical aspect after resin infiltration and rubber dam isolation removal. A depression can be detected on the microabraded bleached area after infiltration.

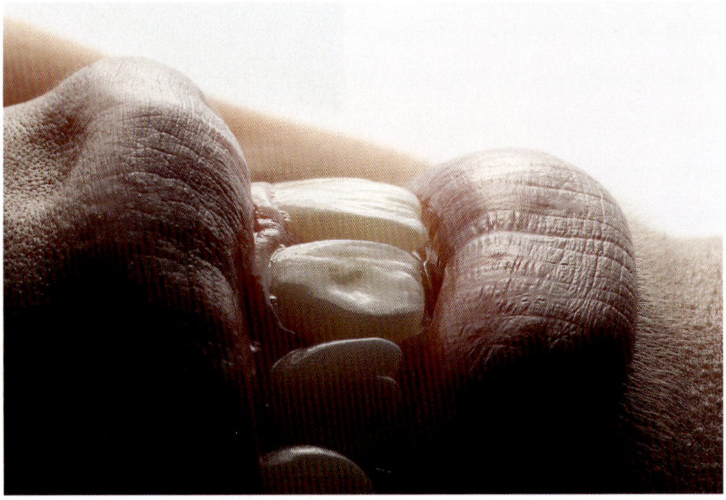

Fig. 34. A lateral view highlights the removal of the tooth structure. The patient was very pleased with the results so far, but she and her parents agreed to continue with the restorative phase to restore the initial tooth dimensions.

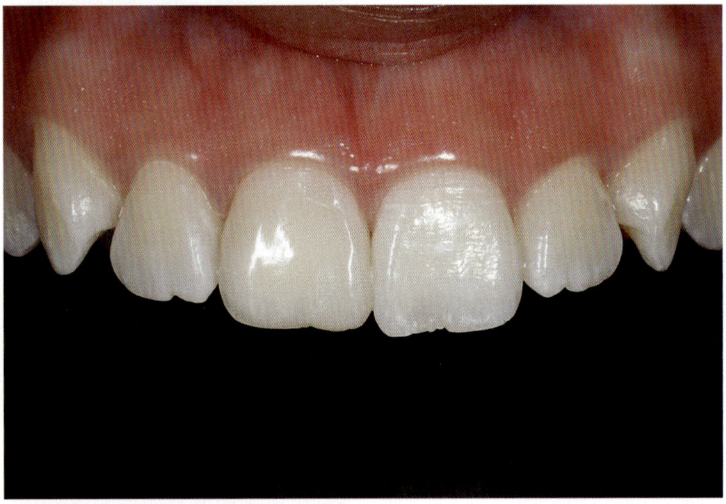

Fig. 35. A resin restoration was performed to restore the volume and shape of the tooth lost with the previous protocols. Intraoral aspect of the restoration.

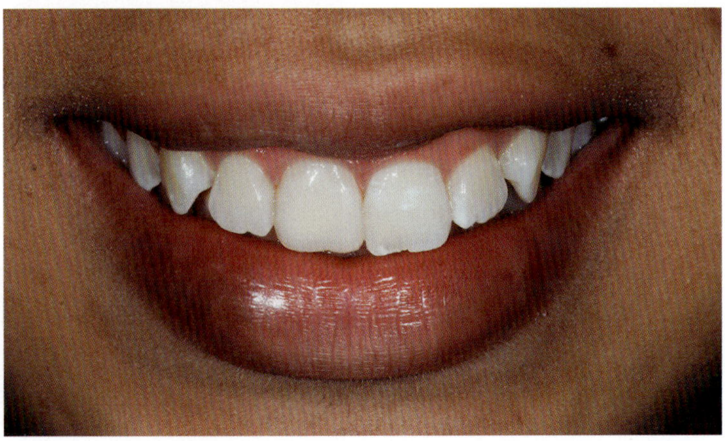

Fig. 36. A resin restoration was performed to restore the volume and shape of the tooth lost with the previous protocols. Smile view of the restored tooth.

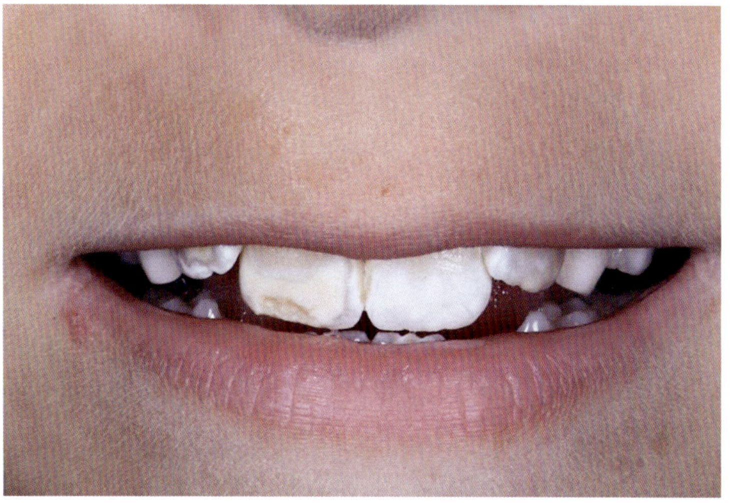

Fig. 37. Clinical aspect of the mild and the severe MIH lesions in case scenario 4, view of the lesion during smiling.

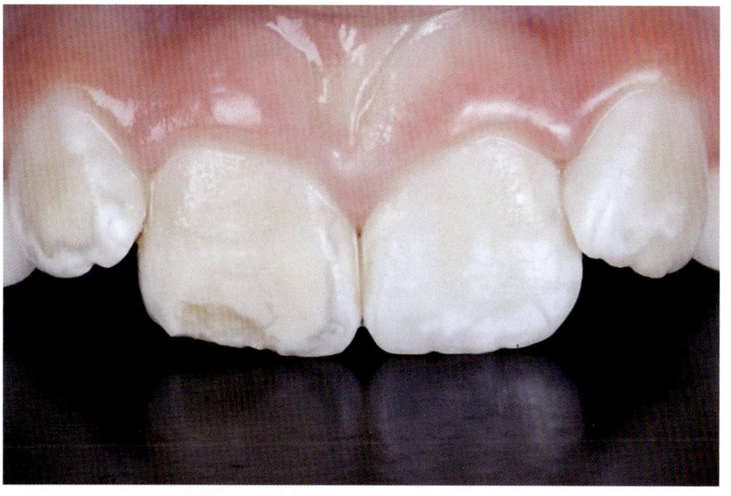

Fig. 38. A closer view of the lesions including the severe lesion that was restored. The removal of tissue in this particular case for the right central incisor reached dentin due to the characteristics of the altered enamel. It is important to highlight that the enamel surrounding the restoration was sound for proper adhesion.

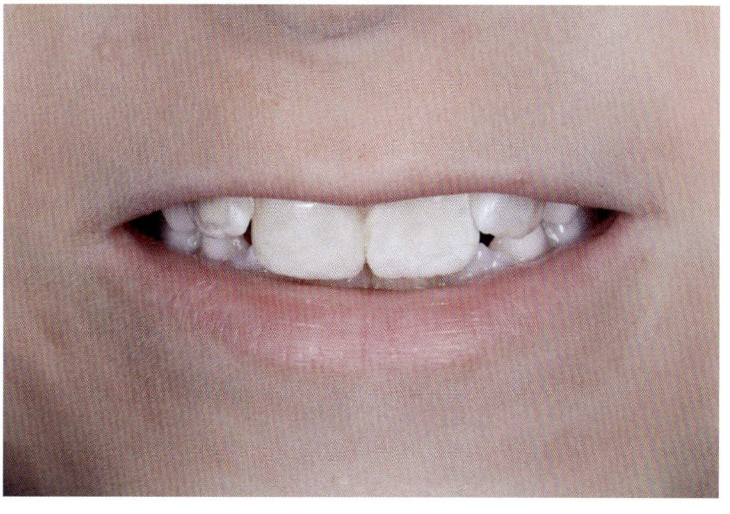

Fig. 39. Final intraoral aspect of the restored tooth. Esthetics was improved, and the patient was pleased with the results.

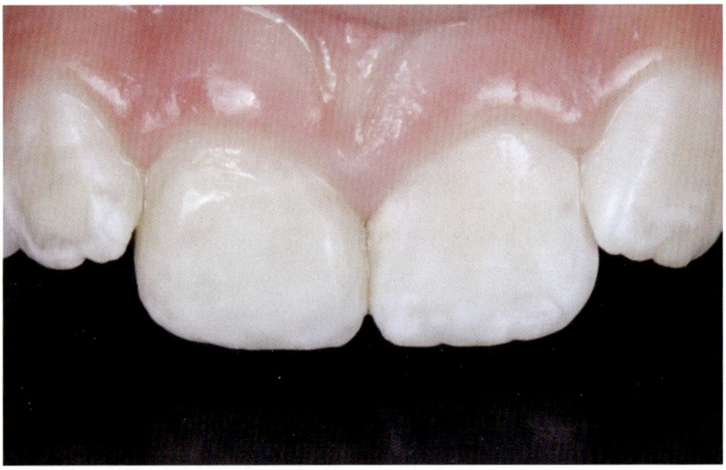

Fig. 40. Final extraoral aspect of the restored tooth. Future protocols might address the mild lesion present.

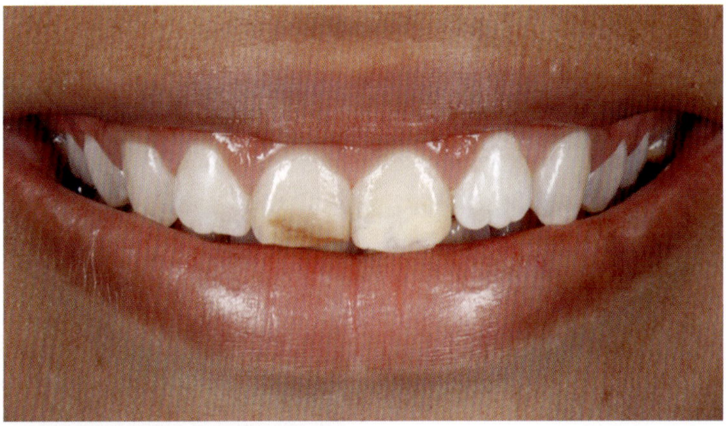

Fig. 41. Clinical aspect of the mild and the severe MIH lesions in case scenario 5. It is worth mentioning that the removal of tissue in this particular case for the right central incisor reached dentin due to the characteristics of the altered enamel. The enamel surrounding the restoration was sound for proper adhesion in that particular tooth. For the left central incisor, tissue removal did not reach dentin. Affected enamel was covered with composite resin, and adhesion to the sound surrounding enamel was granted.

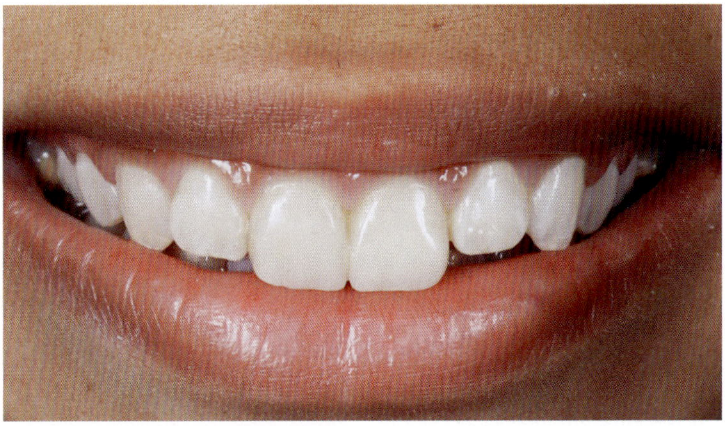

Fig. 42. Final aspect of the restored teeth. Esthetics was improved, and the patient was happy with the results.

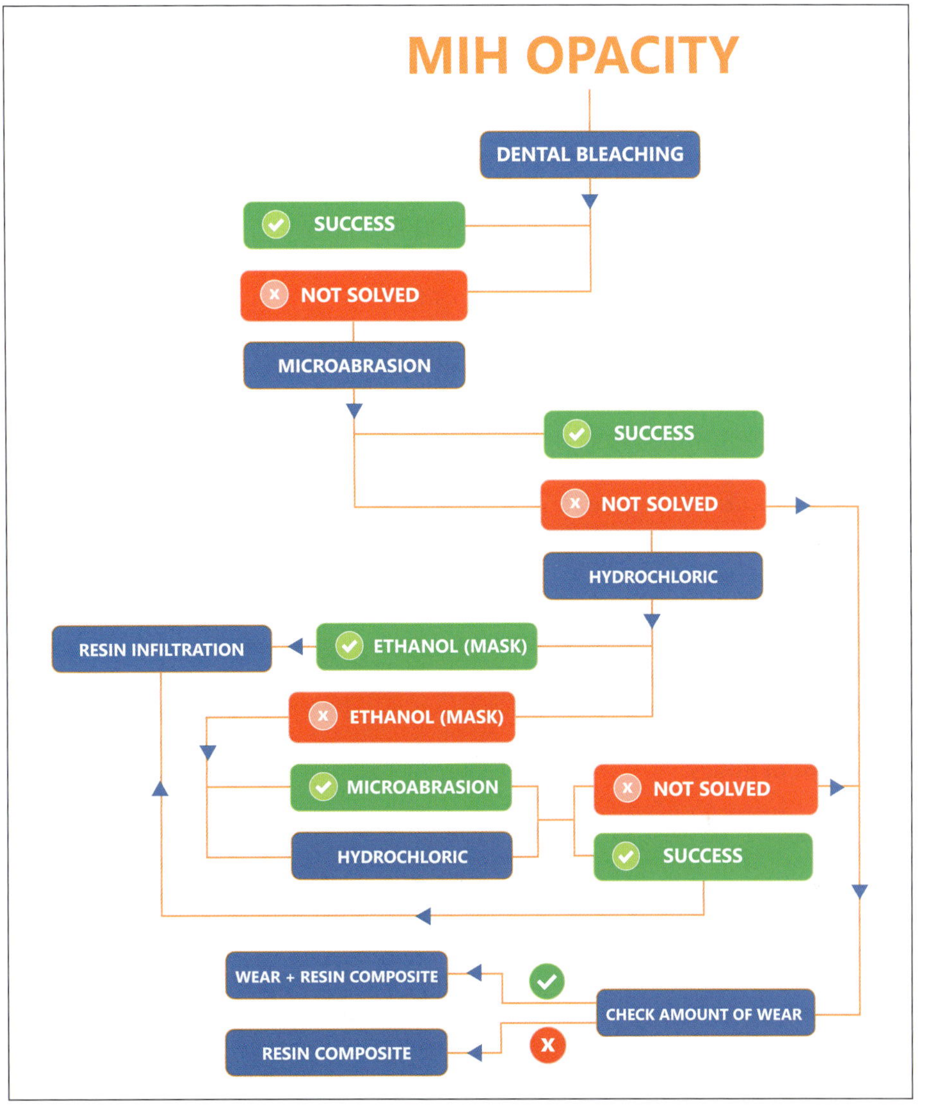

Fig. 43. Flowchart of the treatment options for re-establishing the esthetics of incisors in patients with MIH.

Conclusion

Esthetic issues associated with MIH should be addressed by considering the unique characteristics of each clinical case. A suggested decision-making process is to always start with the least invasive treatments. Thus, in cases where the opacity is white, tooth whitening can mask the opacity. However, when this approach is unsuccessful or when the opacity is yellow-brown, another alternative is microabrasion. In most cases, microabrasion alone will not achieve an esthetic result and can be combined with hydrochloric acid erosion to remove the superficial layer of enamel. An important clinical criterion indicating sufficient enamel removal is the masking of opacity after the application of ethanol. If this masking is not achieved, further enamel removal is necessary, which can be done through additional acid application, microabrasion, or even using a diamond bur. Mild and moderate lesions typically require the removal of the external enamel layer to make the lesion accessible for treatment protocols. If the opacity is masked after ethanol application and the tooth has not lost its anatomical shape, infiltrants are applied for at least 15 min for a better result. If the tooth has lost its anatomy due to wear or the stain is not masked, composite resins with opacifying properties can be used (shown in Fig. 43). For severe lesions, a combination of protocols may be necessary, and these may ultimately lead to restorative treatments. In conclusion, treatment options ought to be based on the principles of minimal intervention, the clinical expertise of the dentist, cost-effectiveness, patient's preference, and the expected longevity of the treatments.

Statement of Ethics

The authors state that subjects (or guardians) provided written informed consent for publishing images related to their dental treatment illustrated in this text.

Conflict of Interest Statement

The authors have no conflicts of interest to declare.

Funding Sources

There was no funding for the present manuscript.

Author Contributions

Jefferson Pires da Silva Júnior – contribution with data harvesting (case report), writing, agrees and approved the text. Rafael Pinto de Mendonça – contribution with data harvesting (case report), agrees and approved the text. Rafael Santos Rocha – contribution with data harvesting (case report), writing, agrees and approved the text. Daniela Rios Honório – study design, writing, agrees and approved the text. Eduardo Bresciani – study design, data harvesting, writing, agrees and approved the text.

References

1 Mittal N. Phenotypes of enamel hypomineralization and molar incisor hypomineralization in permanent dentition: identification, quantification and proposal for classification. J Clin Pediatr Dent. 2016 Jun;40(5):367–74.

2 Almulhim B. Molar and incisor hypomineralization. JNMA J Nepal Med Assoc. 2021 Mar;59(235):295–302.

3 Fearne J, Anderson P, Davis GR. 3D X-ray microscopic study of the extent of variations in enamel density in first permanent molars with idiopathic enamel hypomineralisation. Br Dent J. 2004 May;196(10):634–8.

4 Denis M, Atlan A, Vennat E, Tirlet G, Attal JP. White defects on enamel: Diagnosis and anatomopathology – two essential factors for proper treatment (part 1). Int Orthod. 2013 Jun;11(2): 139–65.

5 Schwendicke F, Elhennawy K, Reda S, Bekes K, Manton DJ, Krois J. Global burden of molar incisor hypomineralization. J Dent. 2018 Jan;68:10–8.

6 Bandeira Lopes L, Machado V, Botelho J, Haubek D. Molar-incisor hypomineralization: an umbrella review. Acta Odontol Scand. 2021 Jul;79(5):359–69.

7 Inchingolo AM, Inchingolo AD, Viapiano F, Ciocia AM, Ferrara I, Netti A, et al. Treatment approaches to molar incisor hypomineralization: a systematic review. J Clin Med. 2023 Nov;12(22):7194.

8 Sundfeld D, da Silva L, Kluppel OJ, Santin GC, de Oliveira R, Pacheco RR, et al. Molar incisor hypomineralization: etiology, clinical aspects, and a restorative treatment case report. Oper Dent. 2020 Jul;45(4):343–51.

9 Athayde G dos S, Reis PPG dos, Jorge RC, Americano GCA, Fidalgo TK da S, Soviero VM. Impact of masking hypomineralization opacities in anterior teeth on the esthetic perception of children and parents: a randomized controlled clinical trial. J Dent. 2022 Aug; 123:104168.

10 Fragelli C, Barbosa TS, Bussaneli DG, Restrepo M, Cordeiro RCL, Santos-Pinto L. Aesthetic perception in children with molar incisor hypomineralization. Eur Arch Paediatr Dent. 2021 Apr;22(2): 227–34.
11 Marouane O, Chtioui F. Transillumination-aided infiltration: A diagnostic concept for treating enamel opacities. J Esthet Restor Dent. 2020 Jul;32(5):451–6.
12 Brescia AV, Montesani L, Fusaroli D, Docimo R, Di Gennaro G. Management of enamel defects with resin infiltration techniques: two years follow up retrospective study. Children (Basel). 2022 Sep;9(9):1365.
13 Giannetti L, Murri Dello Diago A, Corciolani E, Spinas E. Deep infiltration for the treatment of hypomineralized enamel lesions in a patient with molar incisor hypomineralization: a clinical case. J Biol Regul Homeost Agents. 2018 May-Jun;32(3):751–4.
14 Lygidakis NA, Garot E, Somani C, Taylor GD, Rouas P, Wong FSL. Best clinical practice guidance for clinicians dealing with children presenting with molar-incisor-hypomineralisation (MIH): an updated European Academy of Paediatric Dentistry policy document. Eur Arch Paediatr Dent. 2022 Feb;23(1):3–21.
15 Marouane O, Douki N. Démarche diagnostique et thérapeutique pour la gestion des taches blanches de l'émail. Le Fil Dentaire. 2019;1:1.
16 Amrollahi N, Hashemi S, Heidari Z. Impact of molar incisor hypomineralization on oral health-related quality of life in 8–10 years old children: a systematic review and meta-analysis. J Evid Based Dent Pract. 2023 Sep;23(3):101889.
17 Dias FMCS, Gradella CMF, Ferreira MC, Oliveira LB. Molar-incisor hypomineralization: parent's and children's impact perceptions on the oral health-related quality of life. Eur Arch Paediatr Dent. 2021 Apr;22(2):273–82.
18 Fragelli C, Barbosa TS, Bussaneli DG, Restrepo M, Cordeiro RCL, Santos-Pinto L. Aesthetic perception in children with molar incisor hypomineralization. Eur Arch Paediatr Dent. 2021 Apr;22(2): 227–34.
19 Militi A, Sicari F, Portelli M, Merlo EM, Terranova A, Frisone F, et al. Psychological and social effects of oral health and dental aesthetic in adolescence and early adulthood: an observational study. Int J Environ Res Public Health. 2021 Aug;18(17):9022.
20 Hasmun N, Lawson J, Vettore M, Elcock C, Zaitoun H, Rodd H. Change in oral health-related quality of life following minimally invasive aesthetic treatment for children with molar incisor hypomineralisation: a prospective study. Dent J (Basel). 2018 Nov;6(4):61.
21 Attal JP, Atlan A, Denis M, Vennat E, Tirlet G. White spots on enamel: treatment protocol by superficial or deep infiltration (part 2). Int Orthod. 2014 Mar;12(1):1–31.
22 Brescia AV, Montesani L, Fusaroli D, Docimo R, Di Gennaro G. Management of enamel defects with resin infiltration techniques: two years follow up retrospective study. Children. 2022 Sep; 9(9):1365.
23 Bhandari R, Thakur S, Singhal P, Chauhan D, Jayam C, Jain T. In vivo comparative evaluation of esthetics after microabrasion and microabrasion followed by casein phosphopeptide-amorphous calcium fluoride phosphate on molar incisor hypomineralization-affected incisors. Contemp Clin Dent. 2019;10(1):9.
24 Vieira A, Emerenciano N, Moda M, Silva Ú, Fagundes T, Danelon M, et al. Treatment of molar-incisor hypomineralization: a case report of 11-year clinical follow-up. Oper Dent. 2023 Mar;48(2): 121–9.
25 Sundfeld D, da Silva L, Kluppel O, Santin G, de Oliveira R, Pacheco R, et al. Molar incisor hypomineralization: etiology, clinical aspects, and a restorative treatment case report. Oper Dent. 2020 Jul;45(4):343–51.
26 Baroni C, Mazzoni A, Breschi L. Molar incisor hypomineralization: supplementary, restorative, orthodontic, and esthetic long-term treatment. Quintessence Int. 2019;50(5):412–7.
27 Serna-Muñoz C, Martínez-Beneyto Y, Pérez-Silva A, Poza-Pascual A, Ibáñez-López FJ, Ortiz-Ruiz AJ. Perception, knowledge, and attitudes towards molar incisor hypomineralization among Spanish dentists: a cross-sectional study. BMC Oral Health. 2020 Dec;20(1):260.
28 Weber KR, Wierichs RJ, Meyer-Lueckel H, Flury S. Restoration of teeth affected by molar-incisor hypomineralisation: a systematic review. Swiss Dent J. 2021 Dec;131(12):988–97.
29 Krämer N, Bui Khac NHN, Lücker S, Stachniss V, Frankenberger R. Bonding strategies for MIH-affected enamel and dentin. Dent Mater. 2018 Feb;34(2): 331–40.
30 Chay PL, Manton DJ, Palamara JEA. The effect of resin infiltration and oxidative pre-treatment on microshear bond strength of resin composite to hypomineralised enamel. Int J Paediatr Dent. 2014 Jul;24(4):252–67.
31 Rolim TZC, da Costa TRF, Wambier LM, Chibinski AC, Wambier DS, da Silva Assunção LR, et al. Adhesive restoration of molars affected by molar incisor hypomineralization: a randomized clinical trial. Clin Oral Investig. 2021 Mar; 25(3):1513–24.

Eduardo Bresciani
Department of Restorative Dentistry, Institute of Science and Technology of São José dos Campos, São Paulo State University (Unesp)
Av Eng Francisco Jose Longo 777
São José dos Campos 12245-000 (Brazil)
eduardo.bresciani@unesp.br

Published online: July 1, 2024
Rios D, Santos-Pinto L (eds): Molar Incisor Hypomineralisation: New Perceptions. Monogr Oral Sci. Basel, Karger, 2024, vol 32, pp 236–260 (DOI: 10.1159/000538890)

Restorative Therapy of MIH-Affected Molars

Fernanda Lyrio Mendonça[a] Isabella Claro Grizzo[b]
Catarina Ribeiro Barros de Alencar[c] Daniela Rios[b]

[a]Bahiana School of Medicine and Public Health, Salvador, Brazil; [b]Department of Paediatric Dentistry, Orthodontics and Public Health, Bauru School of Dentistry, University of São Paulo, Bauru, Brazil; [c]Faculty of Nursing and Medicine Nova Esperança, João Pessoa, Brazil

Abstract

One fourth of teeth affected by molar incisor hypomineralisation (MIH) have required or will require treatment due to pain, sensitivity, or posteruptive breakdown. Restorative treatment becomes necessary in cases of severe MIH, characterized by posteruptive breakdown, which exhibits a wide range of clinical characteristics. Until approximately 20 years ago, all techniques, materials, and research were developed for treating caries lesions, not hypomineralisation. Research attempting to evaluate approaches to MIH treatment is recent and inconclusive. Therefore, there is still insufficient high-quality scientific evidence to establish a definitive clinical protocol for treating this condition. Recommendations based on best clinical practices can be provided rather than conclusions supported by a high level of evidence. To assist in clinical judgment regarding the best treatment strategy, eligible therapeutic options for restoring MIH-affected molars will be presented based on the strength and adhesive potential of the remaining hypomineralised enamel. The literature presents options for restorative materials ranging from direct alternatives such as glass ionomer cement and resin composite, through prefabricated devices, such as stainless-steel crowns and orthobands, to indirect restoration alternatives. However, it is essential to understand the indications of each restorative alternative and to know the restorative techniques, many of which are specifically developed to mitigate the difficulties encountered with the use of conventional techniques. Emphasis will be placed on the importance of adopting a personalized approach to restorative decision-making, considering the philosophy of minimal intervention dentistry and potential benefits for the patient's well-being and the family's needs.

Introduction

Oral health issues present a significant global health challenge, impacting approximately 35% of the world's population. Unfortunately, a considerable portion of those affected does not receive the ideal treatment [1]. This lack of access to treatment can be attributed to various factors. Furthermore, the absence of adequate oral health care has adverse effects on individuals' well-being and quality of life [1]. For instance, children experiencing dental pain may encounter compromised academic performance, while adults often witness a decline in workplace productivity. Consequently, society bears a substantial burden due to the widespread prevalence of untreated oral health problems [2].

When it comes to molar incisor hypomineralisation (MIH), the challenge becomes even more complex due to its multifaceted nature as an enamel defect, which introduces diagnostic complexities, thereby complicating treatment decisions [3]. This complexity is further heightened by the high prevalence of MIH across the globe. According to a study conducted by Schwendicke et al. [4] in 2018, the current prevalence stands at approximately 13.1% (11.8–14.5%).

Clinically, molars affected by MIH exhibit enamel with demarcated opacities, reflecting a structural composition characterized by a low mineral content and a high organic content [5, 6]. The mechanical stability of these opacities in the oral environment is contingent upon the degree of hypomineralisation; they may either maintain stability or become fragile, in the last case, predisposing them to posteruptive breakdown (PEB) [7, 8]. The stability of these opacities can elicit patient complaints regarding aesthetics, and some individuals may also experience hypersensitivity [9], topics that have been addressed in previous chapters. On the other hand, in cases of PEB, categorized as severe instances of MIH, there is a need to restore both the tooth's structure and function [10].

The clinical presentation variability of each MIH-affected tooth complicates the establishment of a standardized treatment protocol [3]. The determination of the most suitable restorative treatment involves careful consideration of factors, such as the child's age, emotional maturity, MIH severity, presence of hypersensitivity, and patient/parental preferences and expectations [11]. Deciding on the optimal technique and material is particularly challenging when teeth exhibit extensive structural loss. In general, students and professionals, both general practitioners and specialists, face difficulties in diagnosis, but their main complaints are related to treatment [12–16]. In most studies, the conclusion emphasizes the need for more information and training for the treatment of MIH [12–16].

This chapter delves into various treatment alternatives for molars affected by MIH and posteruptive enamel loss. The discussion on the various possible alternatives for rehabilitating molars severely compromised by MIH will be guided by the most robust available scientific evidence and by clinical expertise from specialists. Furthermore, the treatment possibilities will be presented comprehensively, highlighting their strengths and weaknesses. A particular emphasis will be placed on the importance of adopting a personalized approach to restorative decision-making, taking into account potential benefits for the patient's well-being and the family's specific needs. Recognizing the significance of family input ensures enhanced engagement, commitment, and cooperation throughout the treatment process [17].

Is There Reliable Scientific Evidence for Treating MIH-Affected Molars?

A previous study that estimated the global prevalence of MIH reported that 27.4% (23.5–31.7%) of these teeth did or will require the need for treatment due to pain, sensitivity, or PEB [4]. For first permanent molars with MIH and the need for restorative treatment, it has been proposed to use different materials, such as glass ionomer cement (GIC), composite resins (CRs), stainless-steel crowns (SSCs), and full crowns [18].

Despite the high-quality restorative materials currently available on the market, both in terms of composition and physical properties, treating molars affected by MIH remains a clinical challenge, even for specialized and experienced professionals. The assessment of available evidence on the treatment of teeth with MIH reveals limitations in supporting the effectiveness of treatments. These limitations stem from the methodological quality and risk of bias present in systematic reviews, as well as the overall quality of primary studies, which often lack long-term follow-up, among other constraints [3, 8, 19].

Though different treatments have been proposed for MIH with PEB, there is still not enough scientific evidence of good quality to establish a definitive clinical protocol for the treatment of this condition. Therefore, recommendations stemming from best clinical practices offer an alternative guidance for MIH treatment, particularly in the absence of treatments grounded in higher levels of evidence [20]. To assist in the clinical judgment of the best treatment strategy, the eligible therapeutic options to restore affected molars will be presented below according to the strength and adhesive potential of the remaining dental structure.

Insights on Important Steps of Restorative Treatment of Molars with MIH

How to Control the Painful Stimulus to Perform the Restorative Procedure?

Ultrastructural characteristics of MIH teeth lead to chronic pulp inflammation that has the potential to reduce the anesthetic effect and cause a painful experience for the patient during the treatment even after the use of anesthesia [21, 22]. In this sense, in cases of increased dental hypersensitivity, pre-emptive analgesia is favorable for the anesthesia of teeth with MIH prior to restorative procedures [23]. Pre-emptive analgesia is the use of analgesic therapy prior to a clinical procedure to prevent or reduce transoperative and postoperative hypersensitivity, commonly used in third molar extraction and endodontic treatment [24].

Vicioni-Marques et al. [23] evaluated the effectiveness of pre-emptive analgesia in children with severe MIH, posteruptive enamel breakdown, and hypersensitivity. Ibuprofen (10 mg/kg child weight) or placebo was administered, followed by infiltrative anesthesia and restoration with resin composite. The authors stated that dental hypersensitivity was reduced both during and after the procedure, providing increased comfort to the patient and ostensibly reducing anxiety, which contribute to an improved technique, thus increasing the chances of clinical success. However, the use of anti-inflammatory medication before the clinical procedure should not be carried out indiscriminately, but rather judiciously, specifically in patients experiencing chronic pain due to MIH. This pain can be identified through both the anamnesis and sensitivity tests involving air and percussion on the affected tooth.

Regarding the anesthetic solution to be used, a recent randomized controlled trial was conducted to compare articaine 4% with lidocaine 2% in terms of injection pain and effectiveness of anesthesia when treating permanent mandibular first molars affected by MIH. The results suggest that articaine 4% injection was more painful than lidocaine 2%, but both solutions were effective in anesthetizing permanent mandibular first molars in a sample of 20 children [25].

Despite these findings, it is important to highlight that few studies have been conducted so far to elucidate issues related to pain management during restorative treatment of teeth with MIH, and further investigations are necessary.

How Much Decayed and Undecayed Tissue Must Be Removed before Inserting the Restorative Material?

Patients with MIH posteruptive enamel breakdown require special care, both due to the presence of the alteration that brings an uncertain dental outcome on its own and because they are initially treated in childhood. Thus, it is essential to embrace a holistic approach to oral health care, known as minimal intervention dentistry (MID), which incorporates minimally invasive operative skills. MID, as implied by its name, is a philosophy that prioritizes preserving as much tooth structure as possible [26]. It emphasizes the early detection of carious lesions and the remineralisation of enamel and dentin through effective caries control measures [26]. Additionally, it advocates for minimal invasive operative interventions when necessary, promoting the concept of repair over replacement for restorations to minimize intervention [26]. The primary goal is to sustain the functionality of teeth for as long as possible [26].

To minimize the risk of pulp exposure in teeth affected by posteruptive enamel breakdown, adopting a minimally invasive approach during the removal of carious lesions is crucial [27]. Therefore, it is imperative to opt for selective removal of carious tissue [26]. This involves completely removing carious tissue from adjacent surfaces to ensure optimal adhesion of the restorative material, while selectively removing carious tissue from the pulp and axial surfaces. The selection of tissue for removal is guided by the characteristics of dentin [28]. The focus is on removing infected dentin, which is pliable and easily extracted, while leaving the affected dentin, which is resistant to cutting and has a leathery consistency [29].

In this context, the atraumatic restorative treatment (ART) concept is also recommended [30, 31]. ART results in low levels of discomfort/pain and dental anxiety associated with MIH [22, 32, 33]. The most user-friendly steps of the ART include the avoidance of anesthesia and the elimination of rotary instruments. However, in the case of children with MIH and dentin hypersensitivity, anesthesia may be required. It is important to note that the use of anesthesia is not contraindicated by the ART technique; rather, it is evident that for the majority of teeth, treatment can be performed without the need for anesthesia [30, 31]. Even in cases where the ART is not employed, the use of manual instruments for caries lesion removal can be a viable alternative to enhance patient comfort and improve the tactile sensation for the operator.

It is essential to consider that in the presence of posteruptive enamel breakdown, teeth affected by MIH may not necessarily exhibit caries lesions, as their causal factor is the biofilm imbalance due to sugar exposure [34]. When there is no lesion, within the philosophy of minimal intervention, remaining hypomineralised tissue removal is not required. However, in this chapter, the removal of opacities around the enamel loss to enhance the adhesion of the restorative material will be discussed.

Recommended Restorative Techniques according to the Strength and Adhesive Potential of the Remaining Dental Structure

Even when restricted to severe cases of MIH, there is a wide range of clinical characteristics, making it challenging to generalize treatment recommendations. The current literature highlights the analysis of lost structure and hypersensitivity as primary criteria [3, 35]. Nevertheless, the conditions of the remaining structure are equally, if not more, important, as enamel characteristics will determine the level of adhesion for the restorative material. Didactically, treatment options will be divided based on the strength and adhesive potential of the remaining dental structure, but for all of them, the discussion about the characteristics of remaining enamel will be addressed (shown in Fig. 1–3). Regarding hypersensitivity, data suggest that 34.7% of children with MIH and PEB experience sensitivity, which results from exposed dentin and/or hypomineralised remaining enamel [9, 35]. Ideally, the optimal solution would involve covering both dentin and hypomineralised remaining enamel with the restoration (shown in Fig. 4), but this is not always feasible. Depending on the treatment, in the event of

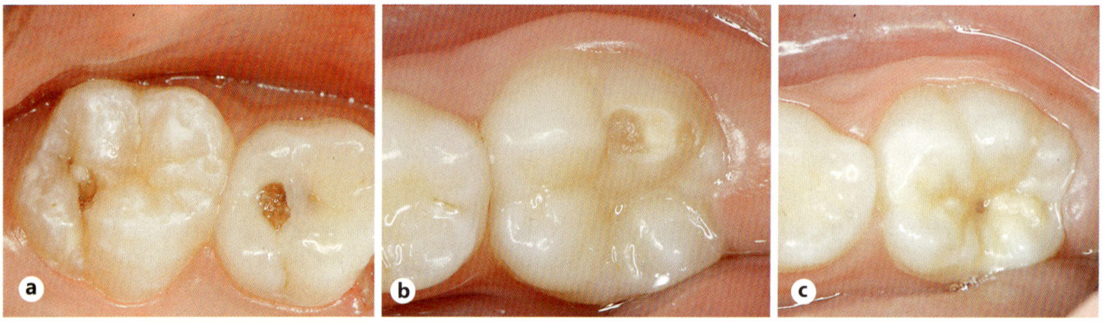

Fig. 1. In all presented MIH-affected teeth, the demarcated opacity covers less than one-third of the surface with PEB. In these instances, removing the opacities might be considered as a good option to enhance adhesion, as the enamel removal is minor and will not significantly impact tooth strength.

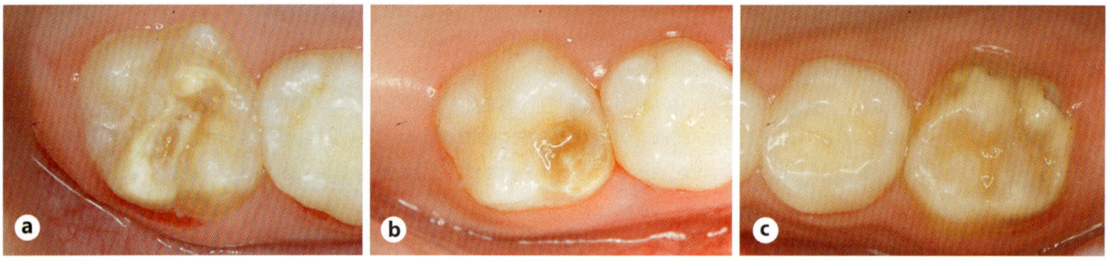

Fig. 2. In all presented MIH-affected teeth, the demarcated opacity covers up to two-thirds of the surface with PEB. In these instances, the removal of opacities may impact tooth strength. Therefore, a careful analysis should be conducted before considering opacity removal to enhance adhesion.

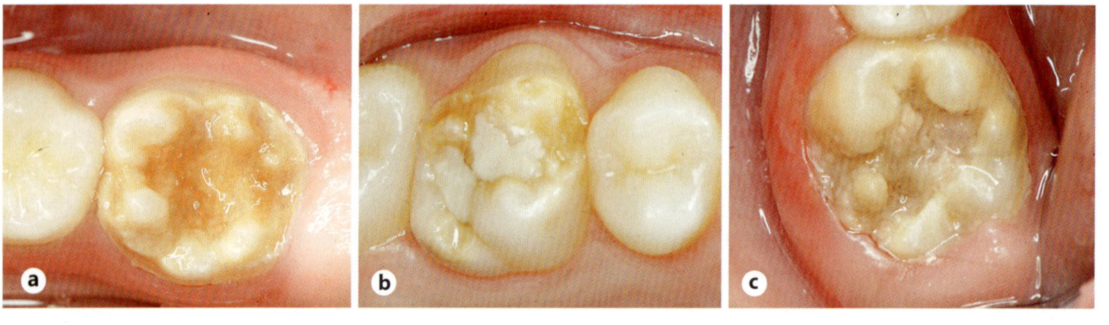

Fig. 3. In all presented MIH-affected teeth, the demarcated opacity covers more than two-thirds and the PEB affects more than two tooth surfaces. In these instances, removing the opacities will significantly affect tooth strength. In addition, pulp can be exposed and biological spaces within the periodontal ligament might be intruded upon when conducting hypomineralised enamel removal. Therefore, the opacity removal should be avoided.

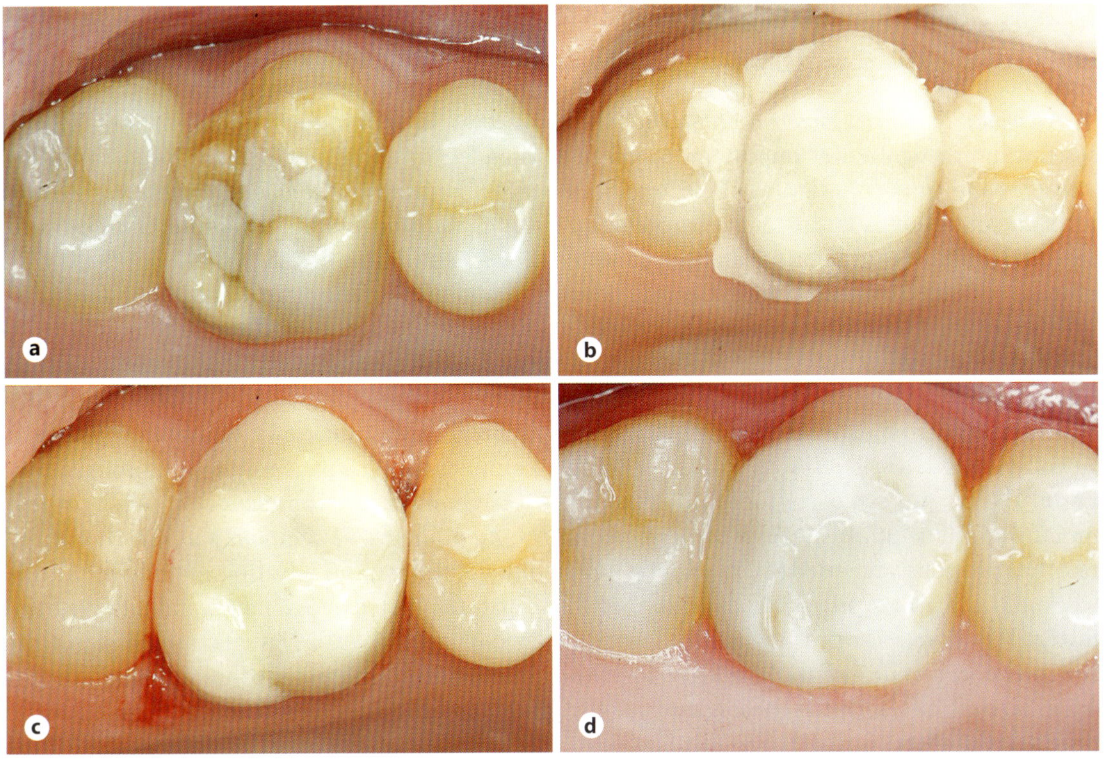

Fig. 4. A 12-year-old patient presented with an MIH-affected molar, featuring PEB. The patient's main complaint was pain while chewing, consuming cold or sweet foods, and during tooth brushing (**a**). The selected treatment approach involved the utilization of the simplified occlusal replica-adapted technique with GIC (**b**). The concluding phase of the treatment reveals that all enamel surfaces were covered with GIC. Subsequently, the patient no longer experienced any pain (**c**). A 4-year follow-up demonstrates the continued success of the case, with acceptable restoration and no pain compliant (**d**).

the impossibility of covering all the remaining enamel, this can be associated with mild MIH approaches for hypersensitivity.

Teeth with a Maximum of Two Surfaces Lost, Not Involving More than Half of the Area Subjected to Mechanical Forces

A. Restoration with Adhesive Materials

When the remaining tooth structure of the MIH-affected molars is not significantly compromised due to posteruptive enamel breakdown and/or caries lesion, conventional restorations with adhesive materials are recommended [3]. However, there are varying philosophies in the literature regarding the longevity of restorative materials, especially GIC. Some authors regard it as a temporary material, while others advocate its use as a permanent restoration option. Given that no material lasts a lifetime, how can we distinguish between a temporary and a definitive restoration? This reflection is crucial because GIC restorations are considered temporary by most authors studying MIH, while CR restorations are deemed permanent [3, 35–37]. Yet, there is no long-term clinical study directly comparing these two types of materials under identical conditions. On the other hand, there is a randomized clinical trial for caries lesion treatment that found no difference in the survival rate between these materials after 6 years of follow-up [38].

A1. Glass Ionomer Cement Restorations. GIC systems are recognized as important dental restorative and luting materials. These materials form chemical bonds to the tooth structure, are biocompatible, release fluoride, and are capable of replenishing themselves with fluoride ions originating from the oral environment [39].

Grossi et al. [40] evaluated the survival rate of GIC restorations placed using the ART technique in first permanent molars affected by MIH using an encapsulated hybrid restorative system (Equia Forte®). The success of restorations after 12 months of follow-up was 98%, a higher success rate than previously reported by Fragelli et al. [41] who used a high-viscosity GIC that was hand-mixed. Therefore, it is important to highlight that restorative technique and the type of restorative material used influence the success rates of the restorations.

The diversity of commercial brands of restorative GICs can be a problem when it comes to making a choice. The decision made at the time of selection is crucial. For example, a caries-related study evaluated the cost-effectiveness of a high-cost glass ionomer compared to a low-cost one. The results showed that after a follow-up period of 2 years, it was evident that restorations of high cost exhibited better survival rates, demonstrating comparable overall costs in comparison to low-cost GICs [42]. Therefore, the brand should also be taken into consideration when choosing the material. With the aim of assisting clinicians in choosing conventional GICs, a consensus was reached categorizing the laboratory performance of materials in various tests [43]. Eighteen ionomer brands were evaluated, 7 of which did not meet the minimum property requirements to be considered a definitive restorative material [43]. The best glass ionomer classified by this study was Equia Forte, which may explain the excellent results obtained in the study by Grossi et al. [40] and the difference in survival in the study by Fragelli et al. [41].

For the GIC restoration success, it is also important to follow each treatment step recommended by the manufacturer. Special attention might be given for the enamel conditioning (polyacrylic acid) and restoration protection from syneresis and imbibition (shown in Fig. 5).

Considering the critical need for a moisture-free operating field to perform restorations with a resinous material, in cases of partially erupted molars showing caries and/or posteruptive enamel breakdown in combination with insufficient compliance of the patient, the use of conventional GICs has been recommended [8, 44].

A2. Adhesive Restorations with Composite Resins. CR restorations are also an option for restoring teeth affected by MIH that exhibit PEB associated or not with caries lesions [10]. However, the literature is clear in stating that adhesion to hypomineralised enamel compared to sound enamel is limited due to the lower mineral content, high protein content, disorganization of crystals, and increased porosity [5, 6].

In an attempt to enhance the bond strength of CRs into hypomineralised enamel, a pretreatment with 5% sodium hypochlorite was proposed before restoration and the rationale behind this approach is the use of an oxidative/proteolytic agent to promote deproteinization to eliminate any protein content and thereby improve adhesion [45, 46]. However, studies have yielded conflicting results regarding the efficacy of this approach. Some in vitro studies have indicated that the use of sodium hypochlorite did not improve adhesion [47, 48]. On the other hand, a clinical study evaluated the performance of CR restorations associated with deproteinization with 5% sodium hypochlorite, highlighting good results in the retention rate [45]. Although this result appears promising, further clinical studies with a long follow-up period are needed to support this approach.

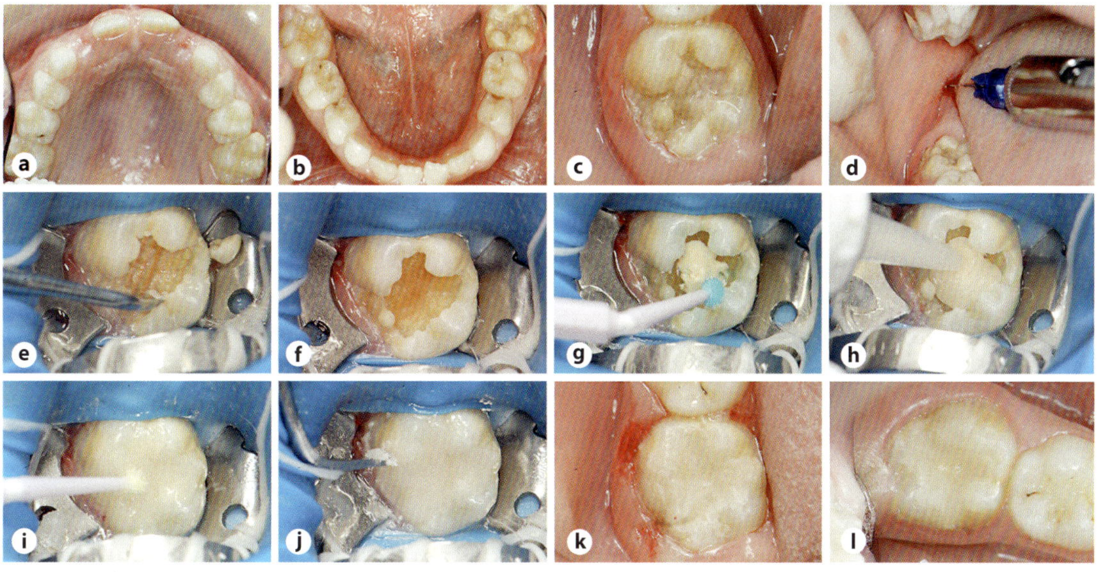

Fig. 5. An 8-year-old patient presented with an MIH-affected molar, featuring PEB and caries lesion. The patient's main complaint was pain. Initial clinical aspect of the patient's teeth, showing MIH in teeth 26 (**a**) and 36 (**b**). Clinical aspect of tooth 36, with yellow-brown demarcated opacity associated with extensive breakdown and caries lesion (**c**). Due to the patient reporting pain, anesthesia of the inferior alveolar nerve was administered (**d**). Selective caries lesion removal with hand instruments (**e**). Tooth aspect after selective caries removal (**f**). Indirect pulp protection with calcium hydroxide liner and application of polyacrilic acid on the dental surface to promote adequate adhesion (**g**). GIC (Equia Forte, GC) was then inserted (**h**), followed by the protection of the restoration surface with a coating agent (Equia Forte Coat, GC) (**i**). Removal of gross excess with hand instruments (**j**). Final clinical aspect of the restoration (**k**). Clinical aspect after 1 year of follow-up (**l**).

Another aspect addressed in the literature involves the complete removal of all hypomineralised opacities in the remaining enamel, aiming to achieve a cavity preparation with healthy margins [49]. Despite the growing interest in identifying optimal approaches for managing MIH-affected teeth [11], only a limited number of clinical studies have compared the effectiveness of noninvasive procedures, which retain hypomineralised tissue, with conventional restorations that involve the removal of all opacities during cavity preparation. In a study conducted by Linner et al. [44], the survival rate of composite restorations with removal and nonremoval of hypomineralised tissue was assessed after a 36-month period. The results revealed a higher success rate for conventional composite restoration (76.2%) in comparison to noninvasive restorations (29.9%). However, these data should be interpreted with caution due to limitations regarding the small sample size and heterogeneity between the groups that could influence results, since treatment decisions were individually determined based on factors such as defect size and cooperation, and did not follow a standardized protocol.

While the survival rate was lower for noninvasive treatment, this approach should not be viewed negatively, as it allowed the preservation of the tooth structure and can be a viable choice for managing patients with hypersensitivity, protecting the hypomineralised surface, and improving the patient's quality of life [44]. Furthermore, a crucial factor to consider when deciding the extent of opacities to remove is that MIH opacities have the potential to affect the entire thickness of all enamel surfaces (shown in Fig. 3) [6]. Complete removal of hypomineralised tissue may pose the risk of pulp exposure [27] and does not ensure adhesion, as seemingly healthy areas in hypomineralised teeth may still exhibit alterations in their ultrastructure [50]. However, in situations where the remaining opacities are minimal, the benefits of enhanced adhesion would outweigh the minor loss of enamel during removal (shown in Fig. 1). Therefore, the best approach is to exercise common sense and avoid generalizing the same procedure for all types of posteruptive loss due to MIH (shown in Fig. 1–3).

The long-term success of the resin restorations also depends on the adhesive system [10]. Bonding strategies for MIH-affected teeth have been evaluated; however, there is no consensus regarding the best adhesive system, whether etch-and-rinse adhesive or self-etch adhesive [10, 46, 48, 49, 51]. Krämer et al. [48] observed in vitro that although adhesion to hypomineralised enamel compared to sound enamel is limited regardless of the adhesive system, the bond strength with an etch-and-rinse adhesive was higher compared to self-etch adhesive. On the other hand, a clinical study demonstrated that although no statistically significant difference was observed, the survival rates were 68% for self-etching adhesive and 54% for total-etch adhesive. In this study, the teeth had initially been restored with GIC, which was partially removed before composite restoration [52]. Universal adhesive has also been proposed as an option for MIH-affected teeth, as this system offers the choice to either perform or omit enamel conditioning with 37% phosphoric acid [53]. Rolim et al. [10] showed that the survival rate of CR restorations using etching before the universal adhesive system in MIH-affected teeth was similar to the self-etching protocol at 12 months. In this study, adhesion was performed in a more resistant enamel since the opaque and fragile hypomineralised tissue was selectively removed. Furthermore, this study also showed that in the self-etch group, there was a reduction in self-reported postoperative sensitivity, suggesting that this system could be a feasible option for MIH-affected teeth. More precise information regarding adhesion to hypomineralised structure can be found in Chapter 17. An important observation that professionals can make in the clinic is to differentiate between adhesive failure and the breakdown of hypomineralised enamel around the restoration (Fig. 6, 7). This distinction can assist researchers in understanding whether material failures are attributed to the material itself or to the application technique. Unlike the treatment of dental caries, the restoration may extend beyond the cavity resulting from PEB to cover the entire tooth, thereby safeguarding the remaining enamel.

Teeth with More than Two Lost Surfaces, Involving More than Half of the Area Subjected to Mechanical Forces

A. Stainless-Steel Crowns

In addition to deficiencies in resin material adhesion, there are three other major challenges related to the rehabilitation of molars with PEB. The first of these is the extent of posteruptive loss, which can affect more than two tooth surfaces, greatly compromising the strength of the tooth structure (shown in Fig. 3). The second challenge is the enamel's resistance around the restoration of the tooth with posteruptive breakdown, which often exhibit opacities and may fracture over time, even after the tooth has been restored (shown in Fig. 6, 7).

Finally, when the patient experiences hypersensitivity, the restoration may not always alleviate the sensitivity, as the material covers the exposed dentin but does not cover the opacities around the restoration (shown in Fig. 4). Due to the presence of porosities, these opacities are unable to protect the pulp-dentin complex, and patients can still experience pain.

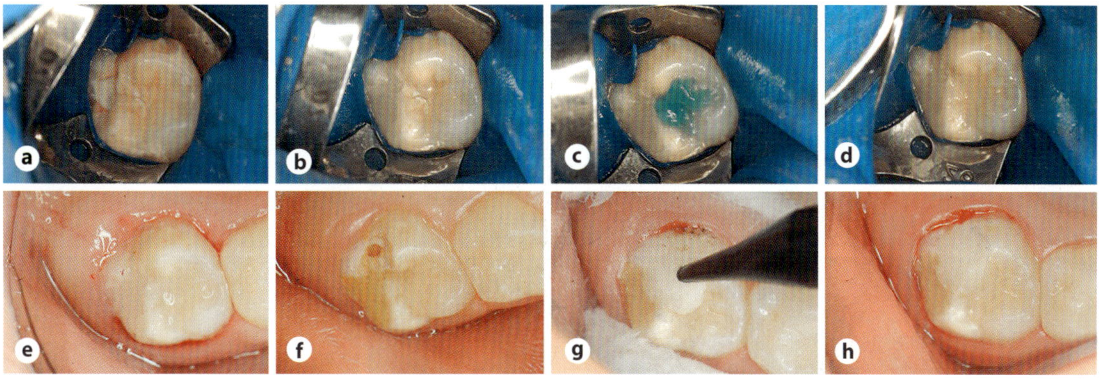

Fig. 6. Initial clinical aspect of tooth 16, showing demarcated opacity in occlusal surface associated with PEB in distal surface (**a**). The PEB area was restored with resin composite (**b**). The occlusal surface that presented demarcated opacity without PEB was conditioned with phosphoric acid and then the resin sealant was applied (**c**). Tooth 16 after the sealant application (**d**). Final clinical aspect, after finishing and polishing (**e**). PEB of the hypomineralised enamel surrounding the restoration (even the sealant and restoration were not capable of avoiding structure loss) (**f**). Restoration repair with GIC (**g**). Final aspect after restoration repair (**h**).

However, when dealing with molars exhibiting loss of structure and hypersensitivity, restorative treatment able to overcome all these challenges is mandatory to improve child's discomfort [11]. Preformed SSCs are a good alternative to restore the shape and function of dental crown but also to improve hypersensitivity by covering areas that just exist demarcated opacities due to MIH [54]. A previous study conducted by Fütterer et al. [55] also demonstrated that the use of SSC had a beneficial effect on patients' oral health. Patients experiencing hypersensitivity who received SSCs reported a reduction in discomfort, subsequently leading to an enhancement in oral hygiene [55].

A prior clinical case report outlined various indications for the use of SSC in MIH-affected teeth such as patients at a high risk of caries who demonstrated poor adherence to follow-up appointments, hypersensitivity relief, and the need to augment the vertical dimension. Although the conventional technique normally recommends tooth preparation for the SSC adaptation [56, 57], the case report proposed a conservative technique without tooth preparation [58].

To deal with the minimum intervention dentistry requirements, a more conservative treatment philosophy known as the Hall technique was indicated to seal caries lesions in primary teeth with the use of SSC and has shown good results in terms of caries arrestment and survival rate [59]. In this treatment, the metal crown is seated over the tooth with no caries lesion removal, no local anesthesia, and no tooth/crown preparation [60]. Although the Hall technique is a philosophy for the treatment of caries lesions for deciduous teeth, the use of SSC without dental preparation for permanent teeth represents a viable, promising, and minimally invasive alternative for severe cases of MIH (shown in Fig. 8) [61, 62]. This procedure has been used, and some authors consider the use of steel crowns without preparing the permanent tooth to be an adaptation of the Hall technique, since there is no removal of tooth structure [35]. However, we do not find this nomenclature appropriate. In the Hall technique, the crown is used to cover the caries lesion, preventing the lesion and biofilm from coming into contact with the sugar, while in the MIH, the steel crown is used to protect the opacities around the posteruptive loss

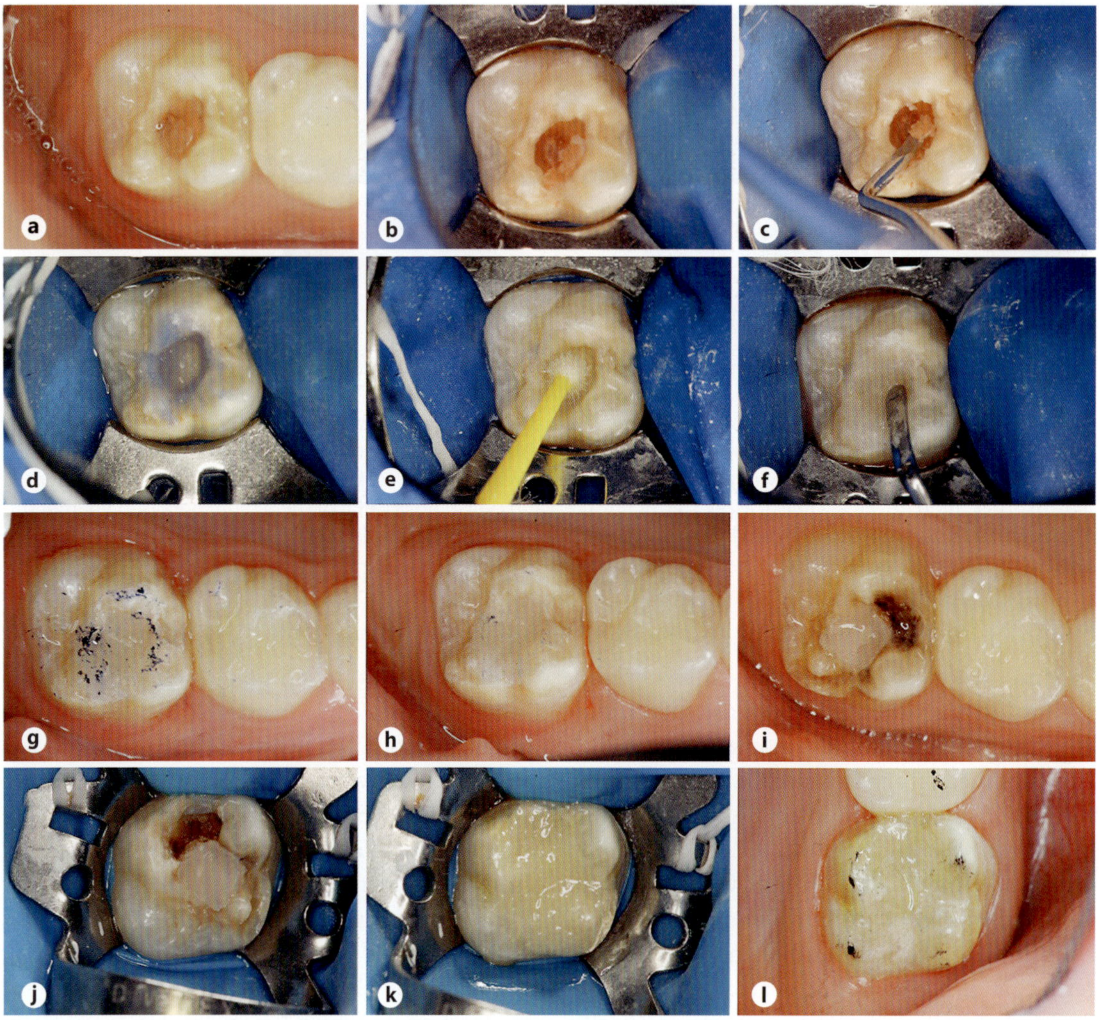

Fig. 7. Initial clinical appearance of tooth 16, which presents a demarcated yellow-brown opacity associated with PEB (**a**). The caries lesion can be observed (**b**). Selective removal of the caries lesion with manual instruments (**c**). Enamel conditioning with phosphoric acid (**d**). Application of a universal adhesive system (**e**). Insertion of CR in increments (**f**). Occlusal adjustment (**g**). Final clinical appearance (it is important to check that there is no premature contact) (**h**). Clinical appearance of the tooth after 1 year of follow-up, noting PEB in the opacity of the enamel around the restoration (**i**). No active caries lesion is observed (**j**). Repair of the restoration with GIC (**k**). Final appearance after restoration repair and occlusal adjustment (**l**).

from breaking, resolve hypersensitivity, and rehabilitate function. In other words, the philosophy that governs the Hall technique, paralysis of the caries lesion, is not used in teeth with MIH; the purpose is to preserve tooth structure and control hypersensitivity.

SSC has easy clinical execution, good cost-benefit ratio when compared to other indirect restorations and high success rate. In addition, the SSC usage promotes the maintenance of a healthy periodontium and length of the dental arch [39]. Farias et al. [61] evaluated the survival

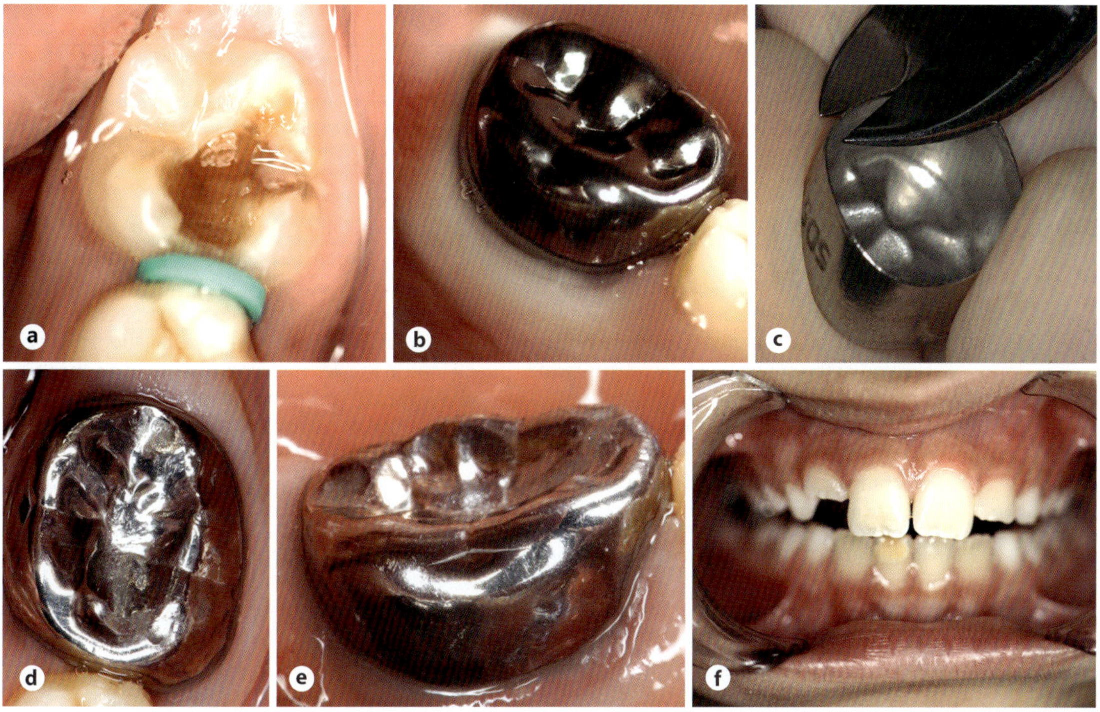

Fig. 8. Tooth 46 with extensive PEB (**a**). Crown test, showing ischemia and need to reduce its height (**b**). Removal of excess from the cervical region of the crown with gold scissors (**c**). Occlusal, vestibular, and lingual view of tooth 46 after the stainless steel crown cementation (**d** and **e**). Final patient occlusion, showing alteration of the vertical dimension (**f**).

of restorations with SSC or CR in first permanent molars with severe MIH. The results have shown that SSC had a significantly higher survival rate than CR over 24 months. The primary outcome was the failure-free survival time, but patient-centered variables were also considered as secondary outcomes. Patients who received SSC reported less discomfort when compared to those who received CR restorations. Regarding the vertical dimension, data from Hall technique studies [63, 64] demonstrated the re-establishment of the vertical dimension within a 4-week period. In MIH-affected teeth, the nonpreparation SSC conservative technique has raised concerns regarding patient openbite. However, Farias et al. [61] observed an initial opening of the bite immediately after crown cementation, which gradually returned to baseline values within the first month.

Despite good performance, the SSC does not have an aesthetic appearance, and the decision regarding treatment should involve the patient's family and consider the satisfaction and expectations of both parents and the child. Therefore, dentists should explain the treatment's durability, reliability, and the importance of preserving tooth structure in order to enhance parental acceptance [58]. Normally, children are not overly concerned about the appearance of SSCs [63, 64]. The clinical steps of this technique are shown in Table 1.

Table 1. How to perform stainless steel crown in molars with severe MIH [58]

	Clinical phase	Recommendation
Session 1	Pulp diagnosis and placement of an elastic separator on the proximal surfaces of the tooth where the crown will be placed	Do not floss in the interproximal space with the elastic separator
Session 2	The second session should be 24 or 48 h after the first Removing the separating elastics Tooth anesthesia and caries lesion selective removal with hand instruments (if necessary) Selection of the crown that best adapts to the tooth to be restored Make cervical adjustments with scissor and polish with stone Cementation should be carried out with glass ionomer for cementation	The crown that best fits the lost tooth structure should be chosen, so that minimal adjustments can be made Prophylaxis before crown installation In addition, immediately after installation, there is a change in the vertical dimension, but this change should not be any more than 3 mm Periodontal biological limits should be observed
Session 3	Recommend checking at 1 week and 1 month to ensure periodontal health and re-establishment of occlusion	

B. Prefabricated Zirconia Crowns

Prefabricated zirconia crowns for permanent molar were recently introduced as an option for restoring teeth severely destroyed by carious lesion or enamel developmental defect in children [65]. The advantage of zirconia crowns over steel ones is aesthetics. The main drawback is the need for dental preparation, as zirconia is rigid, requiring modification of the tooth to fit the prefabricated crown. Therefore, much healthy tooth structure is lost, not respecting the principle of minimal intervention, which is really a problem when considering a permanent tooth.

Currently, according to the World Health Organization, world life expectancy is 73 years. The first permanent molar erupts at around 6 years of age, and fractures due to MIH usually occur in the first years of the tooth's function [66]. Given that this tooth is anticipated to remain functional for at least another 66 years, health care providers who address molar in its early life bear a significant responsibility to conserve as much structure as possible. The final treatment decision should be made by the patient and their family according to their needs. However, for this, they must be informed in a language that allows them to make a conscious choice.

C. Indirect Restorations and Full Crowns

The use of indirect restorations shows excellent clinical performance in cases of MIH [44]. However, as already mentioned, especially during the period when MIH is identified, the child is young, and invasive procedures, with the need of tooth preparation should be avoided to enhance the tooth's longevity, adhering to the philosophy of minimal intervention. Linner et al. [44] reported a 100% success rate for ceramic crowns against 76.2% for conventional resin restoration, 7% for GIC, and 29.9% conservative resin restoration, in a 36-month control period. Singh et al. [67] compared the clinical performance of zirconia, lithium disilicate, and cast metal crowns as full-coverage restorations on MIH-affected first permanent molars. After 24 months, the crowns showed similar clinical success in terms of the criteria used to compare their clinical performance (retention, marginal adaptation, relief from hypersensitivity,

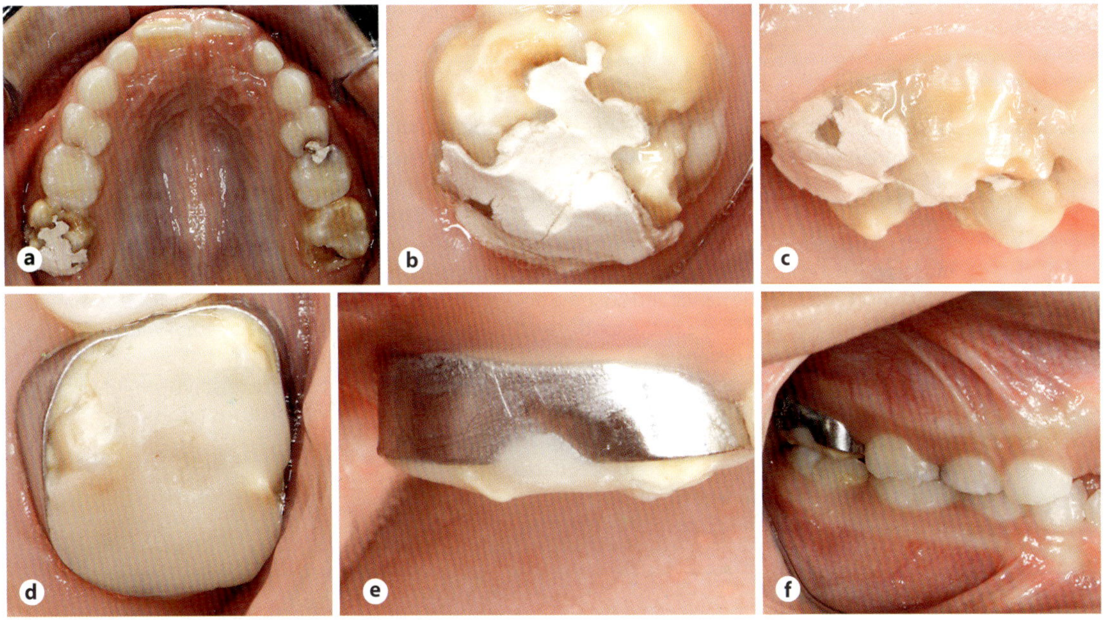

Fig. 9. Initial clinical aspect of the patient's oral condition with dental caries (**a**). Initial clinical aspect of tooth 16, which presents yellow-brown opacities associated with unsatisfactory atypical restoration involving proximal, palatal, and occlusal surfaces (**b**) and loss of subgingival enamel (**c**). Occlusal view of tooth 16 after orthodontic band cementation and glass ionomer restoration (**d**). Lateral view of tooth 16 after orthodontic band cementation (**e**). Final patient occlusion, showing no alteration of the vertical dimension (**f**).

proximal contact, and gingival health), with no statistically significant difference among the three groups. Therefore, the material of the crown does not influence the clinical success, but more studies with a longer follow-up are required to reach a definitive conclusion.

In dental restorations with a need for both durability and a conservative preparation, indirect composite resin restorations (ICRR) may be a possible solution for the treatment of hypomineralised permanent first molars and is midway between direct composite resin restorations (DCRRs) and full crowns [68]. ICRRs are thus an aesthetic alternative to cast metal restorations and preformed metal crowns with minimal microleakage [69]. On the other hand, indirect restorations are considered a conservative solution compared to full crowns and are characterized by greater control over laboratory procedures, systematic preparation, and reshaping of contact points [70].

Hakmi and Dashash [71] compared DCRRs and ICRRs for treating permanent first molars affected by MIH in terms of clinical performance. The results indicated that the clinical success rate was 90% in the ICRR group versus 85% in the DCRR group after 12 months of follow-up without statistically significant differences ($p = 0.218$). Children were significantly more satisfied ($p = 0.0351$) with ICRR than DCRR.

As already mentioned, the age of the child with MIH is a crucial factor to consider when selecting indirect restorations and full crowns, especially in early ages when they might be avoided. Additionally, other important aspects include cost, the child's behavior during the procedure, the extent of opacities in the remaining enamel, patient preferences, and other factors.

Table 2. How to perform orthoband restoration in molars with severe MIH

	Clinical steps	Recommendations
Session 1	Pulp diagnosis and previously separate the proximal regions of with separating elastics one day before the procedure (if necessary)	If it is not possible to complete this step-in advance, orthodontic rubber bands can be applied on the same day as the procedure, provided that the patient is willing to wait for a period of 30 min to 1 h
Session 2	Tooth anesthesia and caries lesion selective removal with hand instruments (if necessary) Selection of orthodontic bands and adapted according to the size and shape of the tooth, respecting the biological distances Application of 10% polyacrylic acid for 15 s Washing and drying the tooth surfaces Orthoband cementation using luting GIC After cementing the bands, the occlusal surfaces should be restored with high-viscosity GIC Occlusal adjustment and protection of the restoration again	In some cases, the tooth only has hypomineralised tissue, which does not need to be removed The material should be inserted using a commercial delivering system, digital pressure with finger might also be performed If you use sealant surface or adhesives for GIC protection, light curing for 20 s is necessary

D. Orthoband Restorations

When MIH-affected teeth experience PEB involving multiple surfaces, employing orthobands followed by GIC restoration could be a viable option to reinforce the dental structure [72] and mitigate the risk of additional fractures [73]. The orthoband serves as a substitute for the lost surface and functions as a protective shield for the subsequent GIC restoration performed after cementation (shown in Fig. 9). The orthoband restoration is also recommended when there is no available size of the SSC that fits the tooth size. The clinical steps of this technique are shown in Table 2.

To date, only one documented case report has addressed its use in MIH-affected molars during a 36-month follow-up period demonstrating favorable performance and improving hypersensitivity [73]. In addition, orthoband has been encouraged as a conservative and temporary therapy [35]. There is currently no scientific evidence supporting the recommendation for the use of orthobands. Clinical randomized studies are urgently needed to evaluate the long-term survival rates of these orthobands, confirming their classification as temporary therapy or potentially changing the indication to permanent. It is equally crucial to investigate their ongoing impact on periodontal health and assess patient acceptance.

Despite reports of using GIC inside the orthoband to fill the PEB, there is a need to explore the application of CR as well. Theoretically, bands could enhance the mechanical strength of the remaining structure, potentially compensating for adhesive deficiencies and improving the restoration's longevity. Two crucial clinical considerations to discuss with patients regarding the potential use of bands involve aesthetic concerns in individuals with wide smiles and challenges in establishing occlusal anatomical alignment when using GIC. Two positive aspects of this therapy include the complete coverage of the tooth crown, encompassing demarcated opacities of the remaining enamel and the straightforward execution of the clinical procedure, which also translates to a low cost. However, there is a lack of clinical research confirming these advantages.

New Treatment Options

Teeth with a Maximum of Two Surfaces Lost, Not Involving More than Half of the Area Subjected to Mechanical Forces

A. Silver-Modified Atraumatic Restorative Treatment

The silver-modified atraumatic restorative treatment (SMART) technique is originally recommended for treating cavitated caries lesions and involves two steps. First, the caries lesion is not removed but is inactivated using silver diamine fluoride (SDF) [74–76]. The second step involves applying a sealant/restoration with high-viscosity GIC [74–76]. The main idea of this treatment is to combine the inactivation of caries lesions with the use of the SDF while restoring the function of the tooth, using GIC [75, 76]. However, there is no consensus regarding the necessity of this technique for caries prevention compared to the use of SDF alone or the use of the ART technique. The literature indicates that the hermetic sealing promoted by the adhesive material cuts off the nutritive supply to the cariogenic biofilm, interrupting the progression of the caries lesion [77], not needing the association between SDF and restorative treatment.

In the case of molars affected by MIH, the objective of the SMART technique may differ, especially in cases where there are no caries lesions. In these situations, the primary advantage of applying SDF would be to reduce hypersensitivity not only in the area of enamel loss but also in the adjacent hypomineralised opacity [78, 79]. The main advantages of this therapy include its technical simplicity and treatment of opacities in the remaining enamel, particularly in terms of sensitivity. On the other hand, disadvantages include dark brown pigmentation in opacities due to SDF. When considering molars severely affected by MIH, the SMART technique may hypothetically result in enamel strengthening, as SDF interacts with calcium and phosphate ions, leading to their precipitation onto the tooth structure [80]. This could diminish the risk of future losses or improve the adhesiveness of restorative materials. However, these aspects require further investigation.

The use of SDF associated or not with glass ionomer restoration is considered a temporary therapy for MIH-affected molars [35]. However, the literature only provides studies on the use of this therapy for sealing and preventing carious lesions, which are not the main issues faced by MIH patients [79]. A recent study compared the clinical effects of SDF and the SMART sealant technique in molars affected by MIH with initial caries lesions and observed that both approaches demonstrated a preventive effect against caries [79]. Similar results were observed in another study, where GIC sealants proved effective in preventing caries lesions in MIH-affected teeth during a 12-month follow-up period [81]. Furthermore, it was observed that the SDF presented an effective desensitization when applied to teeth with hypersensitivity [78].

Resembling other treatment alternatives for MIH, the SMART technique needs to be studied in severely affected molars with PEB to assess various outcomes, such as long-term survival, duration of hypersensitivity relief, cost, and patient acceptance.

Teeth with More than Two Lost Surfaces, Involving More than Half of the Area Subjected to Mechanical Forces

A. Simplified Occlusal Replica-Adapted Technique with GIC

The simplified occlusal replica-adapted technique with GIC, also named RINA technique, can be an efficient indication not only to restore tooth morphology but also to improve hypersensitivity by covering areas that just exist demarcated opacities with a thin layer of GIC [82]. It is important to emphasize that this technique is more patient-friendly, as it does not require prior tooth wear and provides short treatment time, being more

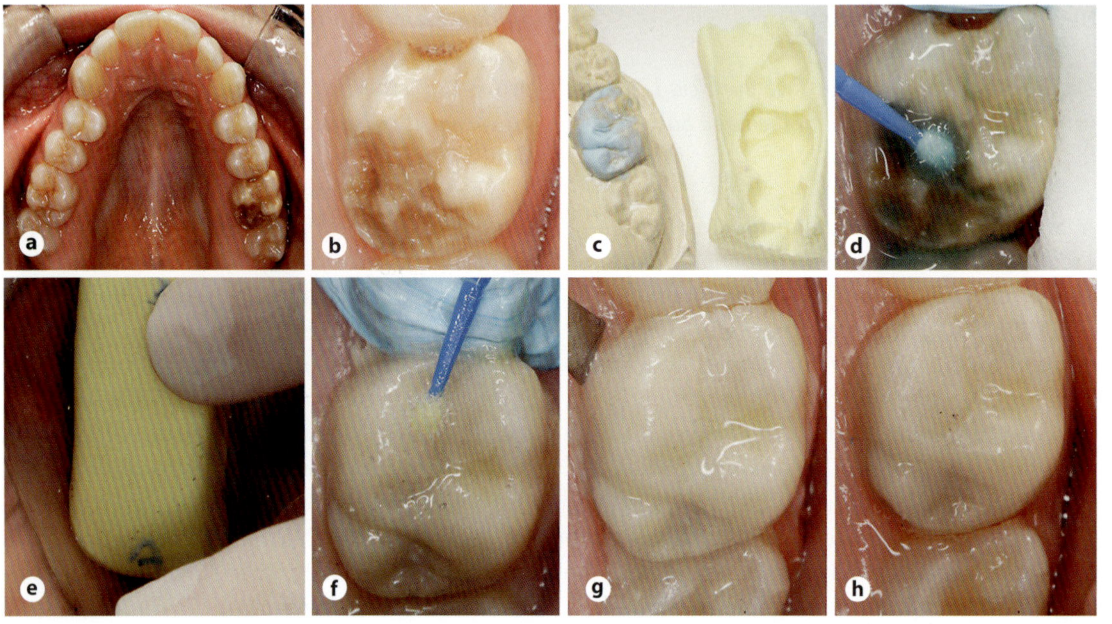

Fig. 10. Initial clinical aspect of the patient's oral condition with no dental caries (**a**). Initial clinical aspect of tooth 26 that presents yellow-brown opacities and PEB on the proximal, palatal, and occlusal surfaces (**b**). Wax-up to replace missing dental structure and silicone impression (**c**). Application of polyacrilic acid on the dental surface (**d**). Silicone impression was filled with GIC (Equia Forte, GC) and applied on tooth 26 (**e**). Protection of the restoration (**f**). Removal of excesses with hand instruments (**g**). Final aspect after finishing and polishing with rotatory instruments (after 24 h) (**h**).

comfortable and suitable for patients who do not present emotional maturity to undergo a more complex rehabilitation procedure [82]. Additionally, this approach aligns with the philosophy of MID, aiming to preserve tooth structure and prevent the cycle of repetitive restorations (shown in Fig. 10). However, there is only one published case report specifically addressing its application in MIH-affected molars, which showed a good performance in 18 months of follow-up [82]. In this case report, the glass ionomer used was considered the best brand in the consensus on glass-ionomer cement thresholds for restorative indications [43]. Therefore, randomized clinical studies with a long follow-up period and comparing different brands of GIC are necessary to determine its survival rate. This technique can also be tested with the use of resin composites, offering additional potential for clinical assessment. The clinical steps of this technique are shown in Table 3.

B. Digital Workflow for Restoring MIH-Affected Molars

The digital workflow has significantly enhanced the diagnosis, planning, and execution of dental treatments [83]. An important milestone in this technological evolution was the adoption of intraoral scanning systems that not only provide better and more precise visualization of dental structures but also offer patients a more comfortable experience compared to conventional impressions [84]. Furthermore, the digital workflow can accelerate some procedures steps, decreasing the patient's chair time and promoting a more efficient clinical practice [83].

Table 3. How to perform the simplified occlusal replica-adapted technique with GIC [82]

	Procedures		Recommendation
Session 1	**Clinical phase** Pulp diagnosis Maxillary and mandibular impressions with alginate or scan	**Laboratory phase** Tooth waxing (with wax, CR, or through digital flow). After that, copy the waxed tooth using silicone (polyvinylsiloxanes) to create the matrix necessary for performing the restoration. In the digital flow, the restoration guide can be printed.	The wax-up should be performed in the missing structure to recover the morphology, extending to the areas that just have demarcated opacities without PEB. Therefore, wax-up covers almost all tooth crown.
Session 2	Tooth anesthesia and caries lesion selective removal with hand instruments (if necessary) Relative isolation with cotton rolls Application of polyacrylic acid to the tooth; washing and drying Manipulation of the GIC and filling to the silicon matrix Positioning the matrix with the GIC in place and waiting for it to cure Removal of the matrix, application of the surface protector, and light curing Removal of excess with manual instruments, occlusal adjustment, and reapplication of the coat		No finishing or polishing with rotatory instruments should be performed in this session
Session 3 (After 24 h)	Finishing and polishing of the restoration with rotating instruments		This procedure should be done under irrigation to avoid surface drying and cracking

Understanding a digital workflow involves more than just handling equipment and technology; it encompasses comprehending the entire process until to obtain a final treatment result. The restorative process, using workflow, can be divided into three stages: digital model, design, and restoration impression. Considering the different systems available on the market, the dentist can just scan and send the file to the laboratory or also add design software within the system itself. Moreover, there are systems that enable dentists to perform in office all the necessary steps, such as conducting digital impressions, utilizing design software to create a restoration, and producing the restoration using an integrated milling machine [83] or resin 3D printer. In the context of MIH, the digital workflow holds promise as it enables more precise monitoring of the dynamic nature of this enamel defect. Storing data facilitates dentists' access to images at any treatment stage and aids in monitoring enamel breakdowns over time. This can serve as a useful tool to demonstrate to parents that the loss of structure can occur in different tooth areas and even after restorative treatment. Furthermore, it can facilitate the creation of a personalized restorative treatment plan, especially in cases where affected teeth display extensive PEB (shown in Fig. 11). For instance, in the simplified occlusal replica-adapted technique with GIC [82], the use of impression material can be replaced with scanning, and the wax-up to restore the missing structure can also be achieved digitally, using dedicated software. However, if the dentist does not have suitable software for this purpose, waxing can be carried out in the conventional way using printed mod-

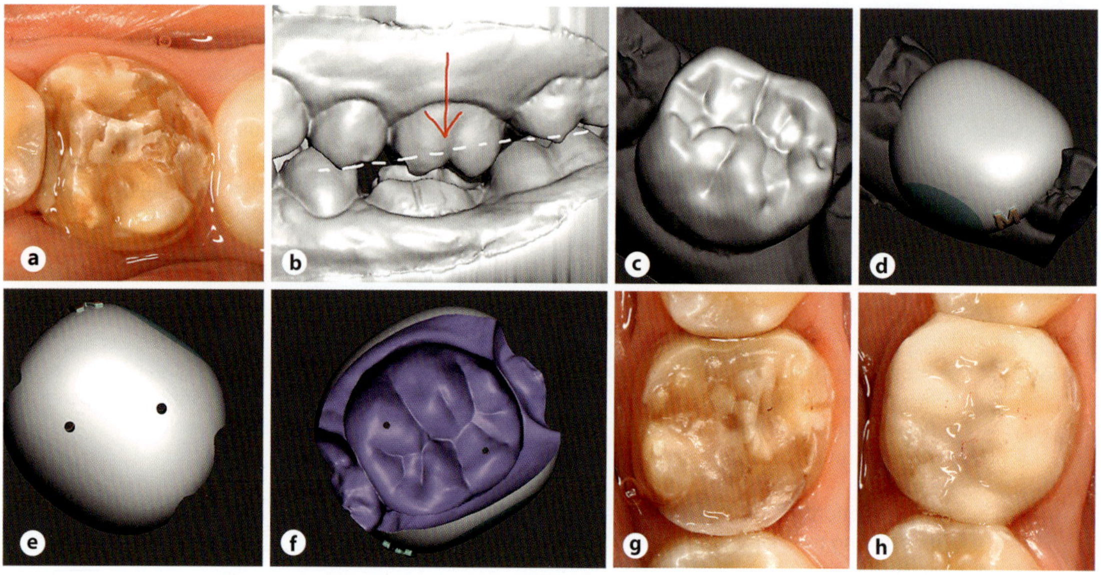

Fig. 11. Initial clinical aspect of tooth 36 (**a**). Digital scanning and waxing up were performed to reconstruct the missing structure of tooth 36 (**b** and **c**). The matrix design included two holes, aligning with the diameter of the injectable resin tip, which was produced through 3D printing (**d–f**). Direct resin restoration of the proximal surfaces (**g**), with subsequent placement of the transparent matrix on the tooth, resin injection, and photopolymerization. The final appearance after initial finishing (**h**).

els. It is worth noting that there is still no clinical study evaluating the use of digital workflow in the restoration of MIH-affected molars. Several aspects need to be assessed, including survival rates, the optimal material (milled or printed), cost considerations, and the learning curve of the technique for professionals.

C. Composite Resin-Injectable Technique

The evolution of adhesive dentistry has led to the recognition of flowable CRs as a viable option for different clinical situations, due to their enhanced physical and mechanical properties, associated with their ease of application [85]. Although there is a lack of randomized clinical study, the injectable CR technique has been performed as a minimally invasive option to restoring teeth, when the wear of the tooth structure is not mandatory [86]. In this technique (shown in Fig. 11), the restoration is carried out directly using a transparent matrix, making the procedure faster and more precise in terms of reestablishing the shape and function of the tooth. For this technique, the dentist must scan both arches to more accurately assess the interocclusal relationship. After that, the waxing of the tooth can be carried out digitally or the models can be printed and waxing carried out in a conventional way. In the sequence, the matrix can be obtained using a transparent silicone or be printed. In the clear matrix, two holes, matching the diameter of the injectable resin tip, should be performed to facilitate the resin injection and the excess material flow. In the clinical phase, the transparent matrix should be positioned, the resin injected, and polymerized. This technique provides an initial insight that must be evaluated before its recommended application.

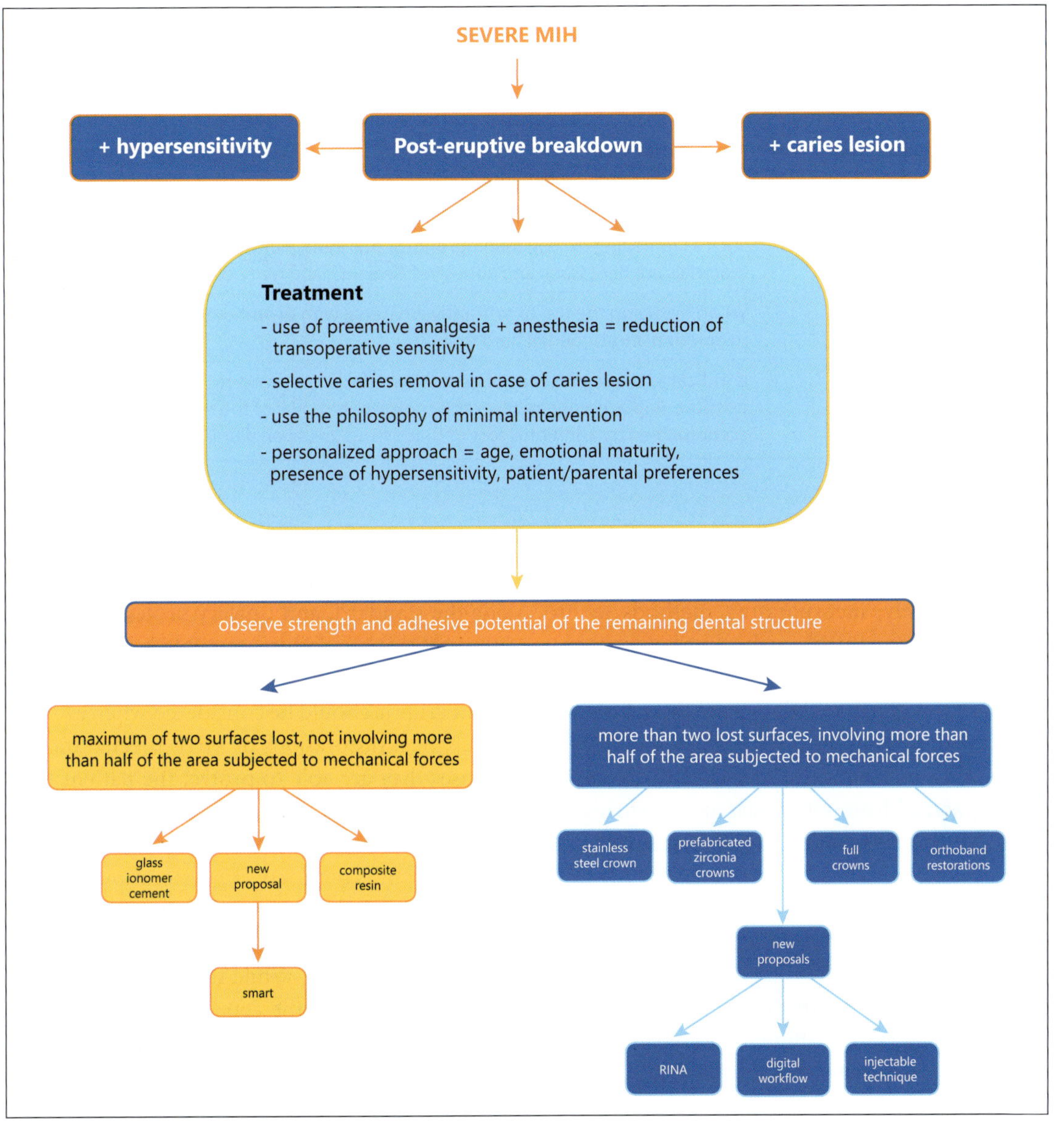

Fig. 12. Flowchart of treatment options for molars severely affected by MIH.

How to Minimize Failures in Restorative Treatment?

To enhance the success of treatments for MIH, clinicians should adopt several strategies. First, accurate diagnosis and comprehensive treatment planning are paramount (shown in Fig. 12). A thorough understanding of the severity and extent of hypomineralisation facilitates the appropriate selection of techniques and materials. Considering the expectations and needs of both the patient and parents is crucial for ensuring com-

Table 4. Four clinical options for dealing with unsatisfactory restorations, arranged in an increasing order of invasiveness [87]

Clinical steps	Recommendations
No treatment (monitoring)	When there is only a minor change in color or marginal imperfections that pose no harm to the patient if left untreated
Refurbishment	When small adjustments are made without causing damage to the tooth structure, such as removing excess, refining, and/or polishing. Furthermore, no restorative materials are necessary, and adhesives, sealants, and glaze can be used if necessary
Repair	When involving the use of restorative material with or without a preparation in the restoration and/or dental hard tissues
Replacement	Is indicated in the presence of generalized or severe problems when the repair is not possible. Replacement involves the complete removal of the restoration, typically accompanied by additional loss of tooth structure, even if unintentional

pliance. Furthermore, the dental professional should possess the expertise to execute procedure steps effectively, incorporating methods to improve moisture control, such as utilizing proper isolation. Additionally, proficiency in managing various types of patient behavior is essential. Last, implementing long-term follow-ups and regular monitoring of restorations is vital to promptly identify and address potential issues, ensuring the durability and effectiveness of the treatment.

Dental Restoration Repair

Since we are dealing with young children, restorations repair and refurbishment are considered feasible alternatives to increase the longevity of restorations and teeth, avoiding the repetitive restorative cycle [3, 8]. Generally, the likelihood of restoration failure increases with time, primarily influenced by chemical and physical factors within the oral cavity [4, 10]. In the case of MIH, this failure may also occur in a shorter time compared to caries lesion restoration, as hypomineralised remaining enamel is fragile and exhibits limited adhesion. Additionally, the restoration of MIH-affected teeth tends to be atypical, encompassing buccal, palatal, and lingual surfaces, and often lacks anatomical design [3, 7]. An important aspect is that atypical restorations are entirely outside the standard, and unwary professionals may interpret this as a failure, possibly leading to premature replacement with crowns. Therefore, different criteria should be considered when evaluating atypical restorations of MIH-affected molars. In cases they are able to protect the patient from pain, maintain function, and preserve dental structure, these are acceptable characteristics, and no treatment is required. If a restoration failure is indeed identified, it is important to initially consider the possibility of noninvasive procedures (shown in Fig. 6, 7). While there is not sufficient evidence regarding the repair of restorations in teeth affected by MIH, when dealing with an unsatisfactory restoration, it is crucial to identify the primary reasons for failure to minimize the likelihood of recurrence and unnecessary tooth wear. Four clinical options for dealing with unsatisfactory restorations are described in Table 4.

Conclusion

Among the diseases and conditions affecting oral health, the perception of MIH as a concern is relatively recent. Consequently, the majority of rehabilitative treatments employed for severe cases of hypomineralised molars are based on what has been developed for the treatment of cavitated caries lesions. Perhaps this is why both the selection and success of treatments have posed significant challenges.

As a result, future studies should concentrate on the development of materials and techniques specifically tailored to the rehabilitative needs of MIH. Moreover, the lack of scientific evidence in this field, which is in a period of intense evolution, should not deter clinicians from rehabilitating their patients to return to function and quality of life by providing them with the alternatives discussed in this chapter.

Ultimately, it is important to adopt a personalized approach to restorative decision-making, taking into account the philosophy of minimal interventional dentistry and the potential benefits for the well-being of the patient and the needs of their family.

Acknowledgment

We extend our thanks to the Bauru School of Dentistry – University of São Paulo, as well as to the parents and patients who place their trust in our work. Additionally, we appreciate the generosity of our partner companies, which provide essential materials, enabling us to conduct effective treatments and research.

Statement of Ethics

We state that the pictures of patients were obtained by patient's written informed consent for publication of the images.

Conflict of Interest Statement

The authors declare no conflicts of interest.

Funding Sources

I.C.G. and F.L.M. receive scholarships provided by FAPESP. D.R. is research funded by CNPq (Productivity Program).

Author Contributions

All authors have made equal contributions to the conception and writing of the work. The final version of the chapter was critically reviewed and approved by the entire research team.

References

1 Peres MA, Macpherson LMD, Weyant RJ, Daly B, Venturelli R, Mathur MR, et al. Oral diseases: a global public health challenge. Lancet. 2019 Jul;394(10194):249–60.

2 Kassebaum NJ, Bernabé E, Dahiya M, Bhandari B, Murray CJ, Marcenes W. Global burden of untreated caries: a systematic review and metaregression. J Dent Res. 2015 May;94(5):650–8.

3 Lygidakis NA, Garot E, Somani C, Taylor GD, Rouas P, Wong FSL. Best clinical practice guidance for clinicians dealing with children presenting with molar-incisor-hypomineralisation (MIH): an updated European Academy of Paediatric Dentistry policy document. Eur Arch Paediatr Dent. 2022 Feb;23(1):3–21.

4 Schwendicke F, Elhennawy K, Reda S, Bekes K, Manton DJ, Krois J. Global burden of molar incisor hypomineralization. J Dent. 2018 Jan;68:10–8.

5 Fagrell TG, Dietz W, Jälevik B, Norén JG. Chemical, mechanical and morphological properties of hypomineralized enamel of permanent first molars. Acta Odontol Scand. 2010 Jul; 68(4):215–22.

6 Crombie FA, Manton DJ, Palamara JE, Zalizniak I, Cochrane NJ, Reynolds EC. Characterisation of developmentally hypomineralised human enamel. J Dent. 2013 Jul;41(7):611–8.

7 Jälevik B. Prevalence and diagnosis of molar-incisor- hypomineralisation (MIH): a systematic review. Eur Arch Paediatr Dent. 2010 Apr;11(2):59–64.

8 Lygidakis NA, Wong F, Jälevik B, Vierrou AM, Alaluusua S, Espelid I. Best clinical practice guidance for clinicians dealing with children presenting with molar-incisor-hypomineralisation (MIH): an EAPD policy document. Eur Arch Paediatr Dent. 2010 Apr;11(2):75–81.

9 Raposo F, de Carvalho Rodrigues AC, Lia ÉN, Leal SC. Prevalence of hypersensitivity in teeth affected by molar-incisor hypomineralization (MIH). Caries Res. 2019;53(4):424–30.

10 Rolim TZC, da Costa TRF, Wambier LN, Chibinsli AC, Wambier DS, Assunção LRS, et al. Adhesive restoration of molars affected by molar incisor hypomineralization: a randomized clinical trial. J Clin Oral Investig. 2021 Mar;25(3): 1513–24.
11 Somani C, Taylor GD, Garot E, Rouas P, Lygidakis NA, Wong FSL. An update of treatment modalities in children and adolescents with teeth affected by molar incisor hypomineralisation (MIH): a systematic review. Eur Arch Paediatr Dent. 2022 Feb;23:39–64.
12 Yehia AM, Abdelaziz AM, Badran A. Knowledge, clinical experience, and perceived need for training regarding molar-incisor hypomineralization among a group of Egyptian dental students: a cross-sectional study. BMC Oral Health. 2022 Aug;22(1):323.
13 Delgado RM, Botelho J, Machado V, Mendes JJ, Lopes LB. Knowledge, perception, and clinical experiences on molar incisor hypomineralization amongst Portuguese dentists. BMC Oral Health. 2022 Jun;22(1):250.
14 Serna-Muñoz C, Martínez-Beneyto Y, Pérez-Silva A, Poza-Pascual A, Ibáñez-López FJ, Ortiz-Ruiz AJ. Perception, knowledge, and attitudes towards molar incisor hypomineralization among Spanish dentists: a cross-sectional study. BMC Oral Health. 2020 Sep;20(1):260.
15 Karkoutly M, Hamza B, Al Batal S, Al Barazi A, Bshara N. Knowledge, perceptions, attitudes, and clinical experiences on molar incisor hypomineralization among Syrian pediatric dentists and general dental practitioners: a cross-sectional study. BMC Oral Health. 2022 Dec;22(1):561.
16 Gómez-Clavel JF, Sánchez-Cruz FY, Santillán-Carlos XP, Nieto-Sánchez MP, Vidal-Gutiérrez X, Pineda ÁEG. Knowledge, experience, and perception of molar incisor hypomineralisation among dentists in the metropolitan area of Mexico City: a cross-sectional study. BMC Oral Health. 2023 Dec;23(1):1018.
17 Maciel R, Salvador D, Azoubel K, Redivivo R, Maciel C, da Franca C, et al. The opinion of children and their parents about four different types of dental restorations in a public health service in Brazil. Eur Arch Paediatr Dent. 2017 Feb;18(1):25–9.
18 Elhennawy K, Schwendicke F. Managing molar-incisor hypomineralization: a systematic review. J Dent. 2016 Dec;55: 16–24.
19 Gevert MV, Soares R, Wambier LM, Ribeiro AE, Avais LS, de Souza JF, et al. How is the quality of the available evidence on molar-incisor hypomineralization treatment? An overview of systematic reviews. Clin Oral Investig. 2022 Oct;26(10):5989–6002.
20 Weber KR, Wierichs RJ, Meyer-Lueckel H, Flury S. Restoration of teeth affected by molar-incisor hypomineralisation: a systematic review. Swiss Dent J. 2021 Dec;131(12):988–97.
21 Fagrell TG, Lingström P, Olsson S, Steiniger F, Norén JG. Bacterial invasion of dentinal tubules beneath apparently intact but hypomineralized enamel in molar teeth with molar incisor hypomineralization. Int J Paediatr Dent. 2008 Sep;18(5):333–40.
22 Rodd HD, Boissonade FM, Day PF. Pulpal status of hypomineralized permanent molars. Pediatr Dent. 2007 Nov-Dec;29(6):514–20.
23 Vicioni-Marques F, Paula-Silva FWG, Carvalho MR, Queiroz AM, Freitas O, Duarte MPF, et al. Preemptive analgesia with ibuprofen increases anesthetic efficacy in children with severe molar: a triple-blind randomized clinical trial. J Appl Oral Sci. 2022 Apr;30:e20210538.
24 Kissin I. Preemptive analgesia: why its effect is not always obvious. Anesthesiology. 1996 May;84(5):1015–9.
25 Haidar M, Raslan N. Comparative study of articaine 4% versus lidocaine 2% in the local anesthesia of permanent mandibular first molars affected by MIH: a randomized controlled trial. Eur Arch Paediatr Dent. 2023 Oct;24(5):621–30.
26 Schwendicke F, Frencken JE, Bjørndal L, Maltz M, Manton DJ, Ricketts D, et al. Managing carious lesions: consensus recommendations on carious tissue removal. Adv Dent Res. 2016 May;28(2): 58–67.
27 Gatón-Hernandéz P, Serrano CR, da Silva LAB, de Castañeda ER, da Silva RAB, Pucinelli CM, et al. Minimally interventive restorative care of teeth with molar incisor hypomineralization and open apex-A 24-month longitudinal study. Int J Paediatr Dent. 2020 Jan; 30(1):4–10.
28 Ricketts D, Innes N, Schwendicke F. Selective removal of carious tissue. Monogr Oral Sci. 2018;27:82–91.
29 Innes NP, Frencken JE, Bjørndal L, Maltz M, Manton DJ, Ricketts D, et al. Managing carious lesions: consensus recommendations on terminology. Adv Dent Res. 2016 May;28(2):49–57.
30 Frencken JE, Liang S, Zhang Q. Survival estimates of atraumatic restorative treatment versus traditional restorative treatment: a systematic review with meta-analyses. Br Dent J. 2021 Apr 21:1–11.
31 Garbim JR, Laux CM, Tedesco TK, Braga MM, Raggio DP. Atraumatic restorative treatment restorations performed in different settings: systematic review and meta-analysis. Aust Dent J. 2021 Dec;66(4):430–43.
32 Frencken JE, Flohil KA, de Baat C. Atraumatic restorative treatment in relatie tot pijn, ongemak en angst voor tandheelkundige behandelingen [Atraumatic restorative treatment in relation to pain, discomfort and dental treatment anxiety]. Ned Tijdschr Tandheelkd. 2014 Jul-Aug;121(7–8):388–93.
33 Simon AK, Bhumika TV, Nair NS. Does atraumatic restorative treatment reduce dental anxiety in children? A systematic review and meta-analysis. Eur J Dent. 2015 Apr-Jun;9(2):304–9.
34 Pitts NB, Twetman S, Fisher J, Marsh PD. Understanding dental caries as a non-communicable disease. Br Dent J. 2021 Dec;231(12):749–53.
35 Bekes K, Steffen R, Krämer N. Update of the molar incisor hypomineralization: Würzburg concept. Eur Arch Paediatr Dent. 2023 Dec;24(6):807–13.
36 Fukuda R, Yoshida Y, Nakayama Y, Okazaki M, Inoue S, Sano H, et al. Bonding efficacy of polyalkenoic acids to hydroxyapatite, enamel and dentin. Biomaterials. 2003 May;24(11):1861–7.
37 Yoshida Y, Van Meerbeek B, Nakayama Y, Snauwaert J, Hellemans L, Lambrechts P, et al. Evidence of chemical bonding at biomaterial-hard tissue interfaces. J Dent Res. 2000 Feb;79(2): 709–14.
38 Gurgan S, Kutuk ZB, Ergin E, Oztas SS, Cakir FY. Clinical performance of a glass ionomer restorative system: a 6-year evaluation. Clin Oral Investig. 2017 Sep; 21(7):2335–43.

39 Croll TP, Nicholson JW. Glass ionomer cements in pediatric dentistry: review of the literature. Pediatr Dent. 2002 Sep-Oct;24(5):423–9.
40 Grossi JA, Cabral RN, Ribeiro APD, Leal SC. Glass hybrid restorations as an alternative for restoring hypomineralized molars in the ART model. BMC Oral Health. 2018 Apr;18(1):65.
41 Fragelli CM, Souza JF, Jeremias F, Cordeiro Rde C, Santos-Pinto L. Molar incisor hypomineralization (MIH): conservative treatment management to restore affected teeth. Braz Oral Res. 2015;29: S1806-83242015000100271.
42 Olegário IC, Ladewig NM, Hesse D, Bonifácio CC, Braga MM, Imparato JCP, et al. Is it worth using low-cost glass ionomer cements for occlusal ART restorations in primary molars? 2-year survival and cost analysis of a randomized clinical trial. J Dent. 2020 Oct;101: 103446.
43 de Lima Navarro MF, Pascotto RC, Borges AFS, Soares CJ, Raggio DP, Rios D, et al. Consensus on glass-ionomer cement thresholds for restorative indications. J Dent. 2021 Apr;107:103609.
44 Linner T, Khazaei Y, Bücher YK, Pfisterer J, Hickel R, Kühnisch J. Comparison of four different treatment strategies in teeth with molar-incisor hypomineralization-related enamel breakdown: a retrospective cohort study. Int J Paediatr Dent. 2020;30(5):597.
45 Sonmez H, Saat S. A clinical evaluation of deproteinization and different cavity designs on resin restoration performance in MIH-affected molars: two-year results. J Clin Pediatr Dent. 2017; 41(5):336–42.
46 Lagarde M, Vennat E, Attal J-P, Dursun E. Strategies to optimize bonding of adhesive materials to molar-incisor hypomineralization- affected enamel: a systematic review. Int J Pediatr Dent. 2020; 30(4):405–20.
47 Gandhi S, Crawford P, Shellis P. The use of a 'bleach-etch-seal' deproteinization technique on MIH affected enamel. Int J Paediatr Dent. 2012 Nov;22(6):427–34.
48 Krämer N, Bui Khac NN, Lücker S, Stachniss V, Frankenberger R. Bonding strategies for MIH-affected enamel and dentin. Dent Mater. 2018 Feb;34(2): 331–40.
49 William V, Messer LB, Burrow MF. Molar incisor hypomineralization: review and recommendations for clinical management. Pediatr Dent. 2006 May-Jun; 28(3):224–32.
50 Bozal CB, Kaplan A, Ortolani A, Cortese SG, Biondi AM. Ultrastructure of the surface of dental enamel with molar incisor hypomineralization (MIH) with and without acid etching. Acta Odontol Latinoam. 2015;28(2):192–8.
51 William V, Burrow MF, Palamara JE, Messer LB. Microshear bond strength of resin composite to teeth affected by molar hypomineralization using 2 adhesive systems. Pediatr Dent. 2006;28(3):233–41.
52 de Souza JF, Fragelli CB, Jeremias F, Paschoal MAB, Santos-Pinto L, de Cássia Loiola Cordeiro R. Eighteen-month clinical performance of composite resin restorations with two different adhesive systems for molars affected by molar incisor hypomineralization. Clin Oral Investig. 2017 Jun;21(5):1725–33.
53 Jang JH, Lee MG, Woo SU, Lee CO, Yi JK, Kim DS. Comparative study of the dentin bond strength of a new universal adhesive. Dent Mater J. 2016;35(4):606–12.
54 Seale NS, Randall R. The use of stainless steel crowns: a systematic literature review. Pediatr Dent. 2015 May-Apr;37(2): 145–60.
55 Fütterer J, Ebel M, Bekes K, Klode C, Hirsch C. Influence of customized therapy for molar incisor hypomineralization on children's oral hygiene and quality of life. Clin Exp Dent Res. 2020 Feb;6(1): 33–43.
56 Kindelan SA, Day P, Nichol R, Willmott N, Fayle SA; British Society of Paediatric Dentistry. UK National Clinical Guidelines in Paediatric Dentistry: stainless steel preformed crowns for primary molars. Int J Paediatr Dent. 2008 Nov;18(1): 20–8.
57 Croll TP. Preformed posterior stainless steel crowns: an update. Compend Contin Educ Dent. 1999 Feb;20(2):89–106.
58 Grizzo IC, Bisaia A, Di Leone CCL, Di Campli FGR, Mendonça FL, Rios D. Revisiting the use of stainless steel crowns for treatment of molar-incisor hypomineralization: a case series. Gen Dent. 2022 Sep-Oct;70(5):62–6.
59 Midani R, Splieth CH, Mustafa Ali M, Schmoeckel J, Mourad SM, Santamaria RM. Success rates of preformed metal crowns placed with the modified and standard hall technique in a paediatric dentistry setting. Int J Paediatr Dent. 2019 Sep;29(5):550–6.
60 Innes NPT, Stirrups DR, Evans DJP, Hall N, Leggate M. A novel technique using preformed metal crowns for managing carious primary molars in general practice – a retrospective analysis. Br Dent J. 2006 Apr;200(8):451–4.
61 de Farias AL, Rojas-Gualdrón DF, Mejía JD, Bussaneli DG, Santos-Pinto L, Restrepo M. Survival of stainless-steel crowns and composite resin restorations in molars affected by molar-incisor hypomineralization (MIH). Int J Paediatr Dent. 2022 Mar;32(2):240–50.
62 Discepolo K, Sultan M. Investigation of adult stainless steel crown longevity as an interim restoration in pediatric patients. Int J Paediatr Dent. 2017 Jul; 27(4):247–54.
63 Bell SJ, Morgan AG, Marshman Z, Rodd HD. Child and parental acceptance of preformed metal crowns. Eur Arch Paediatr Dent. 2010 Oct;11(5):218–24.
64 Akhlaghi N, Hajiahmadi M, Golbidi M. Attitudes of parents and children toward primary molars restoration with stainless steel crown. Contemp Clin Dent. 2017 Jul-Sep;8(3):421–6.
65 Casián-Adem J, Cobos L, Waggoner WF, Fuks AB. Prefabricated zirconia crowns – a solution to treat hypomineralized permanent molars: report of a case. J Clin Pediatr Dent. 2021 Jan;45(1):8–11.
66 World Health Statistics 2023: Monitoring Health for the SDGs, Sustainable Development Goals. Geneva: World Health Organization; 2023.
67 Singh SK, Goyal A, Gauba K, Bhandari S, Kaur S. Full coverage crowns for rehabilitation of MIH affected molars: 24 month randomized clinical trial. Eur Arch Paediatr Dent. 2022 Feb;23(1): 147–58.
68 Feierabend S, Halbleib K, Klaiber B, Hellwig E. Laboratory-made composite resin restorations in children and adolescents with hypoplasia or hypomineralization of teeth. Quintessence Int. 2012 Apr;43(4):305–11.

69 Dhareula A, Goyal A, Gauba K, Bhatia SK, Kapur A, Bhandari S. A clinical and radiographic investigation comparing the efficacy of cast metal and indirect resin onlays in rehabilitation of permanent first molars affected with severe molar incisor hypomineralisation (MIH): a 36-month randomised controlled clinical trial. Eur Arch Paediatr Dent. 2019 Oct;20(5):489–500.
70 Dhareula A, Goya A, Gauba K, Bhatia SK. Esthetic rehabilitation of first permanent molars affected with severe form of molar incisor hypomineralization using indirect composite onlays-a case series. Pediatr Dent J. 2018 August;28(2):62–7
71 Hakmi A, Dashash M. Direct or indirect composite for restoring permanent first molars affected by molar incisor hypomineralisation (MIH): a randomized clinical controlled trial. BDJ Open. 2023 Aug 12;9(1):37.
72 Beretta M, Federici Canova F, Moscati M, Campanella V, Gallusi G. State-of-the-art on MIH. Part. MIH clinical management using ozone. Eur J Paediatr Dent. 2020;21(2):163–6.
73 Bagattoni S, Gozzi I, Lardani L, Piana G, Mazzoni A, Breschi L, et al. Case report of a novel interim approach to prevent early post eruptive enamel breakdown of molar-incisor hypomineralization-affected molars. J Am Dent Assoc. 2021 Jul;152(7):560–6.
74 Hu S, Meyer B, Duggal M. A silver renaissance in dentistry. Eur Arch Paediatr Dent. 2018 Aug;19(4):221–7.
75 Alvear Fa B, Jew JA, Wong A, Young D. Silver modified atraumatic restorative technique (SMART): an alternative caries prevention tool. StomaEduJ. 2016; 3(2):243–9.
76 Modasia, R., Modasia, D. Application of silver diamine fluoride as part of the atraumatic restorative technique. BDJ Student. 2021;28:42–3.
77 Lim ZE, Duncan HF, Moorthy A, McReynolds D. Minimally invasive selective caries removal: a clinical guide. Br Dent J. 2023 Feb;234(4):233–40.
78 Piovesan ÉTA, Alves JB, Ribeiro CDPV, Massignan C, Bezerra ACB, Leal SC. Is silver diamine fluoride effective in reducing dentin hypersensitivity? A systematic review. J Dent Res Dent Clin Dent Prospects. 2023 Spring;17(2): 63–70.
79 Ballikaya E, Ünverdi GE, Cehreli ZC. Management of initial carious lesions of hypomineralized molars (MIH) with silver diamine fluoride or silver-modified atraumatic restorative treatment (SMART): 1-year results of a prospective, randomized clinical trial. Clin Oral Investig. 2022 Feb;26(2):2197–205.
80 Mei ML, Nudelman F, Marzec B, Walker JM, Lo ECM, Walls AW, et al. Formation of fluorohydroxyapatite with silver diamine fluoride. J Dent Res. 2017 Sep;96(10):1122–8.
81 Schraverus MS, Olegário IC, Bonifácio CC, González APR, Pedroza M, Hesse D. Glass ionomer sealants can prevent dental caries but cannot prevent posteruptive breakdown on molars affected by molar incisor hypomineralization: one-year results of a randomized clinical trial. Caries Res. 2021;55(4):301–9.
82 Mendonça FL, Di Leone CCL, Grizzo IC, Cruvinel T, de Oliveira TM, Navarro MFL, et al. Simplified occlusal replica adapted technique with glass ionomer cement for molar-incisor hypomineralization-affected molars: an 18-month follow-up. J Am Dent Assoc. 2020 Sep; 151(9):678–83.
83 Fung L, Brisebois P. Implementing digital dentistry into your esthetic dental practice. Dent Clin North Am. 2020 Oct; 64(4):645–57.
84 Serrano-Velasco D, Martín-Vacas A, Paz-Cortés MM, Giovannini G, Cintora-López P, Aragoneses JM. Intraoral scanners in children: evaluation of the patient perception, reliability and reproducibility, and chairside time – a systematic review. Front Pediatr. 2023 Jun 26;11:1213072.
85 Badr C, Spagnuolo G, Amenta F, Khairallah C, Mahdi SS, Daher E, et al. A two-year. Comparative evaluation of clinical performance of a nanohybrid composite resin to a flowable composite resin. J Funct Biomater. 2021 Sep 9; 12(3):51.
86 Geštakovski D. The injectable composite resin technique: biocopy of a natural tooth – advantages of digital planning. Int J Esthet Dent. 2021 Aug 17;16(3): 280–99.
87 Hickel R, Brüshaver K, Ilie N. Repair of restorations – criteria for decision making and clinical recommendations. Dent Mater. 2013 Jan;29(1):28–50.

Daniela Rios
Department of Paediatric Dentistry, Orthodontics and Public Health
Bauru School of Dentistry, University of São Paulo
Alameda Dr Octávio Pinheiro Brisolla, 9–75, Bauru 17012-101 (Brazil)
danirios@usp.br

Published online: July 1, 2024

Rios D, Santos-Pinto L (eds): Molar Incisor Hypomineralisation: New Perceptions. Monogr Oral Sci. Basel, Karger, 2024, vol 32, pp 261–273 (DOI: 10.1159/000538892)

Orthodontic Analysis behind the Extraction of Hypomineralised First Molars

Daniela Garib[a, b] Daniela Rios[c] Thales Lippi Ciantelli[d] Felicia Miranda[a, b]

[a]Department of Orthodontics, Bauru Dental School, University of São Paulo, Bauru, Brazil; [b]Department of Orthodontics, Hospital of Rehabilitation of Craniofacial Anomalies, University of São Paulo, Bauru, Brazil; [c]Department of Pediatric Dentistry, Bauru Dental School, University of São Paulo, Bauru, Brazil; [d]Department of Orthodontics, UniCPO Faculty (UniCPO), Sorocaba, Brazil

Abstract

This chapter will discuss the orthodontic perspective of extractions of compromised first permanent molars (cFPMs) due to hypomineralisation. The context behind the diagnosis of a poor prognosis of cFPM that would support the planning of extractions will be presented. In addition, the ideal timing for interceptive extraction of cFPM as well as the favorable and unfavorable orthodontic scenarios for extractions in the permanent dentition will be discussed.

Introduction

First permanent molars with poor prognosis due to molar incisor hypomineralisation (MIH) may be candidates for extractions [1]. However, an orthodontic analysis is necessary before the extraction of compromised first permanent molars (cFPMs). The development of the occlusion is influenced by the extraction of the first permanent molars. The success of this intervention will depend on the timing of the interceptive extraction, mainly in the mandibular arch. The sagittal interarch relationship, the presence of dental crowding, tooth agenesis, the presence of third molars, and the stage of dental development need to be assessed before the recommendation of extraction of cFPMs [1–3].

In the permanent dentition, some types of malocclusions present a more favorable scenario for atypical extraction of first permanent molars with poor prognosis. This chapter will discuss the indications and the ideal timing for early extraction of first permanent molars with severe hypomineralisation. The favorable and unfavorable orthodontic scenarios for extractions in permanent dentition will also be presented.

In Which Cases Can the Extraction of Molars with MIH Be Considered as a Treatment Alternative?

MIH is a developmental enamel defect characterized by a range of clinical manifestations [4]. The defect is marked by enamel with elevated organic content, primarily proteins, lower mineral content, and less organized hydroxyapatites compared to unaffected enamel [5, 6]. The extent and intensity of hypomineralisation can vary, resulting in small or extensive creamy-white to yellow-brown demarcated opacities affecting one or all surfaces of the tooth crown [4]. Moreover, the degree of brownish-yellow staining correlates with the enamel's fragility, making it more prone to posteruptive breakdown (PEB) [7]. These fractures may lead to the development of caries lesions in patients with unbalanced dental plaque by cariogenic diet and to atypical restorations that lack typical conformations [8]. It is important to note that MIH does not symmetrically compromise molars; therefore, predicting the number or extent of compromised molars in the case of MIH is not possible [4]. These characteristics can only be determined after the eruption of all four first permanent molars.

Due to the considerable variability in clinical characteristics, establishing a precise cutoff point for considering molar extraction as an alternative treatment for MIH-affected teeth is challenging. Didactically, MIH is categorized as mild when only a localized opacity is present and severe when there are demarcated enamel opacities with PEB, caries lesions, and/or atypical restorations [9]. Both mild and severe MIH cases may involve hypersensitivity [10]. From a practical standpoint, advocating tooth extraction for mild cases is not plausible, as conservative procedures are available, even when accompanied by painful symptoms (refer to Chapter 13). Therefore, for severe MIH cases, tooth extraction can be considered as a treatment alternative [9], if various factors are taken into account, including the number of affected surfaces, adhesion capabilities, the necessity for lifelong treatment, cost implications, and parental preferences.

As discussed in Chapter 17, the adhesion of adhesive systems to the hypomineralised area is deficient [11], resulting in a low survival rate for restorations [12]. This, in turn, necessitates more frequent consultations for repair or replacement of restorations throughout life, children diagnosed with MIH reportedly experience treatment 10 times more frequently than their counterparts without MIH [13]. This fact might ultimately increase the overall cost of treatment. A recent study evaluated the cost-effectiveness of retaining one or more cFPM affected by dental caries or enamel hypomineralisation, compared to timely extraction of them in children aged 8 years. The retention of one or two cFPMs has proven to be a more cost-effective choice compared to the early removal of the same teeth under general anesthesia (GA). Maintaining a cFPM comes with higher costs when compared to its early removal under local anesthesia or, alternatively, the extraction of four cFPMs under GA [14]. As per the findings, extraction becomes a more cost-effective alternative only when performed under local anesthesia or when the removal of four cFPMs is deemed necessary [14]. Conversely, another study highlighted that the most influential factors in cost-effectiveness are the timing of extraction (and the subsequent need for orthodontic alignment, incurring significant costs) and the number of molars requiring treatment per patient [15]. Extraction and orthodontic alignment of the second and third molars consistently emerge as the most cost-effective and efficient option, particularly when more than one molar is affected [15]. In contrast, both resin composite restorations and indirect metal crowns, following temporization using a preformed metal crown, prove to be more expensive and less effective in such scenarios [15]. For single molars where the likelihood of spontaneous alignment is low, resin composite restorations might be considered [15].

There is no evidence in the literature supporting a specific threshold of hypomineralisation severity that indicates extraction. However, the higher the number of surfaces with posteruptive fractures and loss margins in hypomineralised enamel, particularly in the case of yellow-brown discoloration, the higher the likelihood of restoration failures [12]. This may result in repetitive

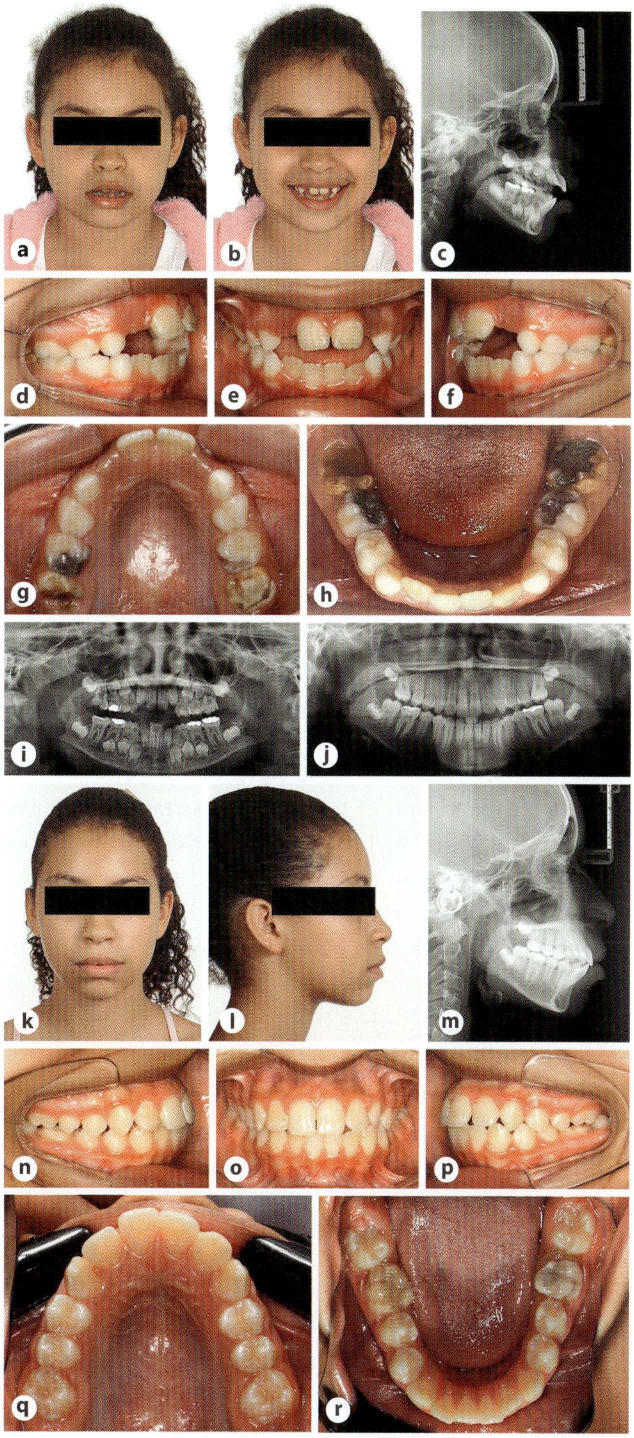

Fig. 1. a–i Initial records of a patient with severely hypomineralised permanent first molars. In the early mixed dentition, a Class I canine relationship was observed bilaterally with an anterior open bite. Interceptive extraction of the maxillary first permanent molars was performed at 8.5 years of age. An interceptive orthodontic treatment was performed to correct the anterior open bite. **j–r** The same patient returned for comprehensive orthodontic treatment at age 12 years. At this time, in the permanent dentition, maxillary second permanent molars had successfully erupted in the place of the permanent first molars. The patient presented with a Class III relationship on the right side, class I on the left side, mandibular dental midline deviation for the left side, and a Class I facial pattern. An asymmetrical extraction of the mandibular right permanent first molar was planned. No extraction was planned for the left side.

restorative cycles and the eventual need for more expensive and complex rehabilitative treatments, such as endodontics, prosthetics, and implants in the long term. Therefore, in this case, the first permanent molar extraction might be an alternative treatment [9, 16].

Given the evidence, the complexity of indicating the extraction of cFPMs as a treatment alternative becomes evident. Initially, it is crucial to analyze the characteristics of the molars individually. Severe structural compromises, posteruptive fractures exposing dentin and affecting the occlusal surface, or compromising two or more surfaces of the tooth, are indications that extraction may be considered as an alternative. Subsequently, it is necessary to consider the patient holistically, taking into account the number of compromised teeth. When all four molars are involved, extraction appears to be a good alternative. Conversely, when only one tooth is compromised, restoration also emerges as a good option, considering the cost-effectiveness. However, this statement holds true only when the extraction is performed at the appropriate time. It is important to highlight that other factors must be considered, such as crowding and the presence and type of malocclusion, as will be discussed next.

Finally, the last factor is shared decision-making, a collaborative process where individuals and their health care providers work together to decide on the best course of action for their care [17]. However, for this person-centered care approach to be effective, individuals must comprehend the risks, benefits, and potential outcomes of different options through dialog and information exchange [18]. Achieving this understanding is a challenging task that heavily relies on the dentist's perspective and the patient's level of health literacy [18]. In the case of a severely affected first permanent molar with MIH, the caregivers of the child must be aware of all the pros and cons of maintaining or extracting the tooth, as well as the favorable and unfavorable orthodontic scenarios, to make an informed decision.

What Is the Ideal Timing for Early Extraction of First Permanent Molars with Severe Hypomineralisation?

When a poor prognosis for the cFPM is established in the mixed dentition, the extraction of the cFPM is followed by a mesial movement of the second and third molar germs (shown in Fig. 1, 2). The space closure occurs spontaneously, and the mesiodistal angulation of second and third molars is acceptable after eruption in the dental arch. However, other factors such as age, the presence or absence of the third molar germ, the angulation of the second molar germ, and location (maxilla or mandible) could affect the spontaneous space closure. Previous studies showed a 50–80% rate of cFPM extraction in patients with MIH [19, 20]. A recent study from the University of Oslo among pediatric patients with the need for cFPM extraction reported that approximately 59% had all four molars extracted, 19% had three, 19% had two, and 3% had one extraction [21]. The treatment decision should be performed among an interdisciplinary team including the general practitioner, the pediatric dentist, and an orthodontist.

The major advantage of cFPM extraction performed in the mixed dentition is that the second molar substitution occurs avoiding costs and burden of care related to frequent restorative procedures in the cFPM. In addition, pain and discomfort related to first molar hypomineralisation are solved with cFPM extraction. The early extraction of cFPM also decreases the frequency of third molar impaction [3]. The presence of the third

Fig. 2. a–l Orthodontic treatment performed in the patient presented in Figure 1. After a 31-month orthodontic treatment period, a bilateral Class I relationship with coincident dental midlines and normal overjet and overbite was observed. No changes were observed in the facial profile. **m–u** A 1.5-year follow-up shows the stability of the occlusal outcomes and of the extraction space closure.

(For figure see next page.)

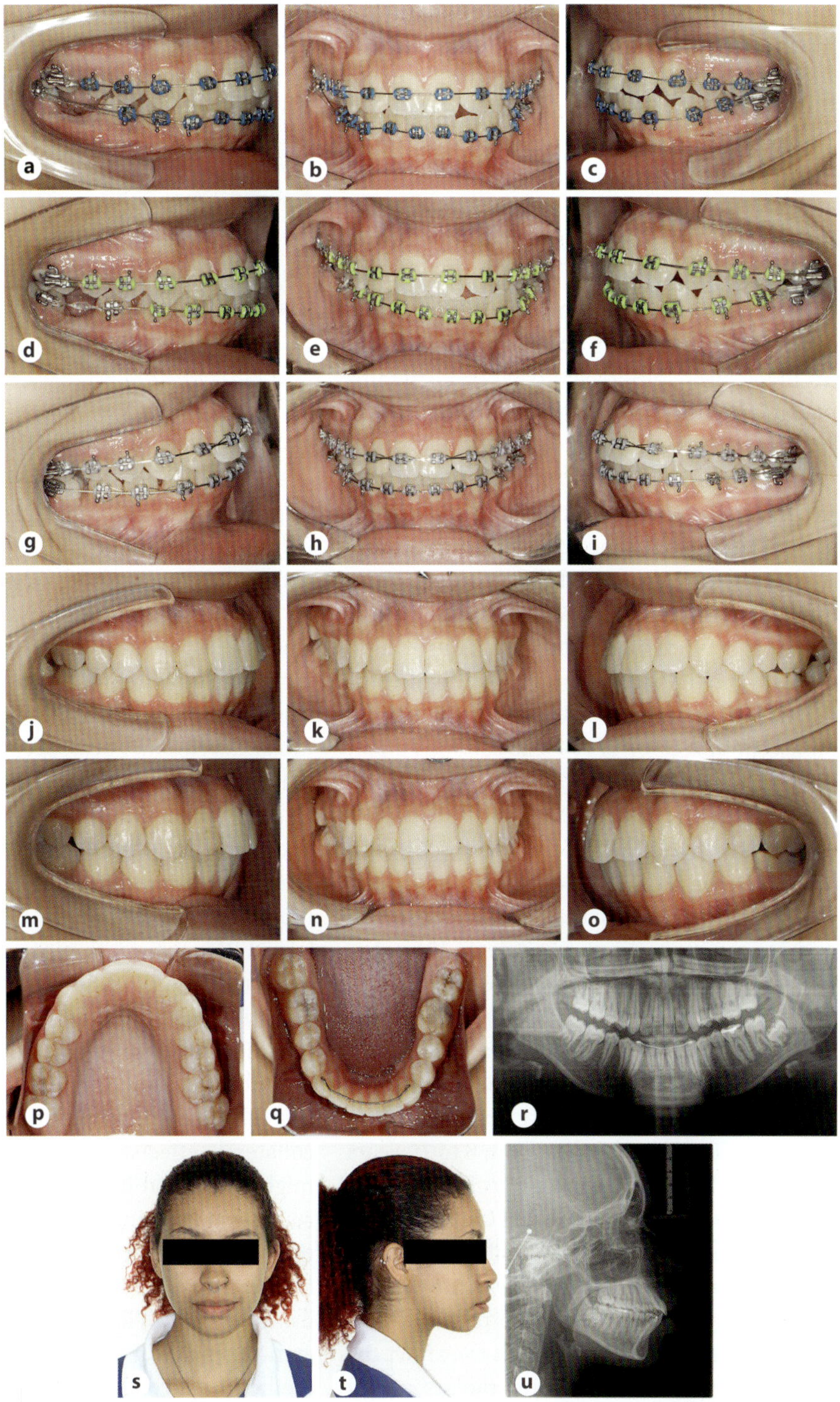

2

molars is favorable during orthodontic planning of extraction of hypomineralised first molars. The extraction or early loss of a first permanent molar tend to accelerate the third molar development on the extraction side [22]. In addition, extraction of first permanent molars may increase the eruption space for the third molars and their angulation [23]. A previous study has demonstrated that extraction of first maxillary permanent molars has a favorable effect on the maxillary second and third permanent molar eruption patterns [24]. In the mandible, changes in the eruption space of third molars were observed; however, no significant changes were observed in the mesiodistal angulation of these teeth [23, 24].

A previous study showed that the success rate of second molar substitution after cFPM extraction with a complete space closure by spontaneous movement in the mixed dentition is 92% in the maxillary arch and 66% in the mandibular arch [25]. In other words, the mandibular arch presents a greater probability of needing a comprehensive orthodontic treatment to close the reminiscent spaces of cFPM extraction. Patient and parents/legal guardians should be aware of this possible future need. In a previous study, following a sample of 27 children (aged 8.2 years) after extractions of cFPM, spontaneous space closure with a favorable dental development was found for the majority of the sample [26]. Approximately 25% of the sample required orthodontic treatment for other reasons than the extraction and approximately 18% required orthodontic treatment because of the extractions [26].

The ideal timing for cFPM extraction in the mixed dentition is the window from 8 to 10 years of age [1, 2]. The dental age for early cFPM extraction, based on the Van der Linden Classification, corresponds to the intertransitional period of the mixed dentition and the second transitional period before the eruption of second premolars. In the mandibular arch, it is advisable to extract the cFPM when mandibular second molars are in stage E of Djemerin with the root bifurcation stage [2]. A panoramic radiograph is recommended at the age of 8.5 to 9 years of age for evaluating the presence of third molars. The presence of third molars is desirable in the hemiarches where the early extraction of cFPM is recommended. However, this assessment needs to be considered with caution once in some cases third molar development can occur later than the optimal age for extraction [26, 27].

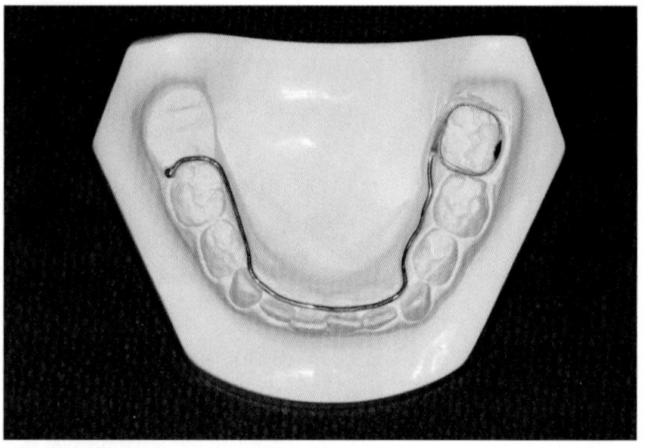

Fig. 3. Modified lingual arch as a cantilever at the extraction side to avoid dental midline deviation.

Early extraction of cFPM can cause some collateral effects in the occlusion, including a slight mesial tipping and rotation of mandibular second molars, an overeruption of the opposing maxillary cFPM, a distal tipping of second premolars, an uprighting of incisors and, finally, a midline deviation when the extraction is asymmetrical [21]. The orthodontist should perform a follow-up of the occlusal development once a year after early cFPM extraction in order to control possible collateral effects. Opposing molar extrusion might be controlled by using a bonded 0.018" round-wire retainer in the lingual aspects of the opposing first permanent molar and second deciduous molars. Midline deviation can be avoided using a modified lingual arch as a cantilever at the extraction side (shown in Fig. 3). With these methods, no compensatory or balancing extraction of sound first molars are recommended.

The occlusion should also be considered before the decision for early extraction of cFPM. The ideal scenario is performing interceptive extractions in patients with normal occlusion or Class I malocclusions. In Class I malocclusions, the early extraction of first permanent molars does not compromise the occlusion development. However, when Class I malocclusions are associated with three special features, cFPM extraction should be avoided during the mixed dentition. The first feature is a severe dental crowding that can be considered when there is a lack of space of 7 mm or more for aligning the permanent incisors in the mandibular dental arch. Severe crowding usually requires tooth extractions in the permanent dentition to solve dental crowding during the orthodontic treatment. In this case, first molar extraction should be avoided during the mixed dentition and postponed to the permanent dentition when the comprehensive orthodontic treatment can be performed. The second feature that is a red flag to avoid early first molar extraction in Class I malocclusions is the biprotrusion of permanent incisors and absence of passive lip seal. Biprotrusion treatment usually involves permanent tooth extraction to move the incisor toward lingual, facilitating lip seal at rest and increasing facial aesthetics. In patients with biprotrusion associated with no passive lip seal, cFPM extraction should also be postponed to the permanent dentition. Finally, Class I malocclusion with multiple tooth agenesis and generalized microdontia is also a contraindication for early cFPM extraction. Patients with this pattern of dental anomalies show a spaced dental arch. The extraction of first permanent molars could increase the complexity of orthodontic mechanics in the permanent dentition, increasing the difficulty to close the spaces during the comprehensive orthodontic treatment.

Skeletal Class II and Class III malocclusions have a challenging decision-making when early FPM extractions are indicated. In Class II patients, before planning for early cFPM extraction, the team should analyze the severity of Class II malocclusion. In moderate/severe Class II malocclusion with an increase overjet (6 mm or more), early extractions should be avoided, in both dental arches. In the maxillary arch, the cFPM extractions should be performed during the permanent dentition to allow the correction of the increased overjet during the comprehensive orthodontic treatment. In the mandibular arch, early extractions of mandibular cFPM could produce an upright of the lower incisors, increasing both the overjet and the overbite and worsening the malocclusion. On the other hand, in mild Class II malocclusions (overjet of 5 mm or less), early cFPM extractions could be accomplished if the malocclusions have the potential to be corrected with other methods than permanent tooth extractions, e.g., functional appliances for mandibular advancement. However, in mild Class II malocclusions, the preferable arch to accomplish early cFPM extractions is the maxillary arch. Early cFPM extractions in the mandibular arch should be avoided in Class II patients to prevent the increasing severity of Class II interarch relationship. Distal migration of mandibular premolars and the uprighting of the mandibular incisors are expected collateral effects of early cFPM extractions, producing a worsening of the malocclusion. When Class II malocclusion is associated with severe dental crowding both in the maxillary and mandibular arch, early cFPM extractions should also be performed in the permanent dentition.

The reasoning for Class III malocclusions is the opposite of Class II malocclusions. Early cFPM extractions in the maxillary arch should be avoided both in mild/moderate and severe Class III cases. In the mandibular arch, early cFPM extractions could be performed in mild Class III cases. In severe Class III cases, where the family accepts the possibility of an orthognathic surgery at the end of the facial growth period, early cFPM extraction can also be accomplished in the mandibular arch. Conversely, in severe Class III cases

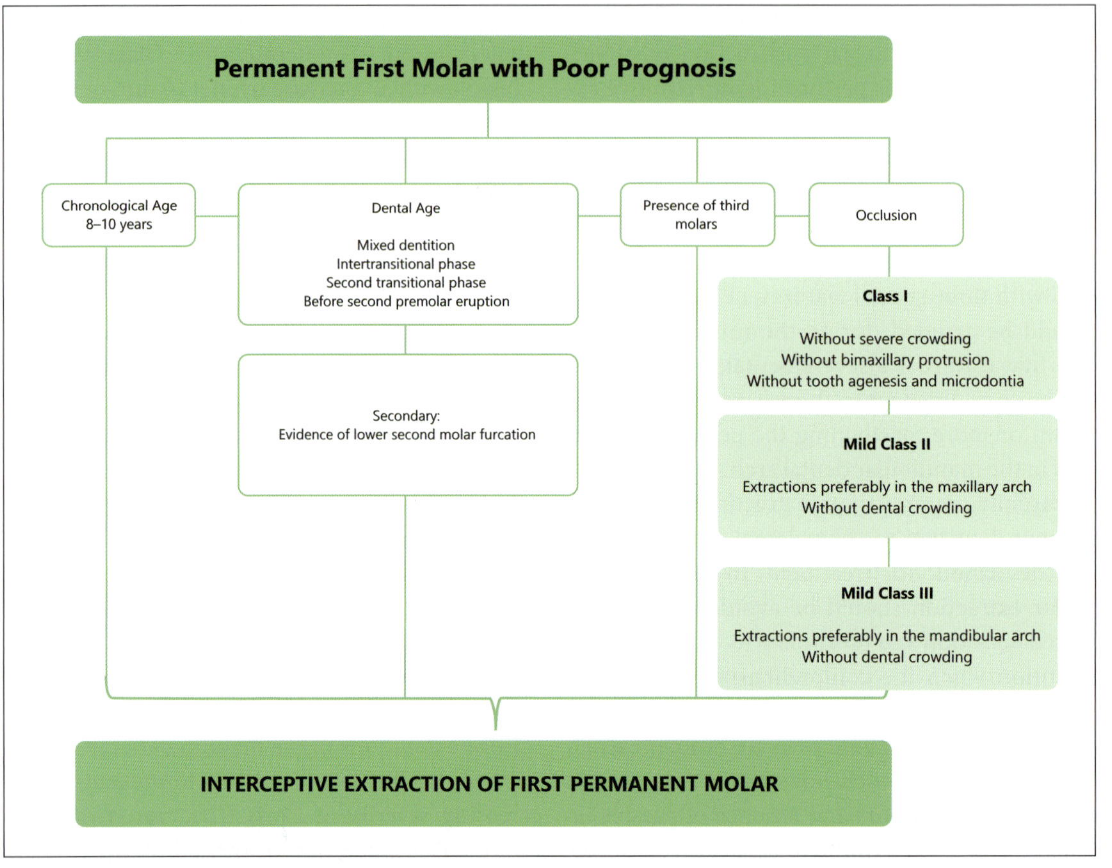

Fig. 4. Orthodontic reasoning guide of early extraction decisions.

where the family would like to avoid orthognathic surgery in the future, the extraction of compromised mandibular first molars should be postponed to the permanent dentition. The reason is that the compensation of Class III malocclusion will need the extraction space for accomplishing the mandibular incisor retraction during the comprehensive orthodontic treatment.

A guide of early extraction decision is shown in Figure 4. The ideal timing for early FPM extraction with poor prognosis due to severe molar hypomineralisation should be the intermediate and late phases of the mixed dentition between 8 and 10 years of age. The timing is more important for the mandibular arch where the success index is decreased compared to the maxillary arch. Before indicating interceptive cFPM extraction, the presence of third molars should be confirmed in the hemiarches with CFPMs. The dental occlusion should also be evaluated. Compromised FPM extraction should be postponed to the permanent dentition in Class I malocclusions with severe dental crowding, with bimaxillary protrusion and lack of passive lip seal, and in cases with multiple missing teeth associated with microdontia. In moderate/severe Class II malocclusions, early FPM extractions should be avoided. In mild Class II malocclusions, early FPM extractions are preferable in the maxillary arch. Finally, in Class III malocclusions, early FPM extraction should always be avoided in the maxillary arch. In the mandibular arch, interceptive cFPM extraction can be indicated in mild cases or in severe cases where a future need of orthognathic surgery is well established and parents/legal guardians are in agreement.

Orthodontically Suitable Cases for Hypomineralised First Permanent Molar Extraction in the Permanent Dentition

Class I Malocclusion with Severe Crowding
In an orthodontic perspective, when considering extractions of first permanent molars, some malocclusions can present greater convenience due to biomechanics of the space closure.

In the presence of a Class I malocclusion with a severe dental crowding in the permanent dentition, orthodontics extractions are often required [28, 29]. The four first or second premolars are often the elective teeth to be extracted during comprehensive orthodontic treatment. However, in the presence of sound premolars, severe crowding, and Class I relationship, the severely compromised first permanent molars could be the ones elected for extractions [30]. In this situation, the space provided by the first molar extractions will be consumed for the alignment of dental crowding. Therefore, a Class I malocclusion associated with severe crowding may represent a favorable scenario for hypomineralised first molar extraction only in the permanent dentition when the space closure will be used to solve dental crowding during comprehensive orthodontic treatment [2, 30]. Previous studies have demonstrated adequate occlusion outcomes after the comprehensive orthodontic treatment with space closure of compromised first molar extraction in Class I malocclusion patients [30, 31]. However, orthodontists, patients, and families should be aware that space closure of the first permanent molars tends to be technically more demanding and can increase treatment time [32].

Class I Malocclusion with Bimaxillary Protrusion
Class I with bimaxillary dentoalveolar protrusion is characterized by protrusive and proclined maxillary and mandibular incisors [33]. Because of the protrusive dentition, a lip protrusion, incompetence, and improper lip seal can be associated with this condition, which negatively affects the facial aesthetics. Therefore, Class I bimaxillary dentoalveolar protrusion often requires extraction of four permanent teeth and great anchorage control to adequately retract the protruded incisors and the lips [34–36]. The extraction of four premolars and the retraction of anterior teeth were shown to be effective in decreasing the incisor protrusion and proclination and lip protuberance [33, 34]. Previous studies demonstrated the possibility of extracting compromised permanent molars instead of sound first premolars in cases of Class I malocclusion with bimaxillary protrusion [37–39]. In cases of hypomineralised first molars associated with Class I malocclusion with bimaxillary protrusion, the first permanent molars could be the elected teeth for extractions. Ideally, the extractions should be performed after the eruption of the second permanent molars and an effective anchorage device should be placed before anterior retraction. In this way, the second permanent molars would be maintained in position, and the extraction spaces would be occupied by the distalization of the anterior dentition.

Class II Malocclusions
Class II malocclusions have many treatment options in the permanent dentition, including with the extraction of two maxillary premolars [40, 41]. During the orthodontic treatment of a Class II malocclusion, the distalization of the maxillary teeth is often necessary to correct the incisor sagittal relationship and the overjet. Extraction of upper teeth can be indicated to promote adequate space for the distalization of anterior teeth, correction of overjet, and achieving a Class I canine relationship [40, 41]. In these cases, anchorage control is essential to promote the correction of

the malocclusion without the side effect of mesial migration of posterior teeth in the maxillary arch. The most common protocol is the extraction of the maxillary first premolars associated with skeletal anchorage to move the anterior teeth posteriorly, avoiding the mesial movement of the posterior segment [42]. Previous findings have demonstrated that Class II malocclusion treated with the extractions of two maxillary first premolars produces adequate occlusal success rates, shorter treatment time, and greater treatment efficiency [42]. Atypical extractions of permanent teeth for treating Class II severe malocclusions have already been described with adequate occlusion outcomes [41, 43–45]. In the presence of sound premolars and severely hypomineralised first molars in the maxilla, the first permanent molars could replace the premolars as the elected teeth to be extracted. Previous studies demonstrated satisfactory occlusal correction after the extraction of maxillary first molars in Class II, division 1 malocclusion [44, 45]. Conversely, premolar extractions in both the maxillary and mandibular arch promotes a more challenging orthodontic treatment in Class II malocclusion cases [46]. This occurs due to a greater orthodontic mechanic difficulty to obtain a satisfactory final occlusal outcome in complete Class II malocclusion treatment with four permanent tooth extraction protocol [46]. In addition, it should be emphasized that permanent teeth extraction in the mandibular arch alone should be avoided in Class II malocclusion cases since it can aggravate these malocclusion features.

Class II, Subdivision

Class II malocclusions can present asymmetrically. In this regard, a Class I relation is observed on one side, while the other side presents a Class II relationship. In face of Class II subdivision cases, asymmetrical extractions of permanent teeth can be chosen as a treatment option [47]. The election of the permanent teeth to be extracted will depend on which dental midline is deviated [47, 48]. In cases with mandibular midline deviation (type 1 Class II subdivision), two premolars are usually extracted in the maxillary arch and one premolar is extracted in the mandibular arch at the Class I side. In cases of maxillary dental midline deviation (type 2), the treatment protocol involves one maxillary premolar extraction on the Class II side [47]. Therefore, in Class II subdivision, the extraction of first permanent molars with poor prognosis can replace the extraction of sound premolars.

Class III Malocclusions

Class III malocclusion treatment in nongrowing patients can be challenging, requiring either orthodontic treatment or orthognathic surgery [49, 50]. In cases with mild skeletal discrepancies and balanced soft-tissue profile, teeth extractions can be used for orthodontic camouflage [51, 52]. In Class III malocclusion, extractions of mandibular first premolars are often indicated to correct the anteroposterior relationship and the anterior crossbite. In the presence of sound premolars, the hypomineralised mandibular first molars could replace the premolars as the elected teeth to be extracted. A previous study reported that the extraction of the mandibular first permanent molars in Class III cases was favorable for the correction of the anterior and posterior relationship [53]. However, mandibular extraction space closure can be technically demanding, and treatment time can be longer than usual. The use of skeletal anchorage, as miniscrews and miniplates, reinforces the anchorage control in the mandibular arch and favors extraction space closure. In addition, extraction on the maxillary arch alone is not recommended in Class III malocclusion cases. In Figures 1 and 2, a case report of a patient with Class III subdivision is presented.

Tooth Agenesis

When tooth agenesis is present in only one dental arch, during the comprehensive orthodontic treatment, the opposite dental arch can be balanced with the extraction of a first permanent molar with poor prognosis. As an example, the presence of severely hypomineralised maxillary first molars may be favorable for extractions when the space of the absent mandibular premolar will be orthodontically closed.

Due to the asymmetric nature of MIH, various scenarios in terms of affected molars and severity may complicate treatment decision. These guidelines cannot be strictly followed in all cases.

Unsuitable Orthodontic Cases for Hypomineralised First Permanent Molar Extraction in the Permanent Dentition

From an orthodontics perspective, there are some specific cases that can be considered unfavorable for the extractions of first permanent molars. Patients with a hypodivergent facial pattern (brachyfacial type) are preferably treated with a nonextraction protocol. This decision is usually related with a significant difficulty in closing extraction spaces in hypodivergent patients due to the strong masticatory muscles. In addition, the space closure tends to increase the overbite that is already increased in hypodivergent patients. Therefore, tooth extractions would demand more complex orthodontic mechanics for controlling the overbite.

Patients with multiple agenesis are also unfavorable for cFPM extractions. Extractions of the severely hypomineralised first molars should be avoided in these cases. A similar approach can be used for patients with generalized diastemas in the dental arch. Closing the diastemas with mechanics during orthodontic treatment coupled with the space closure of first permanent molar extractions would increase the case complexity, the treatment time, and the negative impact on the facial profile.

In cases of cFPM without the recommendation for orthodontic extraction, the space can be maintained for future prosthesis, or the space can be orthodontically closed by moving second molars toward mesial using skeletal anchorage such as miniscrews.

Conclusions

The interceptive extraction of severely hypomineralised first permanent molars can be accomplished in an ideal timeframe around 8–10 years of age, before the eruption of second premolars. Patients with Class I malocclusions without severe dental crowding/bimaxillary protrusion and without missing teeth, including third molars, present a favorable prognosis for the early extraction of cFPMs.

In the permanent dentition, the decision for the extraction with space closure will depend on the anteroposterior interarch relationship, tooth-arch discrepancies, facial growth pattern, and presence of dental anomalies. Missing teeth, hypodivergent facial pattern, and absent third molars may challenge the decision for tooth extraction during the comprehensive orthodontic treatment.

Acknowledgments

The authors thank Dr. Érika Tiemi Kurimori for the assistance with the case report.

Statement of Ethics

Written informed consent was obtained from the individual(s) for the publication of any potentially identifiable images or data included in this chapter.

Conflict of Interest Statement

The authors have no conflict of interest to declare.

Funding Sources

There was no funding for this chapter.

Author Contributions

D.G. (first author): conceptualization, resources, interpretation of data, and writing – original draft. D.R.: conceptualization, resources, interpretation of data, writing – original draft, writing – review and editing. T.L.C.: resources, writing – original draft, writing – review and editing. F.M.: conceptualization, resources, interpretation of data, writing – original draft.

References

1 Cobourne MT, Williams A, Harrison M. National clinical guidelines for the extraction of first permanent molars in children. Br Dent J. 2014;217(11):643–8.
2 Lakhani S, Noble F, Rodd H, Cobourne MT. Management of children with poor prognosis first permanent molars: an interdisciplinary approach is the key. Br Dent J. 2023;234(10):731–6.
3 Ashley P, Noar J. Interceptive extractions for first permanent molars: a clinical protocol. Br Dent J. 2019;227(3):192–5.
4 Weerheijm KL, Jalevik B, Alaluusua S. Molar-incisor hypomineralisation. Caries Res. 2001;35(5):390–1.
5 Mangum JE, Crombie FA, Kilpatrick N, Manton DJ, Hubbard MJ. Surface integrity governs the proteome of hypomineralized enamel. J Dent Res. 2010; 89(10):1160–5.
6 Elhennawy K, Manton DJ, Crombie F, Zaslansky P, Radlanski RJ, Jost-Brinkmann PG, et al. Structural, mechanical and chemical evaluation of molar-incisor hypomineralization-affected enamel: a systematic review. Arch Oral Biol. 2017;83:272–81.
7 Neves AB, Americano GCA, Soares DV, Soviero VM. Breakdown of demarcated opacities related to molar-incisor hypomineralization: a longitudinal study. Clin Oral Investig. 2019;23(2):611–5.
8 Americano GC, Jacobsen PE, Soviero VM, Haubek D. A systematic review on the association between molar incisor hypomineralization and dental caries. Int J Paediatr Dent. 2017;27(1):11–21.
9 Lygidakis NA, Garot E, Somani C, Taylor GD, Rouas P, Wong FSL. Best clinical practice guidance for clinicians dealing with children presenting with molar-incisor-hypomineralisation (MIH): an updated European Academy of Paediatric Dentistry policy document. Eur Arch Paediatr Dent. 2022;23(1):3–21.
10 Raposo F, de Carvalho Rodrigues AC, Lia EN, Leal SC. Prevalence of hypersensitivity in teeth affected by molar-incisor hypomineralization (MIH). Caries Res. 2019;53(4):424–30.
11 Kramer N, Bui Khac NN, Lucker S, Stachniss V, Frankenberger R. Bonding strategies for MIH-affected enamel and dentin. Dent Mater. 2018;34(2):331–40.
12 Linner T, Khazaei Y, Bucher K, Pfisterer J, Hickel R, Kuhnisch J. Comparison of four different treatment strategies in teeth with molar-incisor hypomineralization-related enamel breakdown-A retrospective cohort study. Int J Paediatr Dent. 2020;30(5):597–606.
13 Jalevik B, Klingberg GA. Dental treatment, dental fear and behaviour management problems in children with severe enamel hypomineralization of their permanent first molars. Int J Paediatr Dent. 2002;12(1):24–32.
14 Sanghvi R, Cant A, de Almeida Neves A, Hosey MT, Banerjee A, Pennington M. Should compromised first permanent molar teeth in children be routinely removed? A health economics analysis. Community Dent Oral Epidemiol. 2023;51(5):755–66.
15 Elhennawy K, Jost-Brinkmann PG, Manton DJ, Paris S, Schwendicke F. Managing molars with severe molar-incisor hypomineralization: a cost-effectiveness analysis within German healthcare. J Dent. 2017;63:65–71.
16 Bekes K, Steffen R, Kramer N. Update of the molar incisor hypomineralization: Wurzburg concept. Eur Arch Paediatr Dent. 2023;24(6):807–13.
17 National Institute for Health and Care Excellence. Shared decision making: NICE guideline [NG197]. 2021. Available from: https://www.nice.org.uk/guidance/ng197 (accessed October 2023).
18 Mills I, Scambler S, Neville P, Asimakopoulou K. Developing a person-centred approach in dentistry beyond NHS recall intervals: a commentary. Br Dent J. 2023;235(1):24–8.
19 Humphreys J, Albadri S. Management of molar incisor hypomineralisation (MIH): a 1-year retrospective study in a specialist secondary care centre in the UK. Children (Basel). 2020;7(12):252.
20 AlKhalaf R, Neves AA, Warburton F, Banerjee A, Hosey MT. Management of compromised first permanent molars in a cohort of UK paediatric patients referred to hospital-based services. Int J Paediatr Dent. 2022;32(5):724–36.
21 Brusevold IJ, Kleivene K, Grimsoen B, Skaare AB. Extraction of first permanent molars severely affected by molar incisor hypomineralisation: a retrospective audit. Eur Arch Paediatr Dent. 2022; 23(1):89–95.
22 Yavuz I, Baydas B, Ikbal A, Dagsuyu IM, Ceylan I. Effects of early loss of permanent first molars on the development of third molars. Am J Orthod Dentofacial Orthop. 2006;130(5):634–8.
23 Bayram M, Ozer M, Arici S. Effects of first molar extraction on third molar angulation and eruption space. Oral Surg Oral Med Oral Pathol Oral Radiol Endod. 2009;107(2):e14–20.

24 Langer LJ, Pandis N, Mang de la Rosa MR, Jost-Brinkmann PG, Bartzela TN. Eruption pattern of third molars in orthodontic patients treated with first permanent molar extraction: a longitudinal retrospective evaluation. J Clin Med. 2023;12(3):1060.
25 Teo TK, Ashley PF, Parekh S, Noar J. The evaluation of spontaneous space closure after the extraction of first permanent molars. Eur Arch Paediatr Dent. 2013;14(4):207–12.
26 Jalevik B, Moller M. Evaluation of spontaneous space closure and development of permanent dentition after extraction of hypomineralized permanent first molars. Int J Paediatr Dent. 2007;17(5): 328–35.
27 Santos PB. Why orthodontists need to know about molar incisor hypomineralization. Am J Orthod Dentofacial Orthop. 2024 Mar;165(3):256–61.
28 Konstantonis D, Anthopoulou C, Makou M. Extraction decision and identification of treatment predictors in Class I malocclusions. Prog Orthod. 2013;14:47.
29 Peck S, Peck H. Frequency of tooth extraction in orthodontic treatment. Am J Orthod. 1979;76(5):491–6.
30 Ong DC, Bleakley JE. Compromised first permanent molars: an orthodontic perspective. Aust Dent J. 2010;55(1):2–14; quiz 105.
31 Elhussein M, Jamal H. Molar incisor hypomineralisation-to extract or to restore beyond the optimal age? Children (Basel). 2020;7(8):91.
32 Sandler PJ, Atkinson R, Murray AM. For four sixes. Am J Orthod Dentofacial Orthop. 2000;117(4):418–34.
33 Bills DA, Handelman CS, BeGole EA. Bimaxillary dentoalveolar protrusion: traits and orthodontic correction. Angle Orthod. 2005;75(3):333–9.
34 Langberg BJ, Todd A. Treatment of a Class I malocclusion with severe bimaxillary protrusion. Am J Orthod Dentofacial Orthop. 2004;126(6):739–46.
35 Solem RC, Marasco R, Guiterrez-Pulido L, Nielsen I, Kim SH, Nelson G. Three-dimensional soft-tissue and hard-tissue changes in the treatment of bimaxillary protrusion. Am J Orthod Dentofacial Orthop. 2013;144(2):218–28.
36 Upadhyay M, Yadav S, Nagaraj K, Patil S. Treatment effects of mini-implants for en-masse retraction of anterior teeth in bialveolar dental protrusion patients: a randomized controlled trial. Am J Orthod Dentofacial Orthop. 2008;134(1): 18–29.e1.
37 Abbassy MA, Mitwally RA. Atypical extraction in Class I malocclusion: a case report. J Orthod Sci. 2020;9:9.
38 Chae JM. Unusual extraction treatment of Class I bialveolar protrusion using microimplant anchorage. Angle Orthod. 2007;77(2):367–76.
39 Al-Fraidi A, Afify AR. Unusual treatment of bimaxillary dentoalveolar protrusion via miniscrews and molar extraction. J Orthod Sci. 2012;1(2):51–7.
40 Graber TM, Adams PE. Current orthodontic concepts and techniques. Vol. 11. Philadelphia: WB Saunders Company; 1969.
41 Graber TM. Maxillary second molar extraction in Class II malocclusion. Am J Orthod. 1969;56(4):331–53.
42 Janson G, Barros SE, de Freitas MR, Henriques JF, Pinzan A. Class II treatment efficiency in maxillary premolar extraction and nonextraction protocols. Am J Orthod Dentofacial Orthop. 2007; 132(4):490–8.
43 de Freitas MR, de Lima DV, de Freitas KM, Janson G, Henriques JF. Strategic maxillary second-molar extraction in Class II malocclusion. Am J Orthod Dentofacial Orthop. 2009;136(6):878–86.
44 Booij JW, Kuijpers-Jagtman AM, Bronkhorst EM, Livas C, Ren Y, Kuijpers MAR, et al. Class II Division 1 malocclusion treatment with extraction of maxillary first molars: evaluation of treatment and post-treatment changes by the PAR Index. Orthod Craniofac Res. 2021; 24(1):102–10.
45 Booij JW, Kuijpers-Jagtman AM, Katsaros C. A treatment method for Class II Division 1 patients with extraction of permanent maxillary first molars. World J Orthod. 2009;10(1):41–8.
46 Janson G, Brambilla Ada C, Henriques JF, de Freitas MR, Neves LS. Class II treatment success rate in 2- and 4-premolar extraction protocols. Am J Orthod Dentofacial Orthop. 2004;125(4):472–9.
47 Janson GR, Metaxas A, Woodside DG, de Freitas MR, Pinzan A. Three-dimensional evaluation of skeletal and dental asymmetries in Class II subdivision malocclusions. Am J Orthod Dentofacial Orthop. 2001;119(4):406–18.
48 Janson G, de Lima KJ, Woodside DG, Metaxas A, de Freitas MR, Henriques JF. Class II subdivision malocclusion types and evaluation of their asymmetries. Am J Orthod Dentofacial Orthop. 2007; 131(1):57–66.
49 Alhammadi MS, Almashraqi AA, Khadhi AH, Arishi KA, Alamir AA, Beleges EM, et al. Orthodontic camouflage versus orthodontic-orthognathic surgical treatment in borderline class III malocclusion: a systematic review. Clin Oral Investig. 2022;26(11):6443–55.
50 Winkler MA, Price JO, Foglesong PD, West WH. Biodistribution and plasma survival in mice of anti-melanoma monoclonal antibody cross-linked to OKT3. Cancer Immunol Immunother. 1990;31(5):278–84.
51 Costa Pinho TM, Ustrell Torrent JM, Correia Pinto JG. Orthodontic camouflage in the case of a skeletal class III malocclusion. World J Orthod. 2004; 5(3):213–23.
52 Rabie AB, Wong RW, Min GU. Treatment in borderline Class III malocclusion: orthodontic camouflage (extraction) versus orthognathic surgery. Open Dent J. 2008;2:38–48.
53 Ruellas AC, Baratieri C, Roma MB, Izquierdo Ade M, Boaventura L, Rodrigues CS, et al. Angle Class III malocclusion treated with mandibular first molar extractions. Am J Orthod Dentofacial Orthop. 2012;142(3):384–92.

Felicia Miranda
Department of Orthodontics, Bauru Dental School, University of São Paulo
Alameda Octávio Pinheiro Brisolla 9–75
Bauru 17012-901 (Brazil)
felicia.miranda@usp.br

Published online: July 1, 2024
Rios D, Santos-Pinto L (eds): Molar Incisor Hypomineralisation: New Perceptions. Monogr Oral Sci. Basel, Karger, 2024, vol 32, pp 274–294 (DOI: 10.1159/000539085)

Cost-Effectiveness of Managing MIH Teeth

Renata Paz Leal Pereira[a] Ana Clara Falabello de Lucca[a] Maria Carolina Costa Prestes[a] Thaís Marchezini Reis[a] Daniela Rios[b] Mariana Minatel Braga[a]

[a]Department of Orthodontics and Pediatric Dentistry, Faculty of Dentistry, University of São Paulo, São Paulo, Brazil; [b]Department of Pediatric Dentistry, Orthodontics and Public Health, Bauru School of Dentistry, University of São Paulo, Bauru, Brazil

Abstract

Numerous therapeutic approaches are available for managing molar incisor hypomineralisation (MIH); however, the cost-effectiveness of these strategies is underexplored. Economic evaluations are crucial for determining the optimal treatment approach to individual patients' requirements. We systematically reviewed the literature on the topic to have a more comprehensive discussion about these issues. Systematic searches were carried out. After a two-stage selection, 11 studies were included for synthesis. These studies could be divided into three groups according to the type of information given on costs: assumptions or deductions based on the literature ($n = 6$), cost collection on the available sources ($n = 3$), and cost-effectiveness evaluations ($n = 2$). The economic evidence on MIH management is still scarce and incipient. However, some important findings were produced for this evidence synthesis. A database of costs valuable in different contexts for therapeutic approaches related to MIH and its consequences was created. Furthermore, compiling and digesting the evidence on the cost-effectiveness of different approaches for managing severe MIH cases points out possible directions to be considered in decision-making that should consider these economic outcomes in different contexts and their powers of generalizability and also other aspects of evidence-based practice (e.g., professional and patients' preferences). Finally, there is an imminent need for economic evaluations focused on investigating the potential efficiency of preventive approaches for managing minor-compromised MIH teeth to postpone/avoid the severe consequences, which are more critical, complex, and costly to treat.

Introduction

Several therapeutic options are available to manage molar incisor hypomineralisation (MIH) as a preventive approach, restorations, or extractions. The decision on the appropriate treatment depends on the location of the alteration, the stage of dental development, the severity of the defect, the patient's cooperation and age, and caregivers' and patients' expectations and preferences [1, 2].

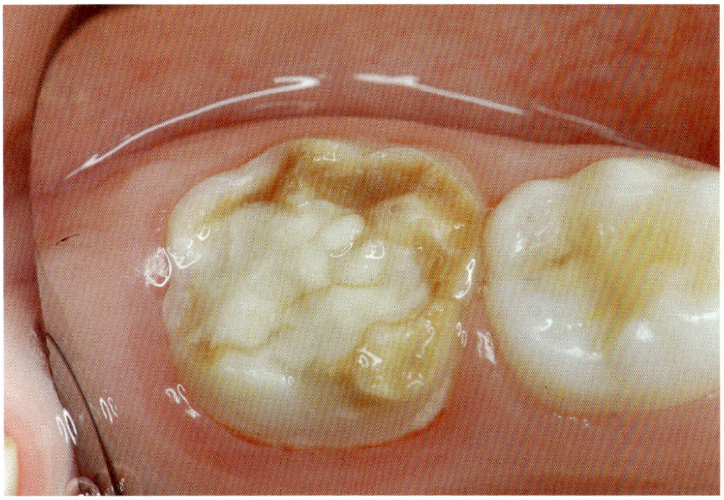

Fig. 1. Permanent molar with severely hypomineralised areas and great structural loss.

Affected MIH teeth often require some interventions and are challenging due to the variation in clinical signs and symptoms associated with such conditions. The presence of posteruptive breakdown, the development of caries lesions, and the risk of hypersensitivity, pain, and aesthetic compromising [1, 3] may result in recurrent retreatments and can cause difficulties in clinical management.

MIH treatment has been based on the principles of prevention before the intervention, although an early operative intervention may be necessary [1] and favorable to the clinical prognosis. Dietary advice, brushing with fluoride dentifrice (with at least 1,000 ppm), and the professional application of topical fluorides can prevent caries lesions in mild and severe cases [1, 2]. Furthermore, for relieving sensitivity, the use of fluorides and casein phosphopeptide-amorphous calcium phosphate lack strong supporting evidence [4]. On the other hand, preventive options may not be sufficiently effective, and other nonoperative and operative adhesive strategies may be necessary (shown in Fig. 1). Specifically for treating affected incisors, aesthetics may significantly impact the child's quality of life and psychosocial status [3, 5, 6] (shown in Fig. 2). Then, aesthetical alternatives may improve optical properties and aesthetics [3, 7, 8]. As adhesion to hypomineralised enamel may be undermined, consequent retreatments and repairs may be necessary [8]. Temporary treatment of the affected teeth may be necessary since definitive restorative treatment should only be given with complete tooth eruption and full patient management. Indirect restorations, such as prefabricated metal crowns, are alternatives to restoring MIH teeth. When restorative treatments are no longer possible, extraction may be an alternative, although it is a more invasive option. Space closure can be achieved spontaneously or through orthodontic alignment [8, 9]. Scheduled extraction is most recommended at the optimal developmental stage after a proper orthodontic evaluation [1, 9].

It is evident that MIH management is a complex task. Such management may, as described, involve regular preventive approaches to complex invasive options, including adjunct orthodontic treatment. Therefore, the choice of appropriate therapy and the moment of intervention has, consequently, both clinical and economic consequences. Contemporary scientific literature has progressively expanded to investigate dental treatments from an extensive per-

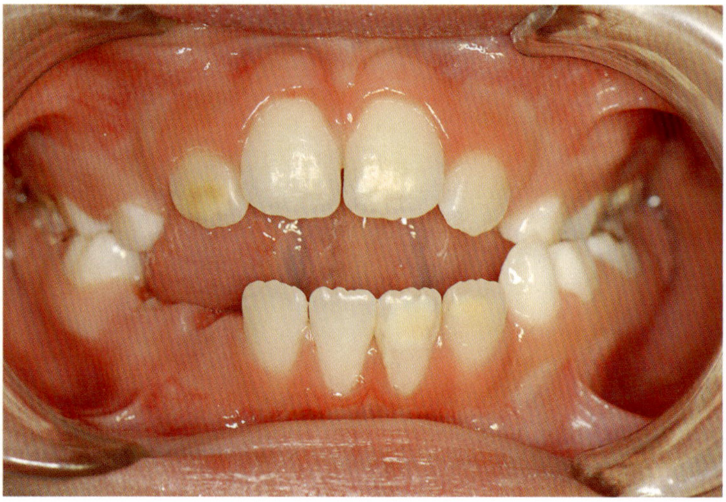

Fig. 2. Demarcated opacity in permanent incisors. The incisors in the image belong to the same patient as the molar shown in Figure 1.

spective, considering treatment longevity and financial consequences derived from that [10, 11]. Thus, conducting a comprehensive conjoint evaluation of relevant costs and health outcomes from the intervention, which could extend over the patient's lifetime, is proper [12]. This consideration is especially important when complex strategies are needed for managing oral health problems, as in the case of MIH.

Therefore, economic evaluations are important to maximize individuals' health effects and well-being with the costs involved [13, 14]. They permit the comparison of two or more alternatives about the paired combination on costs and consequences [11, 15]. Studies in this area are important to guide funds allocation to health promotion and prevention programs [11]. In this sense, this paper will focus on cost-effectiveness issues related to the treatment of MIH patients to discuss the most relevant evidence and the potential impact different approaches may have on individuals and health systems.

Review Methodology

Extensive speculation has been made about the costs of managing MIH and how different strategies may be considered from a financial perspective. Another conceptual hypothesis is that if the noninvasive treatment is implemented earlier, more complex approaches may be avoided, potentially causing savings when the deal is managing MIH. As MIH has been massively discussed nowadays, economic questions have also been in the pipeline. However, we hypothesized that it is still an underinvestigated topic. Therefore, we systematically reviewed the literature to have a more comprehensive discussion about these issues.

We conducted a systematic literature review (registered as PROSPERO: CRD42023462205) to identify the cost-related evidence on different approaches for MIH management. The acronym PICO (Population, Intervention, Control, Outcomes) was used to formulate the focused question and inclusion criteria in this systematic review, in which: (P) individuals with MIH; (I) any approach for management of MIH; (C) none or any comparison for managing MIH; (O) any economic outcome.

An electronic literature search strategy was performed in four databases up to May 8, 2023: Embase, PubMed/Medline, LILACS, Scopus, and Web of Science. Gray literature was conducted in ProQuest Dissertation and Thesis and OpenGrey. No restriction criteria regarding language and publication time were applied. Detailed database search strategy can be found in Appendix 1. Reference lists of included studies were manually searched, and experts on the subject were contacted to recommend additional studies to be included. With a careful analysis of the selected studies, we sought to understand the available evidence on the costs and financial aspects of managing MIH in children.

We included primary studies in which MIH or similar anomalies (hypomineralisation, hypoplasia, etc.) were mentioned in their abstracts. Studies in which we detected no economic mention or no discussion focused on MIH-related conditions were excluded from our sample for analysis.

Besides summarizing the available literature described in the next topics, we also appraised the information regarding the potential risk of bias they could present. For that, the Checklist for Economic Evaluations provided by Joanna Briggs Institute was used for such appraisal [16]. Specifically, for those which included model-based cost-effectiveness evaluations, the risk of bias was assessed using the guidelines for good practice in decision-analytic modeling in health technology assessment [17].

Appraisal of the Available Literature

Of the 65 studies identified, 23 remained as potential sources of information after removal of duplicated records (shown in Fig. 3, Table 1). From these, 11 studies have mentioned any issue with the costs of MIH. Some retrieved studies (n = 6) use the cost as a previous assumption to justify some management strategies for MIH. Given the complexity of MIH, poor patient compliance, difficulties in controlling dental sensitivity, the condition's rarity, and escalated treatment expenses and needs of retreatments, costs of managing MIH have been a priori assumed as high [18, 19] and sometimes, the reason for neglecting this dental condition [18]. Other studies (n = 3) also discussed the cost of treatments used when conducting specific clinical cases, bringing up values collected from cost databases available. Finally, only two studies properly analyzed the cost-effectiveness related to MIH management. Detailed individual study characteristics and such groups described above are presented in Table 1.

Three case reports and case series used the cost variable to justify the selection of treatment strategies for teeth with MIH in children [20–22]. However, no proper data collection or analysis was conducted on such an issue. Other studies mentioned MIH costs in conjunction with such condition description [23] or management [22] into populations. As the main objective of these studies was not a cost evaluation, most of the questions related to costs related to the risk of bias could not be answered properly, reinforcing prior assumptions or deductions, which were not tested, and the information provided was potentially highly biased (Table 2).

All reports were focused on severe conditions of MIH. Such cases enrolled children/adolescents from 6 to 16 years old. Some therapeutic options focused on a surgical approach followed by orthodontic treatment, or autoresolution after extraction at an ideal age are presented in some cases [20–22] (Table 1). Other reports focused on restorative treatment repetitions or severity-associated dental sensitivity/pain [18, 21]. Authors deducted the treatment cost-effectiveness based on previous literature on the issue [12], and the health effects they observed in reported cases [20, 21, 24], also in a cohort of patients followed [22], or a prevalence study of dental anomalies [23]. Besides, given the compromised dental structure observed in severe cases of MIH, they expected a poor survival of treatments and, consequently, deducted increasing costs for

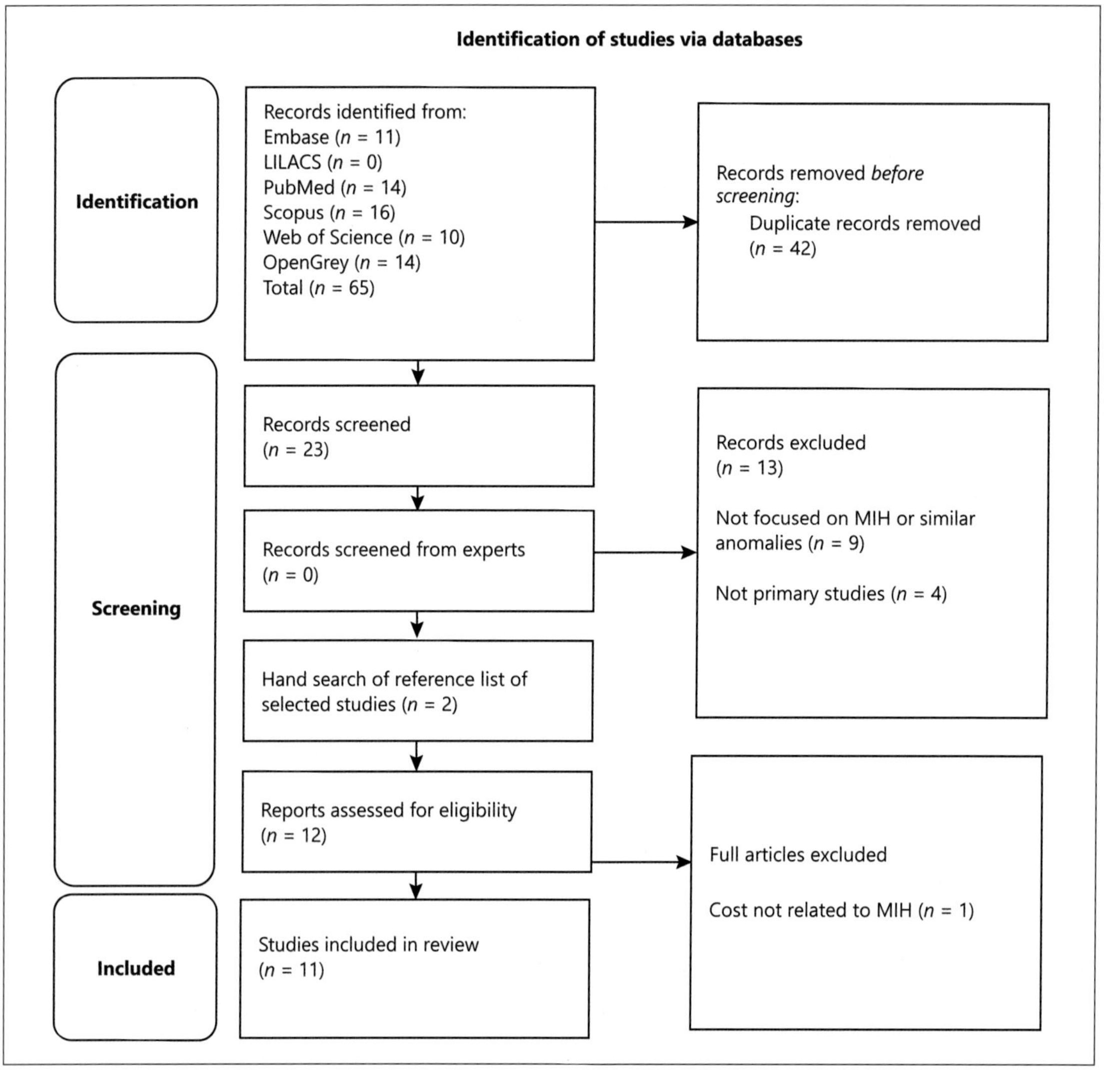

Fig. 3. Flowchart of studies selection considering costs of MIH management as the topic.

managing such conditions due to the need for reinterventions [18, 20–22].

Five studies effectively reported costs related to treating MIH. Three of them only reported costs related to MIH management, and two focused on cost-effectiveness assessment of a base case of severe MIH and potential therapeutic approaches (Table 1). Those studies presented a low risk of bias (shown in Fig. 4).

Two studies considered costs for patients followed for some time, and procedures performed on them were registered and valued [25, 26]. One of them brought descriptive retrospective data of dental treatment under general anesthesia (GA) and, based on that, valued the procedures based on national data [25]. On the other hand, the other prospectively treated the children at in-office appointments and did not specify how costs were

Table 1. Individual characteristics of studies that worked on MIH versus costs, including different study appraisals: assumptions or deductions based on the literature, cost collection on the available databases, and cost-effectiveness evaluations

Study	*n*	Age	Condition	Treatment	Outcome evaluated	Economic data	Economic inference basis	Study assertions
Cost as previous assumption or deducted from clinical cases based on previous literature support								
AlKhalaf et al. (2022) [22]	249	6–11 years	cFPMs in children	Managing cFPMs in children	Number of cases, number of FPMs extracted, mode of anesthesia used in extraction	–	Literature that explores cost-effectiveness [12] and discussion of their findings under the cost-effectiveness and dental service panoramas	*A recent health economic study evaluated the overall costs and effectiveness of retaining cFPMs compared with timely extraction in children effectivenesss [12]. The results of this study have shown that retaining cFPM can be more cost-effective than extraction with spontaneous closure of the gap. The relative cost in that study was influenced by the cost of extraction under GA, and extraction of one or two cFPMs under GA was not cost-effective [12]*
Basalamah and Baroudi (2016) [23]	1,000 (28 MIH)	4–12 years	Hard and soft tissue anomalies	–	Prevalence of dental and oral anomalies	–	A priori authors' assumption of high costs	*It is vital that assessment be carried out periodically to identify these anomalies early in life so that appropriate measures are taken early to mitigate their negative impact and costs of treatment in adult life*
Dhareula et al. (2019) [18]	10	8–14 years (mean 11.4 years)	Moderate to severe MIH, extreme sensitivity to cold (70%), posteruptive breakdown (PEB) (50%), atypical caries (40%), pain (10%)	Preparation with a shoulder margin and onlay placement	Integrity and retention of all treated cases	–	A priori deduction based on the literature associating retreatment and increased cost of treatment [4]	*Poor patient compliance, extreme sensitivity, rarity of the condition and increased treatment costs are some of the factors compounding its management* *Furthermore, as a consequence of frequent loss of restorations due to the problems of adhesion, secondary caries, and successive breakdown of the hypomineralised enamel, these often have to be repeated several times leading to escalated treatment cost*

Table 1 (continued)

Study	*n*	Age	Condition	Treatment	Outcome evaluated	Economic data	Economic inference basis	Study assertions
Elhussein and Jamal (2020) [20]	1	15 years	MIH history of successive restorations Orthodontic needs – class II patient (need of extraction of premolars)	Delayed extraction of FPMs + orthodontic treatment	Space closure fully achieved and orthodontic treatment (time = 16 months)	–	Literature that explores cost-effectiveness [8] and suppositions given the results observed in the clinical cases reported and possible different outcomes (not tested)	*The most cost-effective way of addressing MIH-affected FPMs is extraction, followed by orthodontic space closure when indicated* *This obviates the need for the repeated restorative replacement and saves perfectly healthy premolars from being extracted for space creation in orthodontic treatment in several clinical scenarios* *This approach (extraction) could still be deemed cost effective, as it obviated the need for further dental treatment, i.e., root canal treatment*
Elhussein and Jamal (2020) [20]	1	16 years	MIH History of MIH-affected molar at 9 years Orthodontic needs – class II patient (need of extraction of premolars)	Timely extraction of FPMs No orthodontic treatment	Mesial eruptive position of second permanent molars Several malocclusion features: round tipping of PM; distal tipping of PM; spacing in the arch; excessive retroclination of the lower labial segment – worsened deepbite (sequelae of the early extraction of FPMs)			
Laverde-Giraldo et al. (2021) [21]	1	9 years	MIH Hypersensitivity Unsatisfactory restorations Class I patient	Pain control Fluoride varnish + calcium trisphosphate (Climpro) Phase 2: FPM extraction*	2 PM erupted and well positioned after 1 year	–	Literature that deducted the cost-effectiveness [8] and suppositions given the results observed in the clinical case reported	**Direct restorations represent less costs, but there is a greater need for retreatments. Exodology is a viable and cost-effective therapeutic strategy* [8]. *The systematic review carried out by Elhennawy et al. evaluated the different modalities for the treatment of MIH and concluded that for patients with more than one severely affected molar, extraction followed by orthodontic treatment is the most cost-effective strategy, however, requires greater motivation and commitment from the patient and family* [8]
Feierabend et al. (2012) [19]	8	6–15 years	MIH or hypoplasia	Laboratory-made composite resin restorations for restoring hypoplastic	Longevity of the restorations	–	A priori authors' assumption of high costs independently of cases treated	*Management of children and adolescents with qualitative or quantitative defects of enamel or dentin are often impeded by patient compliance, rare prevalence of disease, lack of evidence, and cost*

Table 1 (continued)

Study	*n*	Age	Condition	Treatment	Outcome evaluated	Economic data	Economic inference basis	Study assertions
Cost effectively collected from any source								
Alshehri et al. (2021) [25]	310	2–16 years	Decayed (D), missing (M), and filled (F) teeth index (dmft [primary dentition]/ DMFT [permanent dentition]) and treatment performed in accordance with the Australian Dental Association (ADA)	Examinations Radiographs Photographs Preventative extractions Oral surgery Pulpotomy restorations Treatment under GA and cost analysis	Cumulative count of treatment mix and cost analysis	Treatment count and cost (direct), indirect, and total costs	Australian Schedule of Dental Services and Glossary (Australian Dental Association, 2021)	*The total cost, consisting of direct and indirect costs, was A$ 313,823 and equated to an approximate mean of A$ 1,554 ± 109 per case* *Upon stratification, for children >7 years old, there was a higher number of dmft/DMFT (count) in the posterior compared with anterior teeth and a high likelihood of MIH in those patients. MIH may affect one in five Australian children [2] or one in six children globally. MIH can affect the first permanent molars that erupt at 6 years of age, and a significant association between MIH and dental caries has been reported. A positive relationship between the extent of hypomineralised second primary molars and carious lesion severity has also been reported.*
Mathu-Muju and Kennedy (2016) [27]	1	12 years	Permanent maxillary first molars extensively decayed	The permanent maxillary first molars were extracted, followed by a period of spontaneous drifting of the dentition Fixed appliances with headgear and elastics were used with a nonextraction approach	2 molars well positioned after 4 years	Costs over a lifetime	American Dental Association's 2013 Survey of Dental Fees	*The final records at 16 years old revealed good alignment, maintenance of a normal overjet and overbite, and a class I molar and canine relationship. The permanent maxillary second molars were occluding with the permanent mandibular first molars, and there has been accelerated eruption of maxillary third molars.* *Management of compromised permanent first molars in young patients presents a challenging diagnostic and treatment dilemma for the dentist. The conventional approach has been to preserve rather than extract teeth. However, understanding that groups of teeth have differing susceptibility to caries means that extraction of one or more significantly compromised permanent first molars does not inevitably lead to further extractions of permanent teeth as the child ages.* *Given the potential prohibitive lifetime costs associated with initiating the costly repair/ replace cycle in a permanent molar, serious consideration should be given to presenting the option of extractions and potential orthodontic treatment to parents*

Table 1 (continued)

Study	*n*	Age	Condition	Treatment	Outcome evaluated	Economic data	Economic inference basis	Study assertions
Zagdwon et al. (2003) [26]	17	6–13 years	Split mouth design using either a preformed metal crown or a cast adhesive coping	Preformed metal crown or a cast adhesive coping	Quality of restorations	Total costs	No information about cost database used Cost components considered: Chairside time cost, materials of preformed metal crowns vs. casts adhesive copings for the restoration	*There were no significant differences between the longevity and success rates for preformed metal crowns and cast adhesive copings for the restoration of first permanent molars affected by either amelogensis imperfecta or severe enamel hypoplasia. Adhesive cast copings conserved more tooth tissue but were more technique sensitive*
Cost collected from databases and analyzed by modeling a base case of MIH								
Elhennawy et al. (2017) [2]	–	6 years	Male with 1, 2, 4 permanent severe MIH-affected molars with vital pulp	Removal and orthodontic alignment, restorative treatment, and indirect restoration	Costs (c) were assessed per patient, effectiveness (e) in mean and tooth retention time (in years)	Tooth retention years/ incremental cost-effectiveness ratios (ICERs)	"German public and private dental fee catalogs, BEMA and GOZ"	*If extraction was performed at the optimal age (9.5/11 years for maxillary/mandibular molars), ex/ortho was most cost-effective (67 years, 446–938 Euro). Comp (51 years, 1,911 Euro) and PMC/IR were dominated (50 years, 2,033 Euro). This cost-effectiveness ratio was also determined when >1 molar was treated. If extraction was performed later, assuming no spontaneous alignment, ex/ortho was more costly than comp, at least when only 1 molar was treated*
Sanghvi et al., 2023 [12]	–	8 years	Male with 1, 2, or 4 cFPMs	Tooth retained with glass-ionomer cement (GIC) restoration; tooth retained with resin composite (RC) restoration; tooth retained with stainless steel crown (SSC); tooth retained with root canal treatment and restoration (RoCT); tooth removed and space closed spontaneously; tooth removed and space closed using fixed orthodontic treatment; tooth removed and space filled with conventional fixed-fixed dental bridge (FDP); tooth removed and space filled with single crown implant (SCI); tooth removed and space filled with a removable partial denture (RPD); tooth removed and patient left with a space	One-way sensitivity analysis was undertaken in which procedure costs were varied systematically to assess the robustness of results to potential underestimation of the cost of dental procedures	QATYs/ICERs	Scottish Statement of Dental Remuneration 2019; Northern Ireland Statement of Dental Remuneration 2018–19; NHS Improvement National Cost Collection Data; Average company prices; Expert opinion	*Regardless of the number of cFPMs, retaining cFPMs was more effective than early removal, generating an additional 2.3 QATYs per cFPM. Early removal of one or two cFPM under GA was more expensive than retention and hence never cost-effective. Retaining a cFPM was more expensive than early removal under local anesthesia or where four cFPMs were extracted under GA. In these cases, retaining cFPMs was cost-effective if a QATY was valued at £100 or £35, respectively.*

Risk of bias

Study	D1	D2	D3	D4	D5	D6	D7	D8	D9	D10	D11
AlKhalaf et al., 2022	+	+	+	+	+	x	+	x	x	x	+
Basalamah and Baroudi, 2016	x	-	x	+	x	+	x	x	x	+	+
Dhareula et al., 2018	+	+	-	+	x	+	x	x	x	x	x
Elhussein and Jamal, 2020	+	+	-	+	x	+	x	x	x	+	+
Feierabend et al., 2012	+	+	x	+	x	x	x	x	x	x	x
Laverde-Giraldo et al., 2021	+	+	-	+	x	+	x	x	x	+	+

D1: Is there a well-defined question?
D2: Is there comprehensive description of alternatives?
D3: Are all important and relevant costs and outcomes for each alternative identified?
D4: Has clinical effectiveness been established?
D5: Are costs and outcomes measured accurately?
D6: Are costs and outcomes valued credibly?
D7: Are costs and outcomes adjusted for differential timing?
D8: Was there an incremental analyses of costs and consequences?
D9: Were sensitivity analysis conducted to investigate uncertainty in estimates of cost or consequences?
D10: Do study results include all issues or concerns to users?
D11: Are the results generalizable to the setting of interest in the review?

x High
- Unclear
+ Low

a

Risk of bias

Study	D1	D2	D3	D4	D5	D6	D7	D8	D9	D10	D11
Alshehri et al., 2021	+	+	+	+	+	+	+	+	x	+	+
Mathu-Muju and Kennedy	+	+	+	-	+	+	+	+	x	+	+
Zagdown, Fayle, and Pollard 2003	+	+	+	+	+	-	+	+	x	+	+

D1: Is there a well-defined question?
D2: Is there comprehensive description of alternatives?
D3: Are all important and relevant costs and outcomes for each alternative identified?
D4: Has clinical effectiveness been established?
D5: Are costs and outcomes measured accurately?
D6: Are costs and outcomes valued credibly?
D7: Are costs and outcomes adjusted for differential timing?
D8: Was there an incremental analyses of costs and consequences?
D9: Were sensitivity analysis conducted to investigate uncertainty in estimates of cost or consequences?
D10: Do study results include all issues or concerns to users?
D11: Are the results generalizable to the setting of interest in the review?

x High
- Unclear
+ Low

b

4

(For legend see next page.)

valued [26]. Finally, another study reported national cost data to contextualize its findings on reported clinical cases, considering different procedures used to manage MIH [27] (Tables 1 and 3). Although costs and effects have been collected in these studies, and some authors have assumed the cost-effectiveness of certain MIH treatments [26, 27], they are not actually combined into a cost-effectiveness analysis.

The only two cost-effectiveness assessments brought complete model-based economic evaluation, simultaneously evaluating and analyzing costs and effects [2, 12] (Table 1). In both, a Markov model was developed to simulate the lifetime. They were published in 2017 [2] and 2023 [12] and conducted in Germany and the United Kingdom (UK) perspectives, respectively. A mixed public-private-payer perspective within German health care was adopted [2], while the other adopted the UK public-payer perspective [12]. As these studies brought the national costs for managing MIH by different approaches, these values were also included in the cost appraisal (Table 2).

A base case of a young child (6 or 8 years old) with compromised first permanent molars (cFPMs) was considered in both models (Table 3). These studies simulated one or more molars severely affected by dental caries or enamel hypomineralisation, and the lifetime is considered the time horizon (shown in Table 3, Fig. 5). Then, costs and effects were accumulated for approximately 60 years. In these models, the strategies of interest can be compared. Different possible clinical paths are represented in the model structure (shown in Fig. 5). For example, after the main intervention, the teeth can be re-restored, treated endodontically, or even removed, as it is illustrated in the upper branch (shown in Fig. 5). On the other hand, after being removed, the child may need (or not) of orthodontic treatment (shown in Fig. 5). These paths can still be changed over time and several times during the lifetime. Then, the Markov models (a mathematical strategy used for these economic analyses) may simulate cycles to simulate these real paths in the mathematical model. Each one of these studies brought different health effects (shown in Table 3). One looked into a more tooth-related view, considering the tooth retention years for modeling [2]. The other included a more qualitative measuring of effect, considering the quality-adjusted tooth years (QATYs) [12].

Fig. 4. Risk of bias assessment using the JBI tool for economic evaluation of information gathered on studies reporting on costs of HMI. **a** Studies informing assumptions or deductions based on the literature. **b** Studies' cost collection in the available sources.

None of the studies met all the criteria from guidelines for good practices in model-based economic evaluations [17]. Still, they met over 80% of the requirements and suggested low risk of bias. The main minor concern was related to comparability to other possible different models available on such topic and/or explanation/justification of some options/results.

Economic Findings and Their Implications

It is noticeable that evidence of the economic impact of MIH and its management is scarce. The literature found is mainly based on previous assumptions of authors, deductions based on indirect evidence, or even suppositions based on preconceptions they construct about MIH management based on primary knowledge about histopathology [28] or even some developing information about the management by itself [8].

Some interesting case reports (or even a series of these cases) explore examples of different ways of leading to this problem, especially exploring severe cases [20, 21], bringing authors' speculation about MIH management costs, exposing, for example, extraction of permanent molars with MIH at an ideal age may be more cost-effective than conservative approaches based on the results of one isolate case or even pair or series of cases. Although case reports

Table 2. Costs (in International Dollars) reported on partial economic evaluations for different approaches for managing MIH

Study	Location	Study design	Prevention	Restorative care				Endodontic treatment	Extraction	Post-extraction interventions		
				Direct restorations-I	Direct restorations-II	Indirect restorations-I	Indirect restorations-II			Orthodontic alignment	Implant insertion	Implant-supported prosthesis
Alshehri et al. (2021)[a] [25]	Australia	Retrospective descriptive study	77.24			319.21[b]	–	142.97[c]	264.31	–	–	–
Elhennawy et al. (2017) [2]	Germany	Modeling	–		80.50	81.25[d]	345.23[e]	237.74[f]	56.59	1,719.30	804.58	–
Mathu-Muju and Kennedy (2016) [27]	Canada/ USA	Case report and review	–		–	366.91[d]	1,319.38[g]	1,212.57	–	–	–	1,702.63
Sanghvi et al. (2023) [12]	United Kingdom	Modeling	–	11.56[h]	12.75[i]	16.35[d]	–	89.25	6.22	367.91	965.34	–
Zagdwon et al. (2003) [26]	England	Prospective clinical trial	–		–	86.87[d]	339.85[j]	–	–	–	–	–

Costs were corrected for inflation based on factors like the consumer price index information, available per country and year at https://databank.worldbank.org/, since the time of collection up to 2023 and converted to International Dollars using the purchase parity power as coefficient (https://data.oecd.org) to make them comparable. I and II symbolize different options of restorations in the same study. [a]All procedures under general anesthesia: additional 225.20 should be added to each treatment because of it. [b]Direct and Indirect restoration. [c]Pulpotomy. [d]Preformed metal crown. [e]Full-metal crown. [f]Root canal treatment assumed three root canals per tooth. [g]Ceramic-fused-to-metal crown. [h]Glass-ionomer cement restoration. [i]Resin composite restoration. [j]Adhesive cast coping.

Table 3. Summary information of cost-effectiveness models used to explore the cost-effectiveness of interventions related to MIH

Study	Elhennawy et al., 2017 [2]		Sanghvi et al., 2023 [12]	
Case base	Six-year-old male with one, two, or four permanent severe MIH-affected molars with vital pulp		8 years with one, two, or four cFPMs	
Time horizon	72 years		62 years	
Perspective	Public and private payer		Public payer	
Origin of effectiveness data	German public and private dental fee catalogs, BEMA and GOZ		Scottish Statement of Dental Remuneration 2019; Northern Ireland Statement of Dental Remuneration 2018–19; NHS Improvement National Cost Collection Data; average company prices; expert opinion	
Health outcome	Tooth retention years		QATYs	
Cost-effectiveness measure	Incremental cost-effectiveness ratios (ICERs)		ICER	
Overall costs 1 MIH molar	**Maintenance**	**Extraction/Ortho**	**Maintenance**	**Extraction/Ortho**
	$376.23	$ 1,612.06 (direct) $ 1,714.98 (indirect)	$ 6.12	$ 161.16
Overall effects 1 MIH molar	**Maintenance**	**Extraction/Ortho**	**Maintenance**	**Extraction/Ortho**
	67 years	51 years (direct) 50 years (indirect)	13.83 QATYs	11.53 QATYs

are an interesting way to generate initial hypotheses or highlight interesting and/or rare clinical cases, they are not considered robust scientific evidence [29]. Furthermore, more controlled and robust investigations are needed to confirm the hypothesis arising [29] and are not sufficient to subside a complete and personalized clinical approach. Even more advanced designs were used to measure the prevalence of MIH at different severities or cohorts of MIH teeth treated, which brought cost issues but did not include cost assessments or reports. Furthermore, these studies did not collect cost-related data or conduct appropriate cost analyses. They have also been based on individuals' (groups') points of view.

Indeed, these studies were not designed to answer such a question, but they ultimately addressed it. Such a way of bringing out cost issues represents an important potential risk of bias as relevant aspects. It is evident in Table 2 that these opinions are not based on a systematic process for addressing the question and may reflect biased impressions. Then, we are not judging the studies but the information on costs that have been vehiculated on them. Finally, case reports may lead to a potential publication bias since unsuccessful cases are not commonly published. In this sense, overestimating potential positive effects and cost assumptions may also be inherent.

Few studies, as reported in the previous section, explored the costs in MIH management or the impact of MIH on costs, and still, fewer appropriately combine the analyses of costs and effects. Moreover, the assumption that the treatment is cost-effective is often made based on partial cost assessment, presuming a hypothetical positive effect or even, on no previous cost assessment, based on an a priori assumption. Then,

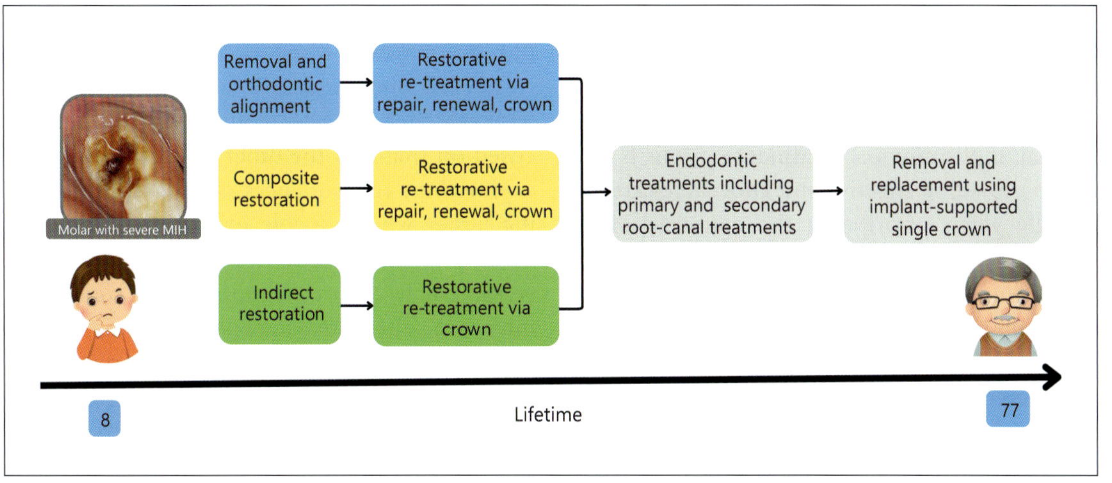

Fig. 5. Comprehensive modeling of MIH molar management. This figure illustrates a detailed model tracking patients and their molars over their lifetime, offering three main pathways for managing molars with MIH: extraction and alignment with or without active orthodontic treatment, retention and restoration using resin composite, and retention and restoration using indirect restorations, crossing from 8 years old to 77 years old (constructed based on information gathered from Elhennawy et al., 2017) [2].

"cost-effectiveness" was sometimes used erroneously, without a real cost-effectiveness evaluation having been carried out.

An appraisal of costs by itself may be interesting. It permits addressing important financial aspects of different treatment options and realities or contexts, as seen in Table 2. In the present paper, it was crucial to consider adjustments for inflation and differences in purchasing power over time and across various countries when comparing the values of different studies from different countries and currencies at different moments [17]. These partial economic evaluations (only focused on costs or inputs) bring out relevant findings, given the methodology adopted, which probably presented a low risk of bias, increasing the certainty of the evidence produced. These studies are concerned with important aspects of an economic evaluation, from the question definition to the appraisal of their results regarding validity, demonstrating mostly clarity and transparency and, consequently, confidence in the data presented. Besides, these findings can be considered a possible information source for feeding further economic models and permit possible sensitivity analyses in further evaluations when other contexts should be tested as a good practice when modeling [17]. That is why, for a global appraisal, you can find a summary report in Table 2, including costs collected for modeling [2, 12], which is deeply discussed further.

On the other hand, isolated cost assessments do not permit weighing both clinical and economic aspects when making decisions [17]. Due to the nature of cost assessments, they are not considered decisive in making decisions on resource allocation since they generally limit themselves to describing costs without presenting information on the associated benefits. A complete economic evaluation, e.g., using the cost-effectiveness models, may permit the combination discussed above [2, 12] (Table 3).

Cost-effectiveness models are a usual methodological strategy to simulate the conditions we could not measure in a primary study due to the long time needed to follow patients. They have often been used for economic evaluations. Such a strategy might provide a solid basis for evaluating and justifying treatment choices in MIH and complex dental conditions. Understanding the financial implications of treatment options is crucial to providing effective and affordable care, especially when prioritizing the conservation of dental tissue. In this sense, this strategy would be very helpful in finding answers like that.

On the other hand, neither the economic models are perfect. Possible shortcomings should be considered, especially when findings are interpreted and extrapolated. As stated previously in this paper, full economic evaluations included in this review are very well designed and present a low risk of bias since they address important aspects related to good practices in modeling for economic evaluations. However, some missed or unclear information on the extrapolation of results and the validity of assuming were detected. That is why, when exploring their results deeply, we will concomitantly point out these possible aspects to be considered by the readers.

One relevant concern when digesting the available evidence (even developing) is related to the spectrum of the disease/anomalies when base cases were chosen (irrespective of the study design). Such findings have been produced only focusing on severe cases of MIH, possibly generating problems of generalizability. Indeed, this is one shortcoming identified in model-based economic evaluations presented. Previous studies have shown that MIH severity did not influence global oral-related quality of life [29]. Potential publication bias for some domains, such as social and emotional well-being, may confound such pooled results [29] and possibly undermine the actual impact of severe conditions on patients' and families' lives. Probably, severe MIH cases are the ones that generate the highest impact on patients and also for professionals and society due to the magnitude of the damage and their consequences, usually linked to pain, the need for complex dental interventions and the costs for managing such consequences appropriately and avoid they become even worst.

On the one hand, this is plausible to justify why evidence has been constantly produced focused on that. On the other hand, no study has explored the consequences and costs of intervening earlier, when possible, in such cases. No studies have investigated the economic impact of preventing such severe conditions, which could be an interesting alternative to reallocating financial resources using a more minimal interventionist model. Additionally, we have to state that one unique study presented costs related to preventive interventions of MIH conditions when recording all procedures, including the preventive approaches, and valued them according to the national public health system [25]. Indeed, the preventive approach is one of the cheapest options compared to other dental interventions related to MIH management (Table 2). Given the Australian scenario explored, prevention corresponds to ratios from 1:1.9 to 1:4 of value invested in the restorative options, which are further steps when posteruptive breakdowns or cavities appear.

A possible reason for the lack of studies on preventive measures for MIH may be the complex nature of the condition, which differs from dental caries in terms of its causal factors. Furthermore, when discussing prevention in the context of MIH, it is essential to clarify that the aim is not necessarily to prevent the enamel defect itself but rather to mitigate undesirable outcomes such as posteruptive breakdown, including associated dental caries.

Although caries preventive strategies are usually cost-effective options for high-risk children [30], not necessarily preventive strategies save money due to interventions and events, which are observed in a longer time horizon or even because secondary or tertiary preventions tend to be more expensive, may be required to treat pre-existent conditions, and reduce harms [31]. Therefore, intervening preventively in less severe MIH conditions, given the purposes discussed above, is a promising idea but an a priori assumption that should be further tested and proved (or not) to ensure a more robust affirmation in that sense.

Different options for restoring MIH teeth have been their costs explored in different studies. Indirect restorations were notably more expensive among restorative options due to additional laboratory costs [26]. Among the indirect options, different indirect therapy options had their costs reported, differing especially on technique preparation and material used. The most commonly reported was the preformed metal crowns. Despite the study methodology presenting a low risk of bias, not only different materials and techniques but also different contexts and valuation processes are inherent in these findings. We can observe that the same treatment (e.g., preformed metal crowns) is differently valued in different contexts, reinforcing the importance of performing economic evaluations in different contexts and testing external validity and transferability when constructing our economic models [17].

Preformed metal crowns cost almost five times more than direct restorations (Table 2). These two approaches were directly compared in one full economic evaluation as two potential alternatives to manage severe cases of MIH [2]. On a lifetime analysis, considering reintervention during patient life, direct and indirect restorations were similar options regarding tooth retention years (health effect), with higher cumulative costs when the indirect techniques were the first option for treatment of MIH molars [2]. Then, we can deduct, in such context, among restorative approaches, that direct restorations would be a more cost-effective option for managing MIH.

Even considering the above exposed, the permanent molar extraction was the most cost-effective strategy compared to direct and indirect restorations when the modeled German context was explored [2] (Table 3). Optimal timing for molar extraction in severe MIH cases may lead to, on average, more than 15 years more in tooth retention (for the first molar until removal and for the second molar after alignment), associated with cost savings from approximately $1,500 to $6,000 in approximately 60 years, given the reduction in the requirement for expensive orthodontic procedures [2]. The ideal range to intervene in the maxilla is 8–10.5 years; in the mandible, it is 10.5–11.5 years [32]. The cost-effectiveness of extraction and subsequent orthodontic treatment is particularly pronounced for maxillary molars and when multiple molars are affected by MIH. If the ideal extraction window has passed, such savings are extremely diminished if one unique tooth is affected [2]. If more teeth are involved, or extraction and potential orthodontic intervention are not viable options, resin composite restorations may be considered a second option. However, no study assessed the cost-effectiveness of different materials for direct restoration of MIH teeth.

In a different context, the UK context, and using qualitative health effects (QATY), differences in cost-effectiveness could be evidenced [12]. In such an evaluation, retaining MIH-affected molars was more cost-effective than early removal, regardless of the number of cFPMs. Therefore, preserving compromised first permanent MIH emerged as the more economically viable approach compared to the early extraction of those molars under GA. Such superiority of tooth maintenance is sustained by a more pronounced health effect (higher QATYs for tooth maintenance) associated with a less costly strategy or a slightly costly strategy for maintaining the tooth/teeth aligned to the societal willingness to pay. Several aspects may explain such different results. One of them is a matter of different contexts that generate serious conditions and influence the effects and costs assumed. Another aspect is the outcome used as a health effect. As stated before, there is a more qualitative effect (QATYs) besides the quantitative one (only tooth retention years) used for this evaluation. This measure is obtained per each affected tooth and is the product of time and utility obtained through the patient's preferences for different tooth health states [33]. For that, the authors undertook a preliminary survey to generate preference weights for several conditions reproduced in the model. Finally, using GA for dental extractions may also generate important differences between the economic evaluations under discussion.

The answer to the question of the cost-effectiveness of a specific intervention will always depend on the individual who receives it and the circumstances in which this happens. Therefore, to understand which population the results found apply to, it is essential to know the ages at baseline and the level of MIH (baseline). The choice of base case age in both studies is appropriate (around 6 to 8 years old) since MIH is detected with the eruption of the first permanent molars and parents, and around this age, children notice the first signs and symptoms of hypersensitivity, posteruptive breakdown, incidence of caries, causing difficulties in achieving pain control, and the possibility of multiple visits for dental care.

Another fundamental aspect of economic evaluation studies is the study's time horizon selection. Considering the natural course of the disease being studied, this horizon should cover a sufficient period to capture relevant results and costs. In MIH cases, adopting a long-term perspective and considering the patient's life expectancy is necessary, given that MIH exhibits changing characteristics over time, resembling the behavior of chronic diseases [34]. In both studies, the time horizon adopted a lifetime time horizon, comprising approximately 70 years, aligning with the life expectancies in their respective regions.

The perspective chosen in these studies is closely linked to the costs included. All the studies considered the payer perspective, encompassing direct and/or indirect costs (specified in each report). The payer perspective typically encompasses health care system expenditures, which, in turn, consider direct costs related to medical care, the intervention itself, and follow-up treatment. Different perspectives were adopted in each case, considering the health systems of each country [2, 12] (Table 3).

Given the considerations above, which should be considered when any situation is supposed to be extrapolated to other contexts and scenarios, the decision to extract teeth severely affected by MIH should be carefully assessed, considering not only the procedure itself but also the long-term implications and the possibility of orthodontic treatment to ensure function aesthetics and additional amounts. These decisions may directly interfere with the cost-effectiveness of MIH strategies. As shown in Table 2, the immediate cost of extraction is not abusive, but addressing postextraction considerations, such as the need for orthodontic interventions to ensure function and aesthetics [25], may significantly change the direction of the results. These economic studies emphasize the importance of considering both clinical and economic aspects when choosing treatment options.

Although generically compromised permanent molars have been considered for the mentioned evaluations, it is possible to extrapolate these results for MIH, given that the clinical conditions are similar. Such methodological options are highly motivated by the absence of data from primary studies, specifically with MIH conditions. Such lack of information limits the economic model of feeding, and such an alternative is a valid approach facing the available evidence up to this moment. The issues addressed in the study, such as treatments and costs, are faced in treating MIH. Therefore, the findings of this study may provide valuable information to guide treatment approaches for MIH, considering the similarities in the clinical and economic concerns involved. Some specificities, such as the longevity of restorations placed on MIH teeth, may be further explored in sensitivity analysis or similar models.

Findings presented and discussed here, even incipient, can inform clinical practices regarding these molars' management while considering patient and payer preferences for maintaining teeth. The choice between the two methods may depend on individual patient characteristics, the dentist's expertise, and cost-effectiveness considerations. Although the accumulated cost may be higher, choosing to restore conservatively may be justified in cases where only one or two teeth are affected by severe enamel defect, such as in MIH cases.

Generalizing results from economic evaluations of health care interventions face limitations and challenges due to potential variations in the design of the intervention or health program and associated costs. Furthermore, several factors complicate the transfer of economic data and evaluation outcomes across regions and countries, such as differences in demographics and epidemiology, variations in conventions and clinical practices among health care systems and professionals, disparities in the distribution and accessibility of health care resources and, differences in payment methods for health care services and interventions. Health preferences are also influenced by cultural factors that vary among countries.

There is considerable divergence among dentists regarding the extraction of severely affected permanent first molars due to MIH. A careful analysis is essential to determine whether extraction is necessary, as it should not be based only on dental and occlusal characteristics [8]. The decision for early extraction should encompass factors beyond personal preferences.

Conclusion

The economic evidence on MIH management is still scarce and incipient. However, some important findings were produced for this evidence synthesis. A database of costs valuable in different contexts for therapeutic approaches related to MIH and its consequences was created. Furthermore, compiling and digesting the evidence on the cost-effectiveness of different approaches for managing severe MIH cases points out possible directions to be considered in decision-making that should consider these economic outcomes in different contexts and its powers of generalizability and also other aspects of evidence-based practice (e.g., professional and patients' preferences). Finally, there is an imminent need for economic evaluations focused on investigating the potential efficiency of preventive approaches for managing minor-compromised MIH teeth to postpone/avoid the severe consequences, which are more critical, complex, and costly to treat.

Appendix 1. Databases and search strategies

Database	Search strategy	Results May 8, 2023
Medline/PubMed	"cost effectiveness analysis"[MeSH Terms] OR "analysis cost effectiveness" OR "cost effectiveness analysis" OR "Cost-Effectiveness" OR "effectiveness cost" OR "cost effectiveness ratio" OR "cost effectiveness ratios" OR "effectiveness ratio cost" OR "ratio cost effectiveness" OR "Costs and Cost Analysis"[MeSH Terms] OR "cost" OR "cost analysis" OR "costs" OR "Cost-effective" OR "Cost Analyses" OR "Cost Measures" OR "Cost Measure" OR "pricing" OR "Affordability" AND "Molar Hypomineralization[MeSH Terms]" OR hypomineralization OR hypocalcification OR hypomaturation OR "mottled enamel" OR "molar-incisor-hypomineralization" OR "Molar Incisor Hypomineralization" OR "cheese molars" OR "Incisor hypomineralization" OR "Molar Hypomineralization"	14

Appendix 1 (continued)

Database	Search strategy	Results May 8, 2023
EMBASE	'analysis cost effectiveness' OR 'cost effectiveness analysis'/exp OR 'cost effectiveness analysis' OR 'cost-effectiveness'/exp OR 'cost-effectiveness' OR 'effectiveness cost' OR 'cost effectiveness ratio'/exp OR 'cost effectiveness ratio' OR 'cost effectiveness ratios' OR 'effectiveness ratio cost' OR 'ratio cost effectiveness' OR 'costs and cost analysis'/exp OR 'costs and cost analysis' OR 'cost'/exp OR 'cost' OR 'cost analysis'/exp OR 'cost analysis' OR 'costs' OR 'cost-effective' OR 'cost analyses' OR 'cost measures' OR 'cost measure' OR 'pricing'/exp OR 'pricing' OR 'affordability'/exp OR 'affordability' AND hypomineralization OR hypocalcification OR hypomaturation OR 'mottled enamel' OR 'molar-incisor-hypomineralization' OR 'molar incisor hypomineralization' OR 'cheese molars' OR 'incisor hypomineralization' OR 'molar hypomineralization'	11
Scopus	"cost effectiveness analysis" OR "analysis cost effectiveness" OR "cost effectiveness analysis" OR "Cost-Effectiveness" OR "effectiveness cost" OR "cost effectiveness ratio" OR "cost effectiveness ratios" OR "effectiveness ratio cost" OR "ratio cost effectiveness" OR "Costs and Cost Analysis" OR "cost" OR "cost analysis" OR "costs" OR "Cost-effective" OR "Cost Analyses" OR "Cost Measures" OR "Cost Measure" OR "pricing" OR "Affordability" AND "Molar Hypomineralization" OR hypomineralization OR hypocalcification OR hypomaturation OR "mottled enamel" OR "molar-incisor-hypomineralization" OR "Molar Incisor Hypomineralization" OR "cheese molars" OR "Incisor hypomineralization" OR "Molar Hypomineralization"	16
Web of Science	"cost effectiveness analysis" OR "analysis cost effectiveness" OR "cost effectiveness analysis" OR "Cost-Effectiveness" OR "effectiveness cost" OR "cost effectiveness ratio" OR "cost effectiveness ratios" OR "effectiveness ratio cost" OR "ratio cost effectiveness" OR "Costs and Cost Analysis" OR "cost" OR "cost analysis" OR "costs" OR "Cost-effective" OR "Cost Analyses" OR "Cost Measures" OR "Cost Measure" OR "pricing" OR "Affordability" AND "Molar Hypomineralization" OR hypomineralization OR hypocalcification OR hypomaturation OR "mottled enamel" OR "molar-incisor-hypomineralization" OR "Molar Incisor Hypomineralization" OR "cheese molars" OR "Incisor hypomineralization" OR "Molar Hypomineralization"	10
LILACS	"cost effectiveness analysis" OR "analysis cost effectiveness" OR "cost effectiveness analysis" OR "Cost-Effectiveness" OR "effectiveness cost" OR "cost effectiveness ratio" OR "cost effectiveness ratios" OR "effectiveness ratio cost" OR "ratio cost effectiveness" OR "Costs and Cost Analysis" OR "cost" OR "cost analysis" OR "costs" OR "Cost-effective" OR "Cost Analyses" OR "Cost Measures" OR "Cost Measure" OR "pricing" OR "Affordability" OR "Avaliação de Custo-Efetividade" OR "Evaluación de Costo-Efectividad" OR "Análise de Custo-Efetividade" OR "Análisis Costo Beneficio" OR "Custos e Análise de Custo" OR "Costos y Análisis de Costo" OR "custo" OR "costo" AND "Molar Hypomineralization" OR hypomineralization OR hypocalcification OR hypomaturation OR "mottled enamel" OR "molar-incisor-hypomineralization" OR "Molar Incisor Hypomineralization" OR "cheese molars" OR "Incisor hypomineralization" OR "Molar Hypomineralization" OR "Hipomineralização Molar" OR "Hipomineralização Incisivo-Molar" OR "Hipomineralização Molar Incisivo" OR "Hipomineralização de Incisivos" OR "Hipomineralización Molar" OR "Hipomineralização do Esmalte Dentário" OR "Hipomineralização Dentária" OR "Hipomineralização do Dente" OR "Hipomineralización del Esmalte Dental"	0

Appendix 1 (continued)

Database	Search strategy	Results May 8, 2023
OpenGrey	("cost effectiveness analysis" OR "analysis cost effectiveness" OR "Costs and Cost Analysis" OR "cost" OR "cost analysis" OR "costs" OR "Cost-effective" OR "Cost Analyses" OR "Cost Measures" OR "Cost Measure" OR "pricing" OR "Affordability") AND ("Molar Hypomineralization" OR hypomineralization OR hypocalcification OR hypomaturation OR "mottled enamel" OR "molar-incisor-hypomineralization" OR "Molar Incisor Hypomineralization" OR "Incisor hypomineralization" OR "Molar Hypomineralization")	14

Search strategies were performed for each database by using specific word combinations and truncations with the support of a librarian.

Statement of Ethics

Patients and their parents or guardians have given their written informed consent, including for publication of nonidentifiable images.

Conflict of Interest Statement

The authors have no conflicts of interest to declare.

Funding Sources

RPLP, ACFL, MCCP, and TMR receive scholarships provided for Coordination for the Improvement of Higher Education Personnel (CAPES). DR and MMB are researchers funded by CNPq (Productivity Program).

Author Contributions

R.P.L.P., D.R., and M.M.B. conceived the chapter and were responsible for overall direction and planning. R.P.L.P., A.C.F.L., M.C.C.P., and T.M.R. performed data collection and risk of bias analyses for the systematic review. R.P.L.P. and M.M.B. wrote the manuscript with input from all authors. All of them revised the final version of the manuscript.

References

1 Somani C, Taylor GD, Garot E, Rouas P, Lygidakis NA, Wong FSL. An update of treatment modalities in children and adolescents with teeth affected by molar incisor hypomineralization (MIH): a systematic review. Eur Arch Paediatr Dent. 2022;23:39–64.

2 Elhennawy K, Jost-Brinkmann PG, Manton DJ, Paris S, Schwendicke F. Managing molars with severe molar-incisor hypomineralization: a cost-effectiveness analysis within German healthcare. J Dent. 2017;63:65–71.

3 Lygidakis NA, Garot E, Somani C, Taylor GD, Rouas P, Wong FSL. Best clinical practice guidance for clinicians dealing with children presenting with molar-incisor-hypomineralisation (MIH): an updated European Academy of Paediatric Dentistry policy document. Eur Arch Paediatr Dent. 2022;23(1):3–21.

4 William V, Messer LB, Burrow MF. Molar incisor hypomineralization: review and recommendations for clinical management. Pediatr Dent. 2006;28(3):224–32.

5 Jälevik B, Klingberg G. Treatment outcomes and dental anxiety in 18-year-olds with MIH, comparisons with healthy controls – a longitudinal study. Int J Paediatr Dent. 2012;22(2):85–91.

6 Hasmun N, Vettore MV, Lawson JA, Elcock C, Zaitoun H, Rodd HD. Determinants of children's oral health-related quality of life following aesthetic treatment of enamel opacities. J Dent. 2020; 98:103372.

7 Crombie F, Manton D, Palamara J, Reynolds E. Resin infiltration of developmentally hypomineralised enamel. Int J Paediatr Dent. 2014;24(1):51–5.
8 Elhennawy K, Schwendicke F. Managing molar-incisor hypomineralization: a systematic review. J Dent. 2016;55:16–24.
9 Eichenberger M, Erb J, Zwahlen M, Schätzle M. The timing of extraction of non-restorable first permanent molars: a systematic review. Eur J Paediatr Dent. 2015;16(4):272–8.
10 Ladewig NM, Camargo LB, Tedesco TK, Floriano I, Gimenez T, Imparato JCP, et al. Management of dental caries among children: a look at the cost-effectiveness. Expert Rev Pharmacoecon Outcomes Res. 2018;18(2):127–34.
11 Rogers HJ, Freitas RD, Beeson MJ, Vernazza CR. Economic evaluations in paediatric dentistry clinical trials. Int J Paediatr Dent. 2020;31(suppl 1):56–65.
12 Sanghvi R, Cant A, de Almeida Neves A, Hosey MT, Banerjee A, Pennington M. Should compromised first permanent molar teeth in children be routinely removed? A health economics analysis. Community Dent Oral Epidemiol. 2023;51(5):755–66.
13 Listl S, Weyant R. For careful consideration: the reporting of health economic evaluations in dentistry. J Public Health Dent. 2019;79(4):273–4.
14 Braga MM, Machado GM, Rocha ES, ViganÓ ME, Pontes LRA, Raggio DP. How can we associate an economic evaluation with a clinical trial? Braz Oral Res. 2020;34(suppl 2):e076.
15 Drummond MF, Sculpher MJ, Torrance GW, O'Brien BJ, Stoddart GL. Methods for the Economic Evaluation of Health Care Programmes. Oxford University Press; 2005.
16 Gomersall JS, Jadotte YT, Xue Y, Lockwood S, Riddle D, Preda A. Conducting systematic reviews of economic evaluations. Int J Evid Based Healthc. 2015; 13(3):170–8.
17 Philips Z, Ginnelly L, Sculpher M, Claxton K, Golder S, Riemsma R, et al. Review of guidelines for good practice in decision-analytic modelling in health technology assessment. Health Technol Assess. 2004;8(36):iii–iv, ix–xi, 1–158.
18 Dhareula A, Goyal A, Gauba K, Bhatia SK, Kapur A, Bhandari S. A clinical and radiographic investigation comparing the efficacy of cast metal and indirect resin onlays in rehabilitation of permanent first molars affected with severe molar incisor hypomineralization (MIH): a 36-month randomized controlled clinical trial. Eur Arch Paediatr Dent. 2019;20(5):489–500.
19 Feierabend S, Halbleib K, Klaiber B, Hellwig E. Laboratory-made composite resin restorations in children and adolescents with hypoplasia or hypomineralization of teeth. Quintessence Int. 2012;43(4):305–11.
20 Elhussein M, Jamal H. Molar incisor hypomineralisation-to extract or to restore beyond the optimal age? Children (Basel). 2020;7(8):91.
21 Laverde-Giraldo M, Mejía-Roldán JD, Jhonson-Giraldo N, Santos-Pinto L, Restrepo Restrepo M. Consideraciones diagnósticas para la exodoncia de primeros molares permanentes severamente afectados por la Hipomineralización de Molares e Incisivos. CES Odontología. 2021;34(2):210–32.
22 AlKhalaf R, Neves AA, Warburton F, Banerjee A, Hosey MT. Management of compromised first permanent molars in a cohort of UK paediatric patients referred to hospital-based services. Int J Paediatr Dent. 2022;32(5):724–36.
23 Basalamah M, Baroudi K. Prevalence of oro-dental anomalies among schoolchildren in Sana'a city, Yemen. East Mediterr Health J. 2016;22(1):33–8.
24 O'Brien B, Gafni A. When do the "dollars" make sense? Toward a conceptual framework for contingent valuation studies in health care. Med Decis Making. 1996;16(3):288–99.
25 Alshehri YFA, Nicholls W, Mai NQ, Park JS, Kruger E. Cross-sectional analysis of dental treatment under general anaesthesia in hospitalized Western Australian children in 2018–19. Aust Health Rev. 2021;45(5):584–90.
26 Zagdwon AM, Fayle SA, Pollard MA. A prospective clinical trial comparing preformed metal crowns and cast restorations for defective first permanent molars. Eur J Paediatr Dent. 2003;4(3):138–42.
27 Mathu-Muju KR, Kennedy DB. Loss of permanent first molars in the mixed dentition: circumstances resulting in extraction and requiring orthodontic management. Pediatr Dent. 2016;38(5):46–53.
28 Jalevik B, Noren JG. Enamel hypomineralization of permanent first molars: a morphological study and survey of possible aetiological factors. Int J Paediatr Dent. 2000;10(4):278–89.
29 Amrollahi N, Hashemi S, Heidari Z. Impact of molar incisor hypomineralization on oral health-related quality of life in 8–10 years old children: a systematic review and meta-analysis. J Evid Based Dent Pract. 2023;23(3):101889.
30 Davidson T, Blomma C, Bagesund M, Krevers B, Vall M, Warnberg Gerdin E, et al. Cost-effectiveness of caries preventive interventions – a systematic review. Acta Odontol Scand. 2021;79(4):309–20.
31 Cohen JT, Neumann PJ, Weinstein MC. Does preventive care save money? Health economics and the presidential candidates. N Engl J Med. 2008;358(7): 661–3.
32 Mazur M, Corridore D, Ndokaj A, Ardan R, Vozza I, Babajko S, et al. MIH and dental caries in children: a systematic review and meta-analysis. Healthcare (Basel). 2023;11(12):1795.
33 Egil E, Yaylali E. Cost-effectiveness analysis of fissure sealants for caries prevention in children. J Public Health Dent. 2023;83(1):43–50.
34 Brazil. Methodological Guideline: Economic Evaluation of Health Evaluation of Health technologies. 2014.

Mariana Minatel Braga
Orthodontics and Pediatric Dentistry Department, Faculty of Dentistry
University of São Paulo
Professor Lineu Prestes Avenue, 2227, São Paulo 05508-000 (Brazil)
mmbraga@usp.br

Published online: July 1, 2024
Rios D, Santos-Pinto L (eds): Molar Incisor Hypomineralisation: New Perceptions. Monogr Oral Sci. Basel, Karger, 2024, vol 32, pp 295–312 (DOI: 10.1159/000538891)

Uses of Internet for Obtaining and Sharing MIH-Related Information

Thiago Cruvinel   Matheus Lotto   Olivia Santana Jorge   Ana Maria Jucá
Tamires Sá Menezes   Jean Ribeiro Leite

Department of Pediatric Dentistry, Orthodontics and Public Health, Bauru School of Dentistry, University of São Paulo, Bauru, Brazil

Abstract

The Internet's increasing prevalence, along with the user-friendly nature of smartphones and the ease of access to virtual spaces, creates a vast and practical domain for digital communication. In this context, obtaining online information plays a crucial role in promoting health and preventing disease, facilitating individual and collaborative decision-making between patients and dental professionals. Digital information resources play a crucial role in providing guidance, support, and knowledge to the public and health care experts on molar incisor hypomineralisation (MIH). This chapter explores various dimensions related to MIH digital information, including a diverse array of digital platforms and the multifaceted landscape of health information-seeking behaviors. This chapter emphasizes the importance of accurate and reliable information dissemination in the digital era. It also sheds light on how understanding the dynamics of digital communication and health information-seeking behavior can improve accessibility and information quality for individuals facing the challenges of MIH.

Introduction

The escalating ubiquity of the Internet, the user-friendly attributes of smartphones, and the readily accessible virtual landscape collectively establish an expansive and pragmatic domain for digital communication [1,2]. Information acquisition, which constitutes a fundamental pillar of health education, assumes paramount significance, serving as a linchpin in endeavors related to health promotion, disease prevention, and collaborative efforts between individuals and health care professionals [3–5].

Digital communication emerges as a potent instrument for elucidating uncertainties and dispelling misconceptions arising from the consumption of erroneous oral health information disseminated online. Consequently, communicators are compelled to substantiate their messages with a sturdy foundation of empirical evidence, thereby endowing their audience with precise and factual knowledge [6]. Paradoxically, it is worth noting that health professionals themselves, occasionally, through digital channels, disseminate inaccurate content, potentially precipitating detrimental health repercussions for the recipients [7].

Within the sphere of oral health, the notable surge in the diagnosis of molar incisor hypomineralisation (MIH) among pediatric patients has engendered a burgeoning discourse among dental professionals and societies globally [8]. In this context, digital informational resources play a pivotal role in offering guidance, support, and essential knowledge to patients, caregivers, and health care practitioners grappling with this condition. This contribution ultimately translates into an enhanced quality of life and improved oral health outcomes.

This chapter is dedicated to expounding facets of MIH-related digital information, encompassing diverse ecosystems and health information-seeking behaviors.

MIH on the Web

Substantial lacunae persist in the realm of scientific research and approaches endorsed by health authorities with the objective of popularizing and broadening their reach across diverse segments of society. Despite the pivotal role played by the media and the Internet in disseminating health-related information, it is noteworthy that numerous online resources tend to accord precedence to popular and extensively debated subjects, relegating lesser-known conditions such as MIH to the periphery. This conundrum begets a dearth of dependable sources for parents, caregivers, and even patients themselves to access comprehensive information about MIH and comprehend its implications. A recent investigation underscored the prevailing low levels of digital literacy regarding the comprehension of online content pertaining to MIH, identifying a paucity of websites offering substantive information on this subject [9].

One of the contributory factors to the limited proliferation of scientific discourse on MIH pertains to its relative novelty, encompassing both terminological nascency and clinical recognition. It has not been long since this condition commenced its journey toward identification and exhaustive scrutiny within the dental community. Consequently, a significant proportion of oral health professionals, as well as the general population, continues to grapple with an incomplete understanding of MIH and its manifold ramifications.

Furthermore, the dearth of awareness surrounding MIH can be ascribed to the specialized nature of the topic. An all-encompassing comprehension of MIH necessitates a profound grasp of dentistry and a multidisciplinary approach that enlists the expertise of specialists in pediatric dentistry, restorative dentistry, and orthodontics [10]. This entails that the promotion of MIH-related knowledge does not enjoy the same prevalence as more widely recognized oral health concerns.

In this context, the quest for information pertaining to MIH on the Internet appears to be markedly influenced by both direct and indirect personal experiences of individuals or caregivers tending to children afflicted by this condition. Direct experiences encompass a spectrum of situations encountered by the affected children themselves, including but not limited to pain, tooth hypersensitivity, traumatic dental injuries, and aesthetic concerns relating to dental structure. Conversely, indirect experiences encompass the pursuit of information catalyzed by the observation of MIH cases in the children of family members and friends as well as an interest piqued by public awareness campaigns or antecedent encounters with literature on the subject [11].

Online Searches and Quality of Content

A recent study has shed light on the low user activity related to MIH on Google, with a gradual growth trend over time [12]. In general, individuals tend to conduct searches related to MIH to gain insights into the condition's definition and differential diagnosis, often comparing it with conditions such as amelogenesis imperfecta and osteogenesis imperfecta. These MIH-related searches using specific dental terminologies are probably carried out by healthcare professionals, particularly dentists, as they seek additional technical information to inform their clinical decision-making when confronted with cases involving enamel defects. This observation may imply that professionals may not possess comprehensive readiness or confidence in diagnosing MIH or distinguishing it from other conditions, potentially leading to delays in achieving accurate diagnoses and, consequently, a higher likelihood of recurrent treatments and crown fractures [13, 14].

In contrast to the increasing number of scientific articles on the subject, websites containing information about MIH remain notably scarce. This suggests that professionals are progressively recognizing the significance of the condition, whereas the broader population still encounters challenges in accessing comprehensive information about MIH. Within this context, most MIH-related websites are authored by general dentists, often lacking in both quality and reliability, making it arduous for the majority of the population to comprehend their content [9].

The interest among Google users in MIH appears substantially lower compared to other prevalent oral conditions. In an effort to substantiate this affirmation, researchers conducted a detailed analysis in September 2023, leveraging Google Trends to examine the search interest over time for specific dental health terms: "molar incisor hypomineralization," "MIH," "tooth decay," "toothache," and "gingivitis." This investigation spanned from 2004 to 2023, focusing solely on searches pertinent to health-related issues on a global scale. The analysis revealed that the levels of public interest in the terms "molar incisor hypomineralization" and its abbreviation "MIH" were minimal, with average relative search volumes (RSV) of 0 and 2, respectively. In contrast, more common dental conditions such as "tooth decay," "toothache," and "gingivitis" captured significantly higher public attention, with their mean RSVs reaching 21, 67, and 44, respectively (as shown in Fig. 1). Google Trends is a tool designed for the analysis of search volumes pertaining to specific topics on Google Search. RSV represents the proportion of a specific search volume in relation to the total volume of Google searches conducted within a specific region at a given time. It is scaled from 0 to 100, with 100 signifying the highest point on the curve [12].

Motivation for Conducting Internet Searches Related to MIH

An individual's inclination to seek health-related information on the Internet is significantly influenced by a myriad of personal and demographic factors, encompassing self-efficacy, emotional responses to risk, perceived risk, trustworthiness, credibility, utility, information quality, age, gender, educational attainment, income level, racial background, and prior experiences [15]. In this context, it has been observed that younger individuals from the predominant racial demographic within their respective regions, as well as women, exhibit a proclivity for heightened consumption of health-related content on the Internet. Moreover, individuals harboring a vested interest in specialized health topics tend to be more attuned to their own needs and motivations, as opposed to those inclined toward general health subjects. Consequently, the veracity of content assumes a relatively diminished role in shaping information-seeking behavior, thereby fostering indiscriminate content consumption [16].

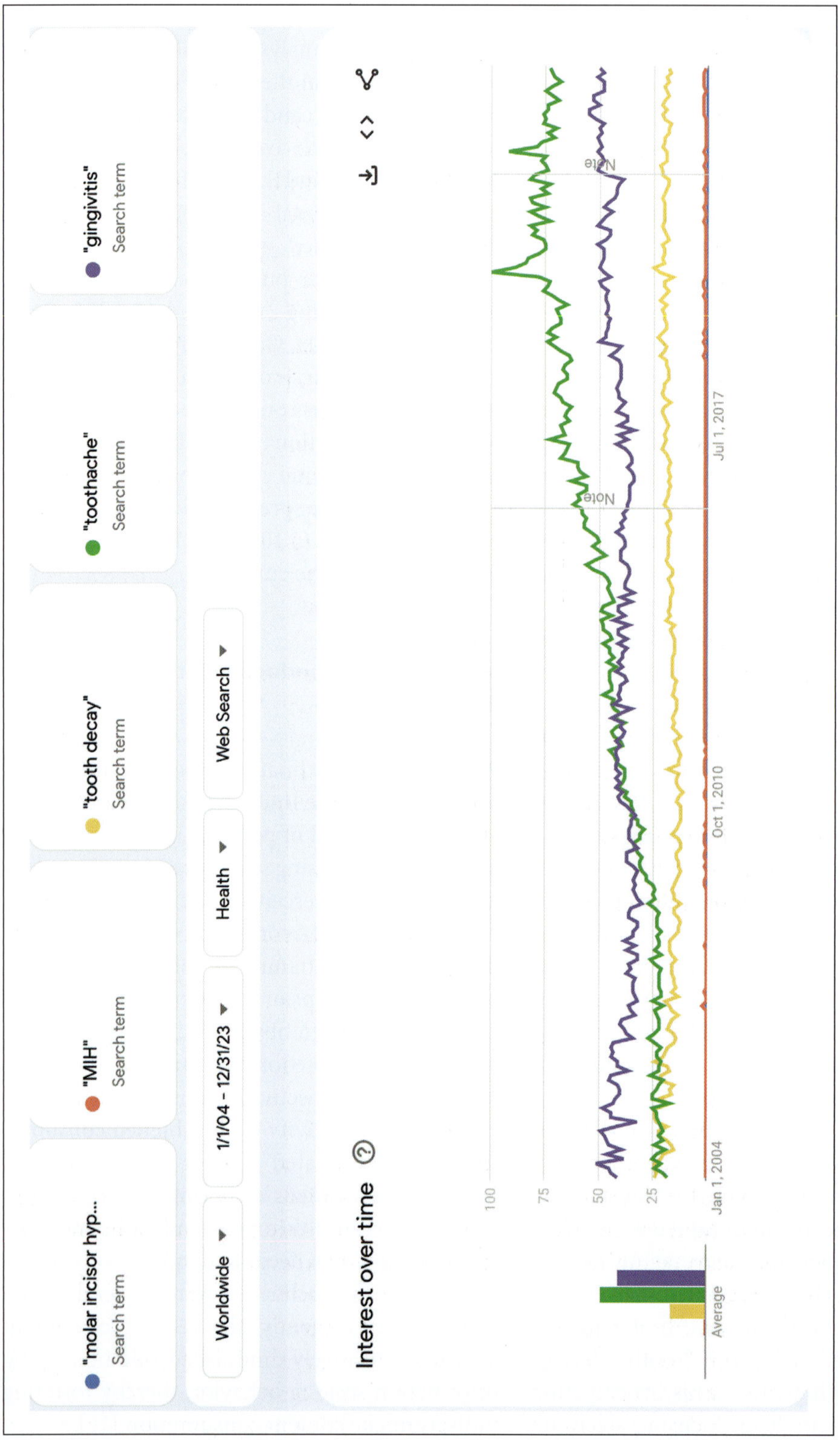

Fig. 1. The fluctuation in RSVs for the search terms "molar incisor hypomineralization," "MIH," "tooth decay," "toothache," and "gingivitis" on Google Search from 2004 to 2023.

The impact of MIH on the quality of life is intricately intertwined with the actions of parents and caregivers seeking comprehensive information within the digital landscape [12, 13]. MIH has been estimated to have a prevalence rate of 14.2% in the global population [17], with approximately 17.5 million new cases emerging each year, of which 27.4% necessitate dental treatment [18]. Existing literature already indicates that when a substantial number of individuals share common signs and symptoms, there is a marked surge in the demand for digital information resources aimed at addressing the adverse implications of this condition [12]. This trend underscores the imperative need to comprehend, manage, and cope with the challenges arising when a condition like MIH impacts a significant portion of the population. Therefore, it becomes paramount to discern the motivators behind searches for MIH-related content to pinpoint areas where efforts to raise awareness about the condition should be concentrated.

A recent phenomenon that has amplified online searches for health-related content is "cyberchondria," defined as the excessive scouring of the web for well-being and health information, often resulting in heightened anxiety and apprehensions [19]. In the context of MIH, the occurrence of this phenomenon is less likely due to the limited popularity of MIH-related content. Among the motivators instigating online searches for MIH-related information, one can underscore the diverse clinical presentations of the condition and, consequently, the multifarious approaches to its treatment. This variability can potentially impact the communication dynamics between dentists and caregivers, prompting the latter to seek supplementary information about MIH for the purpose of confirming the diagnosis or addressing queries pertaining to the condition [9].

The quest for additional information about MIH can also be correlated with factors, such as pain, aesthetics, behavioral concerns, and economic implications. Children afflicted with MIH often necessitate four times as many dental visits compared to their counterparts, engendering financial implications, and affecting the overall quality of life for families, who must prioritize early intervention for the condition [18]. Additionally, children with MIH appear to exhibit more behavioral issues relative to their peers, possibly attributable to the pain and hypersensitivity associated with the condition [20]. Experiences of pain can serve as triggers for Internet searches [21]. In certain instances of MIH, aesthetic impairments manifest, impacting children psychologically, particularly when visible enamel opacities are present on anterior teeth [22], thus motivating web searches for treatment options. Finally, attention should also be accorded to digital searches catalyzed by passive exposure to digital content. In this form of motivation for search, users encounter information inadvertently, develop an interest in the content, and subsequently engage in active web searching. Given that MIH is relatively underpublicized despite its high prevalence and considerable complexity, it can generate interest among individuals who have direct or indirect exposure to these dental alterations [9, 14].

Barriers for Searching Information about MIH

The nomenclature associated with the condition in question is notably extensive and intricate, particularly with the term "hypomineralisation," which may appear unfamiliar to individuals with limited health literacy. Consequently, depending on one's familiarity with the condition and the terminology employed, specific searches for "MIH" are more likely to be predominantly accessed by dental professionals [12].

In this view, several alternative terms have been utilized to refer to MIH, including phrases such as "hypomineralization without fluoride," "demarcated hypomineralized lesion," and "cheese molar." The latter term derives from a clinical characteristic of the condition and holds the potential to facilitate its popularization, aiding comprehension among the general population.

It is noteworthy that the creation of educational content regarding MIH is predominantly conducted in the English language, which poses a barrier to accessing and comprehending the topic for non-English-speaking populations [12]. Additionally, the observation that searches for information about the condition typically emanates from parents or caregivers rather than the affected children themselves may be attributed to imprecise attitudes influenced by established routines and beliefs [23].

Furthermore, it is essential to recognize that the experience associated with MIH can be perplexing. Some individuals may mistakenly believe they have the condition when they do not, while others who do have it may remain unaware. The former scenario is likely less frequent than the latter, particularly considering that MIH remains largely unknown to the general population. Conversely, the presence of MIH is often linked to discomfort, functional challenges, and aesthetic concerns, substantially impacting oral health-related quality of life [24]. These factors can motivate individuals with MIH or their caregivers to conduct searches related to the condition, often utilizing terms such as "yellow spot-on the tooth," "sensitive tooth," "toothache," or "tooth breaking," thereby diverting attention away from the actual condition they may have.

MIH on Social Media

Social media refer to technological platforms that facilitate the creation and dissemination of information and content through virtual channels [25]. They differ fundamentally from traditional media, such as journals, television, books, and radio, due to their infinite content, social orientation, and, most notably, their dependence on individual participation [26]. The advent of social media has dismantled barriers to information access, enabling the majority of individuals to produce and share content on a massive scale. While users of social media primarily seek information for entertainment, social interaction, and personal identification, the ease with which information can be shared with both acquaintances and strangers amplify the visibility of individual choices on these platforms [27].

Internet users have increasingly used social media to express concerns, seek advice, and share their health-related doubts [28]. However, the extensive use of these channels for such purposes raises questions and concerns regarding the quality and accuracy of the content disseminated. First, the democratized nature of social media allows anyone to propagate information, making it challenging to ascertain the authorship of content and whether it adheres to factual accuracy [29]. Second, while promoting individual empowerment and autonomy in health education and decision-making is commendable, the consumption of low-quality content can profoundly influence the reinforcement of detrimental health beliefs [30, 31]. Last, recognizing that students and health care professionals use these platforms to complement their clinical practice [32, 33], inaccurate content can compromise electronic professionalism and amplify the promotion of ineffective protocols, hindering the adoption of individualized health measures [34, 35].

The online landscape of dental information frequently features content of questionable reliability, prompting individuals to base their decisions on personal experiences [36, 37]. Moreover, online platforms often discourage the dissemination of oral health promotion campaigns, hindering the development of vital public health policies. In contrast, messages conveyed by health care professionals tend to wield greater influence in the realm of social media [38].

The consumption of unreliable information exerts a negative impact on individuals' health be-

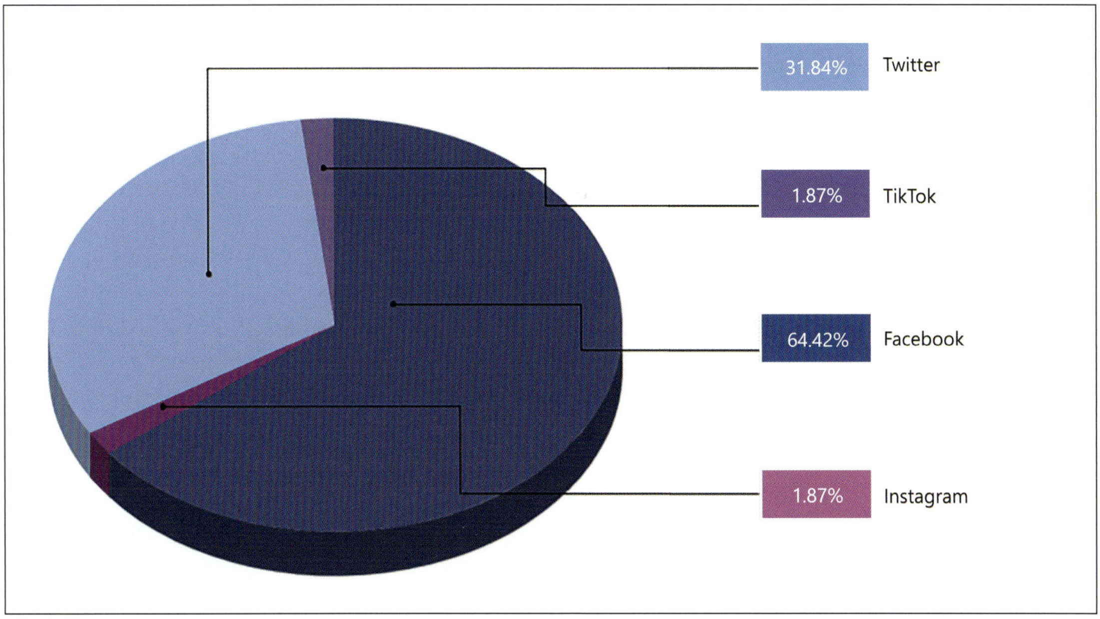

Fig. 2. Distribution of retrieved MIH-related posts according to social media.

haviors [38]. Furthermore, the poor quality of dental content available on the Internet often leads users to empirically address their specific concerns [36, 37]. Therefore, it is imperative to understand how the topic of MIH is presented on social media and who is engaging in these discussions.

In this context, a foundational analysis was conducted in September 2023, where the researchers examined four prominent social media platforms – Facebook, X (previously known as Twitter), Instagram, and TikTok – by searching for the term "molar incisor hypomineralization" directly within their search functionalities. This exploration yielded a total of 267 posts related to the term. A detailed breakdown of the findings highlights that a significant portion of these posts originated from Facebook, accounting for 64.42% of the total, followed closely by X, which contributed 31.84% of the posts. These distributions are graphically represented in Figure 2, offering a clear visualization of the prevalence of discussions surrounding MIH across different social media platforms. However, it is important to highlight that the findings were affected by the terminology used in the research. Incorporating synonyms or terms related to MIH symptoms could provide additional insights for analysis.

The authors conducted a qualitative analysis on the accuracy of post content. To classify a post as containing misinformation, it had to include claims that were clearly incorrect or misleading and lacked scientific basis, potentially leading to the formation of harmful health beliefs among social media users. According to Figure 3, 9.4% of posts spread misinformation, such as incorrectly blaming the cause of MIH on chemical consumption like bisphenol or fluoride. This suggests that MIH misinformation is less common compared to other dental issues such as fluoride use, toothache, amber necklace use, and dental caries [38–41].

Most posts were disseminated by health care professionals (e.g., dentists, health care practitio-

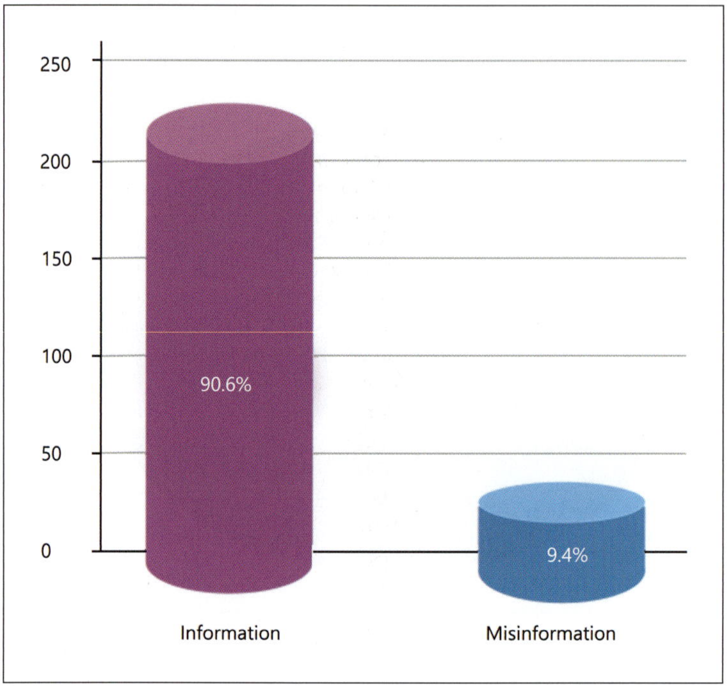

Fig. 3. Detection of misinformation among MIH-related posts.

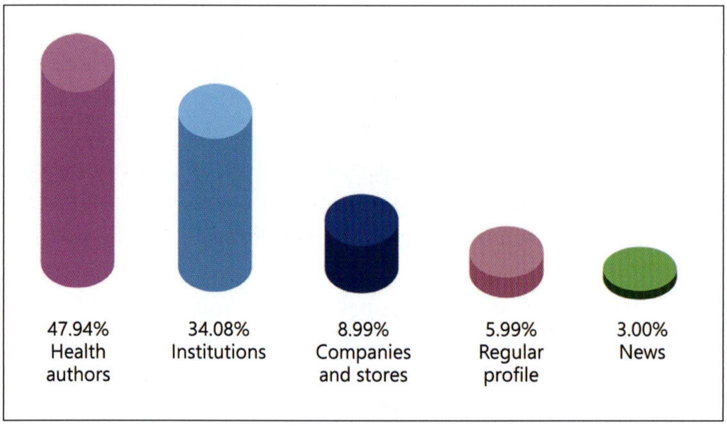

Fig. 4. Categories of authors of posts.

ners, or health communicators) and institutions (e.g., universities and scientific journals). This observation signifies that MIH remains a subject primarily discussed within limited circles, typically associated with health care and scientific contexts (shown in Fig. 4). In other words, MIH has not yet gained widespread attention among the general public, also influenced by the scarcity of digital materials about it on websites.

Chatbots

The advent of interactive chatbots signifies a paradigmatic shift in online health-seeking behavior, a phenomenon that transcends diverse demographic profiles. In essence, these systems adeptly distill extensive textual data from a myriad of sources by leveraging sophisticated mechanisms rooted in natural language processing and large

Table 1. Examples of answers generated by open AI chatbots regarding MIH-related questions

Chatbots	Questions	Answers
ChatGPT	What is MIH?	MIH is a developmental dental condition that primarily affects the molars (back teeth) and incisors (front teeth). It is characterized by the incomplete mineralization or hypomineralization of these teeth, leading to their susceptibility to decay, sensitivity, and other dental problems. MIH typically affects permanent teeth, appearing shortly after eruption, and can cause significant issues for affected individuals. The exact cause of MIH is not fully understood, but it is thought to result from disturbances during tooth development, potentially due to factors, such as genetics, environmental influences, or systemic illnesses during early childhood. This condition can manifest in a range of severity, from mild enamel defects to severe enamel breakdown. Common features of teeth affected by MIH include • Color variation: Affected teeth often appear discolored, ranging from creamy white to yellow or brown. • Enamel defects: The enamel on affected teeth is weakened and may have white or brown spots, rough surfaces, or pits. • Sensitivity: MIH-affected teeth are more sensitive to temperature changes and touch due to the compromised enamel. • Prone to decay: The weakened enamel is more prone to cavities and breakdown, which can lead to pain and discomfort. • Affects specific teeth: MIH primarily affects molars and incisors, but it can also affect canines in some cases. Diagnosis of MIH is typically based on visual examination and clinical evaluation by a dentist. Treatment options depend on the severity of the condition and may include: • Fluoride treatment: Fluoride can help strengthen the enamel and reduce sensitivity. Dentists might recommend fluoride varnishes, gels, or rinses. • Desensitizing agents: Special toothpaste or gels designed for sensitive teeth can help manage discomfort. • Dental sealants: These are protective coatings applied to the teeth's chewing surfaces to help prevent cavities. • Restorative procedures: In more severe cases, restorative treatments like fillings or crowns might be necessary to address decay and protect the affected teeth. • Oral hygiene education: Proper oral hygiene practices, such as regular brushing, flossing, and professional dental cleanings, are essential to prevent further complications. It is important to note that early diagnosis and intervention are crucial in managing MIH and preventing further dental problems. If you suspect you or your child might have MIH, it is recommended to consult a dentist for an accurate diagnosis and appropriate guidance.

Table 1 (continued)

Chatbots	Questions	Answers
	What are the causes of MIH?	MIH is a complex dental condition, and while the exact cause is not fully understood, it is thought to result from a combination of genetic, environmental, and systemic factors. Several factors have been proposed as potential contributors to the development of MIH: • Genetics: There is evidence to suggest that genetic factors play a role in the susceptibility to MIH. Studies have shown a higher prevalence of the condition among individuals with a family history of enamel defects or dental problems. • Environmental factors: Prenatal and early childhood environmental factors can influence tooth development. Factors such as exposure to certain toxins, infections, nutritional deficiencies, and maternal health during pregnancy could potentially impact the development of tooth enamel. • Systemic illnesses: Some systemic health conditions or illnesses during the early developmental stages of teeth (such as infancy and early childhood) may disrupt the formation of tooth enamel. Febrile illnesses, infections, or other health issues might contribute to the development of MIH. • Disturbances during tooth formation: Tooth enamel forms in stages, and any disruptions during these stages can lead to enamel defects. MIH is believed to occur during the mineralization phase of tooth development, resulting in incomplete or structurally weak enamel. • Exposure to environmental factors: Certain environmental factors during early childhood might contribute to the development of MIH. These factors could include exposure to certain chemicals, medications, or dietary components. It is important to note that MIH primarily affects the molars and incisors, which are the first permanent teeth to erupt in the mouth. The timing of the disruption during tooth development and eruption is thought to influence which teeth are affected. Researchers and dental professionals continue to study MIH to better understand its causes and develop effective strategies for prevention and management. Early diagnosis by a dentist is crucial in identifying MIH and providing appropriate guidance for maintaining oral health and preventing further complications.
Chatsonic	What is MIH?	MIH is a common developmental condition that results in enamel defects in the first permanent molar teeth and permanent incisors. It is a systemic origin hypomineralisation that affects one to four permanent first molars and is often associated with affected permanent incisors. Recent data show that MIH is a frequently encountered dental condition worldwide.
	What are the causes of MIH?	The causes of MIH are not fully understood, but several possible factors have been suggested in the literature. These include respiratory tract infections, perinatal complications, dioxins, infections during pregnancy, premature birth, birth complications, and family history of enamel defects. It is important to note that MIH is a systemic origin hypomineralisation that affects the first permanent molars and is often associated with affected permanent incisors. More research is needed to fully understand the exact causes of MIH.

Table 1 (continued)

Chatbots	Questions	Answers
Google Bard	What is MIH?	MIH is a developmental dental defect that affects the permanent first molars and incisors. It is caused by a disruption in the formation of the enamel during tooth development. MIH can cause a variety of problems, including: • Discolored teeth • Brittle teeth • Sensitive teeth • Increased risk of cavities The exact cause of MIH is unknown, but it is thought to be caused by a combination of genetic and environmental factors. Some possible causes of MIH include: • Prematurity • Low birth weight • Infections during pregnancy • Certain medications taken during pregnancy • Certain medical conditions, such as asthma and allergies There is no cure for MIH, but there are a number of treatments available to help manage the symptoms. Treatment options vary depending on the severity of the condition and may include: • Sealants to protect the teeth from cavities • Fillings or crowns to repair damaged teeth • Veneers to improve the appearance of the teeth In severe cases of MIH, it may be necessary to extract the affected teeth. If you have any concerns about MIH, please see a dentist for evaluation and treatment.
	What are the causes of MIH?	The exact cause of MIH is unknown, but it is thought to be caused by a combination of genetic and environmental factors. Some possible causes of MIH include: • Genetic factors: MIH can run in families, suggesting that there is a genetic component to the condition. • Environmental factors: A number of environmental factors have been linked to MIH, including: • Infections during pregnancy, such as cytomegalovirus (CMV) and rubella • Premature birth • Low birth weight • Certain medications taken during pregnancy, such as tetracycline antibiotics • Certain medical conditions, such as asthma and allergies It is important to note that not all children who are exposed to these risk factors will develop MIH. The condition is complex, and there is likely a combination of genetic and environmental factors that contribute to its development. If you have any concerns about your child's risk of developing MIH, please talk to your dentist. They can assess your child's risk factors and provide guidance on how to prevent and manage the condition.

Table 1 (continued)

Chatbots	Questions	Answers
Perplexity	What is MIH?	MIH is a developmental condition that results in enamel defects in the first permanent molars and permanent incisors. It is considered a worldwide problem and usually occurs in children under 10 years old. The condition is caused by the lack of mineralization of enamel during its maturation phase, due to interruption to the function of ameloblasts. Here are some key points about MIH: • MIH is a qualitative developmental defect of enamel that affects at least one first permanent molar • One to four molars, and often also the incisors, could be affected • MIH is a frequently encountered dental condition worldwide • MIH is associated with dental complications that might affect patients' quality of life as well as create treatment challenges to dentists • MIH can cause areas of poorly formed enamel that affect one or more teeth • MIH can be diagnosed by a dentist during a clinical examination • Treatment options for MIH include remineralization, fluoride therapy, resin infiltration, and restorative treatment In conclusion, MIH is a common developmental condition that results in enamel defects in the first permanent molars and permanent incisors. It can be diagnosed by a dentist during a clinical examination and treated with various options depending on the severity of the condition.
	What are the causes of MIH?	MIH is a developmental condition that results in enamel defects in the first permanent molars and permanent incisors. The exact cause of MIH is not fully understood, but multiple possible causes have been suggested in the literature. Here are some of the factors that have been associated with MIH: • Respiratory tract infections during early childhood • Perinatal complications, such as infections during pregnancy, premature birth, and birth complications • Family history of enamel defects • Exposure to dioxins • Prenatal, perinatal, and postnatal issues It is important to note that not all children with these factors develop MIH, and some children with no known risk factors can still develop the condition. Further research is needed to fully understand the causes of MIH.

language models, underpinned by cutting-edge artificial intelligence (AI) technology [42, 43]. Consequently, they furnish individuals with interactive online dialogs that closely emulate human-like interactions [44]. Moreover, users have the capacity to furnish supplementary information pertaining to their geographic location, age, and pertinent variables, thereby facilitating the tailoring of responses to align with their unique requirements. Thus, AI chatbots offer a user-centric and exceedingly personalized search mechanism founded on real-time interactive solutions, holding the potential to substantially enhance public engagement in the consumption of digital health content [45, 46].

In this regard, prior research has consistently showcased the efficacy of chatbot-based interventions in enhancing health care outcomes across various domains, including but not limited to depression management, anxiety alleviation, medication adherence optimization, and dietary support [45, 47–49]. Although previous studies have not specifically examined the capabilities of AI chatbots in disseminating MIH-re-

Table 1 (continued)

Chatbots	Questions	Answers
Youchat	What is MIH?	MIH is a developmental dental condition that affects the enamel of permanent first molars and incisors. It is characterized by a qualitative enamel defect, where the affected teeth have a lower mineral content and are more prone to dental caries (cavities), sensitivity, and other dental problems. MIH typically affects one to four permanent first molars, but it can also involve incisors. The affected teeth may have white, yellow, or brown discoloration, and the enamel may be porous, rough, or fragile. In severe cases, the enamel may be so weak that it can easily chip or break. The exact cause of MIH is still unclear, but it is believed to be a result of a combination of genetic and environmental factors. Some potential risk factors include prenatal or early childhood health factors, such as certain illnesses, medications, or nutritional deficiencies. However, more research is needed to fully understand the etiology of MIH. MIH can have significant impacts on oral health, as the affected teeth are more susceptible to decay and may require extensive dental treatment. Early diagnosis and intervention are important to manage the condition and prevent further complications. Treatment options may include dental sealants, fluoride treatments, restorations (fillings), and, in severe cases, extractions or crowns. It is recommended to consult with a dentist or a pediatric dentist if you suspect that you or your child may have MIH. They can provide a proper diagnosis and develop an appropriate treatment plan based on the individual's specific needs.
	What are the causes of MIH?	The exact causes of MIH are still not fully understood. However, research suggests that a combination of genetic and environmental factors may contribute to the development of MIH. Here are some potential causes that have been identified: • Genetic factors: There is evidence to suggest that genetic factors play a role in the development of MIH. Certain genes may be involved in the formation and mineralization of tooth enamel, and variations in these genes may increase the risk of developing MIH. • Prenatal and early childhood health factors: Certain prenatal and early childhood health factors have been associated with an increased risk of MIH. These factors include prenatal illnesses, premature birth, low birth weight, respiratory infections, high fever, and the use of certain medications during pregnancy or early childhood. • Environmental factors: Environmental factors may also contribute to the development of MIH. Exposure to certain chemicals, toxins, or pollutants during tooth development may affect enamel formation and mineralization. Additionally, nutritional deficiencies, such as a lack of vitamin D or calcium, have been suggested as potential risk factors for MIH. • Systemic illnesses: Some systemic illnesses or conditions, such as asthma, allergies, and gastrointestinal disorders, have been associated with an increased risk of MIH. The exact mechanisms by which these illnesses contribute to MIH are not fully understood, but it is believed that they may disrupt the normal enamel development process.

lated information, certain dental investigations have begun to shed light on their capacity to support informed decision-making in oral health. For instance, a recent qualitative study that examined the responses generated by ChatGPT concerning fluoride consumption demonstrated this chatbot's capacity to provide sufficient and reliable information on this matter [43]. Interestingly, the data generated by these systems can be seamlessly integrated with other digital health tools, rendering them invaluable in the realm of public health for educational purposes concerning oral health care [50].

Table 1 compiles responses from five distinct open chatbots available currently (*ChatGPT*, *Chatsonic*, *Google Bard*, *Perplexity*, and *Youchat*), briefly elucidating their effectiveness as a supportive mechanism for the comprehensive dissemination of relevant MIH information. For that, researchers designed two relevant questions to test and compare the accuracy of chatbots in providing reliable information about the definition and etiology of MIH, namely, "what is molar-incisor hypomineralization?" and "what are the causes of molar-incisor hypomineralization?".

The chatbot responses have shown a satisfactory level of detail in defining MIH. They also summarized key potential causes of MIH as identified by recent systematic reviews and meta-analyses [51, 52], highlighting factors such as perinatal and postnatal influences, birth complications, and genetic factors. However, it is crucial to acknowledge the lack of consensus among researchers on this topic, particularly because the meta-analytic findings are based on the synthesis of studies of low quality. Accordingly, the chatbots discussed additional potential causes for MIH development, including low birth weight, exposure to prenatal medication, and vitamin deficiencies.

Chatbots ideally should be able to debunk prevailing health misinformation besides disseminating accurate and evidence-based information. Regarding this perspective, the current evidence presents conflicting findings. While certain studies underscore chatbots' efficacy in mitigating falsehoods [53, 54], others yield divergent results [55–57]. It is noteworthy that chatbot platforms emphasize the imperative of conscientious utilization on their online platforms, acknowledging the potential for misinformation propagation [58].

This technical constraint is inherent in the developmental characteristics of chatbots. Owing to them reliance on AI algorithms, the precision of chatbots is contingent upon the quality of the training data and the complexity of the queries they encounter. As a result, it is expected that they may exhibit limitations in processing capacity when confronted with intricate open-domain questions, leading to challenges in comprehension, factual accuracy, specificity, and inferential capabilities [59]. A major challenge resides in the imperative to ensure that the AI model undergoes training using an extensive and representative dataset. This endeavor softens potential human-based classification biases and affirms the model's competence in accurately comprehending and generating natural language within a diverse array of contexts.

Another pertinent technical concern pertains to the supervision and maintenance of the chatbots. Undoubtedly, the dependence on outdated content for training purposes invariably results in the generation of obsolete outputs. This aspect can pose a substantial challenge when considering chatbots as a source of information, particularly in light of the rapid evolution of scientific evidence on relevant oral health topics. For example, the most extensively employed generative chatbot, ChatGPT, received its latest substantial update in September 2021 within its open-access iteration, signifying potential limitation in its capacity to address events or advancements transpiring beyond that temporal scope [58]. In this context, scenarios may arise wherein chatbots either refrain from providing corroborative citations for their statements or generate references that exhibit inaccuracies in their content attribution [57].

Finally, an additional technical concern revolves around the implementation of cybersecurity protocols to fortify these models against potential malicious actors who may endeavor to manipulate them for hidden interests. In practical terms, it is incumbent upon governmental authorities to formulate comprehensive regulatory frameworks that oversee the deployment and operationalization of AI-driven chatbots within the public domain [60]. These policies and guidelines should encompass pivotal elements, including the delineation of responsibilities and liabilities associated with chatbot platforms, adherence to ethical principles, the promotion of transparency, the cultivation of collaborative partnerships with stakeholders, the prioritization of data privacy and security, and a commitment to effectively curbing the dissemination of false oral health information [60, 61]. The paramount aim of these regulations is the establishment of a secure and trustworthy environment for the dissemination of oral health content, thus safeguarding the integrity and dependability of this critical service.

Final Considerations

Internet activity can serve as a vital supplementary source of information for driving discussions on public policies about oral health care, treatment, and health literacy. This includes not only raising awareness about the potential consequences of the condition but also equipping professional teams with the tools to provide high-quality dental information to patients [40]. Such initiatives are crucial in mitigating the harm stemming from inadequate MIH care practices among patients.

Professional organizations should intensify their efforts to promote ongoing health education activities, particularly because many dental professionals still possess limited knowledge about the condition [62]. The dissemination of information about MIH should primarily target the dentists responsible for diagnosing and treating this condition, utilizing both digital channels and traditional methods. Additionally, various measures should be developed to enhance public access to quality information, such as the deliberate selection of a common name for the condition, the distribution of specialized materials in various languages, and mass media campaigns to encourage parents and caregivers to seek an early diagnosis for resolute treatments and individualized clinical follow-ups.

It is important to exercise caution when evaluating responses generated by AI chatbots, given their inherent technological limitations. Although some outdated content about MIH may be encountered, it is worth emphasizing that these systems possess the capability to provide reliable and valuable information on this subject. Consequently, dental professionals and associations should acknowledge the significance of these channels as sources of MIH-related information and promote active strategies for the optimal consumption of such content by the public. Moreover, future research efforts should prioritize content management within chatbot platforms, with a focus on the meticulous examination of oral health information and misinformation. This systematic evaluation can offer a more comprehensive understanding of the strengths and limitations of AI chatbots in the context of online oral health information-seeking behavior.

Simultaneously, authorities bear the responsibility of disseminating initiatives aimed at nurturing the necessary skills that enable responsible consumption of online information by recipients. Furthermore, investments in network infrastructure hold pivotal significance in ameliorating digital disparities within countries, thereby ensuring universal access to information and communication technologies and, consequently, the associated societal benefits.

Statement of Ethics

This study did not necessitate approval of the Council of Ethics in Human Research of Bauru School of Dentistry, University of São Paulo. This exemption from the requirement for ethical oversight is attributed to the utilization of publicly accessible data, thus obviating the need for an additional layer of scrutiny, which is typically imposed to safeguard the rights and welfare of human research participants.

Conflict of Interest Statement

The authors have no conflicts of interest to declare.

Funding Sources

This chapter was supported by the São Paulo Research Foundation (grants #2019/11926-8, #2021/07339-0, #2021/10732-5, #2022/08823-5, and #2022/12885-6).

Author Contributions

Thiago Cruvinel contributed to the conception, design, analysis, interpretation, and supervision, and critically revised the manuscript; Matheus Lotto, Olívia Santana Jorge, Ana Maria Jucá, Tamires Sá Menezes, and Jean Ribeiro Leite contributed to the conception, design, analysis, and interpretation, and drafted the manuscript.

References

1 Boulos MNK, Wheeler S, Tavares C, Jones R. How smartphones are changing the face of mobile and participatory healthcare: an overview, with example from eCAALYX. Biomed Eng Online. 2011 Apr 5;10:24.

2 Grewal D, Herhausen D, Ludwig S, Ordenes FV. The future of digital communication research: considering dynamics and multimodality. J Retail. 2022 June;98(2):224–40.

3 Coulter A, Ellins J. Effectiveness of strategies for informing, educating, and involving patients. BMJ. 2007 Jun 7;335(7609):24–7.

4 Stacey D, Légaré F, Lewis K, Barry MJ, Bennett CL, Eden KB, et al. Decision aids for people facing health treatment or screening decisions. Cochrane Database Syst Rev. 2017 Apr 12;4(4):CD001431.

5 Horowitz AM, Kleinman DV. Oral health literacy: a pathway to reducing oral health disparities in Maryland. J Public Health Dent. 2012 Winter;72(suppl 1):S26–30.

6 Lotto M, Strieder AP, Aguirre PEA, Oliveira TM, Machado MAAM, Rios D, et al. Parental-oriented educational mobile messages toa id in the control of early childhood caries in low socioeconomic children: a randomized controlled trial. J Dent. 2020 Oct;101:103456.

7 Lotto M, Jorge OS, Machado MAAM, Cruvinel T. Exploring online oral health misinformation: a content analysis. Braz Oral Res. 2023 May 29;37:e049.

8 Alanzi A, Faridoun A, Kavvadia K, Ghanim A. Dentists' perception, knowledge, and clinical management of molar-incisor-hypomineralisation in Kuwait: a cross-sectional study. BMC Oral Health. 2018 Mar 7;18(1):34.

9 Meade MJ, Dreyer CW. The quality and readability of online molar incisor hypomineralization patient education materials: a systematic analysis. Aust Dent J. 2022 Jun;67(2):159–67.

10 Crombie FA, Manton DJ, Weerheijm KL, Kilpatrick NM. Molar incisor hypomineralization: a survey of members of the Australian and New Zealand Society of Paediatric Dentistry. Aust Dent J. 2008 Jun;53(2):160–66.

11 Aguirre PE, Coelho M, Oliveira T, Rios D, Cruvinel AF, Cruvinel T. What can Google inform us about people's interests regarding dental caries in different populations? Caries Res. 2018 Jan 20; 52(3):177–78.

12 Aguirre PEA, Strieder AP, Lotto M, Oliveira TM, Rios D, Cruvinel AFP, et al. Are the Internet users concerned about molar incisor hypomineralization? An infoveillance study. Int J Paediatr Dent. 2020 Jan;30(1):27–34.

13 Hubbard MJ, Mangum JE, Perez VA, Nervo GJ, Hall RK. Molar hypomineralisation: a call to arms for enamel researchers. Front Physiol. 2017 Aug;8:546.

14 Kühnisch J, Kabary L, Malyk Y, Rothmaier K, Metz I, Hickel R, et al. Relationship between caries experience and demarcated hypomineralised lesions (including MIH) in the permanent dentition of 15-year-olds. Clin Oral Investig. 2018 Jun;22(5):2013–9.

15 Wang X, Shi J, Kong H. Online health information seeking: a review and meta-analysis. Health Commun. 2021 Sep; 36(10):1163–75.

16 Giglietto F, Iannelli L, Valeriani A, Rossi L. "Fake news" is the invention of a liar: how false information circulates within the hybrid news system. Curr Sociol. 2019 Apr 8;67(4):625–42.

17 Bukhari ST, Alhasan HA, Qari MT, Sabbagh HJ, Farsi NM. Prevalence and risk factors of molar incisor hypomineralization in the Middle East: a systematic review and meta-analysis. J Taibah Univ Med Sci. 2022 Dec 31;18(4):696–710.

18 Mazur M, Corridore D, Ndokaj A, Ardan R, Vozza I, Babajko S, et al. MIH and dental caries in children: a systematic review and meta-analysis. Healthcare. 2023 Jun 18;11(12):1795.

19 El-Zayat A, Namnkani SA, Alshareef NA, Mustfa MM, Eminaga NS, Algarni GA. Cyberchondria and its association with smartphone addiction and electronic health literacy among a Saudi population. Saudi J Med Med Sci. 2023 Apr-Jun;11(2):162–8.

20 Cabral RN, Nyvad B, Soviero VLVM, Freitas E, Leal SC. Reliability and validity of a new classification of MIH based on severity. Clin Oral Investig. 2020 Feb; 24(2):727–34.

21 Rizzato VL, Lotto M, Lourenço Neto N, Oliveira TM, Cruvinel T. Digital surveillance: the interests in toothache-related information after the outbreak of Covid-19. Oral Dis. 2022 Nov;28(S2):2432–41.

22 Rodd HD, Graham A, Tajmehr N, Timms L, Hasmun N. Molar incisor hypomineralisation: current knowledge and practice. Int Dent J. 2021 Aug; 71(4):285–91.
23 Lotto M, Strieder AP, Aguirre PEA, Machado MAAM, Rios D, Cruvinel A, et al. Parental perspectives on early childhood caries: a qualitative study. Int J Paediatr Dent. 2020 Jul;30(4):451–8.
24 Alzahrani AY, Najlaa Alamoudi MH, El Meligy OAES. Contemporary understanding of the etiology and management of molar incisor hypomineralization: a literature review. Dent J (Basel). 2023 Jun 23;11(7):157.
25 Aichner T, Grünfelder M, Maurer O, Jegeni D. Twenty-five years of social media: a review of social media applications and definitions from 1994 to 2019. Cyberpsychol Behav Soc Netw. 2021 Apr;24(4):215–22.
26 Kozinets R. Netnography: Redefined. 2nd ed. London: Sage; 2015.
27 Greifeneder R, Jaffe M, Newman E, Schwarz N. The Psychology of Fake News: Accepting, Sharing, and Correcting Misinformation. 1st ed. London: Routledge; 2020.
28 Heaivilin N, Gerbert B, Page JE, Gibbs JL. Public health surveillance of dental pain via Twitter. J Dent Res. 2011 Sep; 90(9):1047–51.
29 Lazer DM, Baum MA, Benkler Y, Berinsky AJ, Greenhil KM, Menczer F, et al. The science of fake news. Science. 2018 Mar 18;359(6380):1094–6.
30 AlMuammar SA, Noorsaeed AS, Alafif RA, Kamal YF, Daghistani GM. The use of Internet and social media for health information and its consequences among the population in Saudi Arabia. Cureus. 2021 Sep 27;13(9):e18388.
31 Zhao Y, Zhang J. Consumer health information seeking in social media: a literature review. Health Info Libr J. 2017 Dec;34(4):268–83.
32 Hsu W-C. Undergraduate students' online health information-seeking behavior during the COVID-19 pandemic. Int J Environ Res Public Health. 2021 Dec 16;18(24):13250.
33 Rolls K, Hansen M, Jackson D, Elliott D. How health care professionals use social media to create virtual communities: an integrative review. J Med Internet Res. 2016 Jun 16;18(6):e166.
34 Kart M, Nandi N. Social media and medical education in the context of the COVID-19 pandemic: scoping review. JMIR Med Educ. 2021 Apr 12;7(2): e25892.
35 Wang Z, Wang S, Zhang Y, Jiang X. Social media usage and online professionalism among registered nurses: a cross-sectional survey. Int J Nurs Stud. 2019 Oct;98:19–26.
36 Aguirre PEA, Coelho MM, Rios D, Machado MAAM, Cruvinel AFP, Cruvinel T. Evaluating the dental caries-related information on Brazilian websites: qualitative study. J Med Internet Res. 2017 Dec 13;19(12):e415.
37 Lotto M, Aguirre PEA, Lourenço-Neto N, Cruvinel AF, Cruvinel T. Is the quality of toothache-related information published in Brazilian websites adequate to assist people in seeking dental treatment? Oral Health Prev Dent. 2020 Apr 1;18(1):301–9.
38 Lotto M, Menezes TS, Hussain IZ, Tsao S-F, Butt ZA, Morita PP, et al. Characterization of false or misleading fluoride content on Instagram: infodemiology study. J Med Internet Res. 2022 May 19;24(5):e37519.
39 Strieder AP, Aguirre PEA, Lotto M, Cruvinel AFP, Cruvinel T. Digital behavior surveillance for monitoring the interests of Google users in amber necklace in different countries. Int J Paediatr Dent. 2019 Sep;29(5):603–14.
40 Lotto M, Aguirre PEA, Rios D, Machado MAAM, Cruvinel AFP, Cruvinel T. Analysis of the interests of Google users on toothache information. PLoS One. 2017 Oct 19;12(10):e0186059.
41 Cruvinel T, Aguirre PEA, Lotto M, Oliveira TM, Rios D, Cruvinel AFP. Digital behavior surveillance: monitoring dental caries and toothache interests of Google users from developing countries. Oral Dis. 2019 Jan;25(1):339–47.
42 Adamopoulou E, Moussiades L. Chatbots: history, technology, and applications. Mach Learn Appl. 2020 Dec;2: 100006.
43 Buldur M, Sezer B. Can artificial intelligence effectively respond to frequently asked questions about fluoride usage and effects? A qualitative study on ChatGPT. Fluoride. 2023 Jun;56(3):201–16.
44 Aggarwal A, Tam CC, Wu D, Li X, Qiao S. Artificial intelligence-based chatbots for promoting health behavioral changes: systematic review. J Med Internet Res. 2023 Feb 24;25:e4078.
45 Abd-Alrazaq A, Rababeh A, Alajlani M, Bewick BM, Househ M. Effectiveness and safety of using chatbots to improve mental health: systematic review and meta-analysis. J Med Internet Res. 2020 Jul 13;22(7):e16021.
46 Singh B, Olds T, Brinsly J, Dumiud D, Virgara R, Matricciani L, et al. Systematic review and meta-analysis of the effectiveness of chatbots on lifestyle behaviours. NPJ Digit Med. 2023 Jun 23;6(1):118.
47 Laranjo L, Dunn AG, Tong HL, Kocaballi AB, Chen J, Bashir R, et al. Conversational agents in healthcare: a systematic review. J Am Med Inform Assoc. 2018;25(9):1248–58.
48 Vaidyam AN, Wisniewski H, Halamka JD, Kashavan MS, Torous JB. Chatbots and conversational agents in mental health: a review of the psychiatric landscape. Can J Psychiatry. 2019 Jul; 64(7):456–64.
49 Oh YJ, Zhang J, Fang M-L, Furuoka Y. A systematic review of artificial intelligence chatbots for promoting physical activity, healthy diet, and weight loss. Int J Behav Phys Act. 2021 Dec 11;18(1): 160.
50 Morita PP, Abhari S, Kaur J, Lotto M, Miranda PASS, Oetomo A. Applying ChatGPT in public health: a SWOT and PASTLE analysis. Front Public Health. 2023 Jul 3;11:1225861.
51 Garot E, Rouas P, Somani C, Taylor D, Wong F, Lygidakis NA. An update of the aetiological factors involved in molar incisor hypomineralisation (MIH): a systematic review and meta-analysis. Eur Arch Paediatr Dent. 2022 Feb; 23(1):23–38.
52 Fatturi AL, Wambier LM, Chibinski AC, Assunção LRS, Brancher JA, Reis A, et al. A systematic review and meta-analysis of systemic exposure associated with molar incisor hypomineralization. Community Dent Oral Epidemiol. 2019 Oct; 47(5):407–15.
53 Miner AS, Laranjo L, Kocaballi AB. Chatbots in the fight against the COVID-19 pandemic. NPJ Digit Med. 2020 May 4;3:65.
54 Johnson SB, King AJ, Warner EL, Aneja S, Kann BH, Bylund CL. Using ChatGPT to evaluate cancer myths and misconceptions: artificial intelligence and cancer information. JNCI Cancer Spectr. 2023 Mar 1;7(2):pkad015.

55 Hsu HY, Hsu KC, Hou SY, Wu CL, Hshie YW, Cheng YD. Examining real-world medication consultations and drug-herb interactions: ChatGPT performance evaluation. JMIR Med Educ. 2023 Aug 21;9:e48433.
56 Danesh A, Pazouki H, Danesh K, Danesh F, Danesh A. The performance of artificial intelligence language models in board-style dental knowledge assessment: a preliminary study on ChatGPT. J Am Dent Assoc. 2023 Nov;154(11): 970–4.
57 Gravel J, D'Amours-Gravel M, Osmanlliu E. Learning to fake it: limited responses and fabricated references provided by ChatGPT for medical questions. Mayo Clin Proc Dig Health. 2023 Sep;1(3):226–34.
58 OpenAI [Internet]. Introducing ChatGPT [cited 2023 Oct 16]. Available from: https://openai.com/blog/chatgpt.
59 Zheng S, Huang J, Chang KCC. Why does ChatGPT fall short in answering questions faithfully? ArXiv. 2023 May 24;2304:10513.
60 De Angelis L, Baglivo F, Arzilli G, Privitera GP, Ferragina P, Tozzi AE, et al. ChatGPT and the rise of large language models: the new AI-driven infodemic threat in public health. Front Public Health. 2023 Apr 25;11:1166120.
61 Wang X, Sanders HM, Liu Y. ChatGPT: promise and challenges for deployment in low- and middle-income countries. Lancet Reg Health West Pac. 2023 Sep 15;41:100905.
62 Seremidi K, Amend S, Krämer N, Gizani S. A cross-sectional survey on knowledge and attitudes of Greek dentists regarding molar incisor hypomineralisation diagnosis and treatment. BMC Oral Health. 2022 Nov 16;22(1):498.

Thiago Cruvinel
Department of Pediatric Dentistry, Orthodontics and Public Health, Bauru School of Dentistry, University of São Paulo
Alameda Dr Octávio Pinheiro Brisolla, 9–75, Vila Universitária
Bauru 17012-901 (Brazil)
thiagocruvinel@fob.usp.br

Author Index

Subject Index